Clinics in Developmental Medicine No. 178
IMPROVING HAND FUNCTION IN
CEREBRAL PALSY

© 2008 Mac Keith Press
30 Furnival Street, London EC4A 1JQ

Editor: Hilary M. Hart
Managing Editor: Caroline Black
Project Manager: Sarah Pearsall

First published in this edition 2008

British Library Cataloguing-in-Publication data
A catalogue record for this book is available from the British Library

ISBN: 978-1-898683-53-7

Typeset by Keystroke, 28 High Street, Tettenhall, Wolverhampton
Printed by The Lavenham Press Ltd, Water Street, Lavenham, Suffolk
Mac Keith Press is supported by Scope

Clinics in Developmental Medicine No. 178

Improving Hand Function in Cerebral Palsy

Theory, evidence and intervention

Edited by

ANN-CHRISTIN ELIASSON
Department of Woman and Child Health, Karolinska Institute,
Stockholm, Sweden

and

PATRICIA A. BURTNER
Department of Pediatrics, Occupational Therapy Graduate
Program, University of New Mexico, Albuquerque, New
Mexico, USA

2008
Mac Keith Press

CONTENTS

AUTHORS' APPOINTMENTS   ix

FOREWORD   xiii
Hans Forssberg

INTRODUCTION   1
Ann-Christin Eliasson and Patricia A. Burtner

1. BRAIN PLASTICITY IN DEVELOPMENT AND DISEASE   13
   Hans Forssberg

2. CORTICAL CONTROL OF HAND FUNCTION   25
   Johann Kuhtz-Buschbeck and Stephan Ulmer

3. NEUROPSYCHOLOGY OF MOVEMENT SEQUENCE LEARNING   43
   Fredrik Ullén

4. NEUROLOGICAL CLASSIFICATION AND NEURORADIOLOGY
   OF CEREBRAL PALSY   61
   Ingeborg Krägeloh-Mann and Martin Staudt

5. NORMAL ANATOMY OF THE UPPER EXTREMITY   79
   Beth Moody Jones

6. MUSCLE ALTERATIONS DUE TO SPASTICITY   101
   Eva Pontén

7. POSTURAL CONTROL FOR REACHING AND HAND SKILLS   109
   Mindy F. Levin and Heidi Sveistrup

8. VISUAL IMPAIRMENT AND CONSEQUENCES FOR HAND
   FUNCTION   124
   Eugenio Mercuri, Andrea Guzzetta and Giovanni Cioni

9. THE ROLE OF SENSATION FOR HAND FUNCTION IN CHILDREN
   WITH CEREBRAL PALSY   134
   Annette Majnemer, Daniel Bourbonnais and Victor Frak

10. TYPICAL AND ATYPICAL DEVELOPMENT OF THE UPPER LIMB
IN CHILDREN   147
Jeanne R. Charles

11. BIMANUAL COORDINATION IN CHILDREN WITH HEMIPLEGIC
CEREBRAL PALSY   160
Andrew M. Gordon and Bert Steenbergen

12. CHOOSING AND USING ASSESSMENTS OF HAND FUNCTION   176
Lena Krumlinde-Sundholm

13. ORTHOPAEDIC INTERVENTION IN THE UPPER EXTREMITY IN
THE CHILD WITH CEREBRAL PALSY: MUSCULOSKELETAL SURGERY   198
L. Andrew Koman, Zhongyu Li and Beth Paterson Smith

14. ORTHOPAEDIC INTERVENTION IN THE MANAGEMENT OF
CEREBRAL PALSY: BOTULINUM TOXINS   213
L. Andrew Koman, Zhongyu Li and Beth Paterson Smith

15. THERAPEUTIC INTERVENTIONS AT THE BODY STRUCTURE AND
FUNCTION LEVEL TO SUPPORT CHILDREN'S UPPER EXTREMITY
FUNCTION   230
Patricia A. Burtner and Janet L. Poole

16. MOTOR LEARNING IN CHILDREN WITH CEREBRAL PALSY:
IMPLICATIONS FOR REHABILITATION   260
Shailesh S. Kantak, Katherine J. Sullivan and Patricia Burtner

17. A COGNITIVE PERSPECTIVE ON INTERVENTION   276
Cognitive orientation to daily occupational performance
(CO-OP) in the child with upper extremity spasticity
A.D. Mandich, H.J. Polatajko and Ann Zilberbrant

18. GOAL-ORIENTED TRAINING OF DAILY ACTIVITIES – A MODEL
FOR INTERVENTION   286
Ann-Christin Eliasson and Birgit Rösblad

19. VOLITION: CHILD-ORIENTED INTERVENTION FOR THE UPPER
EXTREMITY   298
Susan M. Cahill and Gary Kielhofner

20. CONSTRAINT-INDUCED MOVEMENT THERAPY FOR CHILDREN
WITH HEMIPLEGIA   308
Ann-Christin Eliasson and Andrew M. Gordon

21. SELF-CARE AND HAND FUNCTION 320
Anne Henderson and Ann-Christin Eliasson

22. WRITTEN COMMUNICATION: CLINICAL DECISION-MAKING
FOR HANDWRITING IN CHILDREN WITH CEREBRAL PALSY 339
Sonya Murchland, Alison Lane and Jenny Ziviani

23. LEARNING TO PLAY: PROMOTING SKILLS AND QUALITY OF LIFE
IN INDIVIDUALS WITH CEREBRAL PALSY 357
Erna Imperatore Blanche and Susan Hirsch Knox

24. ASSISTIVE TECHNOLOGY DEVICES IN COMPUTER ACTIVITIES 371
Helene Lidström and Maria Borgestig

25. PARTICIPATION – THE ULTIMATE CHALLENGE 385
Jenny Ziviani and Margaret Wallen

26. THE EVIDENCE-BASE FOR UPPER EXTREMITY INTERVENTION
FOR CHILDREN WITH CEREBRAL PALSY 396
Christine Imms

APPENDIX: ASSESSMENTS USED TO MEASURE HAND FUNCTION,
ACTIVITIES AND PARTICIPATION OF CHILDREN WITH CEREBRAL
PALSY 418
Heidi Sanders

INDEX 427

AUTHORS' APPOINTMENTS

Erna Imperatore Blanche   Division of Occupational Science and Occupational Therapy at the School of Dentistry, University of Southern California, Los Angeles, California, USA

Maria Borgestig   Folke Bernadotte regionhabilitering, Department of Women's and Children's Health, Uppsala University Hospital, Uppsala, Sweden

Daniel Bourbonnais   Ecole de réadaptation, Université de Montréal, Montreal, Canada

Patricia A. Burtner   Occupational Therapy Graduate Program, Department of Pediatrics, University of New Mexico, Albuquerque, New Mexico, USA

Susan M. Cahill   Department of Occupational Therapy, College of Applied Health Sciences, University of Illinois at Chicago, Chicago, Illinois, USA

Jeanne R. Charles   Department of Rehabilitation Medicine, Division of Physical Therapy, Emory University School of Medicine, Atlanta, Georgia, USA

Giovanni Cioni   Department of Developmental Neuroscience, Stella Maris Scientific Institute, Pisa; Division of Child Neurology and Psychiatry, University of Pisa, Italy

Ann-Christin Eliasson   Department of Woman and Child Health, Karolinska Institute, Stockholm, Sweden

Victor Frak   Département de kinanthropologie, Université du Québec à Montréal, Montreal, Canada

Andrew M. Gordon   Department of Biobehavioral Sciences, Teachers College, and Department of Rehabilitation Medicine, College of Physicians and Surgeons, Columbia University, New York, USA

Andrea Guzzetta	Department of Developmental Neuroscience, Stella Maris Scientific Institute, Pisa; Division of Child Neurology and Psychiatry, University of Pisa, Pisa, Italy
Anne Henderson	Professor Emeritus, Department of Occupational Therapy, Boston University/Sargent College of Allied Health Professions, Boston, Massachusetts, USA
Christine Imms	School of Occupational Therapy, La Trobe University; Occupational Therapy Department, Royal Children's Hospital; Murdoch Childrens Research Institute, Victoria, Australia
Beth Moody Jones	Langford Sports and Physical Therapy, University of New Mexico, Albuquerque, New Mexico, USA
Shailesh S. Kantak	Motor Behavior and Neurorehabilitation Laboratory, Division of Biokinesiology and Physical Therapy, at the School of Dentistry, University of Southern California, Los Angeles, California, USA
Gary Kielhofner	Department of Occupational Therapy, College of Applied Health Sciences, University of Illinois at Chicago, Chicago, Illinois, USA
Susan Hirsch Knox	Director Emeritus, Therapy in Action, Tarzana, California, USA
L. Andrew Koman	Department of Orthopaedic Surgery, Wake Forest University School of Medicine, Winston-Salem, North Carolina, USA
Ingeborg Krägeloh-Mann	Department of Pediatric and Developmental Neurology, University Children's Hospital, Tübingen, Germany
Lena Krumlinde-Sundholm	Department of Woman and Child Health, Karolinska Institute, Sweden
Johann Kuhtz-Buschbeck	Institute of Physiology, Christian-Albrechts-Universität Kiel, Germany
Alison Lane	School of Health Sciences & Sansom Institute, University of South Australia, Adelaide, South Australia, Australia
Mindy F. Levin	School of Physical and Occupational Therapy, McGill University, Montreal, Quebec, Canada

Zhongyu Li	Department of Orthopaedic Surgery, Wake Forest University School of Medicine, Winston-Salem, North Carolina, USA
Helene Lidström	Division of Occupational Therapy, Department of Neurobiology, Care Sciences and Society, Karolinska Institute, Stockholm, Sweden
Annette Majnemer	School of Physical and Occupational Therapy, Departments of Pediatrics and Neurology and Neurosurgery, McGill University, Montreal, Quebec, Canada
A. D. Mandich	School of Occupational Therapy, Faculty of Health Sciences, University of Western Ontario, London, Ontario, Canada
Eugenio Mercuri	Department of Child Neurology and Psychiatry, Catholic University of Rome, Rome, Italy; Department of Paediatrics and Neonatal Medicine, Hammersmith Hospital, London, UK
Sonya Murchland	Novita Children's Services, Regency Park, South Australia, Australia
Beth Paterson Smith	Department of Orthopaedic Surgery, Wake Forest University School of Medicine, Winston-Salem, North Carolina, USA
H. J. Polatajko	Department of Occupational Therapy, Department of Public Health Sciences, and Graduate Department of Rehabilitation Sciences, Faculty of Medicine, University of Toronto, Toronto, Ontario, Canada
Eva Pontén	Department of Pediatric Orthopaedic Surgery, Karolinska Institute, Stockholm, Sweden
Janet L. Poole	Occupational Therapy Graduate Program, University of New Mexico, Albuquerque, New Mexico, USA
Birgit Rösblad	Department of Community Medicine and Rehabilitation, Physiotherapy, University of Umeå, Sweden
Heidi Sanders	Occupational Therapy Graduate Program, Department of Pediatrics, University of New Mexico, Albuquerque, New Mexico, USA

Martin Staudt   Department of Pediatric and
                          Developmental Neurology, University
                          Children's Hospital Tübingen, Germany
Bert Steenbergen   NICI, Raboud University Nijmegen, Nijmegen,
                          The Netherlands
Katherine J. Sullivan Division of Biokinesiology and Physical
                          Therapy at the School of Dentistry, University
                          of Southern California, Los Angeles,
                          California, USA
Heidi Sveistrup   School of Rehabilitation Sciences, University
                          of Ottawa, Ottawa, Ontario, Canada
Fredrik Ullén   Stockholm Brain Institute, Neuropediatric
                          Research Unit Q2:07, Department of Women
                          and Child Health, Karolinska Institute,
                          Stockholm, Sweden
Stephan Ulmer   Department of Neuroradiology, UKSH
                          Campus Kiel, Kiel, Germany
Margaret Wallen   Children's Hospital at Westmead, Sydney,
                          Australia
Ann Zilberbrant   Occupational Therapist, Montréal, Québec,
                          Canada
Jenny Ziviani   Division of Occupational Therapy, School
                          of Health and Rehabilitation Sciences,
                          University of Queensland, Brisbane, Australia

FOREWORD

Hans Forssberg

Physicians and therapists working in the field of paediatric care and rehabilitation need to be constantly updated in various areas in order to provide the best practice for their patients. This book, written by an impressive group of experts in many fields, will provide the reader with the current knowledge required to manage and treat movement disorders in children with cerebral palsy (CP). Although the book is focused on the upper limb and hand function of these children, much of the knowledge is generic and can be transferred and applied to other sensory-motor functions as well. The book bridges knowledge derived from the basic sciences, clinical assessments and interventions. It reviews current treatments according to evidence-based practice standards, and it applies the World Health Organization (WHO) perspective on function and participation in a practice-oriented manner.

The book stems from remarkable developments that have emerged only over the last two decades. When I started my neuropaediatric career in the 1980s, therapies for CP were based on ideologies created by strong and innovative practitioners. The treatments included fixed schemes of manipulation and movement training, empirically developed throughout their many years of experience. Some of these 'therapy schools' did their best to base their intervention on the neurophysiological knowledge of that time, in which movements depended on various types of reflexes. Some 'therapy schools' even claimed that they could cure CP, if treatment was started at an early age and practised intensively throughout the day. However, there were no studies showing that the therapies had any effect. In brief, 20 years ago, treatment for children with CP had little scientific foundation; it was a non-academic field, resulting in therapies which lacked both a sound theoretical framework and evidence of positive effects.

Since the 1980s, extensive research in basic neuroscience has revealed the structure and function of the sensory and motor systems of the brain and how these systems develop. The reflex-dominated theories of movement control have been replaced by knowledge on how neural circuits and central programmes interact with sensory information, generating and adapting the movements according to the task and environment. During the same time period, the development of powerful technology-based tools, which can look into the living brain and see how it works, has provided detailed information on these sensory-motor circuits in humans. New neuroimaging methods have also allowed detailed descriptions of the patho-neuroanatomy of CP – i.e. which part of the brain is lesioned, which sensory and motor circuits are damaged, and the relation between these lesions and subsequent sensory-motor dysfunctions. The results of these developments are presented in the first section of the book.

The second big change during the last two decades is the shift from empirically driven 'therapy schools' to evidence-based intervention. However, this shift has not yet occurred in all countries, and, in truth, in most countries the shift has been mainly in a way of thinking and has not yet been integrated into practice. As this book describes, there is not yet a solid foundation of evidence-based treatments for movement disorders in CP, but the trend is there. More randomized and controlled studies on various treatments are being published, and there is a clear commitment on the part of therapists, as well as a desire by patients and parents, to use the best available treatment. This shift is a prerequisite for another trend, i.e. allowing parents to play a more active role in choosing and planning the treatment together with the clinicians. In order to discuss and choose treatment methods, the evidence supporting intervention choices has to be well documented. Last, but probably not least, there is strong pressure from health-care authorities to use the money available as effectively as possible, and that requires clear data on the cost effectiveness of treatment outcomes.

A third major shift in paediatric rehabilitation during the last two decades is a change from the traditional medical perspective on neurological impairments, to function, activity and participation according to WHO definitions (International Classification of Functioning, Disability and Health). Children with CP and other neurological impairments can now be categorized based on their function. The pioneering development of the Gross Motor Function Classification System has now been followed by the development of an analogous system for hand function (Manual Ability Classification System). Again, the most important result of these functionally based classifications systems is probably not the ability to classify children in different categories, but rather that they are changing the way of thinking. This will lead to a focus on what the individual child can do – and what it would be possible for the child to do after an intervention. This functional 'mind set' is well represented in most chapters of the book. Several functionally based assessment scales have been developed and validated, and there is now a theoretical framework and an arsenal of methods allowing researchers to perform evidence-based research. New treatment strategies, based on functional goals instead of fixed treatment schemes, can now be developed and tested.

Finally, this book, by including chapters of a very high scientific standard, reflects another important development which has taken place during the last two decades. Therapists, and the therapy profession, have been transformed 'from health workers uncritically using established methods' into true academic professionals critically reviewing their own work. The editors of this book, and most of the contributors, have a professional education as therapists. Ten years ago, there were far fewer scientific scholarly therapists. In many countries, education of therapists has been transferred to the universities and academic positions for teachers and researchers have been created. The establishment of scientifically active therapists, performing evidence-based research from a functional perspective, taking into account new results from basic neuroscience, has immensely accelerated development. By reading this book, the reader will receive up-to-date information about present knowledge in the treatment of children with CP. It will also provide the reader with the opportunity to be part of a dynamically developing field in which many challenges are yet to be resolved.

INTRODUCTION

Ann-Christin Eliasson and Patricia A. Burtner

Previous books in the *Clinics in Developmental Medicine* series addressing the assessment and treatment of children with cerebral palsy have included separate chapters on the development of hand skills. With the emergence of new models and theories of function, disability, motor control and learning in the past two decades, hand function assessment and intervention practices have expanded. Changes in our treatment approaches can be identified in neurorehabilitation, orthopaedic management, and developmental paediatrics, as well as in physical rehabilitation including occupational and physical therapy practices. Thus, a full edition covering the essentials of upper extremity and hand function skills in children with cerebral palsy is needed.

In the first section of this book, selected experts in the fields of neuroimaging, neurology, orthopaedics, anatomy, motor control and motor learning provide theoretical and foundational information regarding the development of hand function in children with cerebral palsy. The second section of this book focuses on current application of this information for clinicians providing assessment and intervention services to improve hand use in this population. Our intent in focusing only on upper extremity and hand function is not to fragment intervention for the individual child, but rather to highlight these current intervention concepts for clinicians and others invested in the well-being of children with cerebral palsy.

Perhaps the greatest influence on our thinking in the past decade has been the World Health Organization's (WHO) revised International Classification of Functioning, Disability and Health (ICF: WHO 2001). Prior to this revision, the focus of intervention was on reducing the child's impairments that interfered with function. As shown in Fig. I.1, the ICF no longer represents a hierarchy of functional levels, but rather an interaction of body functions and structures, activities and participation, which are influenced by the health of the child as well as environmental and personal factors. Such interactive dynamics suggest that environmental interventions may influence a child's activities and participation as readily as body structure and function interventions. It also suggests that perhaps a combination of interventions that integrate different components simultaneously may be most effective. The emphasis of the ICF on the child's participation and activities has led to the development of new assessment instruments and interventions reaching beyond the child's disability, and these include measures and outcomes specific to different environments as well as overall quality of life. The ICF provides a more 'ecological' approach, as described

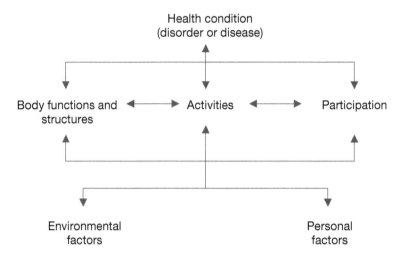

Fig. I.1 Interactions between the components of ICF (WHO 2001: 18).

by Rosenbaum (2004), which widens our perspective beyond the biological dimensions of the child's problems to the health and well-being of the child and family.

What can be learned from theories of motor development?

Another major influence on our thinking over the past two decades can be traced to new theoretical concepts proposed to explain the phenomenon of motor changes as the child develops. Various theories of motor development emerged during the twentieth century due to changing conceptualizations of the role of central nervous system (CNS) maturation and the influence of the environment on the developmental process (see Campbell 2006). Each theory has provided different insights into the development of upper extremity function and the coordination of unimanual and bimanual skills. The Reflex-Hierarchical Model gave us the first ontological description of upper limb or fine motor development. It claimed that 'higher levels' of the CNS were responsible for more complicated behaviours (see Campbell 2006). Within the constructs of this model, the development of hand and arm function was regarded as a result of the maturation of the CNS. Proponents of this model identified motor skills and their normative times of appearance. Within this rule-based model Gesell explained development as a spiralling hierarchy in which development alternated between advancement and regression rather than occurring in a linear fashion. The developmental norms that were established by Gesell and McGraw are used in many developmental assessment tools (Gesell and Amatruda 1947).

From *dynamic systems theory* we have learned that the developmental process is more than a genetically predetermined series of events. Thelen and colleagues (Smith and Thelen 2003) proposed that emerging skills in infants were the result of many local interactions that occur in real time rather than as a result of maturation. Development of motor behaviour emerges as a function of many subsystems within a task context. No one subsystem is the executive of the system; rather the constraints of the task determine the behaviour (Heriza

1991). Therefore dynamic systems theory provides an explanation for the global similarities as well as the individual differences in human development by considering processes of daily activities that are performed by children and how they create developmental change (Smith and Thelen 2003).

Action perception theory proposes that even young babies are very competent beings and that their movement is organized as action in response to their motivation, defined by a goal, and guided by information (von Hofsten 2004). Neonates demonstrate shortly after birth that they can alter their sucking behaviour prospectively by monitoring the flow of the milk (Craig and Lee 1999), and that they can control the gaze and direct it to significant sources of information such as the face and eyes (Farroni et al 2002), as well as direct arm movements toward objects (von Hofsten 1982). However, the development of these actions is highly dependent on the interaction with the environment. Proponents state that perception, cognition and motivation develop as a result of an interaction between neural processes (i.e. cell growth, migration and differentiation) and actions.

Recently the *neuronal group selection theory* was proposed in order to explain the variability in developmental processes. This theory proposes that the brain is 'dynamically organized into variable neuronal networks whose structure and function are selected by development and behavior' (Edelman 1989, Sporns and Edelman 1993, Hadders-Algra 2000: 567). Primary neuronal repertoires, genetically determined, are involved at the beginning of the developmental process. As motor development proceeds, afferent information from the environment results in a repertoire that becomes stable and less variable (Changeux and Danchin 1976, Hadders-Algra 2000). As the infant continues to be exposed to changes in the environment, new and different afferent information results in a secondary, more variable neuronal repertoire adaptive to environmental constraints (Hadders-Algra 2000). Based on these premises, development is not driven solely by *either* genetic determination *or* organization around environment condition/task constraints, but rather by an intertwining of both. In summary, current predominant developmental theory seems to emphasize the interaction between the developing CNS and the environment, considering the maturation of the CNS as only one factor that contributes to the development and coordination of complex movements that are required for an individual to actively explore their environment.

What Does Good versus Poor Upper Extremity and Hand Function Mean for a Child's Independence in Daily Life?

Children with cerebral palsy encounter many practical obstacles when using their hands in daily life (Sköld et al 2004). The hand is typically an effective tool used in almost all life situations. When observing children, one sees wide variations in hand use, from simple gestures to more complex skills, which often involve handling objects with different properties (weights, shapes, textures). Children with cerebral palsy exhibit different degrees of hand limitations, with some having difficulty only with in-hand manipulation, while others have severe impairments making it impossible even to grasp (Krumlinde-Sundholm et al 2007). Regardless of the degree of severity, decreased hand function has an impact on the children's daily activities in self-care, school and engagement in play or leisure activities.

Success in daily activities is typically related to the match between the capabilities of the person and the demands that the activity and the environment impose on the person. When the demands exceed the capability, a discrepancy in task performance occurs (Holm et al 1998). What children want and need to do is different for different children, and it is also related to age. However, hand function is complex and deciding how the intervention should be planned and organized is a difficult process.

Management strategies, therapeutic methods and other interventions for children with cerebral palsy need to be based on knowledge of how the central nervous system controls movement as a result of different types of impairment. But they also need to take account of knowledge of human motor development and motor learning. Therefore this book will include chapters which present the current thinking about the foundations for hand skills as well as information about different types of treatment.

How Do Classification Systems Assist Our Understanding of the Diversity of Disability in Children with Cerebral Palsy?

The diversity of disability greatly influences the choice of treatment for individual children. To provide common terminology for clinicians, children are typically diagnosed with classifications based on location of the lesion, part of the body involved or degree of impairment (Ingram 1964). However, the descriptions are mainly impairment-based and do not provide information about the child's functional abilities in daily life. A new definition of cerebral palsy (CP) focuses on a broader perspective of activity restriction and disability (Rosenbaum et al 2007; see also Chapter 3). In addition, a classification system is now available outlining a clear functional approach: the Gross Motor Function Classification System (GMFCS). This system describes gross motor function in terms of self-initiated movements, with emphasis on function in sitting and walking (Palisano et al 1997). The GMFCS has been important for describing development of gross motor function in children with CP, as well as providing a framework for expectations of intervention. It has been widely adopted internationally, suggesting that it has filled a gap in functional classification (Morris and Bartlett 2004).

Until recently, there was no classification with a functional approach for the use of the hands. The newly developed Manual Ability Classification System (MACS) is designed to classify how children with CP use their hands when handling objects in daily activities (Fig. I.2) (Eliasson et al 2006b). It is important to note that the MACS is independent of typical diagnostic classifications or the GMFCS (Figs I.3 and I.4). By using MACS it will be possible to direct, plan and describe intervention depending on the child's ability to use his or her hands. The MACS will be used in most of the chapters in this book.

The MACS is based on the ICF (WHO 2001). Manual ability has its starting point in upper limb activity and participation but it is also influenced by environmental, personal and contextual factors. The children's ability can be described in terms of five different levels (Fig. I.2). The MACS reports the participation of both hands together and does not aim to distinguish between different capacities of the two hands. It is not designed to classify best capacity, but rather classifies how children actually handle objects in daily life. Objects that are relevant and age-appropriate (for example, eating, dressing, playing, writing objects,

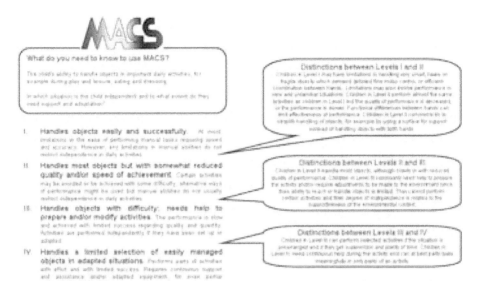

Fig. I.2 MACS leaflet (www.macs.nu).

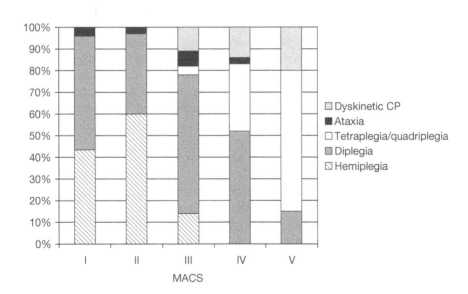

Fig. I.3 Distribution of children across MACS levels according to subtypes of cerebral paresis, based on 168 children aged between 4 and 18 years.

Source: Eliasson AC, Krumlinde-Sundholm L, Rösblad B, Beckung E, Arner M, Öhrvall AM, Rosenbaum P (2006) The Manual Ability Classification System (MACS) for children with cerebral palsy: scale development and evidence of validity and reliability. *Dev Med Child Neurol* 48: 549–554.

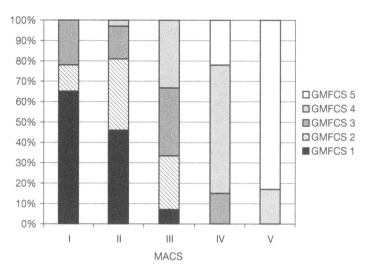

Fig. I.4 Distribution of children across MACS levels in terms of GMFCS level, based on 168 children aged between 4 and 18 years.

Source: Eliasson AC, Krumlinde-Sundholm L, Rösblad B, Beckung E, Arner M, Öhrvall AM, Rosenbaum P (2006) The Manual Ability Classification System (MACS) for children with cerebral palsy: scale development and evidence of validity and reliability. *Dev Med Child Neurol* 48: 549–554.

etc.) are distinct from objects used in advanced skilled activities which require special training for performance, such as playing a musical instrument, and activities closely related to academic skills in school. The MACS also emphasizes manual ability for handling objects in an individual's personal space close to one's body, as distinct from objects that are not within reach, thus minimizing the potential confounding influence of limitations in gross motor function. Distinctions between the levels are based on the quantity and quality of performance and need for assistance or adaptations to perform manual tasks in everyday life. MACS level is independent from diagnosis – for example, children with diplegia appear in several MACS levels (see Fig. I.3). For children with hemiplegia it is their ability to participate in daily activities that places them in a certain level, not the degree of impairment of their hands.

By using the MACS, it is possible not only to describe different functional abilities but also to discuss decision making for treatment and goal setting in a more distinct way for children at different functional levels. First of all, the child's level of independence is classified. Children at MACS levels I and II are independent in most age-related activities, while children at levels III–V need different levels of assistance (see Table I.1). However, this does not mean that children at levels I and II do not need intervention. Often children at level I are uncertain in stressful situations, or when more advanced skills are required. At level II, children are slow and deliberate in their hand use, especially in new and demanding activities; they typically use alternative strategies, especially children with hemiplegia. Intervention may help these children to become more skilled in certain activities or to learn new activities, and lead to increased participation in solitary activities or activities with peers. Thus, treatment might result in a higher level of independence or self-confidence. Children at this level typically compare themselves to peers without disabilities, which can make them feel very different (Sköld et al 2004). Improved fine motor skills have been documented in this group of children after constraint induced movement therapy (Eliasson et al 2003, Charles et al 2006, Hoare et al 2007).

Children at MACS level III need adaptation of the environment, technical aids and a lot of practice to be independent in certain activities. Goals can be directed to independence when there is no time limitation and a good environment. To be able to do things independently sometimes, without the expectation of always performing without assistance, is crucial for this group. By arranging the environment and using adaptations, these children can manage to do a lot.

Children at MACS level IV are typically very dependent on the environment and technical aids to be able to perform parts of activities independently. They usually require the assistance of caregivers to successfully complete activities and participate. The challenge and goal for treatment is to improve these children's activity levels rather than strive for independence. By adapting part of their activities they can complete tasks cooperatively and feel involved in life situations. Their overall performance is highly influenced by their gross motor performance which might vary between GMFCS levels II and V (Fig. I.4). Children at level V have a much reduced level of motor ability but that does not mean they are not able to learn simple actions. To be able to press a bell or activate a music player could be very important.

What is Known about Development of Hand Function in Children with Cerebral Palsy?

In discussing and evaluating treatment it is important to consider the natural history of development, in order to distinguish between changes in the child's development as a result

TABLE I.1
Goals for treatment based on different levels of MACS

Level		Goal for manual skills
I	Handles objects easily and successfully	Improved skill performance and confidence in difficult activities
II	Handles most objects but with somewhat reduced quality and/or speed of achievement	Improved speed, quality and safety by practising age-related activities and more advanced skills
III	Handles objects with difficulty; needs help to prepare and/or modify activities	Independence in additional activities by learning effective strategies and procedure and use of adaptations
IV	Handles a limited selection of easily managed objects in adapted situations	Increased independence in certain selected activities and use of adaptations
V	Does not handle objects and has severely limited ability to perform even simple actions	Add meaningful actions possible to carry out

7

of increasing age and changes arising in response to treatment. Unfortunately, knowledge about the natural history of development of hand function in children with cerebral palsy is limited. In a literature search, only three studies describing upper extremity and hand development were found. The first study reported development of grip patterns and spontaneous use of the hemiplegic hand in a group of 31 children with hemiplegic cerebral palsy (Fedrizzi et al 2003). These children demonstrated only a weak tendency to adopt more advanced grip patterns, and spontaneous use of the hand was stable over time. All scorings were done from video recordings and the children were examined over a 10-year period, starting from under 4 years of age.

The second study included 51 children with cerebral palsy aged between 16 and 60 months enrolled in a study of treatment during the 1990s (Law et al 1997). By recalculating the available data, growth curves were constructed based on four sets of data collected for each child during a 10-month period (Hanna et al 2003). Results suggested that the child's development depended on the severity of hand dysfunction. Children with mild impairment had fairly good development of hand skills, while children with severe impairment at an early age showed a negative trend in their development as measured with the Peabody Fine Motor Development Scales. When the calculations were based on QUEST (Quality of Upper Extremity Skills Test), which measured quality of movement, children showed only minor improvement up to 2–4 years, dependent on severity of hand function.

In contrast to these results, Eliasson and colleagues (2006a) showed improvement in multiple hand function parameters in their follow-up data on ten children with diplegia or hemiplegia 13 years post initial testing, using the Jebsen-Taylor Hand Function Test and a grip-lift task. The first data were collected when the children were 6–8 years old and the second when they were 19–21 years. The Jebsen-Taylor Hand Function Test time scores decreased by 45 per cent from the first to the second data session. Similarly, the overall time to complete the grip-lift task decreased by 22 per cent and the coordination between grasping and lifting, i.e. grip force–load force path ratios, decreased from 1.7 to 1.35 (1 = straight line), suggesting that improvement in hand function occurs over a longer time frame than would commonly be expected.

These studies suggest to us that there is no simple relationship between a child's level of impairment and his or her development of hand skills, i.e. between the ICF levels: Body Function and Activity. Yet, these examples may be understood as follows: the grip patterns (Fedrizzi et al 2003) and the quality of movement (QUEST: Hanna et al 2003) reflect the impairments, which are not easily changed, only seen in experimental research (Eliasson et al 2006a). However it also appears that children can learn effective movement strategies, resulting in increased skills, confirmed by the results of the Jebsen-Taylor Hand Function Test and the Peabody Development Test (Hanna et al 2003, Eliasson et al 2006a). This increase in effective movement outcomes can be interpreted as a reflection of the children having learned to accommodate their deviant grip and movement patterns as they developed to master hand skills in the context of daily activity. This interpretation gives positive evidence for the possibility of improving hand skills by assisting in the motor learning of activities that are relevant for the children.

What is the Current State of the Art of Assessment and Treatment of Upper Extremity and Hand Differences in Children with Cerebral Palsy?

Over the past two decades, new developments in neurorehabilitation, orthopaedics, paediatrics, and occupational and physical therapy have provided new assessments and treatment possibilities specifically designed for children with cerebral palsy. A wide range of intervention methods is used, with some addressing the upper extremity dysfunction itself, while others address the consequences that hand function differences have for the everyday life of the individual concerned. However, little is known about the effect of therapeutic treatment in children and adolescents with cerebral palsy. We continue to struggle with questions such as: what combinations of surgery, pharmacological interventions and therapy are most effective, at what life stage, how often and how long?

Traditionally, the focus of intervention in children with cerebral palsy has been on gross motor function, sitting position, and 'handling', to improve the children's ability in activities of daily living (Bobath and Bobath 1984). This therapeutic approach was based on the assumptions of reflex hierarchical theory and the premise that gross motor abilities have been identified as the prerequisite for fine motor skills (Bobath and Bobath 1984, Gordon 1987). The principles of neurodevelopmental training (NDT) are regularly applied to treatment but, to date, intervention studies focusing on the upper extremity based on this approach have shown minimal improvement (Kluzik et al 1990, Law et al 1991, Fetters and Kluzik 1996, Law et al 1997, Butler and Darrah 2001).

Review of the recent literature lends strong support for the use of occupation-based approaches as opposed to component-driven ones in achieving the ultimate goal of restoring clients' occupational lives (Fisher 1998, Law et al 1998, McLaughlin Gray 1998, Law 2004). In recent years therapists have begun to be guided by the therapeutic approach based on motor learning theories which suggest that motor behaviour emerges through a person's multiple systems interacting with unique task and environmental contexts (Mathiowetz and Bass Haugen 1994). To overcome motor dysfunctions, repeated practice, self-organization and experimentation with varied strategies and tasks are needed, in order for the individual to find the optimal solutions to motor problems encountered and to develop performance skills. Through such repetition it has been argued that an individual's ability to perform tasks develops over time (Schmidt and Wrisberg 2000). These motor control/motor learning and occupation-based (also referred to as task-oriented) approaches will be the focus for treatment in this book.

In recent years there have also been new developments in impairment-based interventions, such as hand surgery, botulinum toxin, etc. These interventions are theoretically linked to biomechanical and neurophysiological principles for restoring the balance between spastic and antagonist muscles. This is an important aspect of treatment, giving the children possibilities for using the hand as efficiently as possible, and is often the prerequisite for optimal therapeutic hand intervention to improve function. However, there is no simple relationship between decreased symptoms and improved functional ability; the focused effort of children to overcome their limitations is also a key factor. There is a third line of intervention employing strategies to adapt the environment in order to ensure the maximum participation of the child in multiple environmental and life situations. These different levels of intervention are in accordance with the International Classification of Functioning, Disability and Health description of health promotion (ICF: WHO 2001). Thus, the ICF framework is a helpful tool for describing different types of intervention.

The second part of this book, which addresses assessment and intervention, has been organized according to ICF levels. When discussing treatment linked to Body Structure and Function, chapters in this section will cover biomechanical and neurorehabilitative treatments such as upper extremity surgery, botulinum toxin, and use of splints. When discussing treatment linked to Activity and Participation, the focus is on interventions that incorporate meaningful activity for the child and are based on recent research of the basic mechanisms of hand function and principles of motor learning. The discussion of activity-based interventions will also include specific approaches to promote mastery of activities of daily living (ADL), handwriting and play. Participation in life situations is the overall goal of treatment, but is not always specifically addressed in the treatment prescribed by professionals. To address this participation gap, we have included intervention models which specifically incorporate the context and environments in which children participate. These models are helpful in planning and carrying out the treatment at all ICF levels relevant for the individual child and family. There are several models available: for example, the Canadian Model of Occupational Performance (CMOP) and the Model of Human Occupation (MOHO) Occupational Therapy Intervention Model (OTIPM) (Fisher 1998, Law et al 1998, Kielhofner 2002). Any model can be used to formulate goals for treatment as long as it adopts a family-centred care perspective.

WHAT ARE FAMILY-CENTRED SERVICES AND WHY ARE THEY IMPORTANT?

Although this book is designed to provide current theoretical and clinical information in the area of upper extremity and hand function in children with cerebral palsy, the services provided are successful only with the 'buy-in' of the child and their family. Thus, the evaluation and intervention process becomes a collaborative process, with families as full participants rather than just receivers of services. In family-centred services (FCS), the recommended interventions and targeted outcomes are individualized according to the unique issues of the child and the family.

Rosenbaum and colleagues (1998) provide three principles based on current literature as the foundation for the conceptual and practical FCS framework. These principles are:

1   *Parents know their children best and want the best for their children.* This guiding principle designates families as equal partners in the decision-making process since they have ultimate responsibility for their child's care after the surgical, pharmacological and therapeutic interventions of professionals. However, as Rosenbaum points out, families are supported by professionals to make informed decisions.
2   *Families are different and unique.* This principle reminds us that there are no 'typical' parents or children. Despite similarities between families and children, each family situation is unique, requiring individuality in care. With this in mind service providers

actively listen and clearly communicate on an individualized level with respect for the family's culture, diversity and goals.

3 *Optimal child development occurs within a supportive family and community context: the child is affected by the stress and coping of other family members.* The child with cerebral palsy is recognized as a member of a family system with stresses and coping needs. By recognizing and valuing the psychosocial needs of parents and families, service providers can assist by providing referrals to resources that support the family, which in turn affects the child's well-being (Rosenbaum 2004).

Concluding remarks

This book represents an overview of the current state of the art in practice for children with cerebral palsy who experience upper extremity and hand function difficulties. It is built on recent theories and evidence. The chapters have been written by a group of distinguished international, interdisciplinary authors. By sharing their expertise, it is hoped that clinicians, children and families in many countries will benefit.

REFERENCES

Bobath K, Bobath B (1984) The neuro-developmental treatment. In: Scrutton D, editor. *Management of the Motor Disorders of Children with Cerebral Palsy.* London: Spastics International Medical Publications, pp. 6–19.

Butler C, Darrah J (2001) Effects of neurodevelopmental treatment (NDT) for cerebral palsy. *Dev Med Child Neurol* 43: 772–784.

Campbell SK (2006) The child's development of functional movement. In: Campbell SK, Vander Linden DW, Palisano RJ, editors. *Physical Therapy for Children, 3rd edn.* St Louis, MO: Sanders Elsevier, pp. 33–76.

Changeux J-P, Danchin A (1976) Selective stabilization of developing synapses as a mechanism for the specification of neuronal networks. *Nature* 264: 705–712.

Charles, J, Wolf, SL, Schneider, J, Gordon, AM (2006) Efficacy of a child-friendly form of constraint-induced movement therapy in hemiplegic cerebral palsy: a randomized control trial. *Dev Med Child Neurol* 48: 635–642.

Craig CM, Lee DN (1999) Neonatal control of sucking pressure evidence for an intrinsic tau-guide. *Exp Brain Res* 124: 371–382.

Edelman GM (1989) *Neural Darwinism: The Theory of Neuronal Group Selection.* Oxford: Oxford University Press.

Eliasson AC, Bonnier B, Krumlinde-Sundholm L (2003) Clinical experience of constraint induced movement therapy in adolescents with hemiplegic cerebral palsy – a day camp model. *Dev Med Child Neurol* 45: 357–359. (Letter.)

Eliasson AC, Forssberg H, Ya-Ching Hung, Gordon AM (2006a) Development of hand function and precision grip control in individuals with cerebral palsy: a 13 year follow up. *Pediatrics* 118: 1226–1236.

Eliasson AC, Krumlinde-Sundholm L, Rösblad B, Beckung E, Arner M, Öhrvall AM, Rosenbaum P (2006b) The Manual Ability Classification System (MACS) for children with cerebral palsy: scale development and evidence of validity and reliability. *Dev Med Child Neurol* 48: 549–554.

Farroni T, Csibra G, Simion F, Johnson MH (2002) Eye contact detection in humans from birth. *Proc Natl Acad Sci USA* 99: 9602–9605.

Fedrizzi E, Pagliano E, Andreucci E, Oleari G (2003) Hand function in children with hemiplegic cerebral palsy: prospective follow-up and functional outcome in adolescence. *Dev Med Child Neurol* 45: 85–91.

Fetters L, Kluzik J (1996) The effects of neurodevelopmental treatment versus practice of reaching of children with spastic cerebral palsy. *Phys Ther* 76: 346–358.

Fisher AG (1998) Uniting practice and theory in an occupational framework: Eleanor Clarke Slagle Lecture. *Am J Occup Ther* 52: 509–521.

Gesell A, Amatruda CS (1947) *Developmental Diagnosis, 2nd edn.* New York: Paul B Hober.

Gordon J (1987) Skill acquisition: assumptions underlying physical therapy intervention: theoretical and historical perspectives. In: Carr J, Shepard R, Gordon J, Gentile AM, Held JM, editors. *Movement Science Foundations for Physical Therapy in Rehabilitation*. Rockville, MD: Aspen Publications, pp. 1–24.

Hadders-Algra M (2000) The neuronal group selection theory: a framework to explain variation in normal motor development. *Dev Med Child Neurol* 42: 566–572.

Hanna SE, Law MC, Rosenbaum PL, King GA, Walter SD, Pollock N, Russell DJ (2003) Development of hand function among children with cerebral palsy: growth curve analysis for ages 16 to 70 months. *Dev Med Child Neurol* 45: 448–455.

Heriza CB (1991) Implications of a dynamical systems approach to understanding infant kicking behavior. *Phys Ther* 71: 222–235.

Hoare BJ, Wasiak J, Imms C, Carey L (2007) Constraint-induced movement therapy in the treatment of the upper limb in children with hemiplegic cerebral palsy (Review). *The Cochrane Library*. Issue 2.

Holm MB, Rogers JC, Stone RG (1998) Person task interventions: decision making guide. In: Neistadt ME, Crepeau EB, editors. *Willard and Spackman's Occupational Therapy, 9th edn*. Philadelphia: Lippincott, pp. 471–498.

Ingram TTS, editor (1964) *Paediatric Aspects of Cerebral Palsy*. London: Livingstone.

Kielhofner G, editor (2002) *A Model of Human Occupation: Theory and Application, 3rd edn*. Baltimore, MD: Lippincott Williams & Wilkins.

Kluzik J, Fetters L, Coryell J (1990) Quantification of control: a primary study of effects of neurodevelopmental treatment on reaching in children with spastic cerebral palsy. *Phys Ther* 70: 65–77.

Krumlinde-Sundholm L, Holmefur M, Kottorp A, Eliasson AC (2007) The Assisting Hand Assessment: current evidence of validity, reliability and responsiveness to change. *Dev Med Child Neurol* 51: 259–264.

Law M (2004) Occupational therapy: depth, innovation and courage. *Aust Occup Ther J* 51: 117–118.

Law M, Cadman D, Rosenbaum P, Walter S, Russel D, DeMatteo C (1991) Neurodevelopmental therapy and upper extremity inhibitive casting for children with cerebral palsy. *Dev Med Child Neurol* 33: 379–387.

Law M, Russel D, Ploock N, Rosenbaum P, Walter S, King G (1997) A comparison of intensive neurodevelopmental therapy plus casting and a regular occupational therapy program for children with cerebral palsy. *Dev Med Child Neurol* 39: 664–670.

Law M, Baptiste S, Carswell A, McColl MA, Polatajko HJ, Pollock N (1998) *Canadian Occupational Performance Measure*. Canada: CAOT.

McLaughlin Gray J (1998) Uniting practice and theory in an occupational framework. 1998 Eleanor Clarke Slagle Lecture. *Am J Occup Ther* 52: 354–364.

Mathiowetz V, Bass Haugen J (1994) Motor behavior research: implications for therapeutic approaches to CNS dysfunction. *Am J Occup Ther* 48: 733–745.

Morris C, Bartlett D (2004) Gross Motor Function Classification System: impact and utility. *Dev Med Child Neurol* 46: 60–65.

Palisano R, Rosenbaum P, Walter S, Russell D, Wood E, Galuppi B (1997) Development and reliability of a system to classify gross motor function in children with cerebral palsy. *Dev Med Child Neurol* 39: 214–223.

Rosenbaum P (2004) Families and service providers forging effective connections and why it matters. In: Scrutton D, Damiano D, Mayston M, editors. *Management of Motor Disorders of Children with Cerebral Palsy*. Clinics in Developmental Medicine 161. London: Mac Keith Press, pp. 22–31.

Rosenbaum P, King S, Law M, King G, Evans J (1998) Family-centered services: a conceptual framework and research review. *Phys Occup Ther Ped* 18: 1–20.

Rosenbaum P, Paneth N, Leviton A, Goldstein M, Bax M, Damiano D, Dan B, Jacobsson B (2007) A report: the definition and classification of cerebral palsy. April 2006. *Dev Med Child Neurol* 109 (Suppl): 8–14.

Schmidt RA, Wrisberg CA (2000) *Motor Learning and Performance. A Problem-based Learning Approach, 2nd edn*. Champaign, IL: Human Kinetics.

Sköld A, Eliasson AC, Josefsson S (2004) Performing bimanual activities – the experience of young persons with children with hemiplegic cerebral palsy. *Am J Occup Ther* 58: 416–425.

Smith LB, Thelen E (2003) Development as a dynamic system. *Trends Cog Sci* 7: 343–348.

Sporns O, Edelman GM (1993) Solving Bernstein's problem: a proposal for the development of coordinated movement by selection. *Child Dev* 64: 960–981.

von Hofsten C (1982) Eye hand coordination in the newborn. *Dev Psych* 18: 450–461.

von Hofsten C (2004) An action perspective on motor development. *Trends Cog Sci* 8: 266–272.

World Health Organization (2001) *International Classification of Functioning, Disability and Health*. Geneva: World Health Organization.

1
BRAIN PLASTICITY IN DEVELOPMENT AND DISEASE

Hans Forssberg

Introduction

The term brain plasticity was introduced around 100 years ago. It is used to describe how the structure and function of neural circuits are modified (1) during development, (2) by experience and learning, and (3) in response to brain lesions. In the middle of the last century, Donald Hebb postulated that cortical neural connections, i.e. synapses, are strengthened and remodelled by experience (Hebb et al 1994). He also showed that rats reared in the rich environment of his own house were much better learners and had better memory capacity than rats living in laboratory cages. The molecular mechanisms behind neural plasticity are complex and not yet fully understood, but numerous studies have shown various mechanisms underlying the activity-dependent modification of synaptic connectivity, including increased number of synapses by changed turnover of dendritic spines, long-term potentiation (LTP) and long-term depression (LDP) (Calverley and Jones 1990, Jenkins et al 1990, Buonomano and Merzenich 1998, Feldman et al 1999, Luscher et al 2000, Trachtenberg et al 2002, Malenka 2003). The latter two mechanisms are important for storage of information in the central nervous system (CNS) and involve several neurotransmitter systems, including gluta-mate (NMDA and AMPA receptors) and GABA (Myers et al 2000), as well as the monoamine systems (dopamine, noradrenalin and serotonin), which are involved by modulating the transmission in the other neurotransmitter systems (Bao et al 2001, Gu 2002).

Neuroimaging methods used to study brain plasticity

The first studies on neural plasticity were performed in experiments on animals. More recently, the development of new powerful imaging techniques has made it possible to study neural plasticity in the human brain as well. Magnetic resonance imaging (MRI) is the most widely used method and enables studies on both structure and function. Volume-based morphometry (VBM) can measure the volumes of critical grey or white matter structures, while diffusion tensor imaging (DTI) measures the integrity of the white matter, i.e. myelinization, size and order of nerve fibres in the neural pathways. By special algo-rithms of the DTI signal, the tracts of the neural fibres can be estimated (trajectography). In functional MRI (fMRI) the synaptic activity in local neural circuits is indirectly measured. In reality it is changes in the blood oxygenation (BOLD signal) that are recorded. Increased metabolism in neurons that are synaptically active induces increased flow of oxygenated blood.

TABLE 1.1
Neuroimaging methods used to study the structure and function of the human brain

Method	Level	Indicates
MRI	Anatomical structures – grey or white matter	The volume of defined nuclei or cortical areas (measured by VBM)
DTI	Movement of water molecules	Integrity of the white matter, myelinization and size of nerve fibres
fMRI	Blood oxygen level (BOLD)	Changes in regional blood flow due to synaptic activity
PET	Molecular level, radioactive ligands	Binding to receptors involved in neurotransmission
TMS	Connectivity from cortex to muscle	Cortical areas (maps) activating specific muscles (EMG recordings)
MEG	Magnetic field from active cortical circuits	Cortical neuronal activity with high temporal resolution

fMRI = functional magnetic resonance imaging; DTI = diffusion tensor imaging; PET = positron emission tomography; TMS = transcranial magnetic stimulation: MEG = magnetic encephalography

In PET studies, radiolabelled agonists or antagonists are used as ligands. When injected, these attach to available receptors and transporters involved in the chemical transmission between pre- and postsynaptic neurons. PET thus measures the availability of these receptors, i.e. a function of the number of receptors and the endogenous release of the transmitter substance. PET can also be used to measure metabolism and blood flow to specific regions.

TMS is a non-invasive technique in which a focused magnetic field pulse, passing through the cranium, is used to evoke electrical discharges of cortical neurons. By stimulating over the motor cortex, the motor area (map) evoking EMG responses in recorded muscles can be defined. With MEG (or multi-electrode EEG) the electrical activation of neural circuits involved in specific actions can be localized with high time resolution.

Plasticity in the developing brain
One of the first descriptions of neural plasticity during development was by Hubel and Wiesel, winning them the Nobel Prize (Hubel and Wiesel 1970, Le Vay et al 1980). They studied the ocular dominance columns in the visual cortex of kittens and monkeys. The visual cortex receives information from both eyes. The right and left eye columns are normally evenly distributed in the primary visual cortex. This organization is not present at birth and takes several weeks to develop in kittens. When Hubel and Wiesel interfered in the development by suturing the eyelid of one eye, thereby only allowing vision from the other eye, the result was an uneven distribution of ocular dominance columns. The columns innervated by the seeing eye expanded at the expense of the non-seeing eye.

These experiments revealed two important principles which have been confirmed in several systems in many different species, including humans. First of all, development of the CNS is not predetermined, but depends on interaction with external factors. Secondly, development is dependent on the activity in the neural circuits. Nerve cells and neural circuits that are frequently used strengthen their connections, while those that are not used are weakened. The phrase 'use or lose' reflects this principle and indicates how an exuberant number of nerve cells and neural pathways which exist in early phases of development are discarded because they are not used. Interestingly, these exuberant neurons and pathways that typically disappear during development may remain after central lesions or peripheral damage blocking the sensory inflow. When there is no competition from lesioned neural circuits, these nerve cells and pathways have less competition and will be used and can survive.

There seems to be an extensive capacity for cross-modal plasticity between auditory and visual areas as a result of lesions/disturbances in early childhood. For example, in congenitally blind humans, speech and auditory processes may activate the visual cortex, and, indeed, blind people localize sound sources better than sighted people (Weeks et al 2000, Roder et al 2002). Sign language activates different brain regions in deaf and hearing individuals (Bavelier et al 2001). After unilateral lesions of the corticospinal system in the human fetus, leading to hemiplegic cerebral palsy, there seem to be exuberant ipsilateral pathways that are maintained and that connect the (undamaged) ipsilateral motor cortex to the (paretic) upper extremity (Carr 1996, Vandermeeren et al 2003b, Staudt et al 2004, Staudt 2007).

Plasticity in the somatosensory system

Studies on cortical synaptic plasticity are partly based on 'cortical maps', i.e. representations of different sensory and motor systems at the primary sensory and motor cortices (Buonomano and Merzenich 1998). In animals, it is possible to investigate the cutaneous innervation of the primary sensory cortex from the hand, by stimulating the fingers and recording from cortical neurons by microelectrodes. Using this procedure, a map of the cortical area that is innervated from each finger can be produced. In monkeys, it was possible to show that the cortical map of the fingers changed after training (Fig. 1.1). In one study, monkeys used two fingers in a tactile discrimination task daily for 5–20 minutes over three weeks (Jenkins et al 1990). The maps of the two fingers that had been used expanded, while those from the fingers not used shrank. These results revealed that more cortical nerve cells were activated by the fingers that had been used frequently, i.e. *use-dependent plasticity*. A similar phenomenon has been described in blind Braille readers, in whom the maps of the 'reading finger' expanded (Pascual-Leone and Torres 1993). Indeed, the plasticity seems to be quite dynamic since the maps fluctuate with the daily reading activity (Sadato et al 1998).

Studies on amputees have shown that absent sensory input may change the cortical maps as well (Pascual-Leone et al 1996). In such cases there is a lack of activity, and other neural circuits that are active can take over cortical nerve cells that are no longer used. In individuals with low amputations, the cortical representation of the remaining upper part of the arm had expanded and occupied the area originally used for the distal part of the arm. In individuals with high amputations, the representation of the face had been extended to

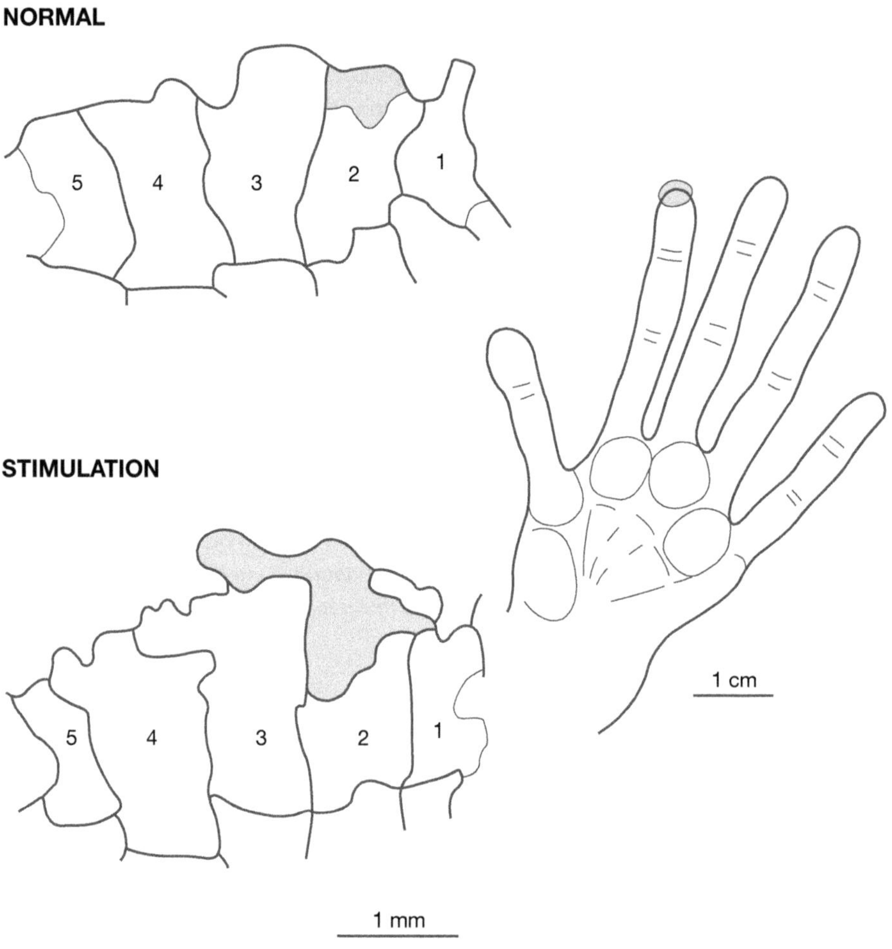

NORMAL

STIMULATION

1 cm

1 mm

Fig. 1.1 Cortical maps of the primary sensory cortex in non-human primates before (normal) and after tactile stimulation of the tip of the index finger. The innervation maps showing the cortical sensory neural representation of the fingers are produced by striking the skin of each finger and at the same time recording from the sensory cortex. The area of the stimulated part of the index finger is indicated by stippling in the schematic area of the hand, and in the two drawings of the cortical maps. Note that after a period of differentiated stimulation of the tip, there was a substantial enlargement of the cortical map of the index finger, in particular of the stimulated area.

Source: Jenkins WM, Merzenich MM, Ochs MT, Allard T, Guic-Robles E (1990) Functional reorganization of primary somatosensory cortex in adult owl monkeys after behaviorally controlled tactile stimulation. *Journal of Neurophysiology* 63: 82–104 (used with permission).

the lost arm and hand areas. Sensation of 'the phantom hand' could in some cases be elicited by touching the face or the upper arm in these patients (Flor et al 1998), which indicates that the perception of the body scheme partly remains although innervated from other parts of the body.

16

Plasticity in the motor system
Similar forms of the neural plasticity seen in the sensory system are also present in the motor cortex. Nudo studied the cortical maps of the upper limbs in monkeys before and after training in specific motor tasks (Nudo et al 1996a, Nudo 1999). In this case the cortical neurons are stimulated by TMS and the muscle activity is recorded by EMG. When the monkeys picked up pellets from a small cup for 15 minutes every day during a 10-day period, the cortical representation of the finger muscles used to pick up the pellet was enlarged, while it was reduced for more proximal muscles of the arm. When the same monkeys trained in another motor task, which required repeated movements of the wrist and elbow, the representation for these more proximal muscles increased, while the distal finger muscle representation was reduced. Thus, when a movement is performed repeatedly, the synaptic connectivity is strengthened in the cortical circuits activating the muscles required for the movement, leading to expanded cortical motor maps for these muscles.

Several studies have shown similar activity-dependent plastic changes in the human motor cortex. In badminton players, the hand of the racket arm has been shown to have a larger cortical representation compared with the other hand. Several studies have been performed with professional musicians, who spend extensive time in motor skill training. One study reported increased cortical sensory-motor representation of the fingers of the left hand in string players, with correlations found between cortical map size and the age at which the player began to play (Elbert et al 1995, Pantev et al 2001). This indicates an interaction between age and activity – the earlier the musician began training and the more intensive the training, the larger the effects. A similar effect on the myelinization of the corticospinal tract has recently been shown in professional piano players in a DTI study (Bengtsson et al 2005). DTI measures the white matter characteristics in the neural pathways. A high anisotropy indicates large and well myelinated nerve fibres, which are known to give fast conduction velocities and fatigue resistance. In this study, the pianists had higher anisotropy in the corticospinal tract through the internal capsule than control participants. This difference could have been due to a genetic disposition among the pianists, actually allowing them to be more technically skilled. However, within the pianist group the anisotropy correlated positively to the amount of training the pianist received before 11 years of age. This suggests that intensive training during childhood, during the period when the corticospinal system is myelinated, may influence the organization, and probably also the function, of the pathways.

Learning of new motor skills
The plastic changes of the maps in the sensory and motor cortices mentioned above were caused by sensory input or enhanced motor activity. The fingers, the hand or the arm were used more frequently than normal, but also the same movement patterns were used repeatedly. This form of practice is different from learning and practising new motor skills. Initially the new movement has to be carefully learned. With time, the movement can be performed more fluently, until it becomes automatized and performed without the person paying attention to the different sequences of the movement. After a longer training time even complicated movements can be automatized, e.g. a secretary can type perfectly while

talking with somebody else. The learning process can be divided into two phases: an early learning phase with rapid improvement of performance, beginning from the first training sessions; and a second more extended phase including several training sessions for days/weeks during which a gradual improvement proceeds and the movement becomes automatized (Ungerleider et al 2002). During the early learning phase there is a consolidation of the learned movement. This means that the movement is improved and stabilized during the rest period between training sessions, partly during sleep. If the rest period is disturbed (e.g. no sleep) the consolidation of the movement is negatively influenced (Shadmehr and Holcomb 1997, Karni et al 1998, Fischer et al 2002).

The brain activity changes underlying learning of new motor skills have been studied in humans by means of fMRI. The results suggest that in general the same areas are synaptically active both during the early learning phases and after the movement has become automatized (Wu et al 2004). Thus, there is no support for a previous hypothesis that new circuits and new areas are activated when the movement becomes automatized. On the other hand, the amount of neural activity decreased as the movement became more automatized. In an attempt to make a simple neural model of motor learning, Ungerleider and coworkers (Ungerleider et al 2002) suggested that there are two different categories of motor learning. One includes learning of new motor programmes (e.g. new sequences of finger tapping). The other involves adaptation of already existing motor programmes to new forms of movement patterns or to a new environment. When new motor programmes are learned (category 1), a large neural network is involved including sensory and motor cortices in the frontal and parietal lobes, basal ganglia and cerebellum. The whole network is active in the beginning of the learning. In later phases the basal ganglia continue to be active, while the activity in the cerebellum ceases. Interestingly, the opposite occurs when the motor learning involves adaptation (category 2). A cortico-cerebellar network continues to be active, while the activity in the basal ganglia is reduced during later phases.

In one of the earliest motor learning studies, changes in the motor cortex were studied in healthy adults before and after a four-week training period (Karni et al 1995). The research paradigm required participants to learn a specific sequence in which they opposed different fingers against the thumb in a specific order. After each training week the learned sequence could be performed faster. The fMRI recordings indicated increased activity in the motor cortex when the learned sequence was performed, as compared to a different, not learned sequence. This study indicated that there might be plastic changes taking place also in the primary motor cortex during learning of motor sequences. However, it has so far not been confirmed by other researchers, and it does not tally with later studies showing a general reduction in activity after the learned sequence has been automatized. Although the new imaging techniques have allowed us to study what is happening in the brain during motor learning, we are still only in the early stages of understanding the interplay between various networks and how the information of the learned motor skills is stored.

In addition to changes of synaptic activity during motor performance after training, there seem to be structural changes in the grey matter. In a recent study in healthy adults, participants were instructed to learn a classic three-ball cascade over a period of three months (Draganski et al 2004). The brain changes in the participants were investigated by MR volumetry before and after the training period learning a new motor skill. Results showed volumetric expansion in the grey matter of these individuals in certain areas of the temporal and parietal lobes. The expansion correlated with the skills the participants learned, indicating a growth of the neural circuits that are used. The grey matter areas which were changed in this study are not directly involved in motor coordination and motor planning, but have important roles in receiving and integrating visual and somatosensory information that serves as a foundation for subsequent motor programming.

Plasticity of the young damaged brain
The plasticity present during development and during learning and training is probably also an important factor supporting rehabilitation after a brain lesion. Nudo and colleagues (Nudo et al 1996b, Nudo 1999) have shown that recovery of motor functions after a cortical lesion in monkeys is dependent upon extension and expansion of the cortical maps post-lesion. Monkeys who were trained after lesions in the hand area of the primary motor cortex exhibited a better recovery than those who were not, and also had a larger expansion of their cortical map. This and other experimental studies give hope, since they show that specific training produces both functional improvements and structural reorganization of the motor cortex. Several clinical imaging studies in adult patients have shown considerable neural reorganization post-stroke (Hallett 2001). In the acute phase of stroke rehabilitation, changes have a multifactor background and thus attributing progress solely to the training is difficult. However, there are now several training studies showing good results also during the chronic phase of the stroke, when most other factors are no longer present. The functional improvements in these individuals are associated with changed brain activity as measured by fMRI (Lindberg et al 2007).

Brain lesions affecting the sensory-motor system during development often result in different types of motor dysfunction compared with those that are seen in the case of adult brains with similar lesions. During development, various neural systems are competing for synaptic space. In the absence of competing circuits, due to lesions or altered neural activity, other neural circuits and pathways, which typically disappear during development, may remain and become functionally active. Whether the outcome of early lesions in children results in better or worse function than in adults is not obvious, however. In some cases outcomes are better, in others worse (Kolb and Whishaw 1998, Kolb et al 2000).

One clinical example is the brain development in children with an early (fetal) lesion in one hemisphere leading to hemiplegic cerebral palsy. Recent studies by several groups using TMS and fMRI in children with hemiplegic cerebral palsy have shown that the cortical circuits and the corticospinal pathways from the motor cortex to the hand muscles do not develop as they do in typically developing children (Carr et al 1993, Carr 1996, Vandermeeren et al 2003a, 2003b, Staudt et al 2004). When a small lesion mainly affecting the primary sensory-motor cortex occurs in these children, secondary motor areas in the premotor cortex and supplementary motor cortex typically take over arm/hand functions (see Fig. 1.2). These areas also have neurons projecting to the spinal cord through the corticospinal system. After a large lesion, however, which also includes these secondary motor areas, hand motor control is transferred over to the undamaged hemisphere on the

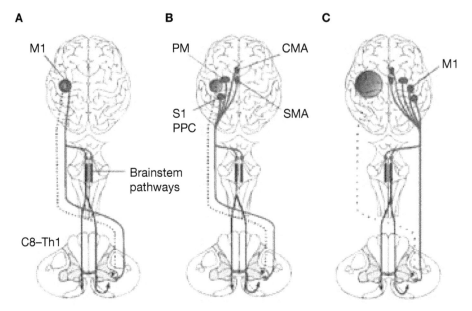

A B C

M1

PM CMA

M1

S1 SMA
PPC

Brainstem
pathways

C8–Th1

Fig. 1.2 Major principles of neural reorganization of the cortical hand motor system after early congenital lesions resulting in hemiplegic cerebral palsy of varying degrees of severity. After a small lesion limited to parts of the primary sensory-motor cortex (A), recovery involves adjacent perilesional areas. After a larger lesion in the same area (B), direct control of hand movements migrates to other frontal motor cortical areas (premotor cortex, supplementary motor area, cingulate motor area), conveyed to the spinal cord via parts of the corticospinal pathways originating from these areas. An even larger lesion, including these other frontal motor areas (C), initiates, in some cases, a transition of direct motor control to the contralateral undamaged hemisphere. In this case, otherwise exuberant ipsilateral corticospinal pathways remain and are used to convey motor signals to the spinal cord.

Source: Adapted from Vandermeeren et al 2003b.

ipsilateral side of the paretic hand. In such cases, motor control is probably exerted through remaining exuberant ipsilateral connections from the primary cortex to the hand muscles.

Interestingly, these plastic changes are not solely beneficial, but may give some problems during bimanual tasks. In children with hemiplegic cerebral palsy, there is a clear relationship between the presence of ipsilateral corticospinal pathways and mirror movements. These may be very disturbing, in particular in bimanual movements, when the two hands have different tasks and are required to move differently to successfully perform desired skills.

Clinical considerations
Knowledge about use-dependent neural plasticity has already influenced theories and thinking around rehabilitation of individuals with functional limitations due to lesions in the nervous system. Although it has already had an influence on clinical interventions, greater implementation in clinical practice is essential for advancing rehabilitation in the future.

A lesion in the CNS of an individual will have a direct effect on the neural circuits involved in the sensory-motor control of, for example, his or her hand dexterity. However, in addition, as a secondary effect, the actual hand which is affected will not be used to the same extent as that of a peer without a disability. According to what we now know about use-dependent plasticity, circuits that are intact, but not used, will be down-regulated by decreased synaptic strength. By stimulating the child to use the limb, the down-regulation of the circuits might be prevented and the synaptic connectivity strengthened. This strengthening of synaptic connectivity is actually precisely what is done in various forms of constraint-induced movement therapy (CIMT) in children and adults with hemiplegia (Taub and Wolf 1997). The CIMT method was first developed for adults post-stroke in whom the neural circuits developed during childhood and were used until the stroke occurred. Training of the hand in the chronic phase after the stroke may thus restore the neural circuits that had been down-regulated by the patients not using the limb (Lindberg et al 2007).

In children with hemiplegic cerebral palsy, the condition is somewhat different, since there is no, or different, activity in the undamaged neural circuits due to the limb not being used or used in a non-typical way. In certain conditions this also leads to a non-typical organization of the descending motor pathways (see above and Fig. 1.2). However, in less severe lesions, when the motor control remains in the affected hemisphere, it is not known to what extent the cortical infrastructure in non-lesioned areas is influenced by not being used during development. There are now several studies in hemiplegic cerebral palsy showing that periods of intense training and use of the affected hand improve the motor function of the hand (Eliasson et al 2005, Bonnier et al 2006, Charles et al 2006). Thus, it seems that the basic infrastructure of cortical neural circuits essential for sensory-motor control is still in place, although it has not been used during typical development. The 'glove' or the 'sling' used to prevent movement of the dominant hand is, of course, the obvious means to stimulate the person to use the affected hand. In the future, new training methods in which the actual hand can be trained by some other means will probably be developed.

In general, the existence of use-dependent neural plasticity prompts us to stimulate self-initiated active movements and to develop training programmes that involve the affected limb and prevent non-use. One longstanding clinical question is: how important is it to start early training and treatment? The first studies on the visual system described 'critical periods' during the first few weeks after birth when activity in the visual pathways was needed in order to support proper development of the ocular columns. More recent studies on cortical sensory and motor maps describe dynamic mechanisms functioning well also in adults. These results indicate that therapy based on activity-dependent plasticity can be used at all ages. This concept has also been demonstrated by the effects of constraint-induced movement therapy in both children and adults. However, the neural plasticity that takes place during development, and in response to task-specific activity in the sensory and motor system, is probably important for accurate development of the neural circuits. This would seem to indicate the importance of early intervention, aiming at encouraging the infant with signs of hemiplegia to use the affected arm. Early intervention has been part of the treatment in many schools of therapy, but so far we lack any clinical evidence that age is critical for starting the intervention. However, with our new knowledge of use-dependent plasticity during development and after CNS damage, there are now good theoretical grounds for initiating studies on the effectiveness of early intervention.

The emerging imaging data on brain activity during different phases of motor learning are fascinating and indicate that the learning of new motor sequences engages the ordinary sensory-motor parts of the brain, and that the level of activity is reduced after the movements have been automatized. Clinically, it might be useful to divide intervention into two categories: (1) the learning of new motor skills – for example, moving the fingers in a special sequence, e.g. playing a tune on the piano; and (2) already existing, but impaired, motor skills – for example, moving only one finger quickly up and down, e.g. playing the same note. The former is dependent on developing a higher order motor programme including temporal and spatial parameters. The latter is mainly dependent on the already existing infrastructure of the neural circuits, which might be underdeveloped by not being used. While the training of the latter might improve connectivity in the existing neural circuits and improve motor capacity of finger movement in any motor task, the motor learning programmes seem to be very task-specific with little transfer to other programmes. In clinical terms, this means that it is important that the motor learning and training are task-specific. Patients should be instructed to specifically train the motor behaviour that needs to be achieved.

REFERENCES

Bao S, Chan VT, Merzenich MM (2001) Cortical remodelling induced by activity of ventral tegmental dopamine neurons. *Nature* 412: 79–83.

Bavelier D, Brozinsky C, Tomann A, Mitchell T, Neville H, Liu G (2001) Impact of early deafness and early exposure to sign language on the cerebral organization for motion processing. *J Neurosci* 21: 8931–8942.

Bengtsson SL, Nagy Z, Skare S, Forsman L, Forssberg H, Ullen F (2005) Extensive piano practicing has regionally specific effects on white matter development. *Nat Neurosci* 8: 1148–1150.

Bonnier B, Eliasson AC, Krumlinde-Sundholm L (2006) Effects of constraint-induced movement therapy in adolescents with hemiplegic cerebral palsy: a day camp model. *Scand J Occup Ther* 13: 13–22.

Buonomano DV, Merzenich MM (1998) Cortical plasticity: from synapses to maps. *Annu Rev Neurosci* 21: 149–186.

Calverley RK, Jones DG (1990) Contributions of dendritic spines and perforated synapses to synaptic plasticity. *Brain Res Rev* 15: 215–249.

Carr LJ (1996) Development and reorganization of descending motor pathways in children with hemiplegic cerebral palsy. *Acta Paediatrica* Suppl 416: 53–57.

Carr LJ, Harrison LM, Evans AL, Stephens JA (1993) Patterns of central motor reorganisation in hemiplegic cerebral palsy. *Brain* 116: 1223–1247.

Charles J, Charles J, Wolf SL, Schneider J, Gordon AM (2006) Efficacy of a child-friendly form of constraint-induced movement therapy in hemiplegic cerebral palsy: a randomized control trial. *Dev Med Child Neurol* 48: 635–642.

Draganski B, Gaser C, Busch V, Schuierer G, Bogdahn U, May A (2004) Neuroplasticity: changes in grey matter induced by training. *Nature* 427: 311–312.

Elbert T, Pantev C, Wienbruch C, Rockstroh B, Taub E (1995) Increased cortical representation of the fingers of the left hand in string players. *Science* 270: 305–307.

Eliasson AC, Krumlinde-Sundholm L, Shaw K, Wang C (2005) Effects of constraint-induced movement therapy in young children with hemiplegic cerebral palsy: an adapted model. *Dev Med Child Neurol* 47: 266–275.

Feldman DE, Nicoll RA, Malenka RC (1999) Synaptic plasticity at thalamocortical synapses in developing rat somatosensory cortex: LTP, LTD, and silent synapses. *J Neurobiol* 41: 92–101.

Fischer S, Hallschmid M, Elsner AL, Born J (2002) Sleep forms memory for finger skills. *Proc Natl Acad Sci* 99: 11987–11991.

Flor H, Elbert T, Muhlnickel W, Pantev C, Wienbruch C, Taub E (1998) Cortical reorganization and phantom phenomena in congenital and traumatic upper-extremity amputees. *Exp Brain Res* 119: 205–212.

Gu Q (2002) Neuromodulatory transmitter systems in the cortex and their role in cortical plasticity. *Neuroscience* 111: 815–835.

Hallett M (2001) Plasticity of the human motor cortex and recovery from stroke. *Brain Res Rev* 36: 169–174.

Hebb DO, Martinez JL, Glickman SE (1994) The organization of behavior – a neuropsychological theory. *Contemp Psychol* 39: 1018–1020.

Hubel DH, Wiesel TN (1970) The period of susceptibility to the physiological effects of unilateral eye closure in kittens. *J Physiol* 206: 419–436.

Jenkins WM, Merzenich MM, Ochs MT, Allard T, Guic-Robles E (1990) Functional reorganization of primary somatosensory cortex in adult owl monkeys after behaviorally controlled tactile stimulation. *J Neurophys* 63: 82–104.

Karni A, Meyer G, Jezzard P, Adams MM, Turner R, Ungerleider LG (1995) Functional MRI evidence for adult motor cortex plasticity during motor skill learning. *Nature* 377: 155–158.

Karni A, Meyer G, Rey-Hipolito C, Jezzard P, Adams MM, Turner R, Ungerleider LG (1998) The acquisition of skilled motor performance: fast and slow experience-driven changes in primary motor cortex. *Proc Natl Acad Sci* 95: 861–868.

Kolb B, Whishaw IQ (1998) Brain plasticity and behavior. *Annu Rev Psychol* 49: 43–64.

Kolb B, Cioe J, Whishaw IQ (2000) Is there an optimal age for recovery from motor cortex lesions? II. Behavioural and anatomical consequences of unilateral motor cortex lesions in perinatal, infant, and adult rats. *Restor Neurol Neurosci* 17: 61–70.

Le Vay S, Wiesel TN, Hubel DH (1980) The development of ocular dominance columns in normal and visually deprived monkeys. *J Comp Neurol* 191: 1–51.

Lindberg PG, Schmitz C, Engardt M, Forssberg H, Borg J (2007) Use-dependent up- and down-regulation of sensorimotor brain circuits in stroke patients. *Neurorehabil Neural Repair* 21: 315–326.

Luscher C, Nicoll RA, Malenka RC, Muller D (2000) Synaptic plasticity and dynamic modulation of the postsynaptic membrane. *Nat Neurosci* 3: 545–550.

Malenka RC (2003) The long-term potential of LTP. *Nat Rev Neurosci* 4: 923–926.

Myers WA, Churchill JD, Muja N, Garraghty PE (2000) Role of NMDA receptors in adult primate cortical somatosensory plasticity. *J Comp Neurol* 418: 373–382.

Nudo RJ (1999) Recovery after damage to motor cortical areas. *Curr Opin Neurobiol* 9: 740–747.

Nudo RJ, Milliken GW, Jenkins WM, Merzenich MM (1996a) Use-dependent alterations of movement representations in primary motor cortex of adult squirrel monkeys. *J Neurosci* 16: 785–807.

Nudo RJ, Wise BM, SiFuentes F, Milliken GW (1996b) Neural substrates for the effects of rehabilitative training on motor recovery after ischemic infarct. *Science* 272: 1791–1794.

Pantev C, Engelien A, Candia V, Elbert T (2001) Representational cortex in musicians. Plastic alterations in response to musical practice. *Ann NY Acad Sci* 930: 300–314.

Pascual-Leone A, Torres F (1993) Plasticity of the sensorimotor cortex representation of the reading finger in Braille readers. *Brain* 116: 39–52.

Pascual-Leone A, Peris M, Tormos JM, Pascual AP, Catala MD (1996) Reorganization of human cortical motor output maps following traumatic forearm amputation. *NeuroReport* 7: 2068–2070.

Roder B, Stock O, Bien S, Neville H, Rosler F (2002) Speech processing activates visual cortex in congenitally blind humans. *Eur J Neurosci* 16: 930–936.

Sadato N, Pascual-Leone A, Grafman J, Deiber MP, Ibanez V, Hallett M (1998) Neural networks for Braille reading by the blind. *Brain* 121: 1213–1229.

Shadmehr R, Holcomb HH (1997) Neural correlates of motor memory consolidation. *Science* 277: 821–825.

Staudt M (2007) (Re-)organization of the developing human brain following periventricular white matter lesions. *Neurosci Biobehav Rev* 31: 1150–1156.

Staudt M, Gerloff C, Grodd W, Holthausen H, Niemann G, Krageloh-Mann I (2004) Reorganization in congenital hemiparesis acquired at different gestational ages. *Ann Neurol* 56: 854–863.

Taub E, Wolf SL (1997) Constraint induced movement techniques to facilitate upper extremity use in stroke patients. *Top Stroke Rehabil* 3: 38–60.

Trachtenberg JT, Chen BE, Knott GW, Feng G, Sanes JR, Welker E, Svoboda K (2002) Long-term in vivo imaging of experience-dependent synaptic plasticity in adult cortex. *Nature* 420: 788–794.

Ungerleider LG, Doyon J, Karni A (2002) Imaging brain plasticity during motor skill learning. *Neurobiol Learn Mem* 78: 553–564.

Vandermeeren Y, Bastings E, Fadiga L, Olivier E (2003a) Long-latency motor evoked potentials in congenital hemiplegia. *Clin Neurophysiol* 114: 1808–1818.

Vandermeeren Y, Sebire G, Grandin CB, Thonnard JL, Schlogel X, De Volder AG (2003b) Functional reorganization of brain in children affected with congenital hemiplegia: fMRI study. *Neuroimage* 20: 289–301.

Weeks R, Horwitz B, Aziz-Sultan A, Tian B, Wessinger CM, Cohen LG, Hallett M, Rauschecker JP (2000) A positron emission tomographic study of auditory localization in the congenitally blind. *J Neurosci* 20: 2664–2672.

Wu T, Kansaku K, Hallett M (2004) How self-initiated memorized movements become automatic: a functional MRI study. *J Neurophysiol* 91: 1690–1698.

2
CORTICAL CONTROL OF HAND FUNCTION

Johann Kuhtz-Buschbeck and Stephan Ulmer

Gestures, writing, painting, music, the use of tools – all these activities require skilled use of the hands. It is the control of the spinal motoneurons by the cerebral cortex that endows the human hand with its remarkable motor repertoire. After an overview of the anatomy and neurophysiology of the motor control system, we will discuss the physiological cortical control of hand movements in the context of three tasks: simple and complex finger movements, grasping with a precision grip, and prehension movements. The effects that focal lesions of the corticospinal tract can have on these functional hand movements are briefly outlined in the last part of the chapter.

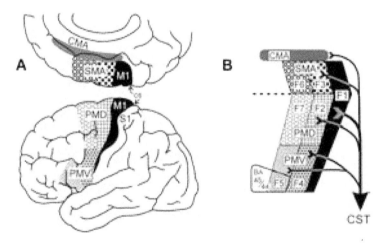

Fig. 2.1 Cortical motor areas. **A.** Medial (upside down) and lateral view of the left hemisphere. Most of the primary motor cortex (M1) is buried in the central sulcus (cs). The supplementary (SMA) and cingulate (CMA) motor areas are located on the medial surface. The lateral premotor cortex (PM) is subdivided into a dorsal (PMD) and a ventral part (PMV). The primary somatosensory cortex S1 is indicated as well. **B.** Parcellation into areas F1–F7 on a scheme of the 'unfolded' cortical motor regions. The SMA, PMD, PMV are each subdivided into two areas. M1 is designated F1. In contrast to F1–F5, areas F6 ('pre-SMA') and F7 ('anterior PMD') have few, if any, corticospinal projections (CST, arrows). F1 (= M1) corresponds to Brodmann's area 4 (BA 4); F2–F4, F6 and F7 correspond to BA 6. Area F5 overlaps with BA 44/45, i.e. the Broca region.

Source: Adapted with permission from Geyer et al 2000.

The motor control system – an overview

Humans have four cortical primary and secondary motor areas (Fig. 2.1A) which contribute to the control of hand movements (Roland and Zilles 1996): (1) the primary motor cortex, M1, also termed Brodmann's area 4 (BA 4; area F1); (2) the supplementary motor area (SMA; areas F3, F6), corresponding to the medial part of Brodmann's area 6 (BA 6); (3) the lateral premotor cortex (PM), which includes the part of BA 6 on the cerebral convexity, and which is subdivided into a ventral (PMV; areas F4, F5) and a dorsal (PMD; areas F2, F7) portion; (4) the cingulate motor area (CMA), located in the cortex lining the cingulate sulcus. All four areas contain somatotopically organized maps of the body, and send mono- or oligosynaptic corticospinal projections to the motoneurons supplying hand muscles (Dum and Strick 2002). Intracortical microstimulation of these regions elicits muscular contractions (Rouiller and Olivier 2004). M1 as the main motor output region has the highest excitability and the most direct effects on the motoneurons. The SMA, PM and CMA as secondary motor areas are mutually interconnected and linked to M1. Neuroimaging studies have demonstrated activity of these four regions during the planning and/or execution of voluntary hand movements. Their further parcellation into the areas F1–F7 (Fig. 2.1B) is based on anatomical and neurophysiological studies in non-human primates, but comparable counterparts exist in humans (Geyer et al 2000). While the anterior areas F6 and F7 are connected with the prefrontal lobe, the more posterior regions F1–F4 receive their main cortical input from the posterior parietal lobe, and F5 from both sources (Rizzolatti and Luppino 2001, Dum and Strick 2005). Parieto-frontal connections form neuroanatomic

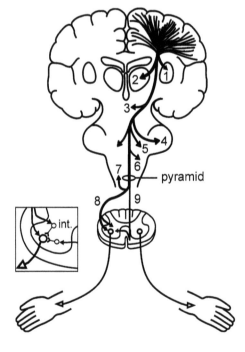

Fig. 2.2 Corticospinal tract (CST). Axons descending from the cortical motor areas send collaterals to the basal ganglia (1), thalamus (2), red nucleus (3), pontine nuclei (4), left and right reticular formation (5), inferior olive (6) and dorsal column nuclei (7). Some fibres terminate in these regions. Approximately one million axons pass through the medullar pyramid. About 90 per cent of them cross to the contralateral side and form the lateral CST (8), and 10 per cent continue ipsilaterally as anterior CST (9). Most CST axons terminate on spinal interneurons (insert: int.), whereas the cortico-motoneuronal fibres project monosynaptically to the motoneurons of intrinsic and extrinsic hand muscles (see Chapter 5 for anatomical details).

circuits (see Fig. 2.9, p. 36) which are involved in sensorimotor transformations during reaching and grasping (Luppino and Rizzolatti 2000).

About 40 per cent of the corticospinal projections originate from the primary motor cortex (F1), another ~30 per cent stem from secondary motor areas (F2–F5 and CMA), and the rest come from postcentral sensory areas (Rouiller 1996, Geyer et al 2000). The axons of the corticospinal tract (CST) descend through the internal capsule, pass through the cerebral peduncles, continue into the pons, and form the pyramid, a distinctive anterior eminence of the medulla. About 90 per cent of the axons cross the midline and continue as lateral CST in the lateral funiculus of the spinal cord, while the remaining 10 per cent of uncrossed fibres continue ipsilaterally as the anterior CST (Fig. 2.2). The motoneurons that supply the extrinsic and intrinsic hand muscles are located in cigar-shaped motor nuclei in the lateral part of the ventral horn of the cervical spinal cord (lamina IX), while those innervating proximal limb and trunk muscles are located more medially (Martin 2005). Motoneurons of intrinsic hand muscles have few, if any, recurrent axon collaterals inducing Renshaw inhibition (Lemon 1993). There is some evidence of skeletofusimotor innervation of forearm muscles in man, i.e. of beta-motoneurons that supply both intra- and extrafusal muscle fibres via branching axons (Kakuda et al 1998). This type of innervation may facilitate the control of rapid alternating finger movements (Illert et al 1996). The axons of all motoneurons leave the spinal cord via the ventral rami of the C5–T1 spinal nerves (C, cervical; T, thoracic), which join to form the brachial plexus with its posterior, lateral and medial cords. The radial and axillary (and other) nerves arise from the posterior cord, the ulnar nerve from the medial cord, whereas both lateral and medial cords give origin to roots of the median nerve.

The CST is not an exclusive connection between the cortical motor areas and the motoneurons (Porter and Lemon 1993). On their way to the spinal cord, the CST axons give off collaterals to the basal ganglia, thalamus, red nucleus, pontine nuclei, reticular formation, inferior olive, and cranial nerve nuclei (Fig. 2.2). Some axons innervate the dorsal column nuclei, where they participate in the modulation of ascending afferent information. Only a fraction of the CST axons, namely the corticomotoneuronal fibres, establish direct monosynaptic connections with the spinal motoneurons supplying hand muscles (Lemon 1993). These fibres stem mainly from M1. Most corticospinal projections originating from secondary motor areas have an indirect rather than a direct influence on the motoneurons (Rouiller 1996). They terminate on spinal interneurons, where they influence the transmission of afferent signals and modulate spinal reflex pathways (e.g. suppress Ia-afferent inhibition). In this way the secondary motor areas determine the global frame of the movement, while the direct corticomotoneuronal projections originating from M1 break the synergies that are performed by spinal circuits, and determine the fine morphology of the movement (Luppino and Rizzolatti 2000). Although secondary motor areas, too, have some direct links to spinal motoneurons (Dum and Strick 2002), they cannot replace the function of M1 in fine motor control. However, they do in fact influence motor commands of M1 via their strong projections to this region.

All cortical motor areas project to the basal ganglia and cerebellum, which are parts of control loops (Porter and Lemon 1993). The basal ganglia are intercalated in a loop of connections from the cortex and back to the cortex via the thalamus. Congenital lesions of the basal ganglia may result in dyskinetic cerebral palsy with disorders of movement and muscle tone (see Chapter 1 for details). These children have trouble holding themselves in an upright steady position and often show involuntary motion. The cerebellum monitors motor commands coming down from the cortex to the pontine nuclei, and collects sensory information ascending from the spinal cord. It sends information to the brainstem, and back to cortical motor areas via the cerebellar nuclei and the ventrolateral thalamus. The cerebellum helps to regulate posture and movement, and is involved in some forms of motor learning. Besides the CST, the rubrospinal tract reaches the motor nuclei supplying muscles of the distal extremity. However, this pathway is not very well developed in humans, so probably it cannot compensate adequately or even take over the function of the CST after lesions (Nathan and Smith 1982). Reticulo- and vestibulospinal pathways innervate medial interneurons in the spinal cord, which connect with motoneurons that control the proximal and axial musculature, and thereby contribute to balance, posture and locomotion, but not to digit movements.

Neural control of hand movements
The activity of cortical areas during hand movements has now been studied with neuroimaging techniques for about two decades. Typically, besides the primary sensorimotor cortex (M1/S1), secondary motor and parietal areas are activated in a task-dependent manner, as will be illustrated with results of recent functional magnetic resonance imaging (fMRI) studies and experiments in non-human primates. We will also outline the development of two functional tasks, namely the precision grip-lift and prehension movements.

SIMPLE AND COMPLEX REPETITIVE FINGER MOVEMENTS

Tasks and brain activity
Fig. 2.3 shows the brain activity of right-handed individuals who repetitively performed simple and complex finger movements with the dominant or the non-dominant hand (Kuhtz-Buschbeck et al 2003). The complex task was a sequential finger-to-thumb opposition movement involving all five fingers, similar to pressing a series of keys on a musical instrument in a certain order. In the simple task, an object was just repetitively compressed between thumb, index and middle finger. Two principal aspects are evident: first, more regions are active during the complex than during the simple task. When the right hand performs the simple movement (Fig. 2.3A), the left primary sensorimotor cortex (M1/S1) and the right cerebellum are engaged. During the complex finger movement, the SMA, left cerebellum and right parietal cortex (BA 7) are recruited additionally (Fig. 2.3B). The second aspect concerns hand dominance: more regions are active during movements of the left hand compared to the right hand. Both complex and simple movements of the non-dominant left hand involve bilateral activity of secondary motor areas and posterior parietal regions, in addition to contralateral M1/S1 activity (Fig. 2.3C, D). Hence, the participation of cortical areas during finger movements depends both on the complexity of the task and on hand dominance.

28

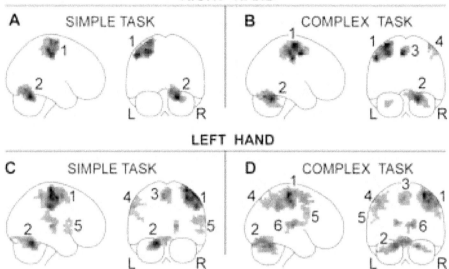

RIGHT HAND

A SIMPLE TASK

B COMPLEX TASK

LEFT HAND

C SIMPLE TASK

D COMPLEX TASK

Fig. 2.3 Brain activity during simple and complex finger movements, performed with the dominant (**A, B**) and the non-dominant hand (**C, D**). In the simple task, a flexible cube was repetitively compressed between thumb, index and middle finger. The complex task was a sequential finger-to-thumb opposition movement involving all five fingers. The figure shows lateral and frontal look-through projections of the brain activations. Numbers indicate clusters of active voxels in M1/S1 (1), cerebellum (2), SMA/CMA (3), posterior parietal lobe (4), PMV (5) and the thalamus (6). Some clusters extend to adjacent regions which are not numbered. The fMRI data were collected from 12 right-handed healthy volunteers; statistical threshold for significant activity Z > 3.09 (L, left; R, right hemisphere).

Source: Adapted with permission from Kuhtz-Buschbeck et al 2003.

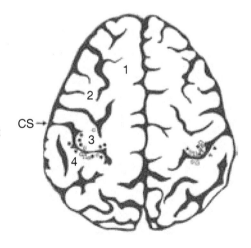

Fig. 2.4 Location of the motor hand area in the precentral gyrus. It has the shape of an inverted omega in the schematic drawing of an axial slice. Symbols represent foci of brain activity, which were recorded with fMRI during repetitive opening/closing of the left and right hand in ten healthy volunteers. Numbers indicate the superior (1) and middle (2) frontal gyrus, the precentral (3) and the postcentral gyrus (4) (CS, central sulcus).

Source: Adapted with permission from Yousry et al 1997.

29

Activity of M1

A third aspect concerns the extent of activation in the primary sensorimotor cortex (M1/S1). One might expect more widespread activity during the complex task, because it involves more fingers than the simple movement. However, the differences are not significant. This similar and congruent activation can be explained by the functional organization of the primary motor cortex M1. Reflecting the richness of manipulatory behaviour, the representation of the hand in M1 is disproportionately large. It is often characterized by an anatomical landmark (Yousry et al 1997), a knob-like structure of the precentral gyrus that is shaped like an omega in the axial plane (Fig. 2.4). When, in non-human primates, a small stimulation electrode is moved in this area, contractions of a given hand muscle can be evoked at various spatially separated foci (Schieber 2001). Accordingly, movements of one finger recruit a set of neurons that are distributed throughout the entire M1 hand area. It can therefore be expected that the neuronal populations that are active during tasks involving different fingers overlap extensively. The M1 hand region does not contain well-ordered demarcated point-to-point representations of the muscles of the thumb, index, middle, ring, little finger, wrist and so on, as the well-known figure of the 'homunculus' might suggest. Instead, each finger is represented in multiple discontinuous zones (Schieber and Santello 2004). A somatotopic gradient is superimposed on these scattered zones, so the thumb is represented stronger laterally and the little finger stronger medially. Horizontal interconnections interlink the neurons extensively. Such a network of intermingled and overlapping representations in the M1 hand area can facilitate numerous different combinations of hand muscle activity, which generate a rich repertoire of movements (Schieber 2001). Since the movements inevitably generate proprioceptive and cutaneous afferent feedback, the adjacent primary sensory cortex is of course activated as well.

NEURAL CONTROL OF THE PRECISION GRIP

Grip-lift task

A person who picks up a soft raspberry will most likely use a precision grip. This grip is characterized by opposition of the thumb to the index finger and is used for fine manipulation of objects. Dexterous manipulation is based on the ability to precisely control the movements and forces of the fingertips, so that the object is neither crushed, nor does it slip out of the fingers. This behaviour has been extensively studied with the precision grip-lift task (Fig. 2.5A), where individuals grasp an object equipped with force transducers between thumb and index finger, lift it from a support and hold it (Johansson 1996). The fingertip forces are measured, i.e. the grip force (perpendicular to the grip surface of the object) and the load force (lift force, tangential to the surface). The precision grip-lift task is composed of several phases: first, the tips of the digits are positioned on the grip surfaces to establish a stable grasp. Then, grip force and load force increase in parallel during the loading phase, which ends when the object starts to move (lift-off). An appropriate force output during the loading phase is generated by anticipatory control mechanisms, based on sensorimotor memory representations acquired during previous manipulations (Gordon et al 1993, Salimi et al 2000). Hence, the forces will increase more rapidly when the object is expected to be heavy,

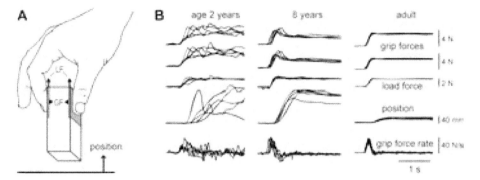

Fig. 2.5 Precision grip-lift task. **A.** An instrumented object is used to study the isometric fingertip forces during lifts with the precision grip. The load force (LF, tangential to the grip surfaces) and the grip forces (GF, normal force) of the thumb and index finger are measured together with the vertical movement (position) of the object. **B.** Superimposed trials of typical lifts performed by normal children at the age of 2 and 8 years, and by one adult. Grip forces of the thumb and index finger, total load force, object position, and grip force rate are shown as a function of time. The object had a weight of 200 g.

Source: Adapted with permission from Forssberg et al 1991.

and more slowly when the object is expected to be light. Note that this scaling is anticipatory, because explicit information about actual object weight is not available until lift-off. In the subsequent transitional phase, the object is lifted to the desired height, and it is held stationary in the air in the static phase.

Developmental aspects

The precision grip first emerges around 10 months of age, so that children become able to pick little sweets out of small wells with individuated thumb and index finger movements (Eyre et al 2000). However, young children produce highly variable forces that increase discontinuously (multiple force rate peaks) during the precision grip-lift task, which are in contrast to the invariant smooth and parallel force profiles of adults (Fig. 2.5B). The large variability may serve as a probing strategy, which allows the nervous system to explore various movement patterns and to select the most efficient ones. Young children have not yet developed efficient anticipatory control mechanisms, and probably have to rely more on sensory feedback during object manipulation. The mature grip-lift synergy with smooth pre-programmed parallel changes in the grip and load forces gradually evolves during the first decade of life (Forssberg et al 1991, 1992). This development has been related to the structural maturation of the central nervous system (Armand et al 1996).

Experimental studies in monkeys indicate that monosynaptic corticomotoneuronal (CM) projections are needed to perform skilful, relatively independent finger movements, e.g. of the thumb and index finger during the precision grip (Lemon 1993). These CM projections provide the possibility for the direct selective voluntary activation of hand muscles. Species with sparse CM connections (e.g. prosimians) are less dexterous than species (e.g. Old World monkeys, humans) with numerous such connections (Lemon and Griffiths

2005). The postnatal development of CM connections has been studied with histological and electrophysiological methods in macaques (Armand et al 1997, Olivier et al 1997). Very few corticospinal axons reach the hand motor nuclei in lamina IX of the cervical spinal cord in newborn macaques. This region is gradually invaded by CST fibres during the next months, and monosynaptic CM connections are established around 5 months of age. At that time, the monkeys begin to move their fingers independently, e.g. when grooming other animals. In man, corticomotoneuronal projections may develop earlier (Martin 2005). Surprisingly, Eyre and coworkers (2000) found evidence for monosynaptic CM projections already in human neonates in a study using transcranial magnetic stimulation (TMS), clearly before the emergence of the precision grip. Therefore the presence of CM connections appears to be necessary, but not sufficient for the control of dexterous independent finger movements. Other authors have suggested that the development of hand motor skills during childhood may be correlated with the maturation of fast CST axons (Müller and Hömberg 1992, Fietzek et al 2000). Increases in axon diameter, myelination and conduction velocity continue until adolescence (Paus et al 1999).

Cortical control of precision grip tasks
The maturation of cortical control mechanisms may also determine the development of the grip-lift synergy and other hand motor skills during childhood. Studies of age-dependent cortical activation are, however, scarce (Halder et al 2007). At present, we are beginning to understand the complex functional organization of the cortical areas involved in the control of fine digit actions in adult subjects. Recent neuroimaging studies indicate that sets of bilateral fronto-parietal areas are recruited in a task-dependent manner when humans apply finely controlled fingertip forces to objects (Ehrsson et al 2000, 2003, Schmitz et al 2005). A further fMRI study investigated the control of static precision grip forces (Kuhtz-Buschbeck et al 2001). In this study, normal volunteers grasped, lifted and held a small object (weight 200 g) with a precision grip of the dominant right hand. In one condition, they used their normal, naturally scaled grip force to hold the object. This force is adjusted automatically to the object's weight and surface characteristics (roughness, curvature). It is a certain safety margin greater than the critical threshold at which the object would slip out of the fingers (Johansson 1996). In the second condition, the object was held gently, using the least possible grip force. Since the safety margin was reduced as much as possible, precise force control was needed to avoid slipping. Such a gentle grip force is used when readily deformable or fragile items are manipulated (e.g. a dried flower). In a third condition, the force was intentionally increased to hold the object with a firmer grip. In all conditions, the object was put down and released after 30 seconds of holding.

As one main result, we found that brain activity during static holding did not just increase in parallel with force. Instead, the SMA and CMA were significantly more active during the gentle force condition than during either of the other two conditions (normal/firm), despite weaker contractions of the hand muscles (Fig. 2.6). The SMA may control spinal and intracortical inhibitory interneurons that precisely keep the motoneuronal activity at the desired level during gentle grasping (Toma et al 1999). In addition to the SMA/CMA, the left M1/S1, PMV, and left posterior parietal cortex were also more strongly activated

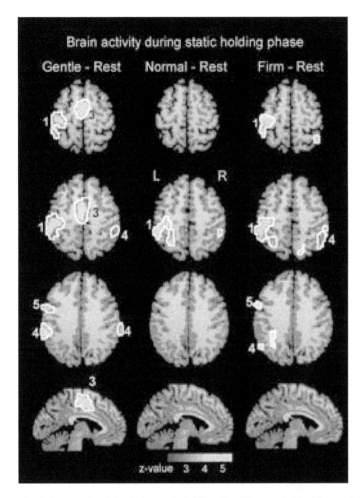

Fig. 2.6 Cortical activity during static holding. An object was held with a precision grip between the right thumb and index finger. The images show regions which were active during holding with gentle (left column), normal (middle column) and firm (right column) grip force. Numbers (compare Fig. 2.3) indicate activity in M1/S1 (1), SMA/CMA (3), the posterior parietal lobe (4), and PMV (5) (L, left; R, right hemisphere). Cerebellar activity could not be measured due to technical reasons. The fMRI data were collected from eight healthy right-handed volunteers; statistical threshold for significant activity Z > 3.09.

Source: Adapted with permission from Kuhtz-Buschbeck et al 2001.

during gentle grasping than they were during normal grasping. These regions seem to be specifically involved in dexterous scaling of the fingertip forces.

Secondly, we found a conspicuous temporal modulation of brain activity during the grip–lift–hold–release sequence. Regardless of the force condition, the activity increased transiently during the dynamic phases (grip-lift, release), while it was weaker during static holding (Fig. 2.7A). This is evident from the mean fMRI signal profiles of the SMA and left M1/S1, but similar transient increases associated with the dynamic phases were found in other areas as well (left S1, bilateral PMV/PMD, CMA, posterior parietal cortex). The temporal modulation reflects the changing involvement of corticospinal control mechanisms and cutaneous afferent input. The excitability of corticospinal neurons innervating distal hand muscles is high just before and during the initial grip-lift phase, as Lemon et al (1995) demonstrated with transcranial magnetic brain stimulation. There is an intense signalling in tactile afferents from the fingertips at initial contact and object release, while low afferent firing rates prevail during static holding (Johansson 1996). Note that due to the inherent temporal lag of the hemodynamic response and the low time resolution of the fMRI technique, the curves (Fig. 2.7B) represent a delayed and temporally smoothed counterpart of the neuronal firing pattern.

Although grasping and lifting an object with a precision grip of the right hand seems to be a rather simple task, other recent fMRI studies confirm that it involves not only the 'classical' motor regions (M1, PM, SMA). The cortex lining the left intraparietal sulcus is implicated in the control of lifting, and right intraparietal areas support the coordination of grip and load forces (Ehrsson et al 2003). Bilateral prefrontal and posterior parietal regions and the ipsilateral PMV may be more active in precision grip than in a power grip task, although the latter involves more force (Ehrsson et al 2000). Schmitz et al (2005) found activations in the right inferior frontal gyrus (BA 44), left parietal operculum and right supramarginal gyrus when objects of changing weight were lifted with a precision grip of the right hand. Unpredictable weight changes were associated with conspicuous activity in the right inferior frontal cortex. Taken together, a network of fronto-parietal areas is involved in a task-dependent manner during precision grip tasks.

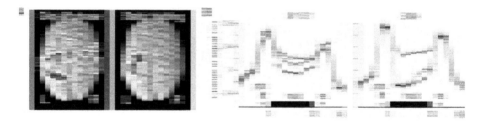

Fig. 2.7 Temporal modulation of cortical activity in a precision grip task. An object was grasped, lifted and held with a precision grip of the right hand, and released. **A.** Brain activity in the 'dynamic' grip-lift phase was more widespread and higher than during static holding. The participants used their normal, automatically scaled grip force. **B.** fMRI signal profiles of activation in the left M1/S1 and SMA. The curves show the modulation of the signal during the gentle (open circles), normal (black circles) and firm (open squares) grip force conditions. The dynamic phases (grip-lift; rel., release) are marked with asterisks, the static phase with a black bar. Error bars indicate standard error. Otherwise as in Fig. 2.6.

Source: Adapted with permission from Kuhtz-Buschbeck et al 2001.

Development of prehension
Reaching out to grasp an object includes two motor components: hand transport and grip formation. The transport component (reaching), which brings the hand to the target, involves contractions of mainly proximal muscles acting on the shoulder and elbow joints. Grip formation pre-shapes the fingers according to the size and shape of the target object (Jeannerod 1986). Well synchronized with hand transport, the fingers first open and then start to close in anticipation of the encounter with the object, so that the finger pads contact it at appropriate sites at the end of the reach (Fig. 2.8A). Hence, efficient unimanual prehension requires the smooth integration of both components in a unified action (Grosskopf and Kuhtz-Buschbeck 2006). Similar to the development of the grip-lift synergy, this mature pattern gradually evolves during childhood. The first goal-directed reaches, around the age of 4 months, display circuitous trajectories and consist of several movement units, i.e. acceleration–deceleration sequences (Konczak and Dichgans 1997). By the age of 1 year, children start to shape their grip according to the object size, but the grip aperture is exaggerated (von Hofsten and Rönnqvist 1988). Reaching movements with more linear trajectories, which consist of one movement unit, develop until the third year.

Analyses of intersegmental limb dynamics revealed concurrent changes in the temporal pattern of the torques acting on the upper arm and forearm, with a better integration of gravitational and reactive torques into movement execution (Konczak et al 1997). In other words, the motor control system learns to anticipate and to utilize effects that self-generated movements have on limb dynamics – e.g. when an active anterior flexion of the shoulder joint induces a reactive extension of the elbow. Gradual improvements continue throughout the first decade of life (Kuhtz-Buschbeck et al 1998), resulting in adult-like stereotyped kinematic profiles with a smooth coordination of hand transport and grip formation at the age of 12 years (Fig. 2.8B).

Cortical control of prehension
According to the visuo-motor channel hypothesis, the two components of prehension are controlled by two distinct input-output systems (Jeannerod et al 1995). The first system uses visual information about the intrinsic properties of the target object (size, shape) and controls the distal muscles in order to pre-shape the hand. This process implies a visuo-motor transformation that may be accomplished by a neuronal circuit formed by the anterior intraparietal cortex (AIP) and area F5 of the PMV (Fig. 2.9). Area F5 accommodates 'grasping neurons' that code specific types of prehension, such as precision grip, tripod grip, whole hand prehension (Luppino and Rizzolatti 2000). It projects both to the spinal cord and to M1, which can steer the appropriate finger movements via CM connections. While focal lesions of M1 cause paresis and severe impairment of individuated finger movements (Lang and Schieber 2003), lesions and/or inactivations of AIP and F5 specifically disrupt pre-shaping during prehension, whereas individuated finger movements are not affected (Binkofski et al 1998, Fogassi et al 2001). It has been postulated that AIP provides F5 with not just one, but multiple descriptions of object affordances, because objects are grasped in

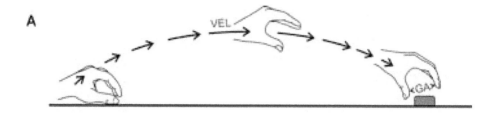

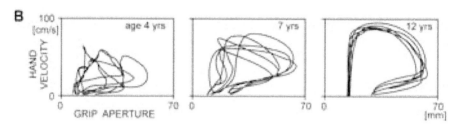

Fig. 2.8 Reach-to-grasp movements. **A.** Hand transport is described with the movement path (arrows) and the spatial velocity (VEL) of the reaching hand (longer arrows = higher velocity). Grasping is described by measuring the grip aperture (GA) of the fingers. The largest grip aperture is reached during the deceleration phase of hand transport. **B.** Kinematic profiles of prehension at the age of 4, 7 and 12 years. The hand velocity is plotted against the grip aperture in three normal children of different ages. For each child, five to six typical trials are superimposed.

Source: Adapted with permission from Kuhtz-Buschbeck et al 1998.

different ways depending on the intended action (e.g. a knife in order to cut, to stab, or to pass it to another person). The appropriate grasp is selected on the basis of prefrontal input, which reaches F5 via area F6 and informs about the current goal and the appropriate timing of the action (Rizzolatti and Luppino 2001).

The second visuo-motor channel is focused on object location and controls hand transport, i.e. the movements of the shoulder and elbow which bring the hand to the target.

Fig. 2.9 Visuomotor stream for grip formation. The anterior intraparietal area (AIP) integrates visual input (VIS) informing about an object's intrinsic properties (size, shape), and somatosensory information (S1). AIP projects to area F5 of the ventral premotor cortex, PMV. Neurons in AIP and F5 code size, shape and orientation of objects, and the specific types of grip that are necessary to grasp them. F5 is connected with the primary motor cortex (M1), which controls the finger movements.

Source: Adapted with permission from Jeannerod et al 1995.

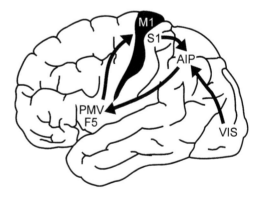

Two other parieto-frontal circuits seem to be involved (Luppino and Rizzolatti 2000): the ventral intraparietal region (VIP) and area F4 of the PMV are reciprocally connected and contain neurons that encode peripersonal space and transform object locations into appropriate movements towards them. Area F2 (posterior PMD), which is linked to the MIP region in the intraparietal sulcus, uses both somatosensory and visual information to plan arm movements. Also area F7 may code object locations in space for coordinated arm–body movements (Geyer et al 2000).

In summary, reaching and grasping involve the transformation of visual information about objects and object location into a goal-directed action. Posterior parietal regions and the secondary motor areas F2–F5 are linked by reciprocal connections that form parieto-frontal circuits, each of which seems to be dedicated to specific aspects of this sensorimotor transformation (Rizzolatti and Luppino 2001). The rostral areas F6 and F7 are connected to the prefrontal cortex and convey inputs concerning action goals, timing of action, and memory of past action (Picard and Strick 2001). The primary motor cortex (F1) receives input from areas F2–F5 and controls differentiated finger movements via its direct

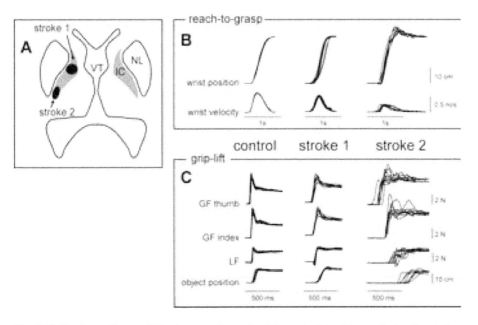

Fig. 2.10 Hand coordination following capsular stroke. Kinematic data of two patients after strokes of the anterior (stroke 1) or posterior part (stroke 2) of the caudal limb of the internal capsule, and of a control participant. **A.** Superimposed on a schematic representation of an axial slice, the focal ischemic lesions are indicated as black dots (IC, internal capsule; VT, ventricle; NL, nucleus lentiformis). **B.** Position and velocity of the wrist are depicted for several reach-to-grasp trials. In the patient with the posterior lesion (stroke 2), the movements were slowed in the terminal phase, showed vertical hypermetria, and irregular hand paths. **C.** The precision grip-lift trials were irregular with an increase in grip force beyond the optimal level in the patient with stroke 2.

Source: Adapted with permission from Wenzelburger et al 2005.

projections to the motoneurons. Most of these conclusions are based on studies in macaques, but recent brain imaging studies suggest that the organizational principle is similar in humans (Binkofski et al 1999, Culham et al 2003, Stoeckel et al 2003).

Congruent with their role in movement planning, secondary motor areas are also active when individuals mentally rehearse hand movements, without any overt action (Gerardin et al 2000, Kuhtz-Buschbeck et al 2003). Studies of the Bereitschaftspotential (a negativity of the EEG signal preceding movement onset) indicate that the SMA and CMA are involved in the preparation of and readiness for self-initiated movements (Erdler et al 2000). Activity in these regions starts before the onset of a self-initiated finger movement, about 0.5 seconds earlier than M1 activity (Cunnington et al 2003). Furthermore, the SMA is known to coordinate bimanual movements (see Chapter 7 for details).

LESIONS OF THE CORTICOSPINAL TRACT AND HAND FUNCTION
The CST fibres descending from the cortical motor areas to the motoneurons of hand muscles lie in a compact area in the posterior limb of the internal capsule (Morecraft et al 2002), and are frequently damaged in stroke patients. The more posterior a focal lesion of this pathway is located, the more severe are the chronic deficits of motor hand function (Fig. 2.10). Kinematic analyses specifically show that the terminal phases of reach-to-grasp movements and the initial phases of a precision grip-lift task are affected (Wenzelburger et al 2005). These are the phases in which pre-shaping of the hand and grip stabilization occur, with a strong involvement of corticospinal control mechanisms (Lemon et al 1995). Movements of the trunk and shoulder, which can be controlled via cortico-reticulo-spinal pathways, recover better than distal movements. Indirect oligosynaptic connections to the motoneurons of hand muscles may be important for neuro-rehabilitation after selective, experimental lesions of the monosynaptic CM pathway in monkeys, since the precision grip recovers at least partially in these animals (Sasaki et al 2004).

Forssberg and coworkers (1999) reported that individuals with congenital hemiplegia have difficulties establishing a precise synergy between fingertip forces while manipulating objects. The severity of the impairments correlates with the amount of CST dysgenesis (Duque et al 2003). Transcranial magnetic brain stimulation has been very useful for studying the function of the CST in congenital hemiplegia (Carr et al 1993). If at least some corticospinal projections descending from the lesioned brain hemisphere are preserved, hand function will be better than in patients in whom TMS of the affected hemisphere does not elicit any motor response at all (Staudt et al 2002, 2004). The undamaged hemisphere can participate in voluntary control of the affected hand via ipsilaterally descending corticospinal and cortico-reticulo-spinal projections (Carr et al 1993, Ulmer et al 2005). Some CST axons branch and innervate both left and right motor nuclei, which leads to strong mirror movements (Carr 1996). In contrast to congenital brain lesions, the unmasking of ipsilateral CST projections in adult stroke patients seems to be of little significance for recovery (Turton et al 1996, Netz et al 1997). An overview of congenital hemiplegia and other forms of cerebral palsy is presented in Chapter 1, and different patterns of motor reorganization are described.

In summary, evidence from electrophysiological and neuroimaging experiments indicates that the physiological control of hand movements involves not just an upper motor neuron in contralateral M1 and a lower spinal motoneuron, but a set of interconnected cortical areas that can be reorganized after brain damage.

GLOSSARY

Brodmann areas are subdivisions of the human cortex, according to cytoarchitectonic criteria

extrafusal muscle fibres generate the main force during skeletal muscle contractions

extrinsic hand muscles are situated in the forearm and move the wrist and/or the fingers

functional magnetic resonance imaging can detect changes of oxygenation associated with local brain activity

Ia-afferent inhibition is mediated by spinal interneurons and inhibits alpha-motoneurons of antagonistic muscles

internal capsule: area of white matter in the brain, consisting of afferent pathways and descending motor tracts

intersegmental dynamics describes biomechanical interactions of moving limb segments, e.g. of forearm and upper arm

intracortical microstimulation: local stimulation of the cortex with microelectrodes

intrafusal muscle fibres generate very little force, but are receptors that sense changes in muscle length, e.g. stretch

intraparietal sulcus: a prominent groove in the parietal cortex; it is lined by the intraparietal cortex

intrinsic hand muscles are part of the hand and move finger joints

lamina IX: a region of grey matter in the ventral horn of the spinal cord

monosynaptic neuronal pathways have only one intercalated synapse, e.g. the monosynaptic stretch reflex pathway

oligosynaptic pathways consist of several neurons with several intercalated synapses

operculum: a cortical region which covers the insular cortex like a lid

pre-shaping: the formation of the grip that occurs while the hand reaches out for an object

proprioceptive information is mediated, e.g. by joint and muscle receptors, and concerns the own body

Renshaw inhibition: spinal motoneurons inhibit themselves via recurrent axon collaterals and inhibitory interneurons

reticulospinal pathway: a motor tract which travels from the reticular formation of the brainstem

rubrospinal tract: originates in the red nucleus and is an alternative route for the mediation of voluntary movements

somatotopic arrangement: an ordered representation (e.g. hand represented next to arm) of body parts in the brain

trajectory of reaching: the spatial path of the reaching hand

transcranial magnetic stimulation excites the motor cortex by a transient magnetic field inducing electrical current

vestibulospinal tract: originates from the vestibular nuclei of the medulla and reinforces extensor muscle tone

REFERENCES

Armand J, Olivier E, Edgley SA, Lemon RN (1996) The structure and function of the developing corticospinal tract: some key issues. In: Wing AM, Haggard P, Flanagan JR, editors. *Hand and Brain*. San Diego: Academic Press, pp. 125–145.

Armand J, Olivier E, Edgley SA, Lemon RN (1997) Postnatal development of corticospinal projections from motor cortex to the cervical enlargement in the macaque monkey. *J Neurosci* 17: 251–266.

Binkofski F, Dohle C, Posse S, Stephan KM, Hefter H, Seitz RJ, Freund HJ (1998) Human anterior intraparietal area subserves prehension: a combined lesion and functional MRI activation study. *Neurology* 50: 1253–1259.

Binkofski F, Buccino G, Posse S, Seitz RJ, Rizzolatti G, Freund H (1999) A fronto-parietal circuit for object manipulation in man: evidence from an fMRI-study. *Eur J Neurosci* 11: 3276–3286.

Carr LJ (1996) Development and reorganization of descending motor pathways in children with hemiplegic cerebral palsy. *Acta Paediatr Suppl* 416: 53–57.

Carr LJ, Harrison LM, Evans AL, Stephens JA (1993) Patterns of central motor reorganization in hemiplegic cerebral palsy. *Brain* 116 (Pt 5): 1223–1247.

Culham JC, Danckert SL, DeSouza JF, Gati JS, Menon RS, Goodale MA (2003) Visually guided grasping produces fMRI activation in dorsal but not ventral stream brain areas. *Exp Brain Res* 153: 180–189.

Cunnington R, Windischberger C, Deecke L, Moser E (2003) The preparation and readiness for voluntary movement: a high-field event-related fMRI study of the Bereitschafts-BOLD response. *Neuroimage* 20: 404–412.

Dum RP, Strick PL (2002) Motor areas in the frontal lobe of the primate. *Physiol Behav* 77: 677–682.

Dum RP, Strick PL (2005) Frontal lobe inputs to the digit representations of the motor areas on the lateral surface of the hemisphere. *J Neurosci* 25: 1375–1386.

Duque J, Thonnard JL, Vandermeeren Y, Sebire G, Cosnard G, Olivier E (2003) Correlation between impaired dexterity and corticospinal tract dysgenesis in congenital hemiplegia. *Brain* 126: 732–747.

Ehrsson HH, Fagergren A, Jonsson T, Westling G, Johansson RS, Forssberg H (2000) Cortical activity in precision- versus power-grip tasks: an fMRI study. *J Neurophysiol* 83: 528–536.

Ehrsson HH, Fagergren A, Johansson RS, Forssberg H (2003) Evidence for the involvement of the posterior parietal cortex in coordination of fingertip forces for grasp stability in manipulation. *J Neurophysiol* 90: 2978–2986.

Erdler M, Beisteiner R, Mayer D, Kaindl T, Edward V, Windischberger C, Lindinger G, Deecke L (2000) Supplementary motor area activation preceding voluntary movement is detectable with a whole-scalp magnetoencephalography system. *Neuroimage* 11: 697–707.

Eyre JA, Miller S, Clowry GJ, Conway EA, Watts C (2000) Functional corticospinal projections are established prenatally in the human foetus permitting involvement in the development of spinal motor centres. *Brain* 123 (Pt 1): 51–64.

Fietzek UM, Heinen F, Berweck S, Maute S, Hufschmidt A, Schulte-Monting J, Lucking CH, Korinthenberg R (2000) Development of the corticospinal system and hand motor function: central conduction times and motor performance tests. *Dev Med Child Neurol* 42: 220–227.

Fogassi L, Gallese V, Buccino G, Craighero L, Fadiga L, Rizzolatti G (2001) Cortical mechanism for the visual guidance of hand grasping movements in the monkey: a reversible inactivation study. *Brain* 124: 571–586.

Forssberg H, Eliasson AC, Kinoshita H, Johansson RS, Westling G (1991) Development of human precision grip. I: Basic coordination of force. *Exp Brain Res* 85: 451–457.

Forssberg H, Kinoshita H, Eliasson AC, Johansson RS, Westling G, Gordon AM (1992) Development of human precision grip. II. Anticipatory control of isometric forces targeted for object's weight. *Exp Brain Res* 90: 393–398.

Forssberg H, Eliasson AC, Redon-Zouitenn C, Mercuri E, Dubowitz L (1999) Impaired grip-lift synergy in children with unilateral brain lesions. *Brain* 122 (Pt 6): 1157–1168.

Gerardin E, Sirigu A, Lehericy S, Poline JB, Gaymard B, Marsault C, Agid Y, Le Bihan D (2000) Partially overlapping neural networks for real and imagined hand movements. *Cereb Cortex* 10: 1093–1104.

Geyer S, Matelli M, Luppino G, Zilles K (2000) Functional neuroanatomy of the primate isocortical motor system. *Anat Embryol (Berl)* 202: 443–474.

40

Gordon AM, Westling G, Cole KJ, Johansson RS (1993) Memory representations underlying motor commands used during manipulation of common and novel objects. *J Neurophysiol* 69: 1789–1796.

Grosskopf A, Kuhtz-Buschbeck JP (2006) Grasping with the left and right hand: a kinematic study. *Exp Brain Res* 168: 230–240.

Halder P, Brem S, Bucher K, Boujraf S, Summers P, Dietrich T, Kollias S, Martin E, Brandeis D (2007) Electrophysiological and hemodynamic evidence for late maturation of hand power grip and force control under visual feedback. *Hum Brain Mapp* 28: 69–84.

Illert M, Kummel H, Scott JJ (1996) Beta innervation and recurrent inhibition: a hypothesis for manipulatory and postural control. *Pflugers Arch* 432: R61–R67.

Jeannerod M (1986) The formation of finger grip during prehension. A cortically mediated visuomotor pattern. *Behav Brain Res* 19: 99–116.

Jeannerod M, Arbib MA, Rizzolatti G, Sakata H (1995) Grasping objects: the cortical mechanisms of visuomotor transformation. *Trends Neurosci* 18: 314–320.

Johansson RS (1996) Sensory control of dexterous manipulation in humans. In: Wing AM, Haggard P, Flanagan JR, editors. *Hand and Brain*. San Diego: Academic Press, pp. 381–414.

Kakuda N, Miwa T, Nagaoka M (1998) Coupling between single muscle spindle afferent and EMG in human wrist extensor muscles: physiological evidence of skeletofusimotor (beta) innervation. *Electroencephalogr Clin Neurophysiol* 109: 360–363.

Konczak J, Dichgans J (1997) The development toward stereotypic arm kinematics during reaching in the first 3 years of life. *Exp Brain Res* 117: 346–354.

Konczak J, Borutta M, Dichgans J (1997) The development of goal-directed reaching in infants. II. Learning to produce task-adequate patterns of joint torque. *Exp Brain Res* 113: 465–474.

Kuhtz-Buschbeck JP, Stolze H, Johnk K, Boczek-Funcke A, Illert M (1998) Development of prehension movements in children: a kinematic study. *Exp Brain Res* 122: 424–432.

Kuhtz-Buschbeck JP, Ehrsson HH, Forssberg H (2001) Human brain activity in the control of fine static precision grip forces: an fMRI study. *Eur J Neurosci* 14: 382–390.

Kuhtz-Buschbeck JP, Mahnkopf C, Holzknecht C, Siebner H, Ulmer S, Jansen O (2003) Effector-independent representations of simple and complex imagined finger movements: a combined fMRI and TMS study. *Eur J Neurosci* 18: 3375–3387.

Lang CE, Schieber MH (2003) Differential impairment of individuated finger movements in humans after damage to the motor cortex or the corticospinal tract. *J Neurophysiol* 90: 1160–1170.

Lemon RN (1993) The G. L. Brown Prize Lecture. Cortical control of the primate hand. *Exp Physiol* 78: 263–301.

Lemon RN, Griffiths J (2005) Comparing the function of the corticospinal system in different species: organizational differences for motor specialization? *Muscle Nerve* 32: 261–279.

Lemon RN, Johansson RS, Westling G (1995) Corticospinal control during reach, grasp, and precision lift in man. *J Neurosci* 15: 6145–6156.

Luppino G, Rizzolatti G (2000) The organization of the frontal motor cortex. *News Physiol Sci* 15: 219–224.

Martin JH (2005) The corticospinal system: from development to motor control. *Neuroscientist* 11: 161–173.

Morecraft RJ, Herrick JL, Stilwell-Morecraft KS, Louie JL, Schroeder CM, Ottenbacher JG, Schoolfield MW (2002) Localization of arm representation in the corona radiata and internal capsule in the non-human primate. *Brain* 125: 176–198.

Müller K, Hömberg V (1992) Development of speed of repetitive movements in children is determined by structural changes in corticospinal efferents. *Neurosci Lett* 144: 57–60.

Nathan PW, Smith MC (1982) The rubrospinal and central tegmental tracts in man. *Brain* 105: 223–269.

Netz J, Lammers T, Homberg V (1997) Reorganization of motor output in the non-affected hemisphere after stroke. *Brain* 120 (Pt 9): 1579–1586.

Olivier E, Edgley SA, Armand J, Lemon RN (1997) An electrophysiological study of the postnatal development of the corticospinal system in the macaque monkey. *J Neurosci* 17: 267–276.

Paus T, Zijdenbos A, Worsley K, Collins DL, Blumenthal J, Giedd JN, Rapoport JL, Evans AC (1999) Structural maturation of neural pathways in children and adolescents: in vivo study. *Science* 283: 1908–1911.

Picard N, Strick PL (2001) Imaging the premotor areas. *Curr Opin Neurobiol* 11: 663–672.

Porter R, Lemon RN (1993) *Corticospinal Function and Voluntary Movement*. Oxford: Clarendon Press

Rizzolatti G, Luppino G (2001) The cortical motor system. *Neuron* 31: 889–901.

Roland PE, Zilles K (1996) Functions and structures of the motor cortices in humans. *Curr Opin Neurobiol* 6: 773–781.

41

Rouiller EM (1996) Multiple hand representations in the motor cortical areas. In: Wing AM, Haggard P, Flanagan JR, editors. *Hand and Brain*. San Diego: Academic Press, pp. 99–124.

Rouiller EM, Olivier E (2004) Functional recovery after lesions of the primary motor cortex. *Prog Brain Res* 143: 467–475.

Salimi I, Hollender I, Frazier W, Gordon AM (2000) Specificity of internal representations underlying grasping. *J Neurophysiol* 84: 2390–2397.

Sasaki S, Isa T, Pettersson LG, Alstermark B, Naito K, Yoshimura K, Seki K, Ohki Y (2004) Dexterous finger movements in primate without monosynaptic corticomotoneuronal excitation. *J Neurophysiol* 92: 3142–3147.

Schieber MH (2001) Constraints on somatotopic organization in the primary motor cortex. *J Neurophysiol* 86: 2125–2143.

Schieber MH, Santello M (2004) Hand function: peripheral and central constraints on performance. *J Appl Physiol* 96: 2293–2300.

Schmitz C, Jenmalm P, Ehrsson HH, Forssberg H (2005) Brain activity during predictable and unpredictable weight changes when lifting objects. *J Neurophysiol* 93: 1498–1509.

Staudt M, Grodd W, Gerloff C, Erb M, Stitz J, Krageloh-Mann I (2002) Two types of ipsilateral reorganization in congenital hemiparesis: a TMS and fMRI study. *Brain* 125: 2222–2237.

Staudt M, Gerloff C, Grodd W, Holthausen H, Niemann G, Krageloh-Mann I (2004) Reorganization in congenital hemiparesis acquired at different gestational ages. *Ann Neurol* 56: 854–863.

Stoeckel MC, Weder B, Binkofski F, Buccino G, Shah NJ, Seitz RJ (2003) A fronto-parietal circuit for tactile object discrimination: an event-related fMRI study. *Neuroimage* 19: 1103–1114.

Toma K, Honda M, Hanakawa T, Okada T, Fukuyama H, Ikeda A, Nishizawa S, Konishi J, Shibasaki H (1999) Activities of the primary and supplementary motor areas increase in preparation and execution of voluntary muscle relaxation: an event-related fMRI study. *J Neurosci* 19: 3527–3534.

Turton A, Wroe S, Trepte N, Fraser C, Lemon RN (1996) Contralateral and ipsilateral EMG responses to transcranial magnetic stimulation during recovery of arm and hand function after stroke. *Electroencephalogr Clin Neurophysiol* 101: 316–328.

Ulmer S, Moeller F, Brockmann MA, Kuhtz-Buschbeck JP, Stephani U, Jansen O (2005) Living a normal life with the nondominant hemisphere: magnetic resonance findings and clinical outcome for a patient with left-hemispheric hydranencephaly. *Pediatrics* 116: 242–245.

von Hofsten C, Rönnqvist L (1988) Preparation for grasping an object: a developmental study. *J Exp Psychol Hum Percept Perform* 14: 610–621.

Wenzelburger R, Kopper F, Frenzel A, Stolze H, Klebe S, Brossmann A, Kuhtz-Buschbeck J, Golge M, Illert M, Deuschl G (2005) Hand coordination following capsular stroke. *Brain* 128: 64–74.

Yousry TA, Schmid UD, Alkadhi H, Schmidt D, Peraud A, Buettner A, Winkler P (1997) Localization of the motor hand area to a knob on the precentral gyrus. A new landmark. *Brain* 120 (Pt 1): 141–157.

3
NEUROPSYCHOLOGY OF MOVEMENT SEQUENCE LEARNING

Fredrik Ullén

1 Introduction

Performing sequences of movements in the correct order and with adequate timing is essential for human behaviour, from simple everyday skills to some of the most complex activities we are capable of. The focus of this review is on the neuropsychology of movement sequence learning. A special emphasis will be put on current issues concerning ordinal and temporal sequence properties, and on differences between implicit and explicit learning. Unfortunately, confusion has occasionally been created by inconsistent usage of these terms in the literature, and I will therefore start with some definitions.

By the *ordinal structure* of a sequence is meant the serial order of the individual movements comprising the sequence. Taking a piano performance of a simple melody as an example, the ordinal structure is the serial order of key presses, one for each note, on the piano keyboard. This should be clearly distinguished from the *temporal structure* of the sequence, that is, the series of temporal intervals between the onsets of the movements, which in this example is determined by the durations of the notes of the melody.

The term *procedural learning* will be used for improvement of the ability to perform a movement sequence. In practice, procedural learning is typically measured by its effects on overt behaviour. These effects will differ in different training paradigms, e.g. decreases of reaction time in the serial reaction time task (section 2.1) or decreases of number of errors in immediate serial recall paradigms (section 2.2).

It has been more problematic to find a generally accepted definition of implicit, as opposed to explicit, movement sequence learning (for discussions see Shanks and St John 1994, Stadler and Frensch 1997, Stadler and Roediger 1997). I will adopt one classical definition: *implicit learning* is procedural learning occurring without conscious awareness of what is being learned. The precise operational definition of this concept will then vary somewhat from study to study, depending on which awareness test is used to measure conscious sequence knowledge. By *explicit learning* we mean the acquisition of consciously accessible information about the structure of the trained movement sequence. Again, the operational definition will depend on the nature of the employed awareness test. Explicit learning is typically, but not necessarily, accompanied by procedural learning. These definitions of implicit and explicit learning differ from definitions that include constraints on underlying neurocognitive mechanisms – for instance that implicit learning should not involve the declarative memory systems of the medial temporal lobe (Forkstam and

Petersson 2005). Logically, they also differ from definitions (Stadler and Roediger 1997) that equate implicit learning with accidental learning – that is, learning occurring without conscious *intention* to learn. Empirically, it may of course still very well be that practically all situations that involve intentional learning also give rise to explicit learning, as here defined – although see section 5.

As we shall see, recent studies demonstrate that ordinal and temporal, as well as implicit and explicit, movement sequence learning show important differences in their neural control mechanisms. Furthermore, these aspects of sequence learning may be differentially impaired in different patient groups. In relation to cerebral palsy, where motor symptoms are indeed heterogeneous, it therefore seems likely that awareness of these concepts by clinicians may increase their understanding of individual differences in the children with whom they work.

2 Common paradigms in movement sequence learning research

2.1 The Serial Reaction Time Task

The serial reaction time task (SRTT) first appeared in its modern form in a classical study by Nissen and Bullemer (1987). It consists of a series of choice reaction time (RT) trials. In the original version, the stimulus was an asterisk, presented at one of four possible locations on a computer monitor. Four response buttons were used, one under each possible stimulus location. The participant pressed the button under the stimulus, as quickly as possible, and the next stimulus appeared after a fixed response-to-stimulus interval (RSI) of 500 ms. The basic properties of the SRTT, observed already in this first study, can be summarized as follows. First, when stimuli follow a random order, RT decreases over trials are minimal. Second, when stimuli follow a repeating ordinal sequence, procedural learning is seen as a gradual reduction of RT, until the mean RT approaches or undershoots values typical of simple visual RT. If the repeating sequence is replaced with random stimuli at this stage, RT increases dramatically. Third, during initial stages of training, participants often express no awareness of the sequence; yet, procedural learning takes place. Fourth, with prolonged training, participants without neurological impairments typically acquire explicit sequence knowledge. The SRTT can thus be used to study both procedural and explicit learning, and it has become one of the most important standard paradigms in sequence research (for reviews see Clegg et al 1998, Keele et al 2003, Rhodes et al 2004).

2.2 Immediate Serial Recall

In immediate serial recall (ISR) paradigms, a sequence of stimuli is presented and the participant is instructed to recall the entire sequence in the correct order. ISR tasks are central in studies of working memory. In movement sequence research, each stimulus typically represents a particular movement. The recall phase consists of the production of a movement sequence, e.g. a sequence of key presses, corresponding to the presented stimulus sequence. For a general review of ISR paradigms in movement sequence research, see Rhodes et al (2004). We will here focus on the use of ISR paradigms to study learning of ordinal and temporal sequences. In this case, paradigms consisting of repeated ISR trials have been used, where the ordinal or temporal structure of the stimulus sequence is kept constant between trials (sections 4.2 and 4.3). Procedural learning can be quantified as a decrease of the number of errors across trials. For studies of temporal sequence learning, repeated ISR has an important advantage over the SRTT, in that the whole target rhythm is presented before reproduction. The SRTT, in contrast, is a series of RT trials. Variability in inter-response intervals will thus partly be due to intertrial variability in reaction time. For a further discussion of these methodological issues, see section 4.2 and Ullén and Bengtsson (2003).

2.3 THE 2 × N TASK

The 2 × N task was developed by Hikosaka and coworkers to study sequence learning in both the monkey (Hikosaka et al 1995) and humans (Hikosaka et al 1996). It is an explicit ordinal learning task. The target sequences consist of a series of button presses. The response buttons are arranged in a square array. The learning can typically be divided into three phases. During phase 1 of the task, the ordinal structure of the sequence has to be discovered through trial-and-error learning. Visual stimuli consist of square arrays corresponding to the button array, with two circles indicating which buttons should be used for the next two sequence elements. Initially, the order of these two presses has to be guessed, and throughout training, an ordinal error will cause a restart from the beginning of the sequence. If the two buttons are pressed in the correct order the next two-item problem ('set') is presented, until a whole sequence, called a 'hyperset', has been completed. Typically, a hyperset consists of 2 × 5 sets (10 elements) in monkey studies and 2 × 10 (20 elements) in human studies. In phase 2, subjects practise the same hyperset further, mixing errors with successful trials. In phase 3, finally, performance is essentially error-free. Procedural learning is seen as both a decrease of the number of ordinal errors (in phases 1 and 2), and an increase of performance speed.

3 Learning the ordinal structure of a movement sequence

3.1 DISSOCIATING IMPLICIT AND EXPLICIT ORDINAL SEQUENCE LEARNING

Disentangling implicit and explicit processes is challenging, and in the past the existence of independent implicit and explicit systems for ordinal sequence learning has occasionally been questioned (Perruchet and Amorim 1992). However, taken together, a number of behavioural findings from the SRTT make a strong case for the notion that ordinal sequences can be learned implicitly, and that such learning involves processes that are partly different from those underlying explicit learning.

First, procedural learning is observed in patients who demonstrate no explicit sequential knowledge, as determined by verbal reports on detection of regularities, the ability to generate the trained sequence, and/or the ability to recognize the trained sequence. Even when all these awareness measures are combined, some healthy individuals show procedural learning but no sign of explicit knowledge on any measure (Willingham et al 1993). A more pronounced dissociation, due to impaired explicit learning with retained procedural learning, is seen in declarative amnesics such as patients with Korsakoff syndrome (Nissen and

Bullemer 1987), patients with Alzheimer disease (Knopman and Nissen 1987), and healthy individuals with temporary amnesia after scopolamine injection (Nissen et al 1987).

Second, explicit learning with no evidence for procedural learning has been observed. While procedural learning typically precedes explicit learning, a minority of healthy individuals appear to develop explicit sequence knowledge in spite of little or no procedural learning (Willingham et al 1989). Impaired procedural learning in the SRTT with small or no defects in explicit learning has been demonstrated in Parkinson patients (Pascual-Leone et al 1993, Dominey et al 1997, Siegert et al 2006), as well as on a bimanual version of the SRTT in patients with transection or agenesis of the corpus callosum (de Guise et al 1999) and younger children (de Guise and Lassonde 2001). A temporary impairment of procedural, but not explicit, learning in the SRTT has been reported after sleep deprivation (Heuer et al 1998).

A third type of evidence comes from studies using the process dissociation procedure, originally proposed by Jacoby (1991) to separate implicit and explicit processing. The key idea is to design two paradigms: one where the explicit and implicit processes both facilitate performance (the facilitation task), and one where they work antagonistically (the interference task). Destrebecqz and Cleeremans (2001) applied this to the SRTT, using two tasks performed after completed SRTT training. In the facilitation task participants were asked to freely generate trials that resemble the sequence used in the SRTT. Both implicit and explicit sequence knowledge will facilitate this performance. In the interference task, the instruction was to generate sequences, but to avoid quoting from the SRTT sequence. Here, it is assumed, successful performance will rely on explicit sequence knowledge, whereas implicit processes will act as a source of errors, in the form of unintentional reproductions of the SRTT sequence (for a discussion see Jacoby 1991). During training, two different versions of the SRTT were employed: one with RSIs of 250 ms, and one with RSIs reduced to 0 ms. The central finding was a major difference in performance in the interference tasks, depending on the RSI in the preceding SRTT. The two SRTT paradigms thus presumably involved implicit and explicit learning to different degrees. When RSIs were 250 ms, participants were able to suppress reproductions of the SRTT sequences. With an RSI of 0 ms, in contrast, elements of the SRTT sequence were reproduced both in the interference and the facilitation task, suggesting that learning was predominantly implicit in this case (Destrebecqz and Cleeremans 2001).

Fourth, implicit and explicit learning ability in the SRTT appear to follow different developmental trajectories (section 5.1).

Fifth, data from individual difference studies show that explicit, but presumably not implicit, sequence learning is correlated with working memory capacity and IQ (section 6.1).

A detailed discussion of the nature of the ordinal representations acquired in the SRTT is outside the scope of this review. However, two important aspects should be noted in passing. First, learning could be based on the perceptual sequence of stimuli as well as the motor sequence of responses. Learning transfer designs, where these two aspects are altered independently (Willingham et al 1989, Mayr 1996, Seger 1997), as well as designs where the stimulus-response mapping is randomized from trial to trial to allow only perceptual learning (Goschke et al 2001, Dennis et al 2006), indicate that both forms of learning can occur. Second, we focus on the learning of movement sequences with a deterministic ordinal structure. However, it appears likely that the involved learning mechanisms at least partly overlap with those used in learning of probabilistic sequences without a fixed structure, which can also be studied with the SRTT. For an interesting recent discussion of the latter issue, see Lungu et al (2004).

3.2 Neural Correlates of Implicit Ordinal Sequence Learning

Further evidence for the notion that implicit and explicit ordinal sequence learning rely on partially separate systems comes from brain imaging data. Collectively, these studies point to a central role for the basal ganglia in implicit ordinal learning. Activity in the basal ganglia is one of the most consistent findings in neuroimaging studies of implicit ordinal learning (Grafton et al 1995, Rauch et al 1995, Doyon et al 1996, Berns et al 1997, Hazeltine et al 1997, Rauch et al 1997, Peigneux et al 2000, Willingham et al 2002, Schendan et al 2003, Aizenstein et al 2004, Thomas et al 2004). Honda and coworkers (1998) did not find basal ganglia activity in a PET study of SRTT learning but, as noted by the authors, this may have reflected limited implicit learning in that experiment. Determining whether brain activity is specifically related to implicit processing of course confronts similar difficulties to separating implicit and explicit processing on a behavioural level. Several pioneering studies thus confound the implicit–explicit dimension with task-order effects or demands from dual tasks, or rely on the assumption that implicit and explicit processing can be completely dissociated by using different training conditions. One of the strongest pieces of evidence so far for a specific role of the basal ganglia in implicit ordinal learning comes from a recent PET study where the process dissociation procedure was used (Destrebecqz et al 2005). Neural activity in the striatum could be tied directly to implicit processing in a sequence generation task performed immediately after SRTT training. Recent studies have also shown that basal ganglia activity is correlated to implicit learning measures in both children and adults (Thomas et al 2004). Furthermore, as mentioned previously, ordinal SRTT learning is impaired in Parkinson patients (Pascual-Leone et al 1993, Dominey et al 1997, Shin and Ivry 2003, Siegert et al 2006).

Activity patterns in other brain regions during implicit SRTT learning are somewhat less consistent. Regions commonly activated include primary sensorimotor cortex (Grafton et al 1995, 1998, Aizenstein et al 2004); lateral and medial premotor areas (Grafton et al 1995, Rauch et al 1995, Berns et al 1997, Rauch et al 1997, Grafton et al 1998); prefrontal (Schendan et al 2003, Aizenstein et al 2004), parietal (Doyon et al 1996, Rauch et al 1997, Grafton et al 1998, Aizenstein et al 2004) and visual (Rauch et al 1995, 1997, Aizenstein et al 2004) cortical regions; and the cerebellum (Doyon et al 1996, Rauch et al 1997).

A traditional view has been that the primary motor cortex (M1) is mainly controlling patterns of muscle activity, with little involvement in sequential organization and other movement-independent aspects of motor skill. Modern studies challenge that view, indicating direct involvement of M1, e.g. in ordinal sequence learning. Data from human neuroimaging studies using learning transfer designs suggest that M1 activity is related to implicit learning of ordinal sequences using effector-specific representations of sequences of responses (Grafton et al 1998, Bischoff-Grethe et al 2004). Functional reorganizations of motor cortex during implicit ordinal learning in the SRTT, i.e. an enlargement of the representations of hand muscles used in the task within cortical output maps, have been demonstrated using transcranial magnetic stimulation (Pascual-Leone et al 1994). Long-term practice of ordinal sequences is accompanied by long-lasting (months) reorganizations of M1. Karni and coworkers, for example, demonstrated a dramatic and sequence-specific expansion of the extent of the activation in M1 following four weeks of practice of a manual sequence task (Karni et al 1995). Recent data from the monkey, using a variant of the SRTT, provide direct evidence that neurons in M1 have different activity patterns during random and sequential trials after long-term training (> two years) of an ordinal sequence (Matsuzaka et al 2007). For further discussions of the idea that M1 together with the basal ganglia is specifically involved in implicit learning of ordinal response sequences, see Hikosaka et al (2002), Hallett (2005) and Ashe et al (2006).

Transfer data show that sequence representations in the inferior parietal cortex and mesial premotor regions are more abstract in nature (Grafton et al 1998). That activity in the mesial premotor cortex is related to effector-independent aspects of sequence structure is also supported by studies of neuronal activity during sequential tasks in the monkey (Mushiaka et al 1991, Shima and Tanji 1998, 2000, Tanji 2001, Isoda and Tanji 2004). Neurons that fire before the performance of a particular sequence element, regardless of which movement is performed (rank-order selective cells), become increasingly more common in rostral premotor areas. Moving rostrally from primary sensorimotor cortex, representations of ordinal sequences thus appear to be increasingly abstract in nature. An interesting suggestion by Ashe and coauthors (2006) is that a similar gradient for the perceptual representation of sequence structure may be found in parietal areas, with encoding of stimulus-specific properties in the posterior parietal cortex and more stimulus-independent coding in anterior regions.

3.3 NEURAL CORRELATES OF EXPLICIT ORDINAL SEQUENCE LEARNING
As mentioned, a body of data supports a specific role for the basal ganglia and motor cortex in implicit ordinal learning. However, recent neuroimaging studies have also shown a large degree of overlap in brain activity between implicit and explicit learning in the SRTT (Willingham et al 2002, Schendan et al 2003, Aizenstein et al 2004). Most, if not all, of the regions involved in implicit ordinal learning have thus also been found active during explicit ordinal learning.

Several lines of evidence suggest that, among these regions, the prefrontal cortex (PFC) is of particular importance for explicit learning. First, PFC activity is found in neuroimaging studies of explicit learning across a variety of sequential tasks: the SRTT (Grafton et al 1995, Berns et al 1997, Willingham et al 2002, Schendan et al 2003), the 2 × N task (Sakai et al 1998, Bapi et al 2006), as well as other ordinal sequence learning paradigms (Jenkins et al 1994, Toni et al 1998). Second, in the SRTT, PFC activity increases over time as participants progress from initial implicit sequence learning to increased explicit awareness of the sequence (Berns et al 1997). Third, the opposite pattern – i.e. a decreased PFC activity over time – has been observed in tasks, such as the 2 × N task, where learning is explicit from the start and in which the participants gradually acquire a more and more automatic performance of the sequence (Jenkins et al 1994, Sakai et al 1998). Fourth, PFC activity has recently been tied to explicit rather than implicit ordinal processing using the process dissociation procedure (Destrebecqz et al 2005).

An important unresolved question concerns the precise role, or roles, of the PFC for explicit ordinal learning. One possibility is that the PFC activity reflects top-down cognitive control, for instance selective attention to task-relevant stimuli (MacDonald et al 2000, Lau et al 2004). It seems likely, however, that the working memory functions of PFC also are utilized more directly to promote learning, e.g. through sequence rehearsal (Pascual-Leone et al 1993). Indeed, an assumption underlying the application of process dissociation procedures to sequence learning is that successful performance of the exclusion task (section 3.1) requires manipulations of sequential structures in working memory. In line with this, individual differences in explicit, but probably not implicit, learning on the SRTT are correlated with working memory capacity and IQ (section 6). Finally, PFC activity is high during the initial phase of the $2 \times N$ task (Sakai et al 1998, Bapi et al 2006) and other ordinal sequence learning tasks that include trial-and-error learning (Toni et al 1998). This presumably also reflects free generation of new sequential patterns: the PFC is known to be involved in free generation of sequential structures both in pseudo-random tasks (Deiber et al 1991, Frith et al 1991) and in more complex behaviours such as musical improvisation (Bengtsson et al 2007).

In other learning paradigms, such as probabilistic category learning, explicit–implicit dissociations have been found in the declarative memory systems of the medial temporal lobe, which are involved in explicit but not implicit learning (Poldrack et al 2001). For movement sequence learning this may not hold. Many studies have not found activation of the medial temporal lobe, and one recent study in which this region was specifically investigated found increased activity during both implicit and explicit learning in the SRTT (Schendan et al 2003).

4 Learning the temporal structure of a movement sequence

4.1 DIFFERENT TYPES OF TEMPORAL SEQUENCES

Time is a continuous variable. However, different types of temporal structures are handled differently by the brain. Two distinctions are of special relevance in the present context.

First, humans can process a vast range of temporal durations, from milliseconds to years. The focus of the present review is movement timing of durations shorter than 1–1.5 s. A number of findings suggest that the neural mechanisms of this type of timing differ from those handling timing in the multisecond range. In brief, these findings include within-task differences in timing variability at different durations in healthy populations; differential impairment of subsecond and multisecond timing in neurological populations; and differential effects of various drugs on subsecond and multisecond timing (for reviews see Gibbon et al 1997, Lewis and Miall 2003). Furthermore, metaanalyses of neuroimaging studies show that multisecond timing relies more on the PFC and parietal areas than does subsecond timing (Lewis and Miall 2003).

Second, the movement timing system appears to include special mechanisms for the processing of metrical sequences, i.e. sequences where all temporal intervals are small integer multiples of an underlying beat (Essens and Povel 1985). Among the various pieces of evidence supporting this can be mentioned, first, that during free generation of shorter temporal sequences, participants spontaneously produce metrical patterns, dominated by two durations with an approximate 2:1 ratio (Fraisse 1946, Essens and Povel 1985). Second, metrical rhythmic patterns are commonly found in traditional musics of different ethnic groups and cultures all over the world (Sloboda 1985, Wallin et al 2000). Third, in reproduction tasks, participants are more accurate, i.e. the mean reproduced duration is closer to target, as well as less variable when reproducing metrical patterns than when producing non-metrical patterns (Essens and Povel 1985, Sakai et al 1999). Fourth, in a learning study using repeated ISR trials, participants learned metrical patterns easily, whereas improvement on non-metrical patterns was slow or non-significant (Collier and Wright 1995). Fifth, the ability to proportionally scale a temporal sequence, i.e. to change its total duration while preserving the relative durations of the individual intervals, seems limited to metrical sequences (Collier and Wright 1995).

Only one published imaging study (Sakai et al 1999) has so far directly contrasted processing of metrical and non-metrical patterns. An ISR task where the participants were required to maintain the temporal sequence in short-term memory before reproduction was used. Brain activity was measured during this maintenance period. In line with the behavioural findings summarized above, different patterns of brain activity were found for metrical and non-metrical temporal structures, with the right PFC and premotor cortex active only in the latter case. Interestingly, this suggests that timing of non-metrical temporal structures, like suprasecond timing, is more cognitively controlled than is metrical timing.

4.2 IMPLICIT TEMPORAL SEQUENCE LEARNING

Can temporal sequences be learned implicitly? Few studies have addressed this question. Salidis (2001) used an auditory version of the SRTT where the RSIs followed a non-metrical temporal sequence. A decrease of mean RTs was seen, with no signs of explicit rhythm knowledge on awareness tests. Ullén and Bengtsson (2003) found learning of metrical temporal sequences in a repeated ISR paradigm where the ordinal structure of the stimuli was random. Learning was seen also in individuals who verbally reported having detected no regularities in the stimuli.

While these studies indicate that implicit temporal sequence learning is possible, they can be criticized on the same grounds as many studies of implicit ordinal learning: the employed awareness measures may be contaminated with implicit knowledge, as well as being too insensitive to exhaust all explicit knowledge (section 3.1). However, we have recently found stronger evidence for implicit temporal sequence learning using the process dissociation procedure (Karabanov and Ullén 2008). No studies have so far attempted to compare the neural correlates of implicit and explicit temporal sequence learning.

4.3 DISSOCIATING TEMPORAL AND ORDINAL SEQUENCE LEARNING

A second question of interest is whether ordinal and temporal sequential structures can be learned independently, or whether these two aspects of a movement sequence are always learned and represented in an integrated manner. Ullén and Bengtsson (2003) found clear evidence for independent ordinal and temporal learning systems, using the ISR paradigm, in that ordinal sequences could be learned from stimuli where the temporal dimension was random, and vice versa. Furthermore, learning transfer experiments indicated that such learning also resulted in independent representations of the ordinal and temporal structure of the sequences.

When the same question has been addressed with SRTT paradigms, results have been somewhat more variable. Ordinal learning is consistently seen even if the temporal sequence of the RSIs is random (Stadler 1993, 1995, Sakai et al 2002) or uncorrelated with the ordinal sequence (Lee 2000, Shin and Ivry 2002). However, temporal learning with a random ordinal sequence was found by Sakai et al (2002), while Shin and Ivry (2002) did not observe temporal learning when the ordinal sequence was uncorrelated with the temporal sequence. A possible explanation for the discrepancy is that independent temporal sequence learning is difficult in the SRTT: when the ordinal sequence is unpredictable, participants cannot prepare the next response in the sequence, even if they have learned the temporal interval preceding it (Ullén and Bengtsson 2003).

4.4 NEURAL CORRELATES OF TEMPORAL SEQUENCE LEARNING

A relatively large set of neuroimaging studies have investigated neural correlates of voluntary movement timing in the subsecond–second range, using a variety of paradigms such as isochronous tapping (Rao et al 1997, Jäncke et al 2000, Lutz et al 2000, Jantzen et al 2004, Lewis et al 2004, Jantzen et al 2005), ISR of temporal sequences (Penhune et al 1998, Schubotz and von Cramon 2001), performance of overlearned temporal sequences (Bengtsson et al 2004, 2005), and bimanual temporal coordination (Ullén et al 2003). These studies demonstrate that a number of regions, including the presupplementary motor area (preSMA), the supplementary motor area, the lateral premotor cortex, the inferior frontal cortex, the cerebellum, the basal ganglia and the superior temporal cortex, are activated fairly consistently across a range of movement timing tasks (for reviews see Macar et al 2002, Lewis and Miall 2003, Ivry and Spencer 2004). A few studies have directly examined the roles of these and other brain regions for the process of temporal sequence learning itself. All these studies employ explicit learning and visually presented temporal sequences, but otherwise differ in methodological details.

Ramnani and Passingham (2001) used the SRTT and a non-metrical sequence. Regions with increased activity during learning included the preSMA and the rostral division of the dorsal premotor cortex, the inferior frontal cortex, as well as parietal regions and the cerebellum. The PFC was active, but decreased its activity as learning progressed. The SRTT was also used by Sakai et al (2002) to compare ordinal and metrical temporal learning in the same individuals. During temporal learning the ordinal stimulus structure was random, and vice versa. Activity in comparisons between temporal and ordinal learning was relatively sparse, but cerebellar activity was found to be specific for temporal learning. During SRTT training of a combined sequence with a fixed ordinal and metrical temporal structure, in a second experiment, widespread frontal activity was seen in the PFC as well as the mesial and lateral premotor cortices.

Penhune and Doyon (2002) studied long-term training of a non-metrical sequence. The training consisted of repeated sequence presentations during which participants synchronized button presses with the stimuli. Brain activity was recorded on days 1 and 5 of training as well as during delayed recall four weeks later. On day 1, extensive cerebellar activity was found while cortical activity was largely limited to visual regions in the occipital and temporal lobes. Four days later, activity was found in the PFC and preSMA, as well as the basal ganglia, while cerebellar activity had decreased. During delayed recall, activity was predominantly frontal, in the preSMA, the dorsal premotor cortex, and M1. The same type of non-metrical sequences was used in a second study in the same group (Penhune and Doyon 2005), in which the participants were scanned across three blocks of training performed on the same day. During the first training block, activity was found in the cerebellum, the superior temporal cortex, the SMA, the preSMA and the precuneus. In later blocks, cerebellar activity decreased whereas activity increased in M1 and the basal ganglia.

Existing studies are thus fairly consistent in finding learning-related activity in the PFC, the preSMA, and the cerebellum. The PFC activity may, as for ordinal sequences, be related to the fact that the learning was explicit. A decrease in PFC activity when performance becomes more automatic, as seen by Ramnani and Passingham (2001), is also observed during ordinal learning, e.g. in the $2 \times N$ task (section 3.3). Furthermore Penhune et al (1998) found the PFC active during ISR of novel temporal sequences, which may be a task that is similar to the initial stages of explicit learning. The results of Sakai et al (1999) suggest that PFC involvement in temporal learning may also vary with the structure of the sequence, with higher PFC activity during processing of complex non-metrical sequences (section 4.1).

The preSMA appears to have a central role in a broad range of tasks that involve voluntary timing (Macar et al 2002, Lewis and Miall 2003). PreSMA activity has, for example, also been specifically related to temporal control during performance of overlearned spatiotemporal sequences (Bengtsson et al 2004, 2005). Recordings from preSMA neurons during ordinal sequential tasks in the monkey have made it possible to characterize a number of activity patterns (section 3.2). However, without an animal model for temporal sequence control, one can only speculate on how activity in these different neurons, e.g. rank-order selective cells, is modulated during the performance of a temporal sequence.

The cerebellum has been suggested to be a key region for both motor and perceptual timing (Ivry and Keele 1989, Ivry and Spencer 2004). The cerebellar activity during temporal sequence learning is in line with this conception. Deficits in SRTT temporal sequence learning, using a non-metrical eight-element sequence, have also been found in patients with cerebellar damage (Shin and Ivry 2003). In general, a large number of studies using neuroimaging techniques (for reviews see Lewis and Miall 2003, Ivry and Spencer 2004), neurological patients (Ivry et al 1988, Ivry and Keele 1989, Spencer et al 2003, Harrington et al 2004), and transcranial magnetic stimulation (Théoret et al 2001) provide strong support for the view that the cerebellum is important for voluntary timing. Some controversy, however, has surrounded the exact nature of the cerebellar involvement in temporal control, i.e. whether it is directly involved in timekeeping, or whether it performs other computational operations which indirectly affect timing (see Rao et al 2001, Harrington et al

2004), two possibilities which are of course not mutually exclusive. Notably, Penhune and coworkers found a progressive *decrease* of cerebellar activity during training (Penhune and Doyon 2002, 2005), as well as a negative correlation between error measures and cerebellar activity, suggesting that the cerebellum is primarily involved in error correction during initial stages of training (see also Doyon et al 2003). Ramnani and Passingham (2001), on the other hand, found an *increase* of cerebellar activity during training, which could be taken as evidence for a more specific cerebellar role in temporal sequence learning. These interesting discrepancies suggest that the details of cerebellar involvement in temporal sequence learning may differ with different training paradigms.

In summary, temporal sequence learning has been studied in relatively few neuroimaging studies, using different paradigms, and no directly relevant animal data are available. Neural mechanisms have thus to be discussed with some caution at present. In particular, data are wanting with regard to differences in brain activity related to implicit and explicit temporal sequence learning, learning of sequences presented in auditory and other non-visual modalities, and comparisons of sequences with different metrical structure.

5 Developmental aspects of movement sequence learning

Ordinal sequence learning in children has been investigated with the SRTT (Meulemans et al 1998, Thomas and Nelson 2001, Waber et al 2003, Wilson et al 2003, Thomas et al 2004, Berger et al 2005, Vicari et al 2005). These studies demonstrate procedural learning in children as young as 4 years (Thomas and Nelson 2001). Some general differences in the performance of children and adults are consistently seen in this task. First, children show much longer RTs than adults, with higher mean RTs for younger children than for older children (Meulemans et al 1998, Thomas and Nelson 2001, Waber et al 2003, Thomas et al 2004). This phenomenon is not in any way unique to the SRTT and other choice RT tasks: between early childhood and adulthood mean RT in a broad range of elementary cognitive tasks shows an approximately exponential decrease with age (for reviews see Fry and Hale 2000, Jensen 2006). Second, children make more errors, and young children often display a pronounced increase in error frequency during training, indicating faster mental and/or motor fatigue (Meulemans et al 1998, Thomas and Nelson 2001, Waber et al 2003, Thomas et al 2004). Third, children appear to have a larger non-sequence-specific procedural learning effect (RT decrease) than adults during random trials (Meulemans et al 1998, Thomas and Nelson 2001).

A central developmental question in the present context is how implicit and explicit learning in the SRTT vary as a function of age during childhood and adolescence. At present the full answer to that question is lacking, mainly because published studies have used limited age sampling. Another difficult methodological concern is explicit awareness testing of children: their lower verbal abilities might cause misunderstandings of task instructions as well as poor verbalization of acquired explicit knowledge.

A large (n = 422) group of children aged 7 to 11 years was studied with the SRTT as well as psychometrical tests by Waber et al (2003). The sample included both normal children and children with a variety of learning problems. Age was negatively correlated with overall RT, but it was not reported whether it predicted sequence-specific procedural learning. Explicit learning was lower than typically found with adults, and positively correlated with age. Similar results were found by Thomas and Nelson (2001), who compared three groups of children, aged 4, 7 and 10 years. A close-to-significant (p = 0.08) trend for larger procedural learning in the 10-year-olds than in the 7-year-olds was found. The data also suggested that the 4-year-olds showed the least procedural learning, although a different version of the SRTT was used in this group. Clear trends were found for explicit learning, with 50 per cent of the 10-year-olds showing explicit awareness and only one participant among the 4-year-olds. Strikingly, in the latter group, explicit awareness was not seen even when the children were informed about the presence of a sequence before training.

Evidence for faster and larger procedural learning in adults than in 7- to 11-year-old children was found by Thomas and coworkers (2004). No explicit awareness test was administered but a version of the SRTT with alternating random and sequential trials, which reduces explicit learning (Meulemans et al 1998), was used. This was also the first study to compare neural correlates of SRTT learning in children and adults. A substantial overlap in neural activity was found in the two age groups, but children showed higher activity in the basal ganglia, whereas adults had higher activity in premotor regions. Basal ganglia activity also correlated with procedural learning measures for both age groups, suggesting that this region develops a key role for implicit ordinal learning early in ontogeny.

Meulemans et al (1998) compared adults and two groups of children, aged 6 and 10 years. In an ANOVA analysis with RT as dependent variable, age group as between-subject variable, and block type (random or sequential) and trial number as repeated measures variables, no interaction was found between age group and block type. RT differences between random and sequential trials were thus similar in all age groups, which was taken as evidence for a lack of age differences in procedural learning. No participants in this study developed explicit sequence knowledge.

In summary, mechanisms for implicit ordinal learning are thus available early in childhood, but they appear to show some differences compared to the adult system on both the behavioural and neurophysiological levels. More pronounced age differences are seen for explicit ordinal learning, which is less developed in children, in particular young children (< 10 years old). Interestingly, one study reports the opposite pattern, i.e. explicit learning but poor procedural learning, in younger children (< 12 years old) performing a bimanual version of the SRTT (de Guise and Lassonde 2001). The explanation may be that procedural learning in that task required interhemispheric communication, which is limited in children due to callosal immaturity.

6 Individual differences in movement sequence learning ability

As has been clear from the previous discussions, there are considerable individual differences in movement sequence learning ability. These are evident both in implicit and explicit learning measures. A few studies have characterized the sources of these individual differences by administering both sequence learning tasks and psychometric tests to the same participants.

The most consistent finding from these studies is probably that explicit ordinal sequence learning is positively correlated with IQ. Feldman et al (1995) found a correlation (r = 0.28), in a large (n = 485) adult sample, between explicit learning in the SRTT and IQ (Wechsler Adult Intelligence Scale), as well as correlations with numerous other cognitive tasks. In children, IQ (Kaufman Brief Intelligence Test) predicted explicit sequence learning in the previously mentioned study by Waber et al (2003). Unsworth and Engle (2005) found a significant correlation (r = 0.48) between scores on the Raven Progressive Matrices, and procedural SRTT learning with intentional task instructions, during which the participants developed explicit sequence knowledge. Explicit sequence learning was also higher in individuals with high working memory capacity, as quantified by performance on the *operation span task*, which requires manipulation of information in working memory during performance of a secondary task, and which is more correlated with IQ than simple span measures (Turner and Engle 1989). One study by Frensch and Miner (1994) found a relationship between simple forward span measures of short-term memory capacity and procedural learning in the SRTT, which may have been more dependent on whether learning was intentional, than on whether it resulted in explicit ordinal knowledge: in two independent experiments significant correlations of r = 0.57 and r = 0.61, respectively, were found between forward span on a spatial short-term memory task and SRTT procedural learning under intentional task instructions, even though the training only resulted in partial explicit knowledge. Under incidental task instructions correlations were insignificant.

The consistent correlations with different IQ tests and working memory capacity suggest that explicit sequence learning ability is related to psychometric general intelligence (*g*) (Jensen 1998), although a direct demonstration of this using factor analytical techniques would be of importance. The individual difference data are thus in line with the neurophysiological literature suggesting that explicit ordinal learning is dependent on the attentional and working memory-related functions of the PFC (section 3.3), which are regarded as central for *g* (Wilhelm and Engle 2005).

In contrast, the correlation between implicit ordinal learning and IQ (or working memory capacity) is presumably either weakly positive or nil, as indicated by insignificant findings even in studies using large (n > 400) samples. Feldman et al (1995) found no correlation between procedural learning and IQ (r = 0.05; n.s.), although RTs during initial trials correlated negatively with IQ. A negative correlation between IQ and overall RT, but no correlation between IQ and implicit procedural learning, was also found by Waber et al (2003). Similarly, Unsworth and Engle (2005) found no significant relationship between procedural learning and working memory capacity (operation span) or IQ (r = 0.17; n.s.) in participants who lacked explicit awareness. Correlations between short-term memory forward span and implicit SRTT learning varied between r = 0.07 and r = 0.14 (all n.s.) in the study by Frensch and Miner (1994). Implicit SRTT learning indeed shows weak correlation with a broad range of cognitive tasks, suggesting that a large portion of the between-subject variance in this variable is fairly task-specific (Feldman et al 1995).

The negative correlation between IQ and mean RT in the SRTT is, like the previously discussed correlation between age and mean RT, an example of a phenomenon observed with different magnitudes in practically all elementary cognitive tasks. In general, such RT–IQ correlations appear to be almost entirely due to correlations between RT and psychometric *g* (for reviews see Jensen 1998, Deary 2003, Jensen 2006).

7 Conclusion

A large body of research has established that movement sequence learning relies on a network of brain regions, which include the PFC, premotor and primary sensorimotor cortices, parietal and occipital regions, as well as the basal ganglia and the cerebellum. Recent studies have highlighted the specific roles of these regions for different forms of sequence learning. In particular, implicit and explicit learning, as well as learning of ordinal and temporal structures, have been shown to rely on partly different neural circuitry. Convergent evidence from a variety of behavioural and neurophysiological paradigms suggests that fronto-striatal circuits play a specific role for implicit ordinal learning, while the PFC is central for explicit ordinal learning. Implicit temporal sequence learning has been little studied, but the PFC, the preSMA, the cerebellum and parietal regions may be of particular importance for explicit temporal sequence learning. Furthermore, temporal sequence learning mechanisms are sensitive to metrical structure, with more complex sequences relying more on prefrontal control. Developmental and individual difference data further support the distinction between implicit and explicit movement sequence learning systems. The implicit system is thus present early in childhood and appears largely unrelated to cognitive ability, while the explicit system develops later and is correlated with general intelligence.

The motor behaviour of children with cerebral palsy, by nature of their diagnosis, differs from that seen in typically developing children. With regard to movement sequence learning, it appears likely that individual children differ in how the main components of the movement sequence learning system – temporal and ordinal, implicit and explicit – are affected. Awareness of these differences could be of assistance to clinicians when optimizing an intervention programme for a particular child.

ACKNOWLEDGEMENTS

I am grateful to Henrik Ehrsson, Guy Madison and Brigitte Vollmer for comments on an earlier version of this review.

REFERENCES

Aizenstein HJ, Stenger VA, Cochran J, Clark K, Johnson M, Nebes RD, Carter CS (2004) Regional brain activation during concurrent implicit and explicit sequence learning. *Cereb Cortex* 14: 199–208.

Ashe J, Lungu OV, Basford AT, Lu X (2006) Cortical control of motor sequences. *Curr Opin Neurobiol* 16: 213–221.

Bapi RS, Miyapuram KP, Graydon FX, Doya K (2006) fMRI investigation of cortical and subcortical networks in the learning of abstract and effector-specific representations of motor sequences. *Neuroimage* 32: 714–727.

Bengtsson S, Ehrsson HH, Forssberg H, Ullén F (2004) Dissociating brain regions controlling the temporal and ordinal structure of learned movement sequences. *Eur J Neurosci* 19: 2591–2602.

Bengtsson SL, Ehrsson HH, Forssberg H, Ullén F (2005) Effector-independent voluntary timing: behavioural and neuroimaging evidence. *Eur J Neurosci* 22: 3255–3265.

Bengtsson SL, Csíkszentmihályi M, Ullén F (2007) Cortical regions involved in the generation of musical structures during improvisation in pianists. *J Cogn Neurosci* 19: 830–842.

Berger A, Sadeh M, Tzur G, Shuper A, Kornreich L, Inbar D, Cohen IJ, Michowiz S, Yaniv I, Constantini S, Vakil E (2005) Motor and non-motor sequence learning in children and adolescents with cerebellar damage. *J Int Neuropsychol Soc* 11: 482–487.

Berns GS, Cohen JD, Mintun MA (1997) Brain regions responsive to novelty in the absence of awareness. *Science* 276: 1272–1275.

Bischoff-Grethe A, Goedert KM, Willingham DT, Grafton ST (2004) Neural substrates of response-based sequence learning using fMRI. *J Cogn Neurosci* 16: 127–138.

Clegg BA, DiGirolamo GJ, Keele SW (1998) Sequence learning. *Trend Cogn Sci* 2: 275–281.

Collier GL, Wright CE (1995) Temporal rescaling of simple and complex ratios in rhythmic tapping. *J Exp Psychol: Hum Percept Perform* 21: 602–627.

Deary IJ (2003) Reaction time and psychometric intelligence: Jensen's contributions. In: Nyborg H, editor. *The Scientific Study of General Intelligence: A Tribute to Arthur R. Jensen.* Oxford: Pergamon, pp. 53–75.

de Guise E, Lassonde M (2001) Callosal contribution to procedural learning in children. *Dev Neuropsychol* 19: 253–272.

de Guise E, del Pesce M, Foschi N, Quattrini A, Papo I, Lassonde M (1999) Callosal and cortical contribution to procedural learning. *Brain* 122: 1049–1062.

Deiber M-P, Passingham RE, Colebatch JG, Friston KJ, Nixon PD, Frackowiak RSJ (1991) Cortical areas and the selection of movement: a study with positron emission tomography. *Exp Brain Res* 84: 393–402.

Dennis NA, Howard JH, Howard DV (2006) Implicit sequence learning without motor sequencing in young and old adults. *Exp Brain Res* 175: 153–164.

Destrebecqz A, Cleeremans A (2001) Can sequence learning be implicit? New evidence with the process dissociation procedure. *Psychon Bull Rev* 8: 343–350.

Destrebecqz A, Peigneux P, Laureys S, Degueldre C, Del Fiore G, Aerts J, Luxen A, Van Der Linden M, Cleeremans A, Maquet P (2005) The neural correlates of implicit and explicit sequence learning: interacting networks revealed by the process dissociation procedure. *Learn Mem* 12: 480–490.

Dominey PF, Ventre-Dominey J, Broussolle E, Jeannerod M (1997) Analogical transfer is effective in a serial reaction time task in Parkinson's disease: evidence for a dissociable form of sequence learning. *Neuropsychologia* 35: 1–9.

Doyon J, Owen AM, Petrides M, Sziklas V, Evans AC (1996) Functional anatomy of visuomotor skill learning in human subjects examined with positron emission tomography. *Exp Brain Res* 8: 637–648.

Doyon J, Penhune V, Ungerleider LG (2003) Distinct contribution of the cortico-striatal and cortico-cerebellar systems to motor skill learning. *Neuropsychologia* 41: 252–262.

Essens PJ, Povel D-J (1985) Metrical and nonmetrical representations of temporal patterns. *Percept Psychophys* 37: 1–7.

Feldman J, Kerr B, Streissguth AP (1995) Correlational analyses of procedural and declarative learning performance. *Intelligence* 20: 87–114.

Forkstam C, Petersson KM (2005) Towards an explicit account of implicit learning. *Curr Opin Neurol* 18: 435–441.

Fraisse P (1946) Contribution a l'étude du rythme en tant que forme temporelle. *J de Psychologie Normale et Patologique* 39: 283–304.

Frensch PA, Miner CS (1994) Effects of presentation rate and individual differences in short-term memory capacity on an indirect measure of serial learning. *Mem Cognit* 22: 95–110.

Frith CD, Friston KJ, Liddle PF, Frackowiak RSJ (1991) Willed action and the prefrontal cortex in man: a study with PET. *Proc R Soc Lond B* 244: 241–246.

Fry AF, Hale S (2000) Relationships among processing speed, working memory, and fluid intelligence in children. *Biol Psychol* 54: 1–34.

Gibbon J, Malapani C, Dale CL, Gallistel CR (1997) Toward a neurobiology of temporal cognition: advances and challenges. *Curr Opin Neurobiol* 7: 170–184.

Goschke T, Friederici AD, Kotz SA, van Kampen A (2001) Procedural learning in Broca's aphasia: dissociation between the implicit acquisition of spatio-motor and phoneme sequences. *J Cogn Neurosci* 13: 370–388.

Grafton ST, Hazeltine E, Ivry R (1995) Functional anatomy of sequence learning in normal humans. *J Cogn Neurosci* 7: 497–510.

Grafton ST, Hazeltine E, Ivry RB (1998) Abstract and effector-specific representations of motor sequences identified with PET. *J Neurosci* 18: 9420–9428.

Hallett M (2005) Motor learning. In: Freund H-J, Jeannerod M, Hallett M, Leiguarda R, editors. *Higher-order Motor Disorders: From Neuroanatomy and Neurobiology to Clinical Neurology.* Oxford: Oxford University Press, pp. 123–140.

Harrington DL, Lee RR, Boyd LA, Rapcsak SZ, Knight RT (2004) Does the representation of time depend on the cerebellum? Effect of cerebellar stroke. *Brain* 127: 561–574.

Hazeltine E, Grafton ST, Ivry R (1997) Attention and stimulus characteristics determine the locus of motor sequence encoding. A PET study. *Brain* 120: 123–140.

Heuer H, Spijkers W, Kiesswetter E, Schmidtke V (1998) Effects of sleep loss, time of day, and extended mental work on implicit and explicit learning of sequences. *J Exp Psychol: Applied* 4: 139–162.

Hikosaka O, Rand MK, Miyachi S, Miyashita K (1995) Learning of sequential movements in the monkey – process of learning and retention of memory. *J Neurophysiol* 74: 1652–1661.

Hikosaka O, Sakai K, Miyauchi S, Takino R, Sasaki Y, Pütz B (1996) Activation of human pre-supplementary motor area in learning of sequential procedures: a functional MRI study. *J Neurophysiol* 76: 617–621.

Hikosaka O, Nakamura K, Sakai K, Nakahara H (2002) Central mechanisms of motor skill learning. *Curr Opin Neurobiol* 12: 217–222.

Honda M, Deiber MP, Ibanez V, Pascual-Leone A, Zhuang P, Hallet M (1998) Dynamic cortical involvement in implicit and explicit sequence learning: a PET study. *Brain* 121: 2159–2173.

Isoda M, Tanji J (2004) Participation of the primate presupplementary motor area in sequencing multiple saccades. *J Neurophysiol* 92: 653–659.

Ivry R, Keele SW (1989) Timing functions of the cerebellum. *J Cogn Neurosci* 1: 136–152.

Ivry R, Spencer RMC (2004) The neural representation of time. *Curr Opin Neurobiol* 14: 225–232.

Ivry RB, Keele SW, Diener HC (1988) Dissociation of the lateral and medial cerebellum in movement timing and movement execution. *Exp Brain Res* 73: 167–180.

Jacoby LL (1991) A process dissociation framework: separating automatic from intentional uses of memory. *J Mem Lang* 30: 513–541.

Jäncke L, Loose R, Lutz K, Specht K, Shah NJ (2000) Cortical activations during paced finger-tapping applying visual and auditory pacing stimuli. *Cogn Brain Res* 10: 51–66.

Jantzen KJ, Steinberg FL, Kelso JAS (2004) Brain networks underlying human timing behavior are influenced by prior context. *Proc Natl Acad Sci USA* 101: 6815–6820.

Jantzen KJ, Steinberg FL, Kelso JAS (2005) Functional MRI reveals the existence of modality and coordination-dependent timing networks. *Neuroimage* 25: 1031–1042.

Jenkins IH, Brooks DJ, Nixon PD, Frackowiak RS, Passingham RE (1994) Motor sequence learning: a study with positron emission tomography. *J Neurosci* 14: 3775–3790.

Jensen AR (1998) *The g Factor*. Westport: Praeger Publishers.

Jensen AR (2006) *Clocking the Mind: Mental Chronometry and Individual Differences*. Oxford: Elsevier.

Karabanov A, Ullén F (2008) Implicit and explicit learning of temporal sequences studied with the process dissociation procedure. *J Neurophysiol* (in press).

Karni A, Meyer G, Jezzard P, Adams MM, Turner R, Ungerleider LG (1995) Functional MRI evidence for adult motor cortex plasticity during motor skill learning. *Nature* 377: 155–158.

Keele SW, Ivry R, Mayr U, Hazeltine E, Heuer H (2003) The cognitive and neural architecture of sequence representation. *Psychol Rev* 110: 316–339.

Knopman DS, Nissen MJ (1987) Implicit learning in patients with probable Alzheimer's disease. *Neurology* 37: 784–788.

Lau HC, Rogers RD, Ramnani N, Passingham RE (2004) Willed action and attention to the selection of action. *Neuroimage* 21: 1407–1415.

Lee D (2000) Learning of spatial and temporal patterns in sequential hand movements. *Cogn Brain Res* 9: 35–39.

Lewis PA, Miall RC (2003) Distinct systems for automatic and cognitively controlled time measurement: evidence from neuroimaging. *Curr Opin Neurobiol* 13: 250–255.

Lewis PA, Wing AM, Pope PA, Praamstra P, Miall RC (2004) Brain activity correlates differentially with increasing temporal complexity of rhythms during initialisation, synchronisation, and continuation phases of paced finger tapping. *Neuropsychologia* 42: 1301–1312.

Lungu OV, Wachter T, Liu T, Willingham DT, Ashe J (2004) Probability detection mechanisms and motor learning. *Exp Brain Res* 159: 135–150.

Lutz K, Specht K, Shah NJ, Jäncke L (2000) Tapping movements according to regular and irregular visual timing signals investigated with fMRI. *NeuroReport* 11: 1301–1306.

Macar F, Lejeune H, Bonnet M, Ferrara A, Pouthas V, Vidal F, Maquet P (2002) Activation of the supplementary motor area and of attentional networks during temporal processing. *Exp Brain Res* 142: 475–485.

MacDonald AWr, Cohen JD, Stenger VA, Carter CS (2000) Dissociating the role of the dorsolateral prefrontal and anterior cingulate cortex in cognitive control. *Science* 288: 1835–1838.

Matsuzaka Y, Picard N, Strick PL (2007) Skill representation in the primary motor cortex after long-term practice. *J Neurophysiol* 97: 1819–1832.

Mayr U (1996) Spatial attention and implicit sequence learning: evidence for independent learning of spatial and nonspatial sequences. *J Exp Psychol Learn Mem Cogn* 22: 350–364.

Meulemans T, Van der Linden M, Perruchet P (1998) Implicit sequence learning in children. *J Exp Child Psychol* 69: 199–221.

Mushiaka H, Inase M, Tanji J (1991) Neuronal activity in the primate premotor, supplementary, and precentral motor cortex during visually guided and internally determined sequential movements. *J Neurophysiol* 66: 705–718.

Nissen MJ, Bullemer P (1987) Attentional requirements of learning: evidence from performance measures. *Cogn Psychol* 19: 1–32.

Nissen MJ, Knopman DS, Schacter DL (1987) Neurochemical dissociation of memory systems. *Neurology* 37: 789–794.

Pascual-Leone A, Grafman J, Clark K, Stewart M, Massaquoi S, Lou JS, Hallett M (1993) Procedural learning in Parkinson's disease and cerebellar degeneration. *Ann Neurol* 34: 594–602.

Pascual-Leone A, Grafman J, Hallett M (1994) Modulation of cortical motor output maps during development of implicit and explicit knowledge. *Science* 263: 1287–1289.

Peigneux P, Maquet P, Meulemans T, Destrebecqz A, Laureys S, Degueldre C, Delfiore G, Aerts J, Luxen A, Franck G, Van der Linden M, Cleeremans A (2000) Striatum forever, despite sequence learning variability: a random effect analysis of PET data. *Hum Brain Mapp* 10: 179–184.

Penhune VB, Doyon J (2002) Dynamic cortical and subcortical networks in learning and delayed recall of timed motor sequences. *J Neurosci* 22: 1397–1406.

Penhune VB, Doyon J (2005) Cerebellum and M1 interaction during early learning of timed motor sequences. *Neuroimage* 26: 801–812.

Penhune VB, Zatorre RJ, Evans AC (1998) Cerebellar contributions to motor timing: a PET study of auditory and visual rhythm reproduction. *J Cogn Neurosci* 10: 752–765.

Perruchet P, Amorim MA (1992) Conscious knowledge and changes in performance in sequence learning: evidence against dissociation. *J Exp Psychol Learn Mem Cogn* 18: 785–800.

Poldrack RA, Clark J, Pare-Blagoev EJ, Shohamy D, Creso Moyano J, Myers C, Gluck MA (2001) Interactive memory systems in the human brain. *Nature* 414: 546–550.

Ramnani N, Passingham RE (2001) Changes in the human brain during rhythm learning. *J Cogn Neurosci* 13: 952–966.

Rao S, Harrington D, Haaland K, Bobholz J, Cox R, Binder J (1997) Distributed neural systems underlying the timing of movements. *J Neurosci* 17: 5528–5535.

Rao SM, Mayer AR, Harrington DL (2001) The evolution of brain activation during temporal processing. *Nature Neurosci* 4: 317–323.

Rauch SL, Savage CR, Brown HD, Curran T, Alpert NM, Kendrick A, Fischman AJ, Kosslyn SM (1995) A PET investigation of implicit and explicit sequence learning. *Hum Brain Mapp* 3: 271–286.

Rauch SL, Whalen PJ, Savage CR, Curran T, Kendrick A, Brown HD, Bush G, Breiter HC, Rosen BR (1997) Striatal recruitment during an implicit sequence learning task as measured by functional magnetic resonance imaging. *Hum Brain Mapp* 5: 124–132.

Rhodes BJ, Bullock D, Verwey WB, Averbeck BB, Page MP (2004) Learning and production of movement sequences: behavioral, neurophysiological, and modeling perspectives. *Hum Mov Sci* 23: 699–746.

Sakai K, Hikosaka O, Miyauchi S, Takino R, Sasaki Y, Putz B (1998) Transition of brain activation from frontal to parietal areas in visuomotor sequence learning. *J Neurosci* 18: 1827–1840.

Sakai K, Hikosaka O, Miyauchi S, Ryousuke T, Tamada T, Iwata NK, Nielsen M (1999) Neural representation of a rhythm depends on its interval ratio. *J Neurosci* 19: 10074–10081.

Sakai K, Ramnani N, Passingham RE (2002) Learning of sequences of finger movements and timing: frontal lobe and action-oriented representation. *J Neurophysiol* 88: 2035–2046.

Salidis J (2001) Nonconscious temporal cognition: learning rhythms implicitly. *Mem Cognit* 29: 1111–1119.

Schendan HE, Searl MM, Melrose RJ, Stern CE (2003) An fMRI study of the role of the medial temporal lobe in implicit and explicit sequence learning. *Neuron* 37: 1013–1025.

Schubotz RI, von Cramon DY (2001) Interval and ordinal properties of sequences are associated with distinct premotor areas. *Cereb Cortex* 11: 210–222.

Seger CA (1997) Two forms of sequential implicit learning. *Consciousness Cognit* 6: 108–131.

Shanks DR, St John MF (1994) Characteristics of dissociable human learning systems. *Behav Brain Sci* 17: 367–395.

Shima K, Tanji J (1998) Both supplementary and presupplementary motor areas are crucial for the temporal organization of multiple movements. *J Neurophysiol* 80: 3247–3260.

Shima K, Tanji J (2000) Neuronal activity in the supplementary and presupplementary motor areas for temporal organization of multiple movements. *J Neurophysiol* 84: 2148–2160.

Shin JC, Ivry RB (2002) Concurrent learning of temporal and spatial sequences. *J Exp Psychol: Learn Mem Cogn* 28: 445–457.

Shin JC, Ivry RB (2003) Spatial and temporal sequence learning in patients with Parkinson's disease or cerebellar lesions. *J Cogn Neurosci* 18: 1232–1243.

Siegert RJ, Taylor KD, Weatherall M, Abernethy DA (2006) Is implicit sequence learning impaired in Parkinson's disease? A meta-analysis. *Neuropsychology* 20: 490–495.

Sloboda JA (1985) *The Musical Mind: The Cognitive Psychology of Music.* New York: Oxford University Press.

Spencer RM, Zelaznik HN, Diedrichsen J, Ivry RB (2003) Disrupted timing of discontinuous movements by cerebellar lesions. *Science* 300: 1437–1439.

Stadler MA (1993) Implicit serial learning: questions inspired by Hebb (1961). *Mem Cognit* 21: 819–827.

Stadler MA (1995) Role of attention in implicit learning. *J Exp Psychol: Learn Mem Cogn* 21: 674–685.

Stadler MA, Frensch PA, editors (1997) *Handbook of Implicit Learning.* New York: Sage.

Stadler MA, Roediger HL (1997) The question of awareness in research on implicit learning. In: Stadler MA, Frensch PA, editors. *Handbook of Implicit Learning.* New York: Sage, pp. 105–132.

Tanji J (2001) Sequential organization of multiple movements: involvement of cortical motor areas. *Annu Rev Neurosci* 24: 631–651.

Théoret H, Haque J, Pascual-Leone A (2001) Increased variability of paced finger tapping accuracy following repetitive magnetic stimulation of the cerebellum in humans. *Neurosci Lett* 306: 29–32.

Thomas KM, Nelson CA (2001) Serial reaction time learning in preschool- and school-age children. *J Exp Child Psychol* 79: 364–387.

Thomas KM, Hunt RH, Vizueta N, Sommer T, Durston S, Yang Y, Worden MS (2004) Evidence of developmental differences in implicit sequence learning: an fMRI study of children and adults. *J Cogn Neurosci* 16: 1339–1351.

Toni I, Krams M, Turner R, Passingham RE (1998) The time course of changes during motor sequence learning: a whole-brain fMRI study. *Neuroimage* 8: 50–61.

Turner ML, Engle RW (1989) Is working memory capacity task dependent? *J Mem Lang* 28: 127–154.

Ullén F, Bengtsson S (2003) Independent processing of the temporal and ordinal structure of movement sequences. *J Neurophysiol* 90: 3725–3735.

Ullén F, Forssberg H, Ehrsson HH (2003) Neural networks coordinating the hands in time. *J Neurophysiol* 89: 1126–1135.

Unsworth N, Engle RW (2005) Individual differences in working memory capacity and learning: evidence from the serial reaction time task. *Mem Cognit* 33: 213–220.

Vicari S, Finzi A, Menghini D, Marotta L, Baldi S, Petrosini L (2005) Do children with developmental dyslexia have an implicit learning deficit? *J Neurol Neurosurg Psychiatry* 76: 1392–1397.

Waber DP, Marcus DJ, Forbes PW, Bellinger DC, Weiler MD, Sorensen LG, Curran T (2003) Motor sequence learning and reading ability: is poor reading associated with sequencing deficits? *J Exp Child Psychol* 84: 338–354.

Wallin NL, Merker B, Brown S, editors (2000) *The Origins of Music.* Cambridge, MA: MIT Press.

Wilhelm O, Engle RW, editors (2005) *Handbook of Understanding and Measuring Intelligence.* Thousand Oaks, CA: Sage Publications.

Willingham DB, Nissen MJ, Bullemer P (1989) On the development of procedural knowledge. *J Exp Psychol Learn Mem Cogn* 15: 1047–1060.

Willingham DB, Greeley T, Bardone AM (1993) Dissociation in a serial respone time task using a recognition measure: comment on Perruchet and Amorim (1992). *J Exp Psychol Learn Mem Cogn* 19: 1424–1430.

Willingham DB, Salidis J, Gabrieli JDE (2002) Direct comparison of neural systems mediating conscious and unconscious skill learning. *J Neurophysiol* 88: 1451–1460.

Wilson PH, Maruff P, Lum J (2003) Procedural learning in children with developmental coordination disorder. *Hum Mov Sci* 22: 515–526.

4
NEUROLOGICAL CLASSIFICATION AND NEURORADIOLOGY OF CEREBRAL PALSY

Ingeborg Krägeloh-Mann and Martin Staudt

I Neurological classification of cerebral palsy

DEFINITION OF CEREBRAL PALSY AND CLASSIFICATION OF SUBTYPES
The term 'cerebral palsy' (CP) constitutes a useful socio-medical framework for certain motor disabled children with special needs. However, it does not describe a disease entity but comprises a group of disorders with different aetiologies (Mutch et al 1992). A European network of health professionals working in the domain of CP – the SCPE (Surveillance of CP in Europe) – agreed on a definition of CP according to the key elements of current definitions used (SCPE 2000):

- CP is a group of disorders;
- it involves a disorder of motor function, movement and posture;
- it is permanent but not unchanging;
- it is due to a non-progressive lesion or abnormality in the developing/immature brain.

The motor disorder of cerebral palsy is often accompanied by other developmental disorders of performance or behaviour (Rosenbaum et al 2007). Progressive conditions resulting in loss of acquired skills, spinal diseases, and cases where hypotonia is the sole neurological finding are excluded.

This definition is based on clinical phenomenology and clinical history. Additional features such as imaging or laboratory results are not primary inclusion criteria. They are important, however, to further describe CP subgroups with respect to aetiology or pathogenesis.

Overall, the CP rate is between 2 and 2.5 per 1000 live births, indicating that CP is the commonest cause of physical disability in early childhood (SCPE 2002). It is especially prevalent in preterm born children – infants of very low birthweight (VLBW, birthweight < 1500 g) are between 40 and 100 times more likely to have CP than normal birthweight infants.

CP is usually classified into neurologically defined subtypes, e.g. spastic, dyskinetic and ataxic (Hagberg and Hagberg 1993) (Table 4.1, Fig. 4.1).

TABLE 4.1
Neurological classification of CP subtypes (according to Cans et al 2007)

Spastic CP is characterized by:

- increased tone
- pathological reflexes, e.g. increased reflexes or hyperreflexia
- pyramidal signs, e.g. Babinski response
- abnormal pattern of movement and posture

It is subdivided into:

- **unilateral spastic CP** or **US-CP** (formerly hemiplegia or hemiparesis)
- **bilateral spastic CP** or **BS-CP** (diplegia and tetra- or quadriplegia pooled together)

Dyskinetic CP is characterized by:

- involuntary, uncontrolled, recurring, occasionally stereotyped movements
- primitive reflex patterns
- varying muscle tone

It may be subdivided into:

- **dystonic CP** dominated by abnormal posturing, which may give the impression of hypokinesia; easily elicitable tone increase; involuntary movements or distorted voluntary movements, and abnormal postures due to sustained muscle contractions leading to slow rotation, extension or flexion of body parts.
- **choreoathetotic CP** dominated by hyperkinesias; tone is fluctuating but mainly decreased; *chorea* means rapid, involuntary, jerky, often fragmented movements, *athetosis* means slow, constantly changing, writhing or contorting movements.

Ataxic CP is characterized by:

- loss of orderly muscular coordination, so that movements are performed with abnormal force, rhythm and accuracy
- trunk and gait ataxia, which leads to disturbed balance
- past pointing, i.e. over- or undershooting of goal-directed movements
- tremor, mainly a slow intention tremor
- low tone

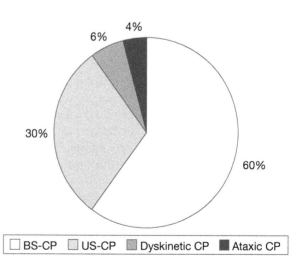

Fig. 4.1 Distribution of CP subtypes

□ BS-CP   □ US-CP   ▨ Dyskinetic CP   ■ Ataxic CP

Spastic CP

Spastic forms are the most predominant by far in CP. They account for around 90 per cent of cases; 1/3 are characterized by unilateral, and 2/3 by bilateral involvement (SCPE 2002). The neurological signs in spastic CP are as follows (Cans et al 2007): increased tone characterized by increased resistance to passive movement which is velocity-dependent (Sanger et al 2003); pathological reflexes, e.g. increased reflexes or hyperreflexia and pyramidal signs, e.g. Babinski response; abnormal pattern of movement and posture, in the lower limbs characterized by equinus foot, crouch gait, hip internal rotation and adduction, in the upper limbs by arms in flexion, hands fisted with thumb adducted or stiff and poorly directed movements of fingers. The severe forms especially often have some dystonic features, which affect hands, face and even trunk, so that the delineation towards dystonic CP is not always clear-cut.

Bilateral spastic CP (BS-CP) is especially prevalent in preterm born children. The overall prevalence is 1.2 per 1000 live births – around 0.5 per 1000 in children with normal birthweight, 10 per 1000 in children with moderately reduced birthweight, and around 40–100 per 1000 live births in very low birthweight children (Krägeloh-Mann et al 1993, Platt et al 2007).

Motor deficit is present in more than 2/3 of children with BS-CP (equivalent to GMFCS III and higher, see below) (Krägeloh-Mann et al 1993, Gorter et al 2004, Himmelmann et al 2007). In around two-thirds hand function is better than leg function. Secondary motor problems with contractures – in equinus position, hip adduction, knee flexion – are frequent, especially in children who do not learn to walk.

Cognitive problems in the sense of learning disability* are encountered especially in children with severe forms of BS-CP (e.g. 20 per cent with learning disability and 70 per cent with severe learning disability (IQ < 70) in the series using functional scores; Krägeloh-Mann et al 1993), whereas in children with milder forms (having leg-dominated motor problems, e.g. 'diplegia', which is mainly associated with GMFCS scores I–III; Gorter et al 2004, Himmelmann et al 2007) around 40 per cent have normal intelligence, 20 per cent have learning disability and 40 per cent have severe learning disability.

Severe cerebral visual problems are encountered especially in children with severe forms of BS-CP, around half of whom are blind or nearly blind; such problems are found in less than 10 per cent of children with milder forms. *Hearing problems* (deaf or nearly deaf) are, however, not frequent, occurring in around 3 per cent (Krägeloh-Mann et al 1993).

Epilepsy is encountered in around half of children with BS-CP; West syndrome in about 10 per cent. Epilepsy is mainly symptomatic; it is related to severity of functional disability and extent and topography of causative lesions – 85 per cent of children with BS-CP who have epilepsy have severe motor disability, 90 per cent have learning disability, and in cases with West syndrome, learning disability is encountered in 100 per cent.

Unilateral spastic CP (US-CP) is reported in the European survey with a prevalence of about 0.6 per 1000 live births (SCPE 2000). It is the typical CP form of the term born child; about 1/3 of cases are preterm born (Himmelmann et al 2005).

---

* North American usage: mental retardation.

Motor deficit in children with US-CP is rarely severe; less than 2 per cent in the population-based series of Uvebrant (1988) could not walk at the age of 5 years; more than half could walk without much restriction, and 30 per cent had a moderate, and 10 per cent a severe limp. In around half of the children hand function was described as quite good with single finger movements possible; only 20 per cent did not have more than holding function. Sensory problems were reported in around 20 per cent – they add to the functional deficit and should be looked for carefully, for example by discrimination tests such as two-point discrimination; younger children can be asked to recognize objects when placed in the normal or the paretic hand. Secondary motor problems with contractures are mainly seen in the paretic foot with equinus position; hip subluxation is not a frequent problem. Hypotrophy of the affected limbs is often seen, but correction of leg length is seldom necessary.

Cognitive problems in the sense of learning difficulties are less often found in children with US-CP than in those with other CP forms. Uvebrant (1988) found mild learning disability in 12 per cent of preterm born children with US-CP; of the term born children in his series 6 per cent had severe learning disability and 13 per cent had mild learning disability. This means that around 85–90 per cent of children wit US-CP do not have cognitive problems in the sense of learning disability.

Severe cerebral visual problems are rare in children with US-CP; they are reported mainly in term born children, occurring in around 5 per cent. Hemianopsia is probably often overlooked as it is well compensated for by the children and only recognized when specifically looked for, though neuroimaging may give a hint.

There is no gross difference in language with hemisphere affected (Carlsson et al 1994, Staudt et al 2003), although children with left hemispheric lesions are reported to be slower in language development (Chilosi et al 2001), which indicates that reorganization of language to the right 'takes some time' but can take place. This happens at the expense, however, of originally right hemispheric functions – visuo-spatial functions can be shown to be mildly deficient, which seems to be related to the degree of right hemispheric language reorganization and not to the overall lesion size (Lidzba et al 2006).

Epilepsy is found in around a third of children with US-CP; 25 per cent of them have severe epilepsy, e.g. drug-resistant (Krägeloh-Mann et al 1993). Epilepsy is mainly symptomatic and more often encountered in US-CP due to cortical malformations or cortical lesions.

Dyskinetic CP

Dyskinetic CP is reported with a prevalence of 0.13 per 1000 live births in the European series (SCPE 2002), which means that 6 per cent of all CP cases have this specific subtype. It occurs especially in term born children (Hagberg and Hagberg 1993, Himmelmann et al 2005). Dyskinetic CP is characterized by involuntary, uncontrolled, recurring, occasionally stereotyped movements; primitive reflex patterns predominate; muscle tone is varying (Cans et al 2007). The European CP network recommends discriminating, if possible, between dystonic and choreoathetotic CP. Dystonic CP is dominated by abnormal posturing and may give the impression of hypokinesia; fluctuating tone is characterized by easily elicitable tone increase; involuntary movements or distorted voluntary movements are typical, and abnormal postures are due to sustained muscle contractions leading to slow rotation, extension or flexion of body parts. Choreoathetotic CP is dominated by hyperkinesias and tone is fluctuating but mainly decreased; *chorea* means rapid involuntary, jerky, often fragmented movements, and *athetosis* means slow, constantly changing, writhing or contorting movements. Pure dyskinetic movement disorders do not show hyperreflexia with clonus or pyramidal signs. But in dyskinetic CP, these spastic signs may be present. Severe BS-CP is very often characterized by additional dyskinetic and more specifically dystonic features. The dominating features should determine the subtype classification. In terms of its clinical functional problems dystonic CP is very close to severe BS-CP, as described above. Children with choreoathetotic CP may be less severely affected and may learn to walk without aids. Children with dyskinetic CP in general are characterized by global movement disorders that also involve facial expression, and have great problems in expressing themselves. They are therefore often misjudged with respect to their cognitive capabilities.

Ataxic CP
Ataxic CP occurs with a prevalence of 0.09 per 1000 live births, i.e. in around 4 per cent of all CP cases (SCPE 2002), mainly in term born children (Hagberg and Hagberg 1993). It is often described as non-progressive cerebellar ataxia. The European network defines ataxic CP as characterized by loss of orderly muscular coordination, so that movements are performed with abnormal force, rhythm and accuracy; typical features are trunk and gait ataxia, which leads to disturbed balance. In the upper limbs a typical feature is past pointing, i.e. over- or undershooting of goal-directed movements; tremor is another common sign, mainly a slow intention tremor. Low tone is also a common feature. Ataxic CP is a heterogeneous condition. Clinical and neuroimaging findings have been systematically reviewed in two studies (Steinlin et al 1993, Esscher et al 1996). Motor development was described as clearly delayed and 10 per cent did not learn to walk independently. Cognitive function was in the domain of learning disability in 2/3, and half of these had severe learning disability; visual problems were described in > 50 per cent, and 20–30 per cent developed epilepsy.

From a clinical viewpoint, the symptoms and signs of CP are not unchanging. The typical neurological signs take time to develop, and it is generally agreed that the child should be at least 3 years of age before the CP diagnosis is established; CP registers accept children definitely only at the age of 5 (SCPE 2000, Stanley et al 2000).

The concept of CP is to some extent artificial, not only because the causes, mechanisms and consequences of the underlying brain pathology are multiple, but also because the age limit of brain immaturity is difficult to define. Usually, there is a distinction between CP of postneonatal onset and CP due to pre-, peri- and neonatal events. Postneonatal CP should be considered separately as causes are usually clearly defined.

FUNCTIONAL SEVERITY IN CEREBRAL PALSY
There is a wide variety of subdivisions within spastic CP:

- hemiplegia, hemiparesis, describing unilateral involvement, with the addition of 'arm- or leg-dominated' to describe topographical involvement;

- diplegia, diparesis, tetraplegia or -paresis or quadriplegia, describing bilateral involvement, the first two terms meaning that legs are more involved than arms, the latter that arms are as much or more involved than legs.

Usually, mild, moderate or severe are gradings which are added to describe functional severity. However, attribution of cases to diplegia versus tetraplegia in different centres may vary by as much as 20 vs 80 to 80 vs 20 (Colver and Sethumadhavan 2003). The SCPE, therefore, recommended using the terms uni- or bilateral spastic CP and describing functional severity in legs and arms according to standardized scores (SCPE 2002, Cans et al 2007) for gross motor function, such as the gross motor function classification system (GMFCS; Palisano et al 1997), and fine motor function (see below), an approach which was internationally accepted (Rosenbaum et al 2007). The combination of functional scores for arms and legs is supposed to give a more reliable assessment of the clinical picture. Higher scores in the legs can indicate what used to be called diplegia or leg-dominated BS-CP (Krägeloh-Mann et al 1993).

The GMFCS, formally assessed with the gross motor function measure (GMFM), has been shown to be very helpful in prognostication about gross motor progress in children with CP (Rosenbaum et al 2002). Motor development curves at each level of the GMFCS predict average development, as illustrated in Fig. 4.2. The main spurt in development is clearly in early childhood up to preschool age. Stability of the GMFCS over time proved to be rather high (73 per cent for all ratings); this was especially true for children initially classified as level I or V and for children older than 6 years (Palisano et al 2006).

UPPER EXTREMITY INVOLVEMENT IN CP
The neurological signs outlined above (under the neurologically defined subtypes of CP) apply in part to upper limb involvement. The following features describe in more detail upper limb involvement in spastic CP. The affected arm is often flexed and hypokinetic during gross motor movements; the spastic hand may show abnormal posturing with features of dystonia (the wrist in ulnar deviation and fingers overextended at the metacarpophalangeal joints) or with tendency to fist clenching at rest. When in use, involvement of the hand is characterized by stiffer, less well directed movements, often with the described dystonic features.

A functional system has been published for upper extremity involvement, called the bimanual fine motor function system (BFMF), which classifies the impairment in each hand separately (Beckung and Hagberg 2002). Another classification system is the manual ability classification system (MACS; Eliasson et al 2006), focusing on children's ability to use their hands in daily activities. MACS has been shown to have good inter-rater reliability between professionals, and also between parents and professionals (see Chapter 12).

66

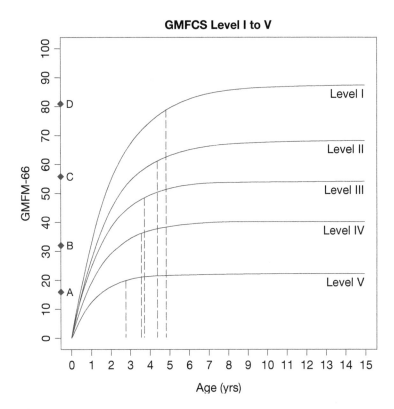

Fig. 4.2 Growth curves.

Source: Rosenbaum et al 2002, with permission from JAMA.

II Neuroradiology of cerebral palsy and upper extremity dysfunction

NEURORADIOLOGICAL FINDINGS IN CHILDREN WITH CEREBRAL PALSY

In the majority of children with cerebral palsy, the underlying brain pathology can be identified by neuroradiological methods. In this respect, magnetic resonance imaging (MRI) is clearly superior to computed tomography (CT) and ultrasound (US).

The multitude of brain pathologies underlying CP can be separated into two major subgroups: (1) malformations, and (2) defective lesions (i.e. lesions characterized by tissue loss and/or gliosis). This subdivision reflects not only differences in the morphology of the brain abnormality, but also different timing periods of their origin (Krägeloh-Mann 2004; Fig. 4.3).

Malformations of the brain can be further subdivided with respect to the developmental phase during which they originate. This subdivision results in a classification of brain malformations into disorders (a) of neuronal proliferation (and/or apoptosis), (b) of neuronal migration, and (c) of cortical organization (Barkovich et al 2001; Fig. 4.3).

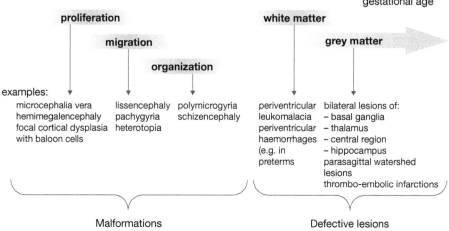

0   24   40 weeks

gestational age

proliferation   **white matter**

migration   **grey matter**

organization

examples:

microcephalia vera	lissencephaly	polymicrogyria
hemimegalencephaly	pachygyria	schizencephaly
focal cortical dysplasia	heterotopia	
with baloon cells		

periventricular leukomalacia / periventricular haemorrhages (e.g. in preterms)

bilateral lesions of:
– basal ganglia
– thalamus
– central region
– hippocampus
parasagittal watershed lesions
thrombo-embolic infarctions

Malformations   Defective lesions

Fig. 4.3 Classification and timing of pre-, peri- or neonatally acquired brain lesions.

Defective lesions can also be further subdivided into (a) those affecting predominantly the periventricular white matter, and (b) those affecting cortical and subcortical grey matter structures. Again, this subdivision reflects different timing periods of the brain injury resulting in the structural defect (Krägeloh-Mann 2004; Fig. 4.3).

A systematic review of studies on MRI in children with CP shows abnormal findings in around 85 per cent, which gave clues to pathogenesis; in only 15 per cent were normal or unspecific findings reported (Krägeloh-Mann and Horber 2007). Periventricular white matter lesions, e.g. periventricular leucomalacia (PVL) or defects following intraventricular haemorrhage, were most frequent (56 per cent), followed by cortical and deep grey matter lesions (18 per cent); brain maldevelopments were comparatively rare, described in only 9 per cent. Brain maldevelopments and grey matter lesions were more often seen in term than in preterm born children with CP (16 vs 2.5 per cent and 33 vs 3.5 per cent), whereas periventricular white matter lesions occurred significantly more often in preterm than in term born children (90 vs 20 per cent).

The topography determines whether a lesion or maldevelopment causes US-CP or BS-CP, i.e. whether the motor system – motor cortex or pyramidal tract – is involved on one side only or on both sides (Fig. 4.4). Topography and extent explain the severity of the clinical picture. BS-CP due to PVL, for example, can be mild (GMFCS I or II), without further developmental problems, or severe (GMFCS V), accompanied by severe learning disability and severe cerebral visual impairment; in the first case PVL constitutes only mild bilateral periventricular gliosis, but in the second severe bilateral and diffuse tissue loss in addition to gliosis explains the more severe motor problems as well as the mental and visual involvement (Fig. 4.4, middle, right). Dyskinetic CP is often caused by bilateral thalamus and basal ganglia lesions; a structure–function relationship is reported here also (Krägeloh-

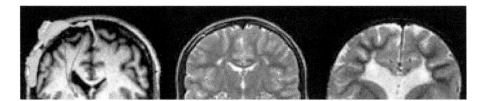

Fig. 4.4 Periventricular lesions of different topography and extent cause US-CP (left, coronal T1w image shows a unilateral posthaemorrhagic periventricular lesion), BS-CP of mild degree (middle, T2w coronal image with mild PVL, e.g. bilateral periventricular circumscribed gliosis), or BS-CP of severe degree (right, T2w coronal image with severe PVL, e.g. bilateral gliosis and extensive tissue loss), as the pyramidal tract (scheme) is affected only on one side or on both sides, here with different severity.

Mann et al 2002). Ataxic CP is different: abnormal MRI findings occur in less than 40 per cent, and in at least half of the cases are not clearly lesional in the sense discussed above; a structure–function relationship is not reported (Steinlin et al 1993).

Guidelines for the diagnosis of CP, therefore, suggest neuroimaging, especially magnetic resonance imaging, as the first diagnostic procedure (after history taking, neurological investigation and investigation for other potential disabilities) (Ashwal et al 2004).

NEURORADIOLOGICAL CORRELATES OF UPPER EXTREMITY INVOLVEMENT IN CP
Dysfunction of the upper extremity in CP results from pathological changes in the neural structures involved in its sensorimotor control (including the motor system, see Chapter 2). In the following, the identification of these structures, and of their somatotopical organization, will be described.

The primary motor cortex (M1) is located in the precentral gyrus and the central sulcus. It is organized in a somatotopic manner, with neurons projecting to the lower extremity located near the interhemispheric fissure, those projecting to the face near the Sylvian fissure, and those projecting to the upper extremity in between. Due to the dense innervation of hand muscles, the precentral gyrus shows a focal thickening at the cortical hand representation. This area has a characteristic appearance, and is therefore called the 'hand knob' area.

On axial MR images, this region can be identified using the characteristic 'omega-' or 'epsilon-sign' of the central sulcus (see Fig. 4.5). On sagittal MR images, the 'hand knob' of the precentral gyrus forms a typical 'hook sign', with the tip of the hook pointing backwards into the central sulcus. More detailed instructions on identification of the central sulcus and its 'hand knob' can be found in Yousry et al (1997).

The primary somatosensory cortex (S1) is the first cortical area to receive somatosensory input from the periphery via the dorsal columns of the spinal cord, the medial lemniscus and the thalamus. It is located in the postcentral gyrus, and shows a somatotopic organization similar to M1. Thus, the primary somatosensory representation of the upper extremity can be identified on MRI using the same methods as described for M1.

In the internal capsule, the cortico-spinal projections from M1 pass through the genu and the posterior limb also in a somatotopical organization, with projections to the face in

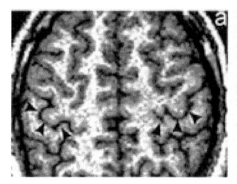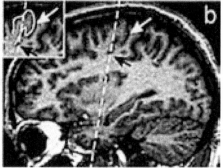

Fig. 4.5 On axial MR images (a) the primary motor representation of the hand can easily be identified by its characteristic knob-like appearance, with the central sulcus showing the configuration of an inverted 'epsilon' or 'omega' (black arrowheads). On sagittal images (b) this 'hand knob' typically has the shape of a hook (see insert), with its tip pointing backwards and downwards into the central sulcus (white arrow).

Source: Adapted from Staudt et al 2000, with permission from Georg Thieme Verlag.

the genu, projections to the upper extremity in the anterior third, and projections to the lower extremity in the middle third of the posterior limb.

After identification of these structures which are critically involved in the sensorimotor control of the hand, the 'upper extremity relevance' of tissue damage can be estimated on structural MRI. With this approach, the severity of structural damage to cortico-spinal pathways could be correlated with motor dysfunction of upper and lower extremities in patients with unilateral and bilateral periventricular lesions (Staudt et al 2000, 2003).

(RE-)ORGANIZATION OF HAND FUNCTIONS AFTER EARLY BRAIN LESIONS
Children with early brain lesions often show surprisingly well-preserved hand functions despite extensive brain lesions, especially in the case of unilateral lesions. This can be explained by the superior reorganizational potential of the developing brain to compensate for such early lesions – the Kennard principle (Kennard 1936). One of the best-known examples of this reorganizational potential is children with congenital hemiparesis in whom hemispherectomies for the control of pharmaco-refractory seizures did not cause any deterioration in hand function. Thus, in these children, the initial lesion (causing the hemiparesis) had apparently induced a take-over of hand motor functions by the contra-lesional hemisphere (Gardner et al 1955). In the recent past, several neurophysiological techniques (e.g. transcranial magnetic stimulation) and neuroimaging methods (e.g. functional magnetic resonance imaging) have been developed which allow a non-invasive assessment of these processes *in vivo*.

METHODS FOR ASSESSING SENSORIMOTOR (RE-)ORGANIZATION
Transcranial magnetic stimulation (TMS) uses short magnetic pulses to induce electric currents in brain tissue. Thus, when TMS is applied over the primary motor cortex (M1), a

volley of action potentials is generated which travels down the cortico-spinal tract, reaches alpha-motoneurons in the spinal cord, and finally elicits a peripheral muscular response. This response can be recorded by surface EMG electrodes attached over the respective target muscle – the so-called motor evoked potential (MEP). MEPs with a short latency (around 20 ms or less) can be regarded as evidence for the presence of direct, monosynaptic, fast-conducting cortico-spinal pathways from the stimulated area (Benecke et al 1991). Thus, when focal coils are used, TMS allows topographic identification of the primary motor representation of a target muscle on the skull surface, as well as assessment of the integrity of cortico-spinal pathways in the case of brain lesions. The spatial accuracy of this technique can be enhanced by the application of neuronavigational systems.

Functional magnetic resonance imaging (fMRI; Fig. 4.6) is a new MR technique which uses local changes of blood oxygenation to visualize brain regions showing activation during certain tasks. For the assessment of upper extremity functions, many different sensory and sensorimotor tasks have been introduced, ranging from simple opening/closing of a hand to complex manipulative tasks. In healthy individuals, all these tasks activate the primary sensorimotor cortex (M1S1) in the contralateral Rolandic cortex (pre- and postcentral gyrus). In addition, especially in the more complex tasks, activation is frequently observed in 'non-primary' sensorimotor areas, such as the supplementary motor area (SMA), the ipsilateral Rolandic cortex, or the cerebellum. In comparison with TMS, fMRI yields superior spatial information (in three dimensions), but cannot differentiate between regions with and without cortico-spinal output.

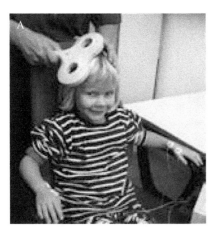 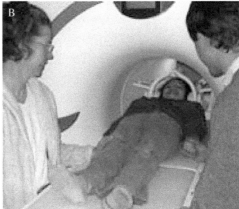

Fig. 4.6 (A) Experimental set-up for the TMS assessment of cortico-spinal projections. A focal 'figure-of-eight' coil is positioned over the motor cortex of the patient. Motor-evoked potentials (MEPs) are recorded bilaterally via surface electromyography from target muscles (here: M. interosseus dorsalis I). (B) Experimental set-up for the fMRI assessment of activation during simple hand movements. Especially in younger children or anxious subjects, repetitive squeezing of the examiner's hand can be a useful approach, because it allows immediate feedback of task performance, and reassures the child by providing hand-to-hand contact.

Source: Staudt et al 2001.

71

TMS in Congenital Hemiparesis

In many patients with congenital hemiparesis, TMS of the contra-lesional hemisphere elicits MEPs not only in the (contralateral) non-paretic hand, but also in the (ipsilateral) paretic hand (Carr et al 1993). Since these MEPs typically show similar latencies, this finding demonstrates that the contra-lesional hemisphere possesses fast-conducting ipsilateral cortico-spinal projections to the paretic hand in these patients. Such ipsilateral pathways have, to date, never been reported for patients with lesions acquired beyond the age of 2 years (Maegaki et al 1995); therefore, they seem to be specific for reorganization after early brain lesions. This phenomenon can be explained by embryological data. Initially, each motor cortex develops bilateral cortico-spinal projections, i.e. projections to both sides of the spinal cord. These bilateral projections apparently compete for their spinal target cells (the alpha-motoneurons), and the ipsilateral projections are gradually withdrawn. In the case of a unilateral brain lesion acquired before or during this phase of brain development, both the ipsilateral and the contralateral projections from the affected hemisphere will be damaged or destroyed, so that in the competition for spinal alpha-motoneurons on the contra-lesional ('paretic') side, the (intact) ipsilateral projections from the contra-lesional hemisphere will be stronger than the (damaged) contralateral projections from the affected hemisphere (Eyre et al 2000, 2001).

These contralateral projections will not be totally withdrawn in all cases, however, so that three types of cortico-spinal (re-)organization in patients with early unilateral brain lesions emerge (Fig. 4.7):

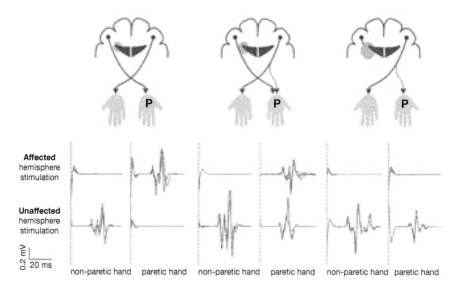

Fig. 4.7 Schematic illustration of the three types of cortico-spinal (re-)organization in patients with early unilateral brain lesions (P = paretic hand; grey circle = lesion), and TMS results from one representative patient from each type (vertical dashed line = time of the TMS stimulus).

Source: Adapted from Staudt et al 2002, with permission from Oxford University Press.

1. Patients with preserved contralateral and no ipsilateral projections
2. Patients with both contralateral and ipsilateral projections
3. Patients without contralateral, but with ipsilateral projections

These types of cortico-spinal (re-)organization show a clear correlation with the severity of structural damage to cortico-spinal pathways, at least in patients with congenital hemiparesis due to unilateral periventricular lesions (Staudt et al 2002).

The quality of hand function achieved by such ipsilateral projections correlates with the developmental stage of the brain during which the insult occurred: in patients with malformations (first and second trimester lesions) and periventricular lesions (early third trimester lesions), this reorganization with ipsilateral projections typically mediates a preserved active grasp function or even some individual finger movements; whereas many patients with cortico-subcortical infarctions (late third trimester lesions) are unable to perform any voluntary movements with their paretic hand despite the presence of ipsilateral projections (Staudt et al 2004a).

Concerning the origin of these ipsilateral projections, the stimulation site for the elicitation of ipsilateral responses is typically identical (< 1 cm distance) to the site for the elicitation of the normal contralateral response in the non-paretic hand (Staudt et al 2002, Vandermeeren et al 2002).

FMRI OF HAND MOVEMENTS IN CONGENITAL HEMIPARESIS

In patients with only *contralateral* cortico-spinal projections (Fig. 4.8, left), active movements of the paretic hand elicit activation in the contralateral Rolandic area, including the (unchanged) primary motor representation of their paretic hand. This activation is typically located in the 'hand knob' area of the Rolandic cortex; thus, no intrahemispheric (re-) organization of the hand motor representation (i.e. a shift of activation to other parts of the affected hemisphere) had occurred, even in patients with quite extensive lesions (Staudt et al 2002, 2004a). Many patients from this subgroup show additional activation in 'non-primary' motor areas, especially in the contra-lesional hemisphere (Fig. 4.8). In patients with periventricular lesions, this co-activation has been demonstrated to be stronger than the co-activation of non-primary motor areas observed in healthy controls (Staudt et al 2002). This additional recruitment of non-primary motor areas is similar to activation patterns reported for good recovery from adult hemiparetic stroke (Weiller et al 1992, 1993).

In patients with only *ipsilateral* cortico-spinal projections (Fig. 4.8, right), active movements of the paretic hand elicit activation in the contra-lesional hemisphere, corresponding to the (reorganized) primary motor representation of their paretic hand. This ipsilateral activation is, again, typically located in the 'hand knob' area of the Rolandic area; thus, in such patients, both hands apparently share a concordant primary motor representation in the contra-lesional hemisphere (Staudt et al 2001). In some patients from this subgroup, this ipsilateral Rolandic activation is the only activation observed (Fig. 4.9).

In the majority of patients, however, additional activation is observed in the Rolandic cortex of the contra-lesional hemisphere – although TMS had detected no cortico-spinal motor tracts originating from these areas (Staudt et al 2002, Vandermeeren et al 2002). A

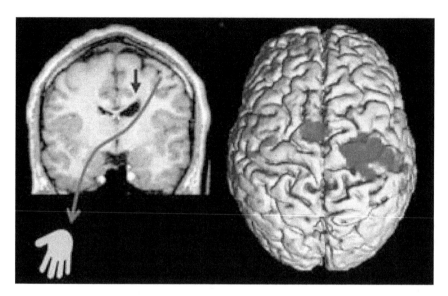

Fig. 4.8 Example of a patient with a unilateral periventricular brain lesion (black arrow) and preserved contralateral cortico-spinal projections from the affected hemisphere to the paretic hand (arrows). fMRI during active movements of the paretic hand reveals activation in the (unchanged) primary sensorimotor cortex (M1S1) of the affected hemisphere and additional activation in a network of 'non-primary' sensorimotor regions, especially in the contra-lesional hemisphere.

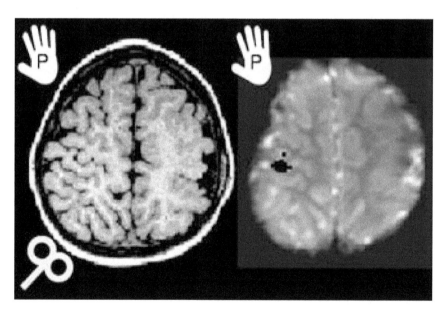

Fig. 4.9 Example of a patient with a unilateral complex malformation and ipsilateral projections from the contra-lesional hemisphere to the paretic hand (right). During active movements with the paretic hand (P), only the ipsilateral 'hand knob' area shows activation (black).

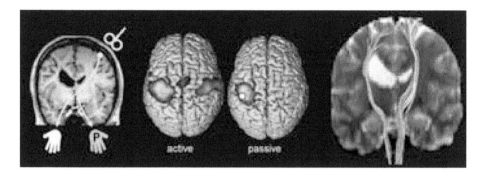

Fig. 4.10 Example of a patient with a unilateral periventricular brain lesion and ipsilateral cortico-spinal projections from the contra-lesional hemisphere to the paretic hand (left). fMRI during active movements of the paretic hand (P) reveals bilateral activation of the Rolandic (pericentral) cortices; during passive movement of the paretic hand, only the contralateral Rolandic area in the affected hemisphere is activated, indicating a contralaterally preserved primary somatosensory (S1) representation of the paretic hand in the affected hemsphere. Accordingly, the white dot represents the topography of the magnetoencephalographically determined S1-representation of the paretic hand. Finally, diffusion tensor tractography (right) visualizes trajectories of somatosensory afferent fibres which bypass the lesion on their way to the Rolandic cortex of the affected hemisphere.

Source: Adapted from Staudt et al 2006, with permission from Lippincott Williams & Wilkins.

similar contralateral activation can be elicited by *passive* movements of the paretic hand, suggesting that the somatosensory representation of the paretic hand is still located in the affected hemisphere. Thus, such patients show a 'hemispheric dissociation' between a (contralaterally preserved) motor and an (ipsilaterally reorganized) somatosensory representation of the paretic hand (Fig. 4.10; Thickbroom et al 2001, Staudt et al 2006).

Finally, in the few patients reported to date with *both contralateral and ipsilateral* cortico-spinal projections, fMRI during active hand movements typically elicited only contralateral activation, again located in the Rolandic area. This suggests that, in patients with this type of cortico-spinal reorganization, the preserved contralateral pathways are predominantly used; however, further studies will be needed to clarify this point.

REFERENCES

Ashwal S, Russman BS, Blasco PA, Miller G, Sandler A, Shevell M, Stevenson R (2004) Practice Parameter: Diagnostic assessment of the child with cerebral palsy. *Neurology* 62: 851–863.

Barkovich AJ, Kuzniecky RI, Jackson GD, Guerrini R, Dobyns WB (2001) Classification system for malformations of cortical development. *Neurology* 57: 2168–2178.

Beckung E, Hagberg G (2002) Neuroimpairments, activity limitations, and participation restrictions in children with cerebral palsy. *Dev Med Child Neurol* 44: 309–316.

Benecke R, Meyer BU, Freund HJ (1991) Reorganisation of descending motor pathways in patients after hemispherectomy and severe hemispheric lesions demonstrated by magnetic brain stimulation. *Exp Brain Res* 83: 419–426.

Cans C, Dolk H, Platt MJ, Colver A, Prasauskiene A, Krägeloh-Mann I (2007) Recommendations from the SCPE collaborative group for defining and classifying cerebral palsy. *Dev Med Child Neurol* Suppl 109, 49: 35–38.

Carlsson G, Uvebrant P, Hugdahi K, et al (1994) Verbal and non-verbal function of children with right- versus left-hemiplegic cerebral palsy of pre- or perinatal origin. *Dev Med Child Neurol* 36: 503–512.

Carr LJ, Harrison LM, Evans AL, Stephens JA (1993) Patterns of central motor reorganization in hemiplegic cerebral palsy. *Brain* 116: 1223–1247.

Chilosi AM, Cipriani P, Bertuccelli B, Pfanner L, Cioni G (2001) Early cognitive and communication development in children with focal brain lesions. *J Child Neurol* 16: 309–316.

Colver A, Sethumadhavan T (2003) The term diplegia should be abandoned. *Arch Dis Child* 88: 286–290.

Eliasson AC, Rösblad B, Krumlinde-Sundholm L, Beckung E, Arner M, Rosenbaum P (2006) Manual Ability Classification System (MACS), for Children with Cerebral Palsy – a field version. *Dev Med Child Neurol* 48: 549–554.

Esscher F, Flodmark O, Hagberg B (1996) Non-progressive ataxia: origins, brain pathology, and impairments in 78 Swedish children. *Dev Med Child Neurol* 38: 285–286.

Evrard P (2001) Pathophysiology of developmental brain damage. *Dev Neurosci* 23: 171–174.

Eyre JA, Miller S, Clowry GJ, Conway EA, Watts C (2000) Functional corticospinal projections are established prenatally in the human foetus permitting involvement in the development of spinal motor centres. *Brain* 123: 51–64.

Eyre JA, Taylor JP, Villagra F, Smith M, Miller S (2001) Evidence of activity-dependent withdrawal of corticospinal projections during human development. *Neurology* 57: 1543–1554.

Farmer SF, Harrison LM, Ingram DA, Stephens JA (1991) Plasticity of central motor pathways in children with hemiplegic cerebral palsy. *Neurology* 41: 1505–1510.

Gardner WJ, Karnosh LJ, McClure JR, Gardner AK (1955) Residual function following hemispherectomy for tumour and for infantile hemiplegia. *Brain* 78: 487–502.

Gorter JW, Rosenbaum PL, Hanna SE, Palisano RJ, Bartlett DJ, Russell DJ, Walter SD, Raina P, Galuppi BE, Wood E (2004) Limb distribution, motor impairment, and functional classification of cerebral palsy. *Dev Med Child Neurol* 46: 461–467.

Hagberg B, Hagberg G (1993) The origins of cerebral palsy. In: David TJ, editor. *Recent Advances in Paediatrics*, No. 11. Edinburgh: Churchill Livingstone, pp. 67–83.

Himmelmann K, Hagberg G, Beckung E, Hagberg B, Uvebrant P (2005) The changing panorama of cerebral palsy in Sweden IX. Prevalence and origin in the birth-year period 1995–1998. *Acta Paediatr* 94: 287–294.

Himmelmann K, Beckung E, Hagberg G, Uvebrant P (2007) Bilateral spastic cerebral palsy – prevalence through four decades, motor function and growth. *Eur J Paediatr Neurol* 11: 215–222.

Holthausen H, Strobl K (1999) Modes of reorganization of the sensorimotor system in children with infantile hemiplegia and after hemispherectomy. *Adv Neurol* 81: 201–220.

Kennard MA (1936) Age and other factors in motor recovery from precentral lesions in monkeys. *Am J Physiol* 115: 137–146.

Krägeloh-Mann I (2004). Imaging of early brain injury and cortical plasticity. *Exp Neurol* 190: S84–S90.

Krägeloh-Mann I, Horber V (2007) The role of magnetic resonance imaging in elucidating the pathogenesis of cerebral palsy: a systematic review. *Dev Med Child Neurol* 49: 144–151.

Krägeloh-Mann I, Hagberg G, Meisner C, Schelp B, Haas G, Edebol Eeg-Olofsson K, Selbmann K, Hagberg B, Michaelis R (1993) Bilateral spastic cerebral palsy – a comparative study between south-west Germany and western Sweden. I. Clinical patterns and disabilities. *Dev Med Child Neurol* 35: 1037–1047.

Krägeloh-Mann I, Helber A, Mader I, Staudt M, Wolff M, Groenendaal F, DeVries L (2002) Bilateral lesions of thalamus and basal ganglia: origin and outcome. *Dev Med Child Neurol* 44: 477–484.

Lidzba K, Staudt M, Wilke M, Krageloh-Mann I (2006) Visuospatial deficits in patients with early left-hemispheric lesions and functional reorganization of language: consequence of lesion or reorganization? *Neuropsychologia* 44: 1088–1094.

Macdonell RA, Jackson GD, Curatolo JM, Abbott DF, Berkovic SF, Carey LM, et al (1999) Motor cortex localization using functional MRI and transcranial magnetic stimulation. *Neurology* 53: 1462–1467.

Maegaki Y, Yamamoto T, Takeshita K (1995) Plasticity of central motor and sensory pathways in a case of unilateral extensive cortical dysplasia: investigation of magnetic resonance imaging, transcranial magnetic stimulation, and short-latency somatosensory evoked potentials. *Neurology* 45: 2255–2261.

Maegaki Y, Maeoka Y, Ishii S, Shiota M, Takeuchi A, Yoshino K, et al (1997) Mechanisms of central motor reorganization in pediatric hemiplegic patients. *Neuropediatrics* 28: 168–174.

Mutch L, Alberman E, Hagberg B, Kodama K, Velickovic Perat M (1992) Cerebral palsy epidemiology: where are we now and where are we going? *Dev Med Child Neurol* 43: 547–555.

Nezu A, Kimura S, Takeshita S, Tanaka M (1999) Functional recovery in hemiplegic cerebral palsy: ipsilateral electromyographic responses to focal transcranial magnetic stimulation. *Brain Dev* 21: 162–165.

Niemann G (2000) A new MRI-based classification. In: Neville B, Goodman R, editors. *Congenital Hemiplegia*. London: Mac Keith Press, pp. 37–52.

Niemann G, Wakat JP, Krägeloh-Mann I (1994) Congenital hemiparesis and periventricular leucomalacia: pathogenic aspects from MRI. *Dev Med Child Neurol* 36: 943–950.

Niemann G, Grodd W, Schöning M (1996) Late remission of congenital hemiparesis: the value of MRI. *Neuropediatrics* 27: 197–201.

Ogawa S, Lee TM, Kay AR, Tank DW (1990) Brain magnetic resonance imaging with contrast dependent on blood oxygenation. *Proc Natl Acad Sci USA* 87: 9868–9872.

Palisano R, Rosenbaum P, Walter S, Russell D, Wood E, Galuppi B (1997) Development and reliability of a system to classify gross motor function in children with cerebral palsy. *Dev Med Child Neurol* 39: 214–223.

Palisano RJ, Cameron D, Rosenbaum PL, Walter SD, Russell D (2006) Stability of the gross motor function classification system. *Dev Med Child Neurol* 48: 424–428.

Platt MJ, Cans C, Johnson A, Surman G, Topp M, Torrioli MG, Krägeloh-Mann I (2007) Trends in cerebral palsy among infants of very low birthweight (<1500g) or born prematurely (<32 weeks) in 16 European centres: a database study. *Lancet* 369: 43–50.

Rosenbaum PL, Walter SD, Hanna SE, Palisano RJ, Russell DJ, Raina P, Wood E, Bartlett DJ, Galuppi BE (2002) Prognosis of gross motor function in cerebral palsy: creation of motor development curves. *JAMA* 288: 1357–1363.

Rosenbaum P, Paneth N, Leviton A, Goldstein M, Bax M (2007) A report: the definition and classification of cerebral palsy April 2006. *Dev Med Child Neurol* Suppl 109, 49: 8–14.

Sanger TD, Delgado MR, Gaebler-Spira D, Hallett M, Mink JW (2003) Task force on childhood motor disorders. Classification and definition of disorders causing hypertonia in childhood. *Pediatrics* 111: e89–e97.

Shimizu T, Nariai T, Maehara T, et al (2000) Enhanced motor cortical excitability in the unaffected hemisphere after hemispherectomy. *Neuroreport* 11: 3077–3084.

Stanley F, Blair E, Alberman E (2000) *Cerebral Palsies: Epidemiology and Causal Pathways.* London: Mac Keith Press.

Staudt M, Niemann G, Grodd W, Krägeloh-Mann I (2000) The pyramidal tract in hemiparesis – relationship of morphology and function in congenital periventricular lesions. *Neuropediatrics* 31: 257–264.

Staudt M, Pieper T, Grodd W, Winkler P, Holthausen H, Krägeloh-Mann I (2001) Functional MRI in a 6-year-old boy with unilateral cortical malformation: concordant representation of both hands in the unaffected hemisphere. *Neuropediatrics* 32: 159–161.

Staudt M, Grodd W, Gerloff C, et al (2002) Two types of ipsilateral reorganization in congenital hemiparesis: a TMS and fMRI study. *Brain* 125: 2222–2237.

Staudt M, Pavlova M, Böhm S, Grodd W, Krägeloh-Mann I (2003) Pyramidal tract damage correlates with motor dysfunction in bilateral periventricular leukomalacia (PVL). *Neuropediatrics* 34: 182–188.

Staudt M, Gerloff C, Grodd W, Holthausen H, Krägeloh-Mann I (2004a) Reorganization in congenital hemiparesis acquired at different gestational ages. *Ann Neurol* 56: 854–863.

Staudt M, Krägeloh-Mann I, Holthausen H, et al (2004b) Searching for motor functions in dysgenic cortex: a clinical TMS and fMRI study. *J Neurosurg* 101: 69–77.

Staudt M, Braun C, Gerloff C, Erb M, Grodd W, Krägeloh-Mann I (2006) Developing somatosensory projections bypass periventricular brain lesions. *Neurology* 67: 522–525.

Steinlin M, Good M, Martin E, et al (1993) Congenital hemiplegia: morphology of cerebral lesions and pathogenetic aspects from MRI. *Neuropediatrics* 24: 224–229.

Surveillance of Cerebral Palsy in Europe (2000) Surveillance of cerebral palsy in Europe: a collaboration of cerebral palsy surveys and registers. *Dev Med Child Neurol* 42: 816–824.

Surveillance of Cerebral Palsy in Europe (2002) Prevalence and characteristics of children with cerebral palsy in Europe. *Dev Med Child Neurol* 44: 633–640.

Thickbroom GW, Byrnes ML, Archer SA, Nagarajan L, Mastaglia FL (2001) Differences in sensory and motor cortical organization following brain injury early in life. *Ann Neurol* 49: 320–327.

Uvebrant P (1988) Hemiplegic cerebral palsy. Aetiology and outcome. *Acta Paediatr Scand*, Suppl 345: 5–100.

Vandermeeren Y, De Volder AG, Bastings E, et al (2002) Functional relevance of motor cortex reorganization in a child with unilateral schizencephaly. *Neuroreport* 13: 1821–1824.

Vandermeeren Y, Sébire G, Grandin CB, et al (2003) Functional reorganization of brain in children affected with congenital hemiplegia: fMRI study. *NeuroImage* 20: 289–301.

Volpe JJ (1995) Hypoxic-ischemic encephalopathy. In: *Neurology of the Newborn*. Philadelphia: Saunders, pp. 211–372.

Weiller C, Chollet F, Friston KJ, Wise RJS, Frackowiak RSJ (1992) Functional reorganization of the brain in recovery from striatocapsular infarction in man. *Ann Neurol* 31: 463–472.

Weiller C, Ramsay SC, Wise RSJ, Friston KJ, Frackowiak RSJ (1993) Individual patterns of functional reorganization in the human cerebral cortex after capsular infarction. *Ann Neurol* 33: 181–189.

Yousry TA, Schmid UD, Alkadhi H, Schmidt D, Peraud A, Buettner A, et al (1997) Localization of the motor hand area to a knob on the precentral gyrus. A new landmark. *Brain* 120: 141–157.

5
NORMAL ANATOMY OF THE UPPER EXTREMITY

Beth Moody Jones

Introduction

The upper limb is characterized by its mobility, range of motion and dexterity. In order to gain this increased mobility, we sacrifice some stability. The hand requires the most intricate of movements to accomplish grasping, fine and gross motor skills. These movements require a coordinated effort of the whole limb.

The limb can be divided into two broad categories: (1) proximal joints and muscles, including the scapula and shoulder, and (2) distal joints and muscles, including the elbow, wrist and hand. Anatomically these areas can be further subdivided into: brachium (arm), antibrachium (forearm), carpus (wrist), pollicus (thumb) and digits (fingers).

The bones of the upper limb include the scapula, clavicle, humerus, ulna, radius, the eight carpal bones, the five metacarpal bones and the 14 phalanges. The upper limb has only one bony attachment to the axial skeleton – the sternoclavicular joint – allowing for greater mobility and function. The sternoclavicular joint has a close relationship with the first rib and therefore the first thoracic vertebra – linking the upper extremity to the cervical/thoracic spine. The nervous tissue that innervates the majority of the upper limb also comes from the cervical region. It is important to recognize that these connections cannot be ignored in evaluation of the upper limb.

Proximal joints and muscles

PROXIMAL JOINTS

The glenohumeral joint is a ball-and-socket synovial joint consisting of the head of the humerus, the glenoid fossa of the scapula and a large, lax, thin joint capsule. The head of the humerus is about three times larger than the glenoid fossa, decreasing the congruency of the joint. This sacrifice of congruency allows for a greater range of motion in the shoulder but it leaves the joint susceptible to degeneration and derangement.

The humerus rests on a very small portion of the inferior glenoid fossa. Passive tension on the capsule, the coracohumeral ligament and the supraspinatus tendon hold the joint in its resting position. Lack of tension in the supraspinatus will eventually lead to joint creep and subluxation. Most of the joint stability is gained from the ligaments and muscles surrounding the joint.

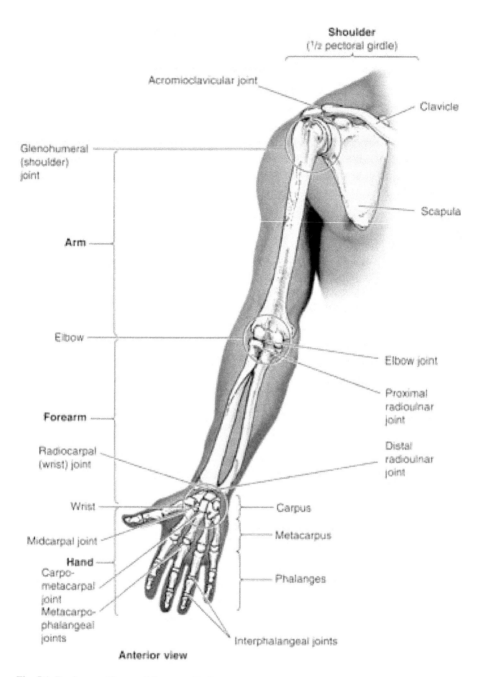

Fig. 5.1 Regions and bones of the upper limb.

Source: Moore and Dalley 2005.

80

The movement available at the shoulder includes flexion/extension around a horizontal axis, medial (internal) rotation/lateral (external) rotation around a vertical axis and abduction/adduction around an anterior/posterior axis. Medial rotation, lateral rotation and extension are thought to be pure glenohumeral movements. Flexion, abduction and adduction require scapular motion to complete. Scapular motion results from motion at the sternoclavicular joint.

The sternoclavicular (SC) joint is a modified synovial sellar joint between the manubrium sternum and the medial end of the clavicle, with an articular disc, joint capsule and ligaments. The fibrocartilage disc and the subclavius muscle as well as a series of very tough ligaments increase the stability of the joint allowing for a very small, but functionally important, amount of movement (Fig. 5.2).

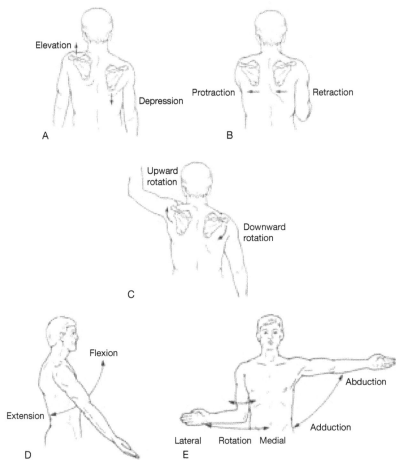

Fig. 5.2 Normal motions of the scapula and glenohumeral joint.

Source: Jenkins 2002.

The acromioclavicular (AC) joint is a plane synovial articulation which has a fairly weak joint capsule. Stability is gained from the attachments of the trapezius and deltoid muscles and a series of very strong ligaments between the clavicle and the coracoid process of the scapula. Movement at the AC joint is comparable to the movement at the SC joint; however, its primary function is to maintain the relationship between the clavicle and the scapula, helping to move the scapula.

Sternoclavicular motion includes protraction/retraction around a vertical axis, elevation and depression around an anterior/posterior axis and upward (lateral) rotation and downward (medial) rotation around an oblique axis that passes through the sternoclavicular joint and infraspinatus fossa of the scapula. The clavicle must be able to spin and glide in all three planes of motion to allow normal kinematics at the shoulder. Movement of the clavicle at the SC joint is translated into movement of the scapula via the long lever arm of the clavicle and via the very stable acromioclavicular joint.

PROXIMAL MUSCLES
There are many different muscles surrounding the glenohumeral, sternoclavicular and acromioclavicular joints. The organization of these muscles relates to their attachments. These groupings include: (1) axioscapular muscles – attaching the scapula to the axial skeleton; (2) scapulohumeral muscles – attaching the humerus to the scapula; and (3) axiohumeral muscles – attaching the humerus directly to the axial skeleton.

Axioscapular muscles
The axioscapular muscles have attachments on the scapula and the axial skeleton. These muscles have an effect at the sternoclavicular joint and so their function will relate to motions of the sternoclavicular joint – that is, protraction/retraction, elevation/depression and scapular rotation. We can further classify this group of muscles based on their location on the axial skeleton, be it anterior or posterior. We can determine the muscle's function based on its location in relationship to the axii of the SC joint (Figs 5.3–5.8).

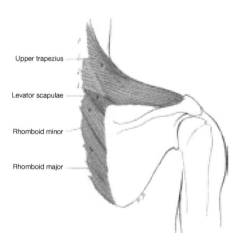

Upper trapezius

Levator scapulae

Rhomboid minor

Rhomboid major

Fig. 5.3 Elevators of the scapula.
Source: Jenkins 2002.

82

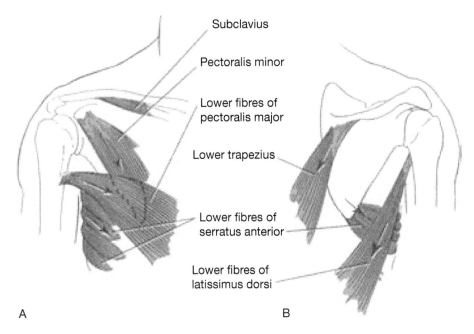

Subclavius

Pectoralis minor

Lower fibres of
pectoralis major

Lower trapezius

Lower fibres of
serratus anterior

Lower fibres of
latissimus dorsi

A   B

Fig. 5.4 Depressors of the scapula.
Source: Jenkins 2002.

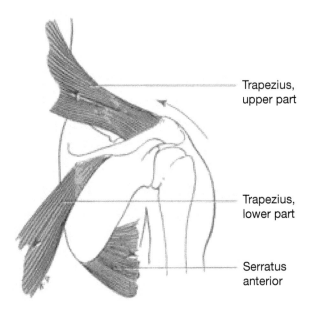

Trapezius,
upper part

Trapezius,
lower part

Serratus
anterior

Fig. 5.5 Upward rotators of the
scapula.
Source: Jenkins 2002.

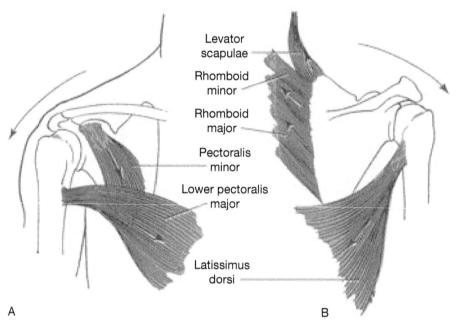

Levator
scapulae

Rhomboid
minor

Rhomboid
major

Pectoralis
minor

Lower pectoralis
major

Latissimus
dorsi

A

B

Fig. 5.6 Downward rotators of the scapula.
Source: Jenkins 2002.

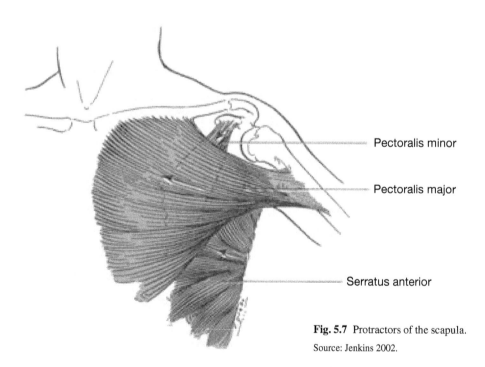

Pectoralis minor

Pectoralis major

Serratus anterior

Fig. 5.7 Protractors of the scapula.
Source: Jenkins 2002.

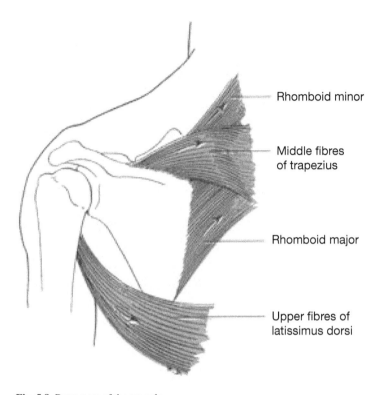

Rhomboid minor

Middle fibres
of trapezius

Rhomboid major

Upper fibres of
latissimus dorsi

Fig. 5.8 Retractors of the scapula.
Source: Jenkins 2002.

Anteriorly these muscles include: pectoralis minor, subclavius and serratus anterior.

Pectoralis minor has a proximal attachment on the third to fifth ribs, and a distal attachment at the coracoid process of the scapula. Its primary actions will include depression, downward rotation and protraction of the scapula. Clinically a tight pectoralis minor may lead to entrapment of the brachial plexus, which passes directly underneath this muscle. Tightness of the pectoralis muscle may also lead to poor position of the glenohumeral joint, causing further alterations of normal mechanics down the upper limb. This can include, but is not limited to, a posture of humeral internal rotation and the appearance of a forward shoulder.

The subclavius muscle is a small muscle which is often forgotten but it plays a key role in stabilizing the sternoclavicular joint. This muscle attaches from the first rib to the mid-clavicle. The function of the subclavius also includes depression of the clavicle and therefore will assist with depression of the scapula.

Serratus anterior is an unusual anterior axioscapular muscle because it has attachments that start anteriorly from the lateral parts of the first to eighth ribs but then end along the anterior surface of the medial scapular border. Serratus anterior is an important stabilizer of the scapula, drawing it close to the axial skeleton. It also assists the trapezius in upward rotation of the scapula and assists pectoralis minor in protraction of the scapula.

The posterior axioscapular muscles include: trapezius, levator scapulae and rhomboid major and rhomboid minor.

Trapezius is a large trapezoid-shaped muscle which has multiple attachments. Proximal attachments include the nuchal ligament in the cervical spine, the external occipital protuberance and the spinous processes of C7–T12. The distal attachments are the clavicle, acromion and spine of the scapula. The muscle fibres of the trapezius allow it to be divided into three parts: the upper, middle and lower regions. All three parts assist the serratus in upward rotation of the scapula. This very important motion is required for the last part of glenohumeral flexion and abduction. Other actions of trapezius include scapular elevation and retraction.

Levator scapulae attaches at the posterior transverse processes of C1–C4 to the medial border of the scapula, superior to the spine of the scapula. The primary function of levator scapulae is to elevate the scapula; however, it also assists in downward rotation of the scapula, dropping the glenoid fossa inferiorly and helping to give the appearance of a lower shoulder. Downward rotation of the scapula leaves the glenohumeral joint vulnerable to subluxation as it changes the normal resting position of the humerus on the lip of the glenoid fossa.

Rhomboid major attaches from the spinous processes of T2–T5 to the medial border of the scapula, inferior to the spine of the scapula down to the inferior angle of the scapula. Rhomboid minor attaches from the spinous processes of C7 and T1 to the medial border of the scapula superior to the spine. Both muscles function as scapular retractors and both will downwardly rotate the scapula.

Scapulohumeral muscles
Scapulohumeral muscles attach the scapula and humerus. These muscles have an effect at the glenohumeral (GH) joint and so their function will relate to motions of the GH joint – that is, flexion/extension, abduction/adduction and medial/lateral rotation. This group of muscles can be classified based on their location on the axial skeleton, be it anterior or posterior. The muscle's function can be determined based on its location in relationship to the axii of the GH joint (Figs 5.9–5.13).

Anteriorly these muscles include: biceps brachii, coracobrachialis and subscapularis.

Biceps brachii has two heads: a short head that has a proximal attachment at the coracoid process of the scapula, and a long head with a proximal attachment on the supraglenoid tubercle of the scapula. The long head has fibres that attach to the glenoid labrum. The glenoid labrum is a fold of connective tissue which is thought to be an extension of the glenohumeral capsule which increases the depth and width of the glenoid fossa. Both heads join together to attach to the tuberosity of the radius and the fascia of the forearm, the bicipital aponeurosis. The biceps brachii has its primary function at the radioulnar joint as the primary supinator of the forearm. It also assists in elbow flexion when the forearm is supinated, especially when power is required. The action of the biceps brachii at the glenohumeral joint is limited but the short head will assist in glenohumeral flexion and the long head will assist in glenohumeral abduction if the primary muscles producing this action are injured. The primary role of the biceps at the glenohumeral joint is to assist in increasing joint stability.

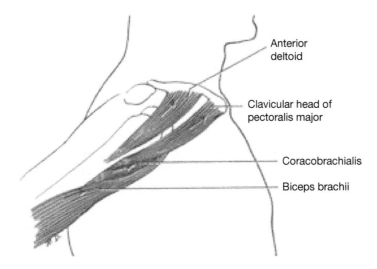

Anterior
deltoid

Clavicular head of
pectoralis major

Coracobrachialis

Biceps brachii

Fig. 5.9 Flexors of the glenohumeral joint.
Source: Jenkins 2002.

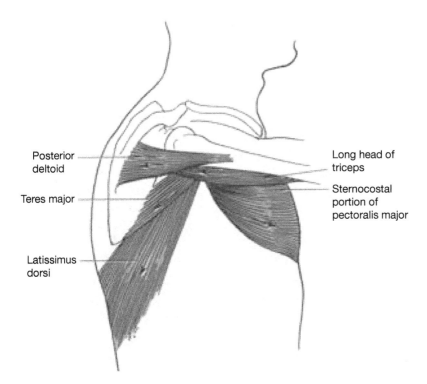

Posterior
deltoid

Teres major

Latissimus
dorsi

Long head of
triceps

Sternocostal
portion of
pectoralis major

Fig. 5.10 Extensors of the glenohumeral joint.
Source: Jenkins 2002.

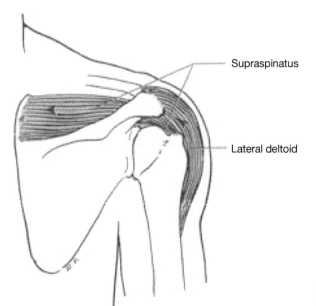

Supraspinatus

Lateral deltoid

Fig. 5.11 Abductors of the arm.
Source: Jenkins 2002.

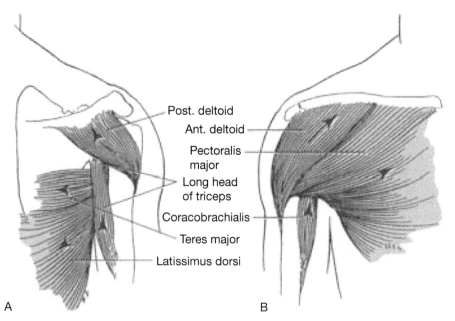

Post. deltoid

Ant. deltoid

Pectoralis major

Long head of triceps

Coracobrachialis

Teres major

Latissimus dorsi

A

B

Fig. 5.12 Adductors of the glenohumeral joint.
Source: Jenkins 2002.

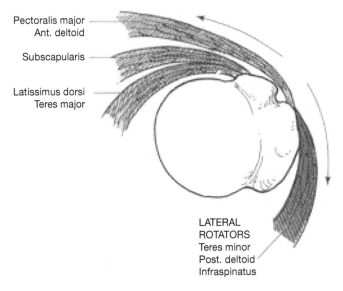

Pectoralis major
Ant. deltoid

Subscapularis

Latissimus dorsi
Teres major

LATERAL
ROTATORS
Teres minor
Post. deltoid
Infraspinatus

Fig. 5.13 Lateral and medial rotators of the glenohumeral joint.

Source: Jenkins 2002.

Coracobrachialis is a small muscle that fuses with the short head of the biceps brachii as it comes off the coracoid process of the scapula. Coracobrachialis has a distal attachment to the middle medial surface of the humerus. The coracobrachialis assists in glenohumeral flexion and adduction. This muscle also assists in increasing glenohumeral stability.

Subscapularis is the anterior portion of the rotator cuff muscle group. Subscapularis has a proximal attachment from the anterior surface of the scapula, the scapular fossa. The distal attachment is to the rotator cuff at the lesser tubercle of the humerus. The muscle's primary actions are glenohumeral medial rotation and adduction. As a rotator cuff muscle it assists in holding the humeral head in the glenoid cavity, increasing the joint stability. The rotator cuff is essential in pulling the glenohumeral joint together, increasing the joint approximation to allow the powerhouse muscles to then move the joint without impingement.

Posteriorly these muscles include: supraspinatus, infraspinatus, teres minor, teres major, long head of the triceps, deltoid.

Supraspinatus is the superior muscle of the rotator cuff muscles. It has a proximal attachment at the supraspinous fossa of the scapula, and a distal attachment to the rotator cuff at the greater tubercle of the humerus. Supraspinatus initiates glenohumeral abduction and then assists the deltoid in completing this motion. As with all muscles of the rotator cuff, it also assists in approximation of the glenohumeral joint to increase its stability.

Infraspinatus is the middle posterior muscle of the rotator cuff, and teres minor is just inferior to it on the lateral border of the scapula. Infraspinatus has a proximal attachment at the infraspinous fossa, and teres minor is at the lateral border of the scapula just below the fossa. Both join together to attach to the rotator cuff at the greater tubercle of the humerus. Both function as the lateral rotators of the glenohumeral joint.

Teres major has a proximal attachment just lateral to that of teres minor along the lateral border of the scapula. It has a distal attachment with latissimus dorsi at the intertubercular grove of the humerus. Because it passes medially and anterior to the humerus it will medially rotate the glenohumeral joint. Other actions include adduction and extension.

The long head of the triceps is one of three heads of a muscle found in the posterior humerus. The long head is the only head that crosses the glenohumeral head and therefore offers some function at the glenohumeral joint. The proximal attachment is the infraglenoid tubercle and glenoid labrum, much like the long head of the biceps brachii except inferior in the glenoid fossa. The long head of the triceps can contribute to shoulder derangement and is a posterior stabilizer of this joint. It also assists in glenohumeral extension and adduction. The remaining functions of the triceps will be covered under distal muscles.

The deltoid is a large medial muscle with three distinct parts. The deltoid has proximal attachments at the clavicle, acromion and spine of the scapula, mirroring the attachments of the trapezius on the medial side. The deltoid has a strong distal attachment on the humerus at the deltoid tuberosity. The three parts offer different functions for this muscle. All three parts will contribute to glenohumeral abduction, and indeed this is the powerhouse for glenohumeral abduction. The anterior part will also assist in glenohumeral flexion and medial rotation, and the posterior part will assist in extension and lateral rotation.

Axiohumeral muscles

Axiohumeral muscles attach the axial skeleton and humerus. These muscles have a primary effect at the glenohumeral joint but can also affect the sternoclavicular joint. They are thought of as the powerhouse muscles of the proximal limb. There is one muscle anterior, the pectoralis major, and one posterior, the latissimus dorsi.

Pectoralis major is a fan-shaped muscle which covers the anterior thoracic wall. This muscle has two heads: the clavicular head which has a proximal attachment from the anterior surface of the clavicle, and the sternocostal head which has proximal attachments from the sternum and the superior six costal cartilages. The heads come together to from one distal attachment on the humerus at the intertubercular grove of the humerus. Action at the sternoclavicular joint includes scapular protraction and depression. Action at the glenohumeral joint is primarily adduction and medial rotation but the clavicular head can assist in glenohumeral flexion and the sternocostal head can assist in extending the glenohumeral joint from an already flexed position.

Latissimus dorsi is a large fan-shaped muscle on the posterior surface of the axilla and lower back. Latissimus dorsi has proximal attachments from the spinous process of the T7–T12, the thoracolumbar fascia, iliac crest and the inferior third and fourth ribs. The latissimus dorsi and the teres major form the posterior axillary fold. The latissimus twists around the teres major inserting along with that muscle into the intertubercular grove of the humerus, just medial to the attachment of the pectoralis major. Action at the glenohumeral joint is extension, medial rotation and adduction. Action at the sternoclavicular joint is minimal but it can assist in downward rotation, depression and retraction of the scapula.

Distal joints and muscles

The distal joints of the upper extremity include the elbow, radioulnar, wrist, and the multiple joints within the hand.

The elbow joint is a hinge synovial joint which incorporates the articulations between the humerus and both the radius and the ulna. The humeroulna articulation is highly congruent due to the trochlear of the ulna. This allows only one type of movement – flexion and extension of the elbow around a horizontal axis. The humeroradial articulation is more mobile, allowing both flexion/extension and supination/pronation as the radius rotates around the annular ligament of the elbow.

The radioulnar joint is a pivoting synovial joint which allows movement of the radius on the ulna. This joint has three areas of articulation: proximal at the elbow as the radius spins or rotates within the annular ligament, distal where the radius rotates around the head of the ulna, and at the interosseous membrane.

Movement at the radioulnar joints is limited to supination and pronation of the forearm around a vertical axis that extends from the radial head to the head of the ulna. When the elbow is flexed and held horizontally, pronation places the palm inferiorly and supination places the palm superiorly.

The wrist joint is comprised of two compound joints: the radiocarpal joint and the midcarpal joint. The radiocarpal joint is created by the articulation of the radius and the proximal carpal bone (scaphoid, lunate and triquetrum). The midcarpal joint is comprised of the articulations of the proximal carpal bones (scaphoid, lunate and triquetrum) with the distal carpal bones (trapezium, trapezoid, capitate and hamate). Movement at the radiocarpal joint includes flexion/extension around a horizontal axis and ulnar (medial) deviation and radial (lateral) deviation around an anterior/posterior axis. Movement at the midcarpal joint is primarily limited to flexion/extension but does contribute to a certain extent to ulnar and radial deviation.

The carpometacarpal (CMC) joints of the digits are located between the distal carpal row and the bases of the second to fifth metacarpal joints. These joints are plane synovial joints allowing only minimal flexion/extension and some gliding to occur. There is more mobility at the fifth CMC with less mobility occurring at each subsequent joint from the fifth in to the second digit.

The thumb is considered the first digit and has its own unique qualities, starting with the CMC joint. The CMC joint of the thumb is comprised of the articulation between the trapezium and the first metacarpal. This is a sellar-shaped articulation allowing two degrees of movement: flexion/extension and abduction/adduction. In addition there is a spin component that can be combined with these planar motions to allow for *opposition*, or the ability of the thumb to cross over the palm of the hand toward the fourth and fifth digits.

The metacarpophalangeal (MCP) joints of all of the digits are between the heads of the metacarpals and the proximal phalanges of digits 1–5. Movement at these joints consists of flexion/extension around a horizontal axis, abduction/adduction around an anterior/posterior axis, and circumduction.

The proximal interphalangeal (PIP) joints and distal interphalangeal (DIP) joints consist of the articulation of the head of the proximal phalanx with the base of the distal phalanx in digits 2–5. Each digit has a PIP and DIP articulation, allowing only flexion/extension around a horizontal axis. The thumb has only two phalanges and therefore will only have an interphalangeal joint (IP).

DISTAL MUSCLES
In this section, we will look at the remaining compartments of the upper limb: the arm, the forearm, and the hand intrinsics.

The arm
The arm can be divided into the anterior compartment and the posterior compartment. The anterior compartment contains the brachialis and the already discussed biceps brachii and the coracobrachialis muscles. The posterior compartment consists of the triceps brachii muscle.

The brachialis muscle is a large flat muscle which has its proximal attachment along the anterior humerus and its distal attachment at the ulnar tuberosity and the coronoid process of the ulna. The brachialis is thought to be the powerhouse for elbow flexion, producing elbow flexion force in all positions of the forearm.

The triceps brachii has three heads: the long head, the lateral head and the medial head. The long head was discussed along with the glenohumeral joint because of its effect at that joint. The lateral and medial heads have their proximal attachment on the posterior humerus. All three heads come together and attach at the proximal end of the olecranon of the ulna. In addition to the particular tasks of the long head, the whole muscle acts as the chief elbow extensor.

The forearm
The forearm can also be divided into anterior and posterior compartments, and the muscles in these compartments are the flexors and the extensors respectively.

THE FLEXORS
The anterior compartment can be further divided into a superficial group and a deep group of muscles. The superficial group includes: pronator teres, flexor carpi radialis (FCR), palmaris longus, flexor carpi ulnaris (FCU) and flexor digitorum superficialis (FDS). The deep group includes: pronator quadratus, flexor pollicis longus (FPL) and flexor digitorum profundus (FDP).

The five muscles of the superficial group, with minor exceptions, all have a common proximal attachment from the medial epicondyle of the humerus. The pronator teres crosses from medial to lateral to attach onto the radius. It is one of the two pronators of the forearm. The flexor carpi radialis has a distal attachment to the base of the second metacarpal. It has a function of flexion and radial deviation at the wrist. Palmaris longus normally attaches to the flexor retinaculum and palmar aponeurosis. It is absent in about 10–12 per cent of the population. It assists in wrist flexion and tenses the palmar aponeurosis. The flexor carpi

92

ulnaris has a distal attachment at the pisiform, the hook of the hamate and the fifth metacarpal. The function of the FCU is flexion and ulnar deviation at the wrist. The flexor digitorum superficialis has a distal attachment at the shafts of the middle phalanges of the second to fifth digits. By crossing the PIP and the MCP, it will assist in flexion at both of these joints. The flexor digitorum superficialis is one of the nine tendons that traverse the carpal tunnel.

The flexor muscles of the deep group can be organized geographically: there is one muscle to the thumb, one to the digits and one to the wrist.

The muscle to the thumb, flexor pollicis longus, has a proximal attachment on the radius and interosseous membrane, and a distal attachment to the base of the distal phalanx of the thumb. It is one of the tendons that traverse the carpal tunnel. Its main action is to flex the distal phalanx of the thumb.

The muscle to the digits is the flexor digitorum profundus (FDP). This muscle has its proximal attachment at the ulna and interosseous membrane, and its distal attachment at the distal phalanx of digits 2–5. Its main action is flexion of the DIP of each of the digits but it will assist in flexion of the PIP and MCP joints. Flexor digitorum profundus is the last set of tendons that traverse the carpal tunnel.

The muscle proximal to the wrist is the pronator quadratus. This muscle has attachments from the ulna to the radius and it is the primary pronating muscle of the forearm.

THE EXTENSORS

The posterior compartment of the forearm is thought of as the extensor compartment. It consists of 12 muscles which can be organized into four categories: muscles to the digits, muscles to the thumb, muscles to the wrist, and 'others'.

Muscles to the digits include extensor indicis, extensor digitorum and extensor digiti minimi. Extensor indicis is a deep muscle with a proximal attachment on the ulna and the interosseous membrane and a distal attachment to the extensor expansion of the second digit. It enables independent extension of the second digit and helps with wrist extension. Extensor digitorum has a proximal attachment from the common extensor origin on the lateral epicondyle of the humerus, and a distal attachment to the extensor expansions of digits 2–5. The main action of the extensor digitorum is to extend the MCP joints of digits 2–5. Because of its attachment to the extensor expansion it will also indirectly extend the phalanges as well. Extensor digiti minimi is another of the muscles that have their proximal attachment at the common extensor tendon on the lateral epicondyle of the humerus. This muscle mimics the extensor indicis by attaching at the extensor expansion of one digit – the fifth. Like the indicis, this will allow for independent extension of this particular digit.

Muscles to the thumb include: extensor pollicis longus, extensor pollicis brevis and abductor pollicis longus. The extensor pollicis longus has a proximal attachment on the ulna and interosseous membrane, and a distal attachment at the base of the distal phalanx of the thumb. Because this muscle crosses over all three joints of the thumb (CMC, MCP and IP), it will extend all three joints. The extensor pollicis brevis has its proximal attachment from the radius and interosseous membrane, and a distal attachment at the base of the proximal phalanx of the thumb. This muscle will extend the CMC and MCP joints of

93

the thumb. The abductor pollicis longus has a proximal attachment from the ulna, radius and interosseous membrane, and a distal attachment to the base of the first metacarpal. This muscle will abduct the thumb and extend the CMC joint.

Muscles to the wrist include: extensor carpi radialis longus (ECRL), extensor carpi radialis brevis (ECRB) and the extensor carpi ulnaris (ECU). All three muscles share a common proximal attachment from the lateral epicondyle area of the humerus. Distally the ECRL attaches to the base of the second metacarpal, the ECRB attaches to the base of the second and third metacarpals and the ECU attaches to the base of the fifth metacarpal. All of these muscles extend the wrist while the ECRL and ECRB assist in radial deviation and the ECU assists in ulnar deviation.

The 'other' muscles include: anconeus, supinator and the brachioradialis. We include these muscles in the extensor group due to the shared radial nerve innervation. Anconeus is a triangular-shaped muscle which has a proximal attachment from the lateral epicondyle of the humerus and a distal attachment on the ulna. Anconeus assists in abducting the forearm during pronation and also helps stabilize and assist in elbow extension. The supinator is a large deep muscle with broad attachments from the lateral epicondyle of the humerus, the radial head and the ulna. This muscle attaches to the posterior side of the radius, just opposite to the attachment of the pronator teres muscle from the anterior compartment. The brachioradialis is a long elbow flexor which divides the anterior and posterior compartments of the forearm. The brachioradialis has attachments from the lateral supracondylar ridge of the humerus to the lateral surface of the radius.

The hand

The intrinsic muscles of the hand can be divided into three groups: the thenar group, the hypothenar group and the central group.

The thenar group forms the thenar eminence of the thumb and includes four muscles: adductor pollicis, flexor pollicis brevis, abductor pollicis brevis, and opponens pollicis. The adductor pollicis is a large muscle deep in the web of the hand. This muscle has attachments from the capitate and the second and third metacarpals to the base of the proximal phalanx of the thumb. It acts to adduct the thumb. The remaining three thenar muscles all have proximal attachments from the flexor retinaculum, scaphoid and trapezium. The opponens has a distal attachment to the first metacarpal and acts to oppose the thenar eminence toward the centre of the palm. The abductor pollicis brevis and the flexor pollicis brevis have distal attachments to the proximal phalanx of the thumb. The abductor abducts and assists in opposition of the thumb, and the flexor will flex the thumb.

The hypothenar group includes three muscles: abductor digiti minimi, flexor digiti minimi and opponens digiti minimi. The abductor digiti minimi has a proximal attachment at the pisiform and a distal attachment to the base of the proximal phalanx of the fifth digit. This muscle abducts the fifth digit and assists the flexor digitorum profundus and flexor digitorum superficialis in flexion of the MCP joint of the fifth digit. The flexor digiti minimi and the opponens digiti minimi have a shared proximal attachment from the hook of the hamate and the flexor retinaculum. The flexor digiti minimi, like the abductor digiti minimi, has a distal attachment to the base of the proximal phalanx and it will also assist in flexion of the MCP of the fifth digit. The opponens digiti minimi has a distal attachment to the metacarpal. Its action will move the fifth metacarpal toward the thenar eminence, bringing the fifth digit into opposition with the thumb.

The last compartment of the hand is the central compartment which holds the lumbricals and the interossei muscles. There are four lumbricals, one arising from each of the flexor digitorum profundus tendons. They have a distal attachment to the lateral side of the extensor expansion (hood) of the second to fifth digits. These muscles will flex the MCP joints while extending the PIP and DIP joints. They also assist the interossei muscles with abduction and adduction of the phalanges. The interossei muscles consist of four dorsal and three palmar muscles. These muscles fill in the space between the metacarpals and have distal attachments to the proximal phalanges and the extensor expansion. The dorsal interossei will abduct the second to fourth digits and the palmar interossei muscles will adduct the second, fourth and fifth digits.

Innervation of the upper limb

The upper limb innervation is primarily supplied via branches of the brachial plexus which is comprised of the anterior spinal nerve roots C5 to T1. While there are many small branches that provide innervation to individual muscles we can divide the upper limb innervation into groups, or areas, which are innervated by the five major branches of the brachial plexus: those from the posterior cord – the axillary nerve and the radial nerve; and those from the medial and lateral cords – the musculocutaneous, median and ulnar nerves (Fig. 5.14).

The axillary nerve is supplied from nerve roots C5 and C6. This nerve is the posterior cord nerve that passes to the posterior compartment of the upper limb. The axillary nerve travels just inferior to the humeral head and through the quadrangular space – an area bounded by the long head of the triceps, teres major, head of the humerus and teres minor. In general terms it can be thought of as the 'nerve of arm abduction' as it provides its primary motor supply to the deltoid muscle (it also innervates the teres minor). The cutaneous sensory end point of the axillary nerve is the skin just above the shoulder.

The radial nerve is the next posterior cord nerve and is comprised of nerve roots C5–T1. It can be generally thought of as the 'nerve of extension'. The radial nerve provides motor fibres to all muscles of the posterior compartments of the arm and forearm. It will provide innervation for the actions of extension of the elbow, wrist, fingers and thumb. It also has some action on supination and elbow flexion through its supply to the 'other' muscles of the posterior compartment – the brachoradialis and supinator. Cutaneous sensory innervation is to the skin of the back of the arm, forearm and hand (Fig. 5.15).

The lateral cord of the brachial plexus gives rise to the musculocutaneous nerve (C5 and C6), or the 'nerve of elbow flexion'. The musculocutaneous nerve gives motor supply to the anterior arm compartment, and cutaneous sensory innervation to the medial side of the forearm (Fig. 5.16).

The lateral and medial cords come together to form the median nerve (C6–T1), or the 'nerve of wrist and finger flexion'. It is also the nerve of forearm pronation, thumb motion and sensation to the hand. The median nerve innervates all of the muscles of the anterior forearm compartment except for one muscle and half a muscle – the flexor carpi ulnaris and the ulnar side of the flexor digitorum profundus are innervated by the other nerve to the hand, the ulnar nerve. The median nerve is the nerve that travels in the carpal tunnel giving motor innervation to all of the thenar muscles except the adductor pollicis. It also provides motor innervation to the two lumbricals that are associated with the second and third digits. The

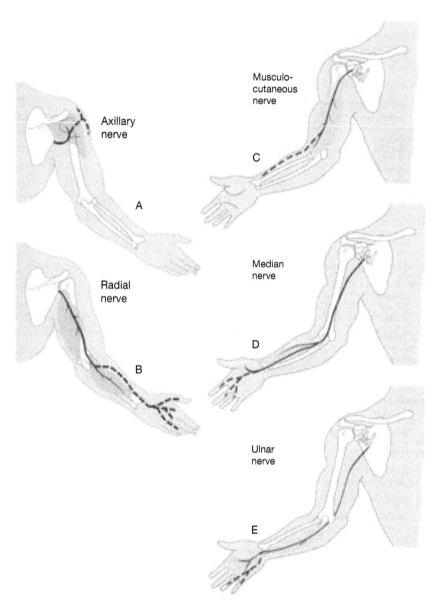

Fig. 5.14 Distribution of the main nerves of the upper limb.

Source: Rosse and Gaddum-Rosse 1997.

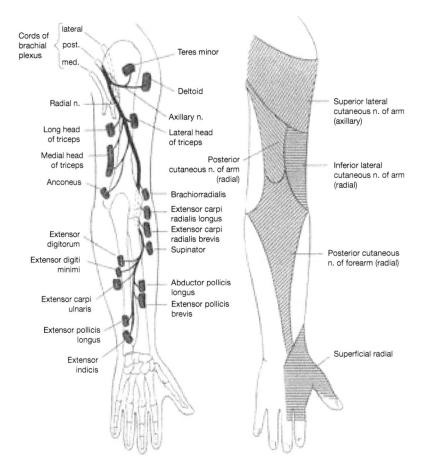

Fig. 5.15 Radial nerve distribution.

Source: Jenkins 2002.

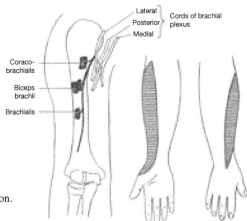

Fig. 5.16 Musculocutaneous nerve distribution.

Source: Jenkins 2002.

97

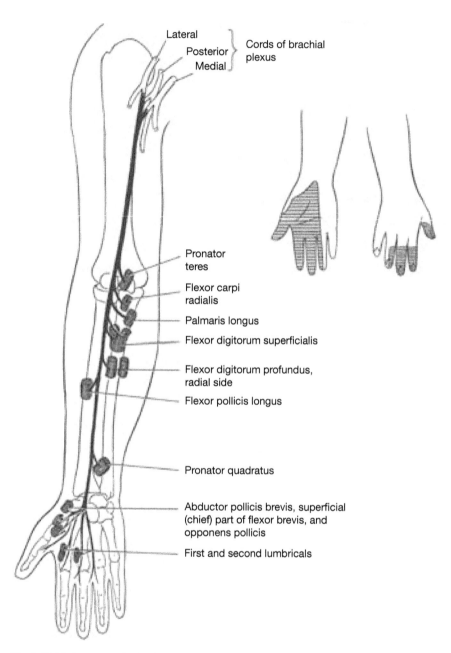

Lateral
Posterior } Cords of brachial
Medial   } plexus

Pronator teres

Flexor carpi radialis

Palmaris longus

Flexor digitorum superficialis

Flexor digitorum profundus, radial side

Flexor pollicis longus

Pronator quadratus

Abductor pollicis brevis, superficial (chief) part of flexor brevis, and opponens pollicis

First and second lumbricals

Fig. 5.17 Median nerve distribution.

Source: Jenkins 2002.

sensory or cutaneous distribution is to the palm of the hand and the palmar side of the second and third digits and the palmar side of the thumb (Fig. 5.17).

The medial cord also supplies the ulnar nerve (C8–T1), which is the 'nerve of the hand intrinsics'. The ulnar nerve supplies the one and a half muscles of the anterior forearm mentioned previously and then traverses to the hand through Guiyon's canal, offering motor innervation to all of the interossei muscles, the hypothenar muscles, the two ulnar lumbricals (to the fourth and fifth digits) and the adductor pollicis. The cutaneous sensory distribution is to the ulnar side of the palm and posterior hand (Fig. 5.18).

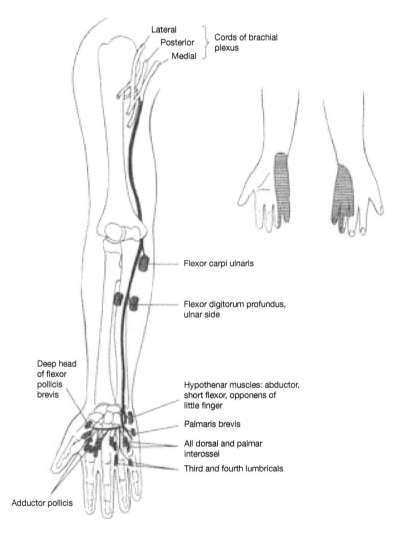

Fig. 5.18 Ulnar nerve distribution.

Source: Jenkins 2002.

99

REFERENCES

Gray H (1995) *Gray's Anatomy: The Anatomical Basis of Medicine and Surgery, 38th edn*. Philadelphia: Churchill Livingstone

Jenkins D (2002) *Hollinshead's Functional Anatomy of the Limbs and Back, 8th edn*. Philadelphia: Saunders.

Levangie PK, Norkin CC (2005) *Joint Structure and Function. A Comprehensive Analysis, 4th edn*. Philadelphia: F.A. Davis.

Moore K, Dalley A (2005) *Clinically Oriented Anatomy, 5th edn*. Philadelphia: Lippincott Williams & Wilkins.

Rosse C, Gaddum-Rosse P (1997) *Hollinshead's Textbook of Anatomy, 5th edn*. Philadelphia: Lippincott-Raven.

6
MUSCLE ALTERATIONS DUE TO SPASTICITY

Eva Pontén

Muscle spasticity is commonly seen in children affected with cerebral palsy (CP). When examining the upper extremity, a common finding is that the flexor muscle/tendon complex is 'short'. The resistance felt when trying to extend the joints is due to either hypertonia of the muscle and/or short/inextensible muscles, or alterations of the ligaments and the joint shape itself. Even though the end result is a 'simple' flexion contracture (Fig. 6.1), the cause is multifaceted and the process is not totally known.

Hypertonia in childhood

The brain damage in children diagnosed with CP may often, after a period of general hypotonia during infancy, result in centrally derived muscle hypertonia. Hypertonia is defined as an increased resistance to passive stretch while the child is attempting to maintain a relaxed state of muscle activity (Sanger et al 2003). The resistance may be caused by spasticity, dystonia or rigidity, often in combination. Spasticity is present when an increased velocity-dependent stretch reflex can be elicited, as shown in Fig. 6.2 (Lance 1981). Dystonia is characterized by an involuntary dysfunctional muscle action during movement or maintenance of posture. Rigidity is defined as resistance to even slow passive movements in both flexion and extension, with no speed threshold. These definitions of tone exclude resistance (or 'stiffness') as a result of fixed contractures – which is a true shortening of the muscle and tendon complex and/or alterations of the three-dimensional structure of the joint and ligaments.

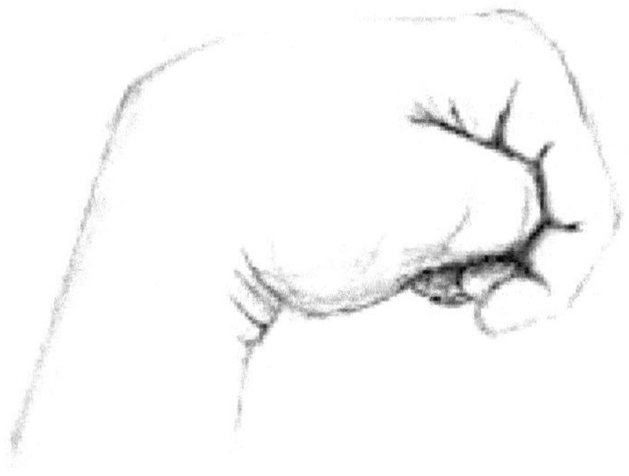

Fig. 6.1 Severe contracture of wrist and finger flexors in the hand of a child with cerebral palsy. Typical pattern is forearm pronation, wrist flexion and ulnar deviation, and thumb flexion and adduction.

Source: Illustration by Sebastian Pontén

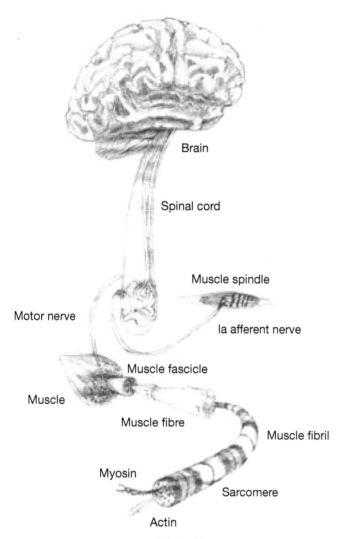

Brain

Spinal cord

Muscle spindle

Motor nerve

Ia afferent nerve

Muscle fascicle

Muscle

Muscle fibre

Muscle fibril

Myosin

Sarcomere

Actin

Fig. 6.2 Overview of the relation between the brain and the muscle structure. The brain damage in CP results in diminished use of the arm, which alters the structure of the muscles. If the arm is used more intensely through training, there are again plastic changes of the muscles. When stretching a muscle, information from the muscle spindle is sent through the Ia muscle afferent nerve fibres to the spinal cord, resulting in a contraction of the muscle. This stretch reflex is normally modulated by many areas in the brain.

Source: Illustration by Sebastian Pontén

Muscle architecture

The muscle itself contributes to the (lack of) balance of the joints and to the contracture formation. The amount of, and the macroscopic arrangement of, the muscle fibres relative to the axis of force generation affect the force output. The measure of this fibre to force-generation relationship is the physiological cross-sectional area (PCSA), and is calculated using the formula: muscle mass x $\cos\theta$/fibre length x density, where θ is the pennation angle of the fibre relative to the force-generating axis. Upper limb muscles all have a pennation angle of less than 20 degrees, which thus has little effect on the muscle output (Zajac 1992). In humans, the sum of the PCSAs of the wrist flexors is larger than that of the extensors (Lieber et al 1990, 1992, Loren et al 1996). Motor control of the wrist and hand is normally balanced by continual eccentric and concentric contractions of both the extensor and flexor muscles. However, in those with cerebral palsy there is a deficient control of the muscles that normally work in concert. The flexors will then have a greater influence on the joint, resulting in a typical position of, for example, a flexed wrist (Fig. 6.1).

In children with hemiplegic CP, the paretic arm is often shorter than the unaffected arm. The circumference of the arm is also smaller, and the amount of fat tissue surrounding the muscles is larger than normal. The PCSA is therefore generally much smaller in the paretic arm than in the less affected arm, which partly explains the weakness in cerebral palsy. Muscle fibre length is also important for the function, as it is the greatest determinant of speed and excursion capacity (Zajac 1992). The longer the muscle fibres, the larger the operating range, which means that short muscle fibres, which may be seen in children with spasticity, result in a decreased range of motion (Lieber and Bodine-Fowler 1993).

Decreased passive extensibility
During deep general anaesthesia, muscles will relax and consequently centrally derived hypertonia of muscles will no longer appear to be present. However, if a patient severely affected with CP is put under general anaesthesia, a decreased range of passive motion still persists in many joints and constitutes true fixed contractures. Fixed contractures of the ankle in hemiplegic CP have been investigated by inducing ischaemia (and thus paralysis) in the legs using a tourniquet. The spastic gastrocnemius and soleus muscles were shown to be shorter/less extensible than the contralateral muscles (Tardieu et al 1982). These observations could be explained by: (a) adhesions between muscles and muscle fibre; (b) few sarcomeres in series; and (c) intracellular alterations.

Adhesions between muscles and muscle fibres
When a limb has been in a cast for a long period of time, the normal gliding movement of the muscles is hampered by increased fibrotic adhesions between the muscle bellies (Järvinen et al 2002). In the child with cerebral palsy, the diminished use of the arm is a relative immobilization, thus often resulting in perimuscular adhesions. In a recent study, the consequences of the adhesions were demonstrated during surgical tenotomies of a relatively overactive flexor carpi ulnaris muscle (FCU) in young individuals with CP.

The force output was measured in the distally detached FCU while the ulnar nerve was stimulated. Different wrist angles changed the force output – even though no part of the muscle crossed the wrist joint. The authors concluded that the force of the contracting FCU was evidently transmitted to other adjacent wrist-flexing muscles by connective tissue adhesions (Smeulders et al 2005, Smeulders and Kreulen 2007).

103

Sarcomeres in series

Studies have suggested that there may be a reduction in the number of sarcomeres in human spastic flexor muscles in the same way as sarcomeres have been shown, in animal studies, to be reduced in a normal muscle that has been immobilized in a shortened position (Tabary et al 1972, Williams and Goldspink 1973, 1978, Tardieu et al 1982, Pontén et al 2007). A sarcomere is the basic contractile unit in the muscle, seen under the microscope as sets of striations in the striated muscle (Figs 6.2 and 6.3). During a contraction the motor proteins actin and myosin interdigitate, making the sarcomere shorter. The amount of actin–myosin overlap (the sarcomere length) affects the power the muscle can exert. If there are few sarcomeres in series, the sarcomeres will be stretched out, resulting in a very short overlap of actin and myosin, and a weaker muscle. Sarcomere lengths of the FCU measured *in vivo* in children with CP have showed a correlation between the length of the sarcomeres and contracture of the wrist. The sarcomeres in the flexor carpi ulnaris muscle are accordingly very long in children with wrist contracture if the wrist is held in neutral (Pontén et al 2007).

Thus, reduction of sarcomeres will, if the sarcomeres are of approximately normal length, result in a shortening of the muscle fibre. Ultrasound measurements of fibre/fascicle length have verified shorter fascicle lengths in the paretic compared to the contralateral gastrocnemius in hemiplegic CP (Mohagheghi et al 2007).

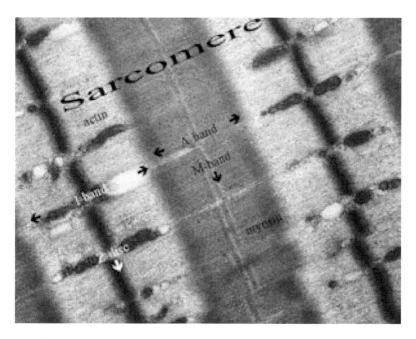

Fig. 6.3 Electron micrograph of skeletal muscle. The A-band, containing myosin, is dissected by the M-band. The I-band, containing actin, is dissected by the Z-disc. A sarcomere stretches between two Z-discs. Titin, a very large spring protein, stretches between the Z-disc and the M-band. During contraction, myosin and actin interdigitate (overlap), seen as the dark band on the border between the A-band and the I-band.

Intracellular alterations

In a normal muscle, when the sarcomere is stretched to about 3.8 mm, passive muscle fibre tension is increased. This passive tension in the muscle is largely constituted by the giant spring protein titin which connects the M-band and the myosins with the Z-band (Fig. 6.3). Titin has different domains which act like springs with different resistance. When the titin molecule is pulled out, it signals different stretching distances to the nuclei (Clark et al 2002). The role of titin in contracture development in individuals with spasticity is under investigation, but is still not clear (Fridén and Lieber 2003, Olsson et al 2006). At sarcomere lengths above 4.5 mm, in a non-spastic muscle, collagen contributes to the resting tension of the muscle fibre.

Spastic single muscle fibres have been shown to be stiffer than normal single fibres (Fridén and Lieber 2003). What precisely causes the passive stiffness is as yet not known. An increased total content of collagen has been found, correlated with the severity of the upper motor neuron syndrome (Booth et al 2001), even though fibrosis between the muscle fibres is rarely seen in sections of human spastic muscle (Marbini et al 2002) (Fig. 6.4).

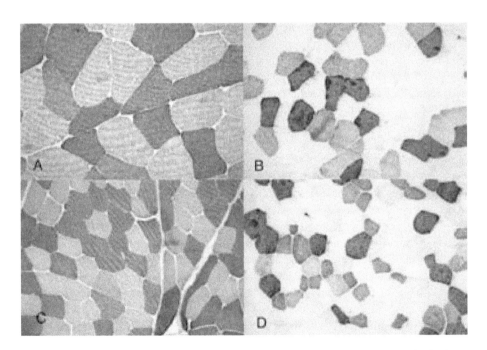

Fig. 6.4 Light micrographs from wrist extensor (extensor carpi radialis brevis, ECRB) and wrist flexor (flexor carpi ulnaris, FCU) from one patient with hemiplegic CP (A and B) and one patient with tetraplegic CP (C and D). N2.261 monoclonal antibody labels type 2A fibres darkly, type 1 lightly, and there is no labelling of type 2X fibres. All micrographs are shown at the same magnification. Note decreased fibre size, increased fibre size variability, and higher proportion of type 2X fibres in flexors compared with extensors, and decreased fibre size in tetraplegic sample.

Source: E Pontén, Umeå University Medical Dissertations. New Series no. 867, 2003.

Myosins

The motor protein myosin is composed of light chains and heavy chains (Fig. 6.2 and Fig. 6.3). Both the speed and the force of the contraction of the individual muscle fibre are determined by which type of myosin heavy chain (MyHC) is present (Pette and Staron 1990, Bottinelli et al 1991, Pette and Staron 2000). Mechanical load of the muscle and changes in the neuromuscular activity can alter the expression of different MyHCs (Pette and Staron 2000). During development, denervation and repair embryonic and fetal MyHCs are expressed (Sartore et al 1982, Schiaffino et al 1988). Muscle cells/muscle fibres can be divided into different groups depending on their MyHC composition. Type 1 fibres contain MyHC I and are slow and fatigue-resistant (formerly 'red' fibres). Type 2 fibres (formerly 'white' fibres) can be subgrouped into fast type 2A fibres which contain MyHC IIa, and type 2X (formerly 2B) fibres which contain the also fast but more fatigable MyHC IIx. Expression of MyHC IIx is rare in normal human limb muscles, and thus type 2X fibres are infrequently found.

Spastic biceps brachii muscles in young adults with CP have been shown to have a higher proportion of type 2X fibres and a larger fibre size variation when compared with controls (Pontén and Stål 2007). Wrist flexors in individuals with CP have, compared to extensors, been shown to have more type 2X fibres, larger fibre area variation and more regeneration, implied by a larger occurrence of developmental MyHCs (Pontén et al 2005) (Fig. 6.4). Also the severity of the cerebral palsy plays a role in the expression of MyHCs. The flexor carpi ulnaris in children with tetraplegic cerebral palsy contains more MyHC IIx and less MyHC I as compared to the amounts seen in children with hemiplegic CP (Pontén et al 2008).

Summary

How do these characteristics of the spastic muscle influence one of the main symptoms experienced by individuals with cerebral palsy – weakness? As mentioned earlier, the physiological cross-sectional area is smaller in individuals with CP and there is an increase in the very fatigable type IIX fibres. These are changes that do result in weakness, but they are secondary to decreased use. More fundamental is the centrally derived functional weakness – for example, due to an inability to recruit higher threshold motor units or to drive lower threshold motor units to higher firing rates (Rose and McGill 2005).

So, in summary, due to altered neuromuscular signalling, immobilization and learned non-use, individuals with spastic muscles have stiffer and shorter muscle fibres expressing faster and more fatigable myosins, adhesions and small muscle bellies. There is also an ongoing regeneration, especially in the flexors. As muscle is a very adaptive tissue, all of these changes may be influenced by activity (e.g. physiotherapy and occupational therapy), and probably influenced differently if the limb is moved passively or actively.

Other treatments may also have beneficial effects on muscle. Oral, intrathecal (e.g. baclofen) and intramuscular (e.g. botulinum toxin) medications diminish spasticity and normalize to some extent the mobility of the limbs. Neurosurgical procedures such as dorsal rhizotomy may reduce spasticity in children with CP, and hand surgery can improve the balance of the joints by tendon transfers or lengthening, thus facilitating use. A combination of different treatments, adapted for each child, will often be most beneficial for improvement of manual skills in daily life.

REFERENCES

Booth CM, Cortina-Borja MJ, Theologis TN (2001) Collagen accumulation in muscles of children with cerebral palsy and correlation with severity of spasticity. *Dev Med Child Neurol* 43: 314–320.

Bottinelli R, Schiaffino S, Reggiani C (1991) Force–velocity relations and myosin heavy chain isoform compositions of skinned fibres from rat skeletal muscle. *J Physiol* 437: 655–672.

Clark KA, McElhinny AS, Beckerle MC, Gregorio CC (2002) Striated muscle cytoarchitecture: an intricate web of form and function. *Annu Rev Cell Dev Biol* 18: 637–706.

Fridén J, Lieber RL (2003) Spastic muscle cells are shorter and stiffer than normal cells. *Muscle Nerve* 27: 157–164.

Järvinen TA, Jozsa L, Kannus P, Järvinen TL, Järvinen M (2002) Organization and distribution of intramuscular connective tissue in normal and immobilized skeletal muscles. An immunohistochemical, polarization and scanning electron microscopic study. *J Muscle Res Cell Motil* 23: 245–254.

Lance JW (1981) Disordered muscle tone and movement. *Clin Exp Neurol* 18: 27–35.

Lieber RL, Fazeli BM, Botte MJ (1990) Architecture of selected wrist flexor and extensor muscles. *J Hand Surg [Am]* 15: 244–250.

Lieber RL, Jacobson MD, Fazeli BM, Abrams RA, Botte MJ (1992) Architecture of selected muscles of the arm and forearm: anatomy and implications for tendon transfer. *J Hand Surg [Am]* 17: 787–798.

Lieber RL, Bodine-Fowler SC (1993) Skeletal muscle mechanics: implications for rehabilitation. *Phys Ther* 73: 844–856.

Loren GJ, Shoemaker SD, Burkholder TJ, Jacobson MD, Fridén J, Lieber RL (1996) Human wrist motors: biomechanical design and application to tendon transfers. *J Biomech* 29: 331–342.

Marbini A, Ferrari A, Cioni G, Bellanova MF, Fusco C, Gemignani F (2002) Immunohistochemical study of muscle biopsy in children with cerebral palsy. *Brain Dev* 24: 63–66.

Mohagheghi AA, Khan T, Meadows TH, Giannikas K, Baltzopoulos V, Maganaris CN (2007) Differences in gastrocnemius muscle architecture between the paretic and non-paretic legs in children with hemiplegic cerebral palsy. *Clin Biomech* 22: 718–724.

Olsson MC, Kruger M, Meyer LH, Ahnlund L, Gransberg L, Linke WA, Larsson L (2006) Fibre type-specific increase in passive muscle tension in spinal cord-injured subjects with spasticity. *J Physiol* 577: 339–352.

Pette D, Staron RS (1990) Cellular and molecular diversities of mammalian skeletal muscle fibers. *Rev Physiol Biochem Pharmacol* 116: 1–76.

Pette D, Staron RS (2000) Myosin isoforms, muscle fiber types, and transitions. *Microsc Res Tech* 50: 500–509.

Pontén EM, Stål PS (2007) Decreased capillarization and a shift to fast myosin heavy chain IIx in the biceps brachii muscle from young adults with spastic paresis. *J Neurol Sci* 253: 25–33.

Pontén E, Fridén J, Thornell LE, Lieber RL (2005) Spastic wrist flexors are more severely affected than wrist extensors in children with cerebral palsy. *Dev Med Child Neurol* 47: 384–389.

Pontén E, Gantelius S, Lieber RL (2007) Intraoperative muscle measurements reveal a relationship between contracture formation and muscle remodeling. *Muscle Nerve* 36: 47–54. Pontén E, Lindstrom M, Kadi F (2008) Higher amount of MyHC IIX in a wrist flexor in tetraplegic compared to hemiplegic cerebral palsy. *J Neurol Sci* 266: 51–56.

Rose J, McGill KC (2005) Neuromuscular activation and motor-unit firing characteristics in cerebral palsy. *Dev Med Child Neurol* 47: 329–336.

Sanger TD, Delgado MR, Gaebler-Spira D, Hallett M, Mink JW (2003) Classification and definition of disorders causing hypertonia in childhood. *Pediatrics* 111: e89–e97.

Sartore S, Gorza L, Schiaffino S (1982) Fetal myosin heavy chains in regenerating muscle. *Nature* 298: 294–296.

Schiaffino S, Ausoni S, Gorza L, Saggin L, Gundersen K, Lomo T (1988) Myosin heavy chain isoforms and velocity of shortening of type 2 skeletal muscle fibres. *Acta Physiol Scand* 134: 575–576.

Smeulders MJ, Kreulen M (2007) Myofascial force transmission and tendon transfer for patients suffering from spastic paresis: a review and some new observations. *J Electromyogr Kinesiol*.

Smeulders MJ, Kreulen M, Hage JJ, Huijing PA, van der Horst CM (2005) Spastic muscle properties are affected by length changes of adjacent structures. *Muscle Nerve* 32: 208–215.

Tabary JC, Tabary C, Tardieu C, Tardieu G, Goldspink G (1972) Physiological and structural changes in the cat's soleus muscle due to immobilization at different lengths by plaster casts. *J Physiol* 224: 231–244.

Tardieu C, Huet de la Tour E, Bret MD, Tardieu G (1982) Muscle hypoextensibility in children with cerebral palsy: I. Clinical and experimental observations. *Arch Phys Med Rehabil* 63: 97–102.

Williams PE, Goldspink G (1973) The effect of immobilization on the longitudinal growth of striated muscle fibres. *J Anat* 116: 45–55.

Williams PE, Goldspink G (1978) Changes in sarcomere length and physiological properties in immobilized muscle. *J Anat* 127: 459–468.

Zajac FE (1992) How musculotendon architecture and joint geometry affect the capacity of muscles to move and exert force on objects: a review with application to arm and forearm tendon transfer design. *J Hand Surg [Am]* 17: 799–804.

7
POSTURAL CONTROL FOR REACHING AND HAND SKILLS

Mindy F. Levin and Heidi Sveistrup

A recognized primary goal of upper limb rehabilitation is to obtain the optimal degree of functioning of the arms and hands when the child is in the sitting position (Boyd et al 2001, Liao et al 2003). Dysfunction of the upper limb and hand is a common and disabling consequence of cerebral palsy (CP) and may be related to problems of postural control. This chapter will review postural control related to arm and hand function during reaching in sitting in typically developing children and those with CP. Areas that need to be addressed in therapeutic approaches to improve upper limb function will be identified.

Numerous interventions have been developed for the physical management of children with cerebral palsy, with many addressing postural control difficulties that affect the child's upper extremity and hand skills (Ketelaar et al 1998, Taub et al 2004; for reviews, see Siebes et al 2002, Steultjens et al 2004). In general, therapeutic approaches have been based on both implicit and explicit assumptions about underlying motor development and/or motor control. For example, neurodevelopmentalists suggest that the development of movements and motor skills results solely from the maturation of the CNS, and thus focus on eliciting and establishing typical movement patterns through therapist-controlled sensorimotor experiences (Piper and Darrah 1984, Bower 1993). However, in recent years, both the assumptions and effectiveness of neurodevelopmental treatment (NDT) approaches to improve motor function have been questioned (Horak 1992, Royeen and DeGangi 1992, Hur 1995, Thelen 1995, Knox and Evans 2002).

More recently, the focus has shifted to a more directly functional, 'task-oriented' approach which targets the learning of motor skills that are meaningful in the child's environment and that are perceived as problematic by either the child or the caregivers (Shepherd 1995, Ketelaar et al 2001). This approach combines the notions of CNS maturation with the dynamic systems theory of motor development and motor control (Bernstein 1967, Gibson 1979, Thelen and Smith 1994, Kelso 1995), with the underlying assumption that the young brain is far more plastic than had previously been thought (see Guralnick 1997) and that functionality emerges from the dynamic interaction between the environment, the performer and the task in the performance of activities (see Shepherd 1995, Wagenaar and van Emmerik 1996, Darrah 1997). A task-oriented approach is thus based on active learning processes within an environment that enables the individual to learn to perform self-initiated actions within naturally occurring constraints (Thelen and Smith 1994). This is in contrast to an alternative approach of learning predetermined movement patterns based on those observed in age-matched typically developing children. Thus, according to this approach, even in the presence of neurological impairment limiting the child's ability to perform a task, the system is encouraged to take advantage of its redundancy and use alternative pathways to produce movements that optimally achieve the goal (Shepherd 1995, Latash and Anson 1996). However, the degree to which the system should be encouraged to use alternative movement patterns (compensation) instead of using movement patterns similar to those observed in typically developing children is still a matter of debate (see below).

Postural control
During early infancy, the head is the major frame of reference in seated postural control, reflected by the dominant cranial-to-caudal order of muscle recruitment (van der Fits et al 1999a). Development of successful reaching in independent sitting emerges at around 8 months (Van der Fits et al 1999a, 1999b), with the ability to modulate direction-specific postural adjustments during reaching emerging at around 9 or 10 months (von Hofsten and Woollacott 1989). Stability in sitting is assured by the development of coactivation of the direction-specific neck and trunk musculature which emerges by the end of the first year of life (Hadders-Algra et al 1996, 1998). About the same time, anticipatory postural adjustments (activity occurring prior to the onset of the arm movement) appear during goal-directed arm movements in anticipation of destabilizing forces (Forssberg and Nashner 1982, Casimiro and Sveistrup 2001). By the age of 15 to 18 months, consistent anticipatory postural muscle activity is observed (van der Fits et al 1999a, 1999b).

The fixed extensor muscle strategy disappears at around 2 years of age (Hadders-Algra et al 1998, van der Heide et al 2003). The frame of reference then moves more caudally, towards the support surface (Berger et al 1995, Hadders-Algra et al 1998), followed, some years later, by a return to a cranial focus at around 3 to 4½ years (Hadders-Algra et al 1998). Another transition period, identified by an increase in movement variability, occurs around age 7 to 9 for reaching patterns (Hay 1979, 1990, Fayt et al 1993, Schneiberg et al 2002). Transition periods are thought to reflect recalibration by the CNS of the influence of various sensory inputs (i.e. vision) on motor behaviour (Shumway-Cook and Woollacott 1985, Kirshenbaum et al 2001).

Children with CP carry out most of their functional activities, such as eating, drawing and playing, while sitting. They often have problems with postural control in sitting, characterized by instability during object manipulation. The postural deficits as characterized by the Gross Motor Function Classification System (GMFCS; Palisano et al 1997) vary greatly across children. This five-level classification system emphasizes sitting (trunk control) and walking, and focuses on function rather than limitations. Children classified in levels I and II are relatively independent reachers without the need for substantial postural assistance. Children in levels III to V require increasing amounts of postural support for reaching. For example, a child in level III may sit on a regular chair but may require pelvic or trunk support to facilitate arm function. A child in level IV will sit on a chair but will need adaptive seating for trunk control and better hand function. Children in level V lack independence in basic head and trunk antigravity postural control, and functional limitations in sitting are not fully compensated even with the use of adaptive equipment.

Postural deficits may result from alterations in descending control due to the early brain lesion (Leonard et al 1990, Brouwer and Ashby 1991, Gibbs et al 1999), as well as musculoskeletal constraints (Burtner et al 1998), and are different depending on the form of CP (Hadders-Algra et al 1999b). In general, the onset of directionally-specific postural trunk muscle activity in children with CP is delayed compared with the typically developing child. Deficits in the sequencing of the activity of multiple muscles have been reported, as well as the presence of high levels of antagonistic muscle coactivation (Nashner et al 1983, Brogren et al 1996, 1998, Burtner et al 1998). A primary problem in the organization of postural adjustments during reaching in children with spastic CP is a reduced capacity to modulate postural output in relation to task-specific conditions (Hadders-Algra et al 1999b).

Two distinct intervention approaches for improving postural control during movement have been proposed. In one approach, postural control and primary movements are viewed as being distinct and controlled separately. Thus, therapeutic interventions from this perspective would be directed specifically toward improving *either* postural control *or* the primary movement, without focusing simultaneously on the other component. The alternative approach argues that postural control and primary movement control are not distinct, suggesting that interventions would focus on the practice of both together rather than on one or the other in isolation (Aruin and Latash 1995, Thelen and Spencer 1998).

USE OF POSITIONING DEVICES FOR THE CHILD WITH POOR HEAD
AND TRUNK CONTROL
Adapted seating plays a significant role in the management of children with CP. Specialized seating has been used to prevent deformity and improve pulmonary function (Nwaobi and Smith 1986), speech and feeding behaviours (Hulme et al 1987a), comfort, and the use of the upper limbs (Hulme et al 1987b, Nwaobi 1987). The optimal sitting position in children with CP is still a matter of dispute with regard to seat inclination (Nwaobi 1987, Myhr and von Wendt 1991, McClenaghan et al 1992, Pope et al 1994, Hadders-Algra et al 1999b) and trunk support (McClenaghan et al 1992, Hadders-Algra et al 1999a, 1999b). Few studies have evaluated whether adaptive sitting leads to improvements in arm motor control, although a tendency to make slower reaching movements by children with severe or moderate CP when additional postural support was provided has been shown. No effect has been reported for kinematic variables describing reaching trajectory, such as the number of movement units, reach duration, or index of curvature (van der Heide et al 2005). Most of these studies report no advantage to changing the seat angle for movement precision, such as directing a light to a target with a joystick (Seeger et al 1984), or for movement smoothness (McPherson et al 1991). One study reported that an anteriorly tilted seat position resulted in decreased speed of arm movement (Nwaobi 1987). However, since seat height and the extent of thigh and foot support may affect reaching distance (Chari and Kirby 1986, Dean and Shepherd 1997), the lack of control of these factors may have introduced an important source of variability in the studies cited.

In the child with severe CP, the impact of specialized seating is variable and individual (e.g. Nwaobi 1987, Myhr and von Wendt 1993). Biomechanical anchoring and segment alignment achieved through external support reduce the number of degrees of freedom the child with severe CP needs to control. This may then free the child to focus on using the hand and upper extremity. The use of external support may, however, limit the development of intrinsic postural control in the severely affected child and result in an ongoing need for postural support. Nevertheless, extrinsic postural support may be used to manage muscle tone and improve comfort and alignment, which in turn may allow greater participation in daily activities (Hulme et al 1987a, 1987b). There is a continuing need to determine the impact of postural support systems on the reduction of impairment and disability and the increase in social participation of children with severe motor impairment.

The goal of specialized seating in the child with milder CP is to optimize body alignment so that the child can make use of the most efficient movement patterns of the arm and hand. Thus, postural stabilization is provided for positioning but not for restraining or decreasing degrees of freedom. Although biomechanical anchoring may be effective in the short term in improving arm reaching and grasping patterns, as for the child with more severe CP, use of this approach may limit the ability to improve postural control.

Arm and trunk movement patterns during reaching and grasping in typically developing children

Few studies have characterized reaching and grasping in typically developing children during early and middle childhood after the age of 3 years (although see Konczak et al 1995, 1997, Kuhtz-Buschbeck et al 1998, Schneiberg et al 2002). These studies have focused on the analysis of movement time, movement segmentation, hand trajectories, temporal aspects of interjoint coordination, head–hand coordination and joint torque (Thelen and Smith 1994, Konczak et al 1995, 1997, Savelsbergh et al 1997, Sveistrup et al, in press). Able-bodied children acquire the ability to co-regulate trunk and arm movements for functional activities over the first ten years of life, with a developmental transition period occurring between the ages of 4 and 7 years (Dellen and Kalverboer 1984, Schellekens et al 1984, Hay 1990). Maturation in descending motor tracts may partially explain the development of skilled reaching in childhood. Specifically, changes in the conduction velocity of the corticospinal tract parallel the gradual improvements in motor skills (Forssberg et al 1991, Müller and Hömberg 1992, Lemon et al 1997).

The kinematics of reaching objects placed in the midline at increasing distances from the trunk have been described for typically developing children aged 4 to 11 years (Schneiberg et al 2002). Movement variables were grouped into four categories reflecting several aspects of reaching kinematics: (1) endpoint trajectory, (2) joint excursions, (3) trunk involvement, and (4) shoulder–elbow movement coordination. These data suggested that different aspects of movement kinematics mature at different rates depending on the task studied. This is consistent with other studies measuring the maturation of different arm and hand tasks in children. For example, the attainment of mature movement patterns or behaviours is reported to occur at around age 8 for the coordination of grip and load forces during precision lifting (Forssberg et al 1991, Kuhtz-Buschbeck et al 1998), age 10 for postural control (Shumway-Cook and Woollacott 1985, Dietz 1992), and age 12 for rapid repetitive hand motions (Müller and Hömberg 1992). Analysis of the change in kinematic variables with age suggested that the maturation of some features of movement (joint excursions, timing of arm and trunk recruitment) generally occurs before others and that the differences depend on the amount of upper body movement involved in the task. In other words, movements requiring the coordination of a greater number of degrees of freedom take longer to mature.

Trunk displacement during reaching close objects, in particular, is part of an immature pattern that disappears after the age of 4 (Schneiberg et al 2002). A different pattern is observed for reaches to objects placed far from the body but still within reach. The immature pattern of large trunk displacement diminishes with age up until the age of 10, after which trunk displacement is no greater than that observed in adults.

Based on findings of arm–trunk coordination in adults, several explanations for the increased involvement of the trunk in near reaches in young typically-developing children may be suggested:

1   Young children may not be able to make appropriate or coordinated joint rotations to minimize trunk involvement due to the lack of maturation of cortical areas involved in sensorimotor integration (Kostoviç et al 1995, Paus et al 1999). This is supported by evidence of an increased dependence on vision in young children (4 years old) for precision grasping (Kuhtz-Buschbeck et al 1998), and it is reported in other studies (Hay 1979, von Hofsten and Rönnqvist 1988, Ferrel et al 2001). Hay and colleagues found that a critical period for perceptuo-motor function, particularly for visually-guided reaching, does not occur until about age 8 (Hay 1979, 1990, Fayt et al 1993).
2   The selection of an appropriate motor strategy for reaching from the vast repertoire of possible strategies occurs with practice (Sporns and Edelman 1993). It is possible that in younger children, the trunk and arm synergies are not completely separated and only after years of practice is this mature pattern established.
3   Another explanation may be the absence of mature feedforward control during reaching so that displacement of the trunk is not adequately prevented when the arm reaches towards the object (Schmitz et al 2002).

Arm and trunk movement patterns during reaching and grasping in children with CP

Several impairments of the arm and hand occur in children with CP. In general, these include weakness, sensory loss, spasticity and muscle shortening (Boyd and Graham 1997, Fehlings et al 2001). These impairments may affect the ability to perform the smooth and coordinated movements needed for successful task accomplishment. Studies have quantified the following variables to characterize reaching deficits: interjoint coordination, movement smoothness (increased number of movement units in the hand trajectory; von Hofsten 1984; Steenbergen et al 2000b, Chang et al 2005), movement speed/time (Chang et al 2005), range of joint movement and presence of compensatory trunk movement (van Thiel et al 1997).

In children with mild to moderate forms of CP, reach velocity increases with age, while there is a negative correlation between reach velocity and age in children with severe CP (van der Heide et al 2005). On the other hand, Chang et al (2005) reported no difference in reach velocity between typically developing children and children with CP, despite prolonged movement time in the latter. Children with CP also have more curved trajectories compared to 5- to 11-year-old typically developing children (Levin and Jobin 1998, van der Heide et al 2005). Reaching movements were characterized by increased trunk movement as well as a lack of smoothness, reduced interjoint coordination between movements of the shoulder and elbow (movement segmentation), decreased angular range of motion of the arm joints, impaired coordination between distal grasping and proximal reaching components, and a lack of flexibility in the selection of hand orientation for grasping (McPherson et al 1991, Steenbergen et al 2000a, 2000b, Volman et al 2002a, 2002b, van Roon et al 2004, Chang et al 2005).

In preliminary work, we have acquired pilot data on reaching movement in a task related to self-feeding in typically developing children and in children with CP. Since self-feeding behaviour begins to develop in early childhood, we compared this behaviour in the two groups of children aged 2–4. The task components analysed during transport of the hand to the food and the grasping of the food were: arm and trunk trajectories, joint angular ranges, interjoint coordination, and trunk movement. The data suggest that even though typically developing children may have accurate hand-to-mouth movement by the age of 4 (Gisel 1991), there is a tendency to use excessive trunk displacement to assist in hand transport toward the food, and to lock the movements of the arm and head to the motion of the trunk to produce a smooth hand trajectory (Fig. 7.1; Schneiberg et al 2003).

Children with mild CP use up to three times the amount of trunk displacement during reaching compared to healthy children of the same age (Fig. 7.2). This excessive use of the trunk, an extra degree of freedom, in the reaching pattern, may influence or delay the development of interjoint coordination between the joints of the reaching arm, and decrease functional reaching behaviour (Ada et al 1994, Cirstea and Levin 2000). Our studies and others of reaching, grasping and eating in children and adolescents with CP report excessive use of trunk displacement for such activities well beyond the age when isolated movements of the arm would be expected to appear in typically developing children, suggesting that trunk displacement is used to compensate for motor deficits in the arm (Van Thiel and Steenbergen 2001, Van Roon et al 2004).

Interventions to improve reaching and grasping
Recent reviews of the effectiveness of therapeutic interventions for improving hand and arm function have failed to demonstrate positive outcomes (Boyd et al 2001, Siebes et al 2002). The lack of positive outcomes could be due to several factors. Two such factors are: (1) the intervention may indeed be ineffective (in terms of approach, or duration or intensity of treatment given); or (2) the intervention may improve function but we lack adequate measurement tools to assess this improvement. Indeed, recent studies in adults and children with hemiparesis have recognized the need to provide evidence of the effectiveness of treatment interventions to improve the quality of arm and hand movement in children with cerebral palsy using objective measures (Chang et al 2005, van der Heide et al 2005).

Surprisingly few prospective studies of therapeutic interventions with objective outcome measures have been reported. Two studies of small numbers of children with spastic CP have used objective measures to quantify changes in the quality of reaching movement

114

Head and trunk rotations in the yaw direction

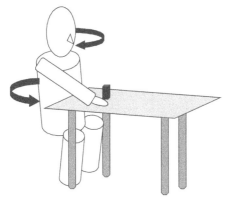

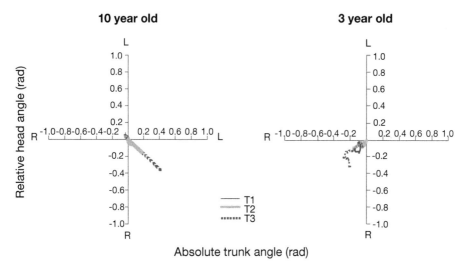

Fig. 7.1 Top: Schematic diagram of head and trunk angles in the yaw direction during reaching with the right arm to grasp a block placed at three distances from the body (T1 = two-thirds arm's length, T2 = arm's length, T3 = one and two-thirds arm's length). Target shown is T2. Bottom: Head yaw angle (relative to the trunk) and absolute trunk yaw angle (relative to space) for reaches to each target in a typically developing 10-year-old child (left) and 3-year-old (right) child. Note that the head and trunk move in opposite directions in the 10-year-old child but in the 3-year-old are locked to and move in the same direction as the reaching right arm.

following a targeted treatment intervention. Fetters and Klusik (1996) exposed eight 10- to 15-year-old children to five days of intensive training of upper limb reaching using either NDT or a motor learning approach. Movement speed was increased after reaching training but these authors concluded that at least two weeks of treatment were required for effective skill retention. Using a case-study approach, Schneiberg et al (2004) evaluated the effect

Hand and trunk trajectories

Child with CP

Typically-developing child

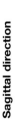

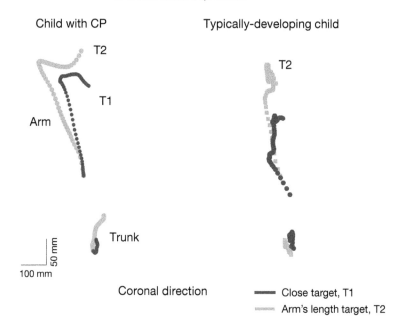

Coronal direction

—— Close target, T1

▬▬▬ Arm's length target, T2

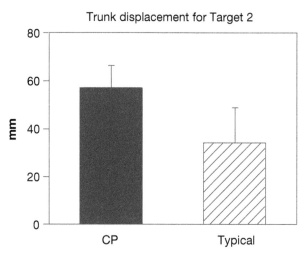

Trunk displacement for Target 2

Fig. 7.2 Hand and trunk trajectories in a 3-year-old child with CP (top left) and a typically developing child of the same age (top right) to a target placed at two-thirds arm's length (black traces, T1) and at arm's length (grey traces, T2). Bottom: Mean (SD) of trunk displacement while reaching to T2 from a group of four children with CP aged 3–5 years old (black bar) compared to nine typically developing children of the same age (hatched bar).

of three weeks of forced-use therapy in three children aged between 2 and 5 years. They found that two of the children improved on a clinical functional upper limb measure (QUEST) and that all three children improved on at least one movement characteristic. However, all three children also increased compensatory trunk movement. Generally, the lack of studies showing objective improvement in the quality of arm movement limits discussion of whether treatment interventions are of any benefit at all to the affected child.

The combination of trunk restraint with reaching and grasping training in children with CP may lead to better arm and hand function than training without limiting trunk movement. This combined treatment approach is based on previous findings that reaching and grasping performed with the affected upper limb can be improved when the child's trunk is passively supported by the therapist or by an external device (e.g. standing shell; Hirschfeld et al 2000), and findings of the benefits of trunk-restraint training in adults with hemiparesis (Michaelsen et al 2006). The excessive trunk displacement observed in adult stroke patients is thought to be compensatory because it allows the patient to bring the hand to the target fairly accurately even when active movements at the affected elbow and shoulder are restricted or impossible (Cirstea and Levin 2000, Michaelsen et al 2001).

Further evidence that the trunk plays a compensatory role in reaching stems from findings that patients who use altered strategies of trunk recruitment do not have a primary deficit in trunk control (Esparza et al 2003) and that arm extension may be improved and trunk use diminished with appropriate interventions such as guided practice (Cirstea et al 2003) and trunk restraint (Michaelsen et al 2001, 2006). Studies have also shown encouraging results such that training with physical restriction of compensatory trunk movement leads to better recovery of 'typical' movement patterns than verbal instruction alone in adults with mild to moderate hemiparesis (Michaelsen et al 2001, 2006). For example, Fig. 7.3 summarizes data on trunk anterior displacement and rotation from two groups of adults with mildly and moderately severe hemiparesis. Each group made 60 repetitions of a reaching movement to a target placed at arm's length in a single session. One group (Fig. 7.3, left) practised the movement while the trunk movement was restricted with a harness. The other group (Fig. 7.3, right) practised the same number of trials without trunk restraint but with the verbal instruction not to move their trunk. The results showed that only the group that practised with the trunk restraint had significant decreases in trunk movements along with improvements in active arm joint ranges, and that these improvements in the reaching pattern were maintained after the period of training. This study and others thus suggest that interventions that focus on decreasing motor compensations may be effective in improving arm and trunk movement patterns.

The use of restriction of excessive trunk movement as a therapy is justified for children over the age of 5, at which time trunk use is expected to decrease during reaching and grasping tasks. Training with a focus on facilitating the effective arm movement pattern while limiting compensatory movements in children with mild CP and good trunk control may lead to significantly greater improvements in arm and hand motor function than the same amount of conventional training alone for reaching and grasping objects located within the length of the arm. This is based on the idea that non-optimal sensory information in children with CP may interfere with the control of movement, as has been previously suggested

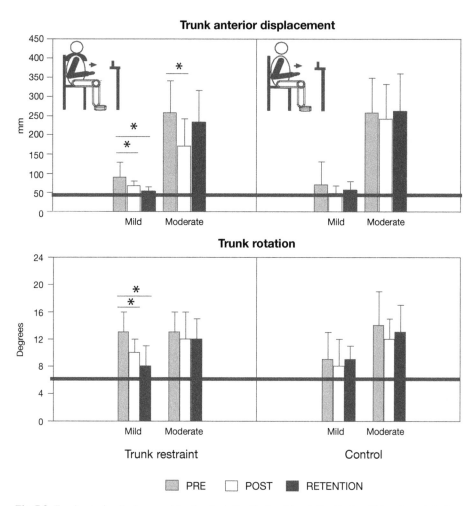

Fig. 7.3 Trunk anterior displacement (top) and rotation (bottom) in adult patients with hemiparesis before (PRE, grey bars) and after (POST, white bars) one session during which patients practised reaching to a target placed at arm's length (n = 60 trials). All measures were done in the absence of trunk restriction. One group (n = 15) practised while the trunk movement was restricted with a harness, and the other group (n = 15) practised with only the verbal instruction not to move the trunk. Data are divided according to severity of motor symptoms. The black horizontal lines indicate the values of normative data from a group of non-disabled control participants matched for age with the stroke group. Values are also shown for data recorded in a 24-hour retention test (black bars).

for deficits of posture (Nashner et al 1983, Hadders-Algra et al 1999a, 1999b) and precision grasping (Eliasson et al 1992, 1995, Gordon and Duff 1999). By restraining the excessive movements of the trunk during reaching and grasping training, more relevant somatosensory input from the arm joints can be provided and used to modulate the reaching pattern. This can be achieved in two ways: by increasing the intensity of the afferent input (Hadders-Algra et al 1999b), or by increasing the frequency of exposure to task-appropriate somatosensory information.

Conclusions

In summary, treatment approaches for the improvement of upper limb function in children with CP are numerous and varied and based on different assumptions about the maturation of the damaged nervous system and its adaptive capacity. Interpretation of the effectiveness of different interventions is often difficult, however, since treatment outcomes are often described in terms of functional task accomplishment which is in turn operationalized as the time to complete a task or the number of tasks completed (Siebes et al 2002). This type of information does not provide an understanding of movement quality (how the task was performed) and, more importantly, whether the movement was made with motor compensations. Interventions that include the restriction of motor compensations while encouraging the nervous system to find new motor solutions to task accomplishment may be more effective in improving upper limb function through the emergence of new motor patterns.

ACKNOWLEDGEMENTS

The authors would like to thank the Quebec Network of Rehabilitation Research (FRSQ) as well as the Canadian Institutes of Health Research for financial support. Mindy Levin holds a Canada Research Chair in Motor Recovery and Rehabilitation.

REFERENCES

Ada L, Canning CG, Carr JH, Kilbreath SL, Shepherd RB (1994) Task specific training of reaching and manipulation. In: Bennett KMB, Castiello U, editors, *Insights into Reach and Grasp Movement.* Amsterdam: Elsevier, pp. 239–264.

Aruin AS, Latash ML (1995) The role of motor action in anticipatory postural adjustments studied with self-induced and externally triggered perturbations. *Exp Brain Res* 106: 291–300.

Berger W, Trippel M, Assaiante C, Zijlstra W, Dietz V (1995) Developmental aspects of equilibrium control during stance: a kinematic and EMG study. *Gait Posture* 3: 149–155.

Bernstein NA (1967) *The Coordination and Regulation of Movements.* London: Pergamon Press.

Bower E (1993) Physiotherapy for cerebral palsy: a historical review. In: Ward CD, editor. *Rehabilitation of Motor Disorders. Ballière Clin Neurol* 2: 29–54.

Boyd RN, Graham HK (1997) Botulinum toxin A in the management of children with cerebral palsy: indications and outcome. *Eur J Neurol* 4 (Suppl 2): 15–22.

Boyd RN, Morris ME, Graham HK (2001) Management of upper limb dysfunction in children with cerebral palsy: a systematic review. *Eur J Neurol* 8 (Suppl 5): 150–166.

Brogren E, Hadders-Algra M, Forssberg H (1996) Postural control in children with spastic diplegia: muscle activity during perturbations in sitting. *Dev Med Child Neurol* 38: 379–388.

Brogren E, Hadders-Algra M, Forssberg H (1998) Postural control in sitting children with cerebral palsy. *Neurosci Biobehav Rev* 22: 291–596.

Brouwer B, Ashby P (1991) Altered corticospinal projections to lower limb motorneurons in subjects with cerebral palsy. *Brain* 114: 1395–1407.

Burtner PA, Qualls C, Woollacott MH (1998) Muscle activation characteristics for stance balance in children with spastic cerebral palsy. *Gait Posture* 41: 748–757.

Casimiro L, Sveistrup H (2001) Feedforward postural adjustments associated with a goal-directed reach produced by infants in the sitting and standing positions. In: Duysens J, Smits-Engelsman BCM, Kigma H, editors.

Control of Posture and Gait. Proceedings of the International Society for Posture and Gait. Brussels: Solvay, pp 22–25.

Chang JJ, Wu TI, Wu WL, Su FC (2005) Kinematical measure for spastic reaching in children with cerebral palsy. *Clin Biomech* 20: 381–388.

Chari VR. Kirby RL (1986) Lower-limb influence on sitting balance while reaching forward. *Arch Phys Med Rehabil* 67: 730–733.

Cirstea MC, Levin MF (2000) Compensatory strategies for reaching in stroke. *Brain* 123: 940–953.

Cirstea MC, Ptito A, Levin MF (2003) Arm reaching improvements with short-term practice depend on the severity of the motor deficit in stroke. *Exp Brain Res* 152: 476–488.

Darrah JD (1997) Clinical reasoning: management of a child with cerebral palsy – comparison of neurodevelopmental and dynamic systems approaches. In: Clinical Reasoning Symposium booklet disseminated at Physical Therapy '97: American Physical Therapy Association. 30 May–2 June. San Diego, CA.

Dean CM, Shepherd RB (1997) Task-related training improves performance of seated reaching tasks after stroke. A randomized controlled trial. *Stroke* 28: 722–728.

Dellen T van, Kalverboer AF (1984) Single movement control and information processing, a developmental study. *Behav Brain Res* 12: 237–238.

Dietz V (1992) Human neuronal control of automatic functional movements: interaction between central program and afferent input. *Physiol Rev* 7: 33–69.

Eliasson AC, Gordon AM, Forssberg H (1992) Impaired anticipatory control of isometric forces during grasping by children with cerebral palsy. *Dev Med Child Neurol* 33: 216–225.

Eliasson AC, Gordon AM, Forssberg H (1995) Tactile control of isometric finger forces during grasping in children with cerebral palsy. *Dev Med Child Neurol* 37: 72–84.

Esparza DY, Archambault P, Winstein CL, Levin MF (2003) Hemispheric specialization in the coordination of arm and trunk movements during pointing in patients with unilateral brain damage. *Exp Brain Res* 148: 488–497.

Fayt C, Minet M, Schepens N (1993) Children's and adults' learning of a visuomanual coordination: role of ongoing visual feedback and of spatial errors as a function of age. *Percept Motor Skills* 77: 659–669.

Fehlings D, Rang M, Glazier J, Steele C (2001) Botulinum toxin type A injections in the spastic upper extremity of children with hemiplegia: child characteristics that predict a positive outcome. *Eur J Neurol* 8 (Suppl 5): 145–149.

Ferrel C, Bard C, Fleury M (2001) Coordination in childhood: modifications of visuomotor representations in 6- to 11-year-old children. *Exp Brain Res* 138: 313–321.

Fetters L, Klusik J (1996) The effects of neurodevelopmental treatment versus practice on the reaching of children with spastic cerebral palsy. *Phys Ther* 76: 346–358.

Forssberg H, Nashner LM (1982) Ontogenetic development of postural control in man: adaptation to altered support and visual conditions during stance. *J Neurosci* 2: 545–552.

Forssberg H, Eliasson AC, Kinoshita H, Johansson RS, Westling G (1991) Development of human precision grip. I. Basic coordination of force. *Exp Brain Res* 85: 451–457.

Gibbs J, Harrison LM, Stephens JA, Evans AL (1999) Cutaneomuscular reflex responses recorded from the lower limb in children and adolescents with cerebral palsy. *Dev Med Child Neurol* 41: 456–464.

Gibson JJ (1979) *The Ecological Approach to Visual Perception.* Boston, MA: Houghton-Mifflin.

Gisel EG (1991) Effect of food textures on the development of chewing in children 6 months to 2 years of age. *Dev Med Child Neurol* 33: 69–79.

Gordon AM, Duff SV (1999) Fingertip forces during object manipulation in children with hemiplegic cerebral palsy. 1. Anticipatory scaling. *Dev Med Child Neurol* 41: 166–175.

Guralnick MJ, editor (1997) *The Effectiveness of Early Intervention: Second Generation Research.* Baltimore, MD: Paul H. Brookes.

Hadders-Algra M, Brogren E, Forssberg H (1996) Ontogeny of postural adjustments during sitting in infancy: variation, selection and modulation. *J Physiol* 493: 273–288.

Hadders-Algra M, Brogren E, Forssberg H (1998) Postural adjustments during sitting at pre-school age: presence of a transient toddling phase. *Dev Med Child Neurol* 40: 436–447.

Hadders-Algra M, van der Fits IBM, Stremmelaar EF, Brogren E (1999a) Periventricular leukomalacia and preterm birth have a detrimental effect on postural adjustments. *Brain* 122: 727–740.

Hadders-Algra M, van der Fits IBM, Stremmelaar EF, Touwen BCL (1999b) Development of postural adjustments during reaching in infants with cerebral palsy. *Dev Med Child Neurol* 41: 766–776.

Hay L (1979) Spatial-temporal analysis of movements in children: motor programs versus feedback in the development of reaching. *J Mot Behav* 11: 189–200.

Hay L (1990) Developmental changes in eye–hand coordination behaviors: preprogramming versus feedback control. In: Bard C, Fleury M, Hay L, editors. *Development of Eye–Hand Coordination across the Lifespan.* Columbia, SC: University of South Carolina Press, pp. 217–244.

Hirschfeld H, Apel I, Isaksson E (2000) Compensating impaired standing postural orientation in cerebral palsy with a standing shell improves voluntary reaching. *Soc Neurosci Abstr* 61.15.

Hoare B, Wasiak J (2005) Constraint induced movement therapy in the treatment of the upper limb in children with spastic hemiplegic cerebral palsy. *Cochrane Database of Systematic Reviews* 4.

Horak FB (1992) Motor control models underlying neurologic rehabilitation of posture in children. In: Forssberg H, Hirschfeld H, editors. *Movement Disorders in Children.* Basel, Switzerland: Karger, pp. 21–30.

Hulme JB, Shaver J, Archer S, Mullette L, Eggert C (1987a) Effects of adaptive seating devices on eating and drinking of children with cerebral palsy. *Am J Occ Ther* 41: 81–89.

Hulme JB, Gallagher T, Walsh J, Niesen S, Waldron D (1987b) Behavioral and postural changes observed with use of adaptive seating by clients with multiple handicaps. *Phys Ther* 67: 1060–1067.

Hur JJ (1995) Review of research on therapeutic interventions for children with cerebral palsy. *Acta Neurol Scand* 91: 423–432.

Kelso JAS (1995) *Dynamic Patterns: The Self-organization of Brain and Behavior.* Cambridge, MA: MIT Press.

Ketelaar M, Vermeer A, Helders PJM (1998) Functional motor abilities of children with cerebral palsy – a systematic literature review of assessment measures. *Clin Rehabil* 12: 369–380.

Ketelaar M, Vermeer A, Hart H, van Petegem-van Beek E, Helders PJM (2001) Effects of functional therapy program on motor abilities in children with cerebral palsy. *Phys Ther* 81: 1534–1545.

Kirshenbaum N, Riach CL, Starkes JL (2001) Non-linear development of postural control. *Exp Brain Res* 140: 420–431.

Knox V, Evans AL (2002) Evaluation of the functional effects of a course of Bobath therapy in children with cerebral palsy: a preliminary study. *Dev Med Child Neurol* 44: 447–460.

Konczak J, Borutta M, Topka H, Dichgans J (1995) The development of goal-directed reaching in infants: hand trajectory formation and joint torque control. *Exp Brain Res* 106: 156?168.

Konczak J, Borutta M, Dichgans J (1997) The development of goal-directed reaching in infants II: Learning to produce task-adequate patterns of joint torque. *Exp Brain Res* 113: 465?474.

Kostoviç I, Juda‰ M, Petanjek Z, ·imié G (1995) Ontogenesis of goal-directed behavior: anatomo-functional considerations. *Int J Psychophysiol* 19: 85?102

Kuhtz-Buschbeck JP, Stolze H, Joehnk K, Boczek-Funke A, Illert M (1998) Development of prehension movements in children: a kinematic study. *Exp Brain Res* 122: 424–432.

Latash ML, Anson JG (1996) What are 'normal movements' in atypical populations? *Behav Brain Sci* 19: 55–106.

Lemon RN, Armand J, Olivier E, Edgley SA (1997) Skilled action and the development of the corticospinal tract in primates. In: Connolly KJ, Forssberg H, editors. *Neurophysiology and Neuropsychology of Motor Development.* Clinics in Developmental Medicine 143/144. London: Mac Keith Press.

Leonard CT, Moritani T, Hirschfeld H, Forssberg H (1990) Deficits in reciprocal inhibition of children with cerebral palsy as revealed by H reflex testing. *Dev Med Child Neurol* 32: 974–984.

Levin MF, Jobin A (1998) Movement segmentation during reaching in children with cerebral palsy. *Can J Rehabil* 11: 215–216.

Liao SF, Yang TF, Hsu TC, Chan RC, Wei TS (2003) Differences in seated postural control in children with spastic cerebral palsy and children who are typically developing. *Am J Phys Med Rehabil* 82: 622–626.

McClenaghan BA, Thombs L, Milner M (1992) Effects of seat surface inclination on postural stability and function of the upper extremities of children with cerebral palsy. *Dev Med Child Neurol* 34: 40–48.

McPherson JJ, Schild R, Spaulding SJ, Barsamian P, Transon C, White SC (1991) Analysis of upper extremity movement in four sitting positions: a comparison of persons with and without cerebral palsy. *Am J Occ Ther* 45: 123–129.

Michaelsen SM, Luta A, Roby-Brami A, Levin MF (2001) Effect of trunk restraint on the recovery of reaching movements in hemiparetic patients. *Stroke* 32: 1875–1883.

Michaelsen SM, Dannenbaum R, Levin MF (2006) Task-specific training with trunk restraint on arm recovery in stroke. Randomised control trial. *Stroke* 37: 186–192.

Müller K, Hömberg V (1992) Development of speed of repetitive movements in children is determined by structural changes in corticospinal efferents. *Neurosci Lett* 144: 57–60.

Myhr U, von Wendt L (1991) Improvement of functional sitting position for children with cerebral palsy. *Dev Med Child Neurol* 33: 246–256.

Myhr U, von Wendt L (1993) Influence of different sitting positions and abduction orthoses on leg muscle activity in children with cerebral palsy. *Dev Med Child Neurol* 35: 870–880.

Nashner LM, Shumway-Cook A, Marin O (1983) Stance postural control in select groups of children with cerebral palsy: deficits in sensory organization and muscular organization. *Exp Brain Res* 49: 393–409.

Nwaobi OM (1987) Seating orientation and upper extremity function in children with cerebral palsy. *Phys Ther* 67: 1209–1212.

Nwaobi OM, Smith PD (1986) Effect of adaptive seating on pulmonary function of children with cerebral palsy. *Dev Med Child Neurol* 28: 351–354.

Palisano R, Rosenbaum P, Walter S, Russell D, Wood E, Galuppi B (1997) Development and reliability of a system to classify gross motor function in children with cerebral palsy. *Dev Med Child Neurol* 39: 214–223.

Paus T, Zijdenbos A, Worsley K, Collins DL, Blumenthal J, Giedd JN, Rapoport JL, Evans AC (1999) Structural maturation of neural pathways in children and adolescents: in vivo study. *Science* 283: 1908–1911.

Piper MC, Darrah J (1984) *Motor Assessment of the Developing Infant.* Philadelphia, PA: W.B. Saunders Co.

Pope PM, Bowes CE, Booth E (1994) Postural control in stitting. The SAM system: evaluation of use over three years. *Dev Med Child Neurol* 38: 241–252.

Royeen CB, DeGangi GA (1992) Use of neurodevelopmental treatment as an intervention: annotated listing of studies 1980–1990. *Percept Motor Skills* 75: 175–194.

Savelsbergh G, von Hofsten C, Jonsson B (1997) The coupling of head, reach and grasp movement in nine months old infant prehension. *Scand J Psych* 38: 325–333.

Schellekens JMH, Kalverboer AF, Scholten CA (1984) The microstructure of tapping movements in children. *J Mot Behav* 16: 20–39.

Schmitz C, Martin N, Assaiante C (2002) Building anticipatory adjustment during childhood: a kinematic and electromyographic analysis of unloading in children from 4 to 8 years of age. *Exp Brain Res* 142: 354–364.

Schneiberg S, Sveistrup H, McFadyen B, McKinley P, Levin MF (2002) The development of coordination for reach-to-grasp movements in children. *Exp Brain Res* 146: 142–154.

Schneiberg S, Chen P, Sveistrup H, McKinley P, McFadyen BJ, Levin MF (2003) Head and trunk coordination during reach to grasp movement in children. *Progress in Motor Control IV*, Caen, France, August.

Schneiberg S, Lamarre C, Bibeau A, Gendron S, Bilodeau N, Levin MF (2004) Kinematic patterns during reach and grasp movement in children with mild cerebral palsy before and after constraint induced therapy (CIT). American Academy of Cerebral Palsy and Developmental Medicine, Los Angeles, September.

Seeger BR, Caudry DJ, O'Mara NA (1984) Hand function in cerebral palsy: the effect of hip-flexion angle. *Dev Med Child Neurol* 26: 601–606.

Shepherd RB (1995) *Physiotherapy in Paediatrics.* Oxford: Butterworth/Heinemann.

Shumway-Cook A, Woollacott MH (1985) The growth of stability: postural control from a developmental perspective. *J Mot Behav* 17: 131–147.

Siebes R, Wijnroks L, Vermeer A (2002) Qualitative analysis of therapeutic motor intervention programs for children with cerebral palsy: an update. *Dev Med Child Neurol* 44: 593–603.

Sporns O, Edelman GM (1993) Solving Bernstein's problem: a proposal for the development of coordinated movement by selection. *Child Dev* 64: 960–981.

Steenbergen B, Hulstijn W, Dortmans S (2000a) Constraints on grip selection in cerebral palsy. Minimizing discomfort. *Exp Brain Res* 134: 385–397.

Steenbergen B, van Thiel E, Hulstijn W, Meulenbroek RGJ (2000b) The coordination of reaching and grasping in spastic hemiparesis. *Hum Mov Sci* 19: 75–105.

Steultjens EMJ, Dekker J, Bouter LM, van de Nes JCM, Lambregts BLM, van den Ende CHM (2004) Occupational therapy for children with cerebral palsy: a systematic review. *Clin Rehabil* 18: 1–14.

Sveistrup H, Schneiberg S, McKinley PM, McFadyen BJ, Levin MF (2008) Head, arm and trunk coordination during reaching in children. *Exp Brain Res*, in press.

Taub E, Landesman Ramey S, DeLuca S, Echols K (2004) Efficacy of constraint-induced movement therapy for children with cerebral palsy with asymmetric motor impairment. *Pediatrics* 113: 305–312.

Thelen E (1995) Motor development: a new synthesis. *Am Psychol* 50: 79–95.

Thelen E, Smith LB (1994) *A Dynamic Systems Approach to the Development of Cognition and Action.* Cambridge, MA: MIT Press.

Thelen E, Spencer JP (1998) Postural control during reaching in young infants: a dynamic systems approach. *Neurosci Biobehav Rev* 22: 507–514.

van der Fits IBM, Klip AWJ, van Eykern LA, Hadders-Algra M (1999a) Postural adjustments during spontaneous and goal-directed arm movements in the first half year of life. *Behav Brain Res* 106: 75–90.

122

van der Fits IBM, Otten E, Klip AWJ, van Eykern LA, Hadders-Algra M (1999b) The development of postural adjustments during reaching in 6- to 18-month-old infants: evidence for two transitions. *Exp Brain Res* 126: 517–528.

van der Heide JC, Otten B, van Eykern LA, Hadders-Algra M (2003) Development of postural adjustments during reaching in sitting children. *Exp Brain Res* 151: 32–45.

van der Heide JC, Fock JM, Otten B, Stremmelaar E, Hadders-Algra M (2005) Kinematic characteristics of reaching movements in preterm children with cerebral palsy. *Ped Res* 57: 883–889.

van Roon D, Steenbergen B, Meulenbroek RGJ (2004) Trunk recruitment during spoon use in tetraparetic cerebral palsy. *Exp Brain Res* 155: 186–195.

van Thiel E, Steenbergen B (2001) Shoulder and hand displacements during hitting, reaching, and grasping movements in hemiparetic cerebral palsy. *Motor Control* 5: 166–182.

van Thiel E, Steenbergen B, Meulebroek RGJ, Hulstijn W (1997) Arm trajectory formation in spastic hemiparesis: a pilot study on shoulder displacement and end-effector paths. In: Colla AM, Masulli F, Morasso P, editors. *Proceedings of the International Graphonomics Society*, Vol 8. Nijmegen: IGS, pp. 47–48.

Volman MJM, Wijnroks A, Vermeer A (2002a) Effect of task context on reaching performance in children with spastic hemiparesis. *Clin Rehabil* 16: 684–692.

Volman MJM, Wijnroks A, Vermeer A (2002b) Bimanual circle drawing in children with spastic hemiparesis: effect of coupling modes on the performance of the impaired and unimpaired arms. *Acta Psychol* 110: 339–356.

von Hofsten C (1984) Developmental changes in the organization of prereaching movements. *Dev Psychol* 20: 378–388.

von Hofsten C, Rönnqvist L (1988) Preparation for grasping an object: a developmental study. *J Exp Psychol* 14: 610–621.

von Hofsten C, Woollacott MH (1989) Postural preparations for reaching in 9-month-old infants. *Neurosci Abstracts* 15: 1199.

Wagenaar RC, van Emmerik REA, editors (1996) Dynamics of movement disorders. *Hum Mov Sci* 15 (Special Issue).

8
VISUAL IMPAIRMENT AND CONSEQUENCES FOR HAND FUNCTION

Eugenio Mercuri, Andrea Guzzetta and Giovanni Cioni

Introduction

As a result of increased knowledge on how to assess various aspects of visual function in infants and young children, in the last decades there has been increasing attention dedicated to the co-occurrence of visual, perceptual and motor impairment in children with brain lesions (Guzzetta et al 2001c). While previous studies mainly reported the prevalence of blindness or severe visual impairment in patients with cerebral palsy, more recent studies have highlighted that various aspects of visual function can be impaired even if there is no severe visual impairment (van Hof-van Duin et al 1998, Mercuri et al 2003, 2004). Abnormal visual fields, visual attention or stereopsis or inability to discriminate movements or colours for example may not produce blindness *per se* but can have a strong impact on the maturation of several aspects of neurodevelopment, such as eye and hand coordination, reaching, or balance (Mercuri et al 1999, Cioni et al 2000). Most of these aspects of visual function can be assessed in the first months after birth (see Atkinson 2000 for a review), but a more comprehensive assessment can be performed in the following months/years, as soon as more cortical aspects of visual function, such as processing more structured visual information or visual attention, become more mature.

Visual disorders in infants and children with brain lesions and cerebral palsy

Using an integrated clinical and imaging approach, a few studies have shown that the prevalence and the severity of visual impairment in the different types of cerebral palsy mainly reflect the extent of brain lesions (Ipata et al 1994, Guzzetta et al 2001a). Blindness and severe visual impairment are more often associated with the most severe forms of cerebral palsy, i.e. spastic or dystonic tetraplegia, and these are generally found in full-term infants with diffuse white matter and cortical damage associated with severe damage of the basal ganglia and thalami, and in preterm infants with cystic periventricular or subcortical leukomalacia (Ipata et al 1994, Mercuri et al 1997, 1999, Cioni et al 2000, Fazzi et al 2004).

Less severe and often isolated abnormalities of specific aspects of visual function are, in contrast, more often associated with less severe forms of cerebral palsy, such as hemiplegia (Fig. 8.1) or diplegia, generally found in full-term infants with more focal brain lesions or with diffuse white matter changes not associated with basal ganglia damage (Ipata et al 1994, Mercuri et al 1996, Guzzetta et al 2001b), and in preterm infants with intraventricular haemorrhage and less severe cystic periventricular leukomalacia (Cioni et al

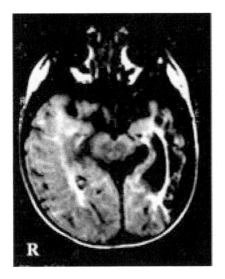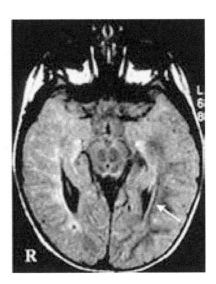

Fig. 8.1 (left) FLAIR axial MR image of child with congenital hemiplegia, reduced visual acuity, absent OKN, and narrowed right field. Large left encephalomalacic lesion involving temporo-occipital cortex and white matter, extending to periventricular regions and optic radiations with cystic and gliotic components. Note left ventricular enlargement and hemispheric hypoplasia, right periatrial white matter involvement. (right) Axial SE T2 MR image of another child with congenital hemiplegia, who had normal acuity, OKN and visual fields. Mild white matter gliosis near the right ventricular wall, involving the optic radiation area, with mild atrial enlargement. Optic radiations are identified on the left by the white arrow.

Source: Guzzetta et al 2001b (modified).

1997, Lanzi et al 1998). In the latter group, the specific location of white matter damage may often give rise to a defect of the lower part of the visual fields (Jacobson et al 2006). This particular type of disorder can significantly contribute to the difficulties children with diplegia experience in walking, especially when walking on irregular ground or when there are obstacles in their way (Dutton et al 2006). At school age, more complex visuo-perceptual disorders can frequently be detected, including abnormal saccadic movements and visual scanning (Fedrizzi et al 1998).

The incidence of visual disorders in children with hemiplegia varies among the different studies, and may reach about three-quarters of cases (Fig. 8.2). Following evidence from studies in adults with acquired hemiplegia, most studies have mainly focused on the assessment of visual fields in school-age patients and only a few recent studies have carried out a wider assessment. These studies suggest that abnormalities of various aspects of visual function are frequent in both children with congenital hemiplegia and those with early-acquired hemiplegia. Acuity is generally normal, while visual fields, visual attention and optokinetic nystagmus (OKN) are more often abnormal, with approximately 80 per cent of children having abnormal results on at least one of these tests (Mercuri et al 1996, Guzzetta et al 2001b). As one would expect, visual fields are often impaired and hemianopia or visual field defects are generally associated with abnormal optic radiations and occipital cortex on brain imaging. In contrast, and contrary to what is observed in adults after a stroke or in

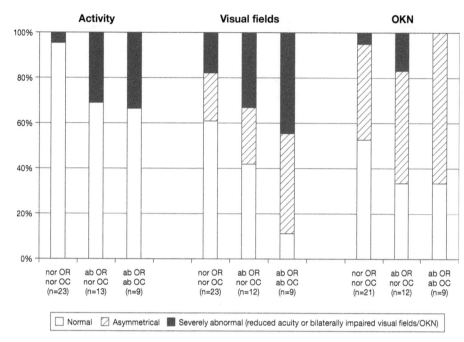

Fig. 8.2 Incidence of abnormal results of visual tests according to visual cortex and optic radiation involvement in 47 children with congenital or early-acquired hemiplegic cerebral palsy.

Source: Guzzetta et al 2001b.

preterm infants with periventricular leukomalacia (Cioni et al 1997), visual fields are often normal in children with involvement of the optic radiations but not of the occipital cortex (see also Fig. 8.1, right), suggesting possible brain plasticity of the immature brain (Guzzetta et al 2001b). OKN abnormalities are also frequent and consist of a directional asymmetrical binocular OKN, with an impairment in the direction towards the predominantly affected hemisphere.

The variability has been thought to reflect differences in the timing of the insult, as previously reported in studies on motor and cognitive difficulties (Cioni et al 1999), but a systematic study from our group has shown that the presence and pattern of visual abnormalities cannot always be predicted by the timing of the insult or the type of lesion observed on MRI (Steinlin et al 1993, Cioni et al 1999).

Finally, children with ataxic CP and cerebellar lesions often have abnormal eye movements, mainly nystagmus, which, when severe, may affect the ability to fix images on the retina and affect visual function and therefore further impair the ability to reach for objects or eye and hand coordination, which are already affected by the ataxic movements (Ipata et al 1994). The high prevalence of visual impairment in cerebral palsy is of great importance for understanding and treating fine manipulation difficulties in these children.

Vision and manipulation in normal development and cerebral palsy

The prominent role of visual guidance in the maturation of hand action and manipulation is now well recognized (Henderson and Pehoski 2006). The linkage between somatosensory perception and vision is considered essential for constructing an accurate representation of the objects in space and for acting in relation to them. This is suggested, for instance, by the observation that early manipulation is more likely to occur and is more refined when the infant simultaneously looks at the manipulated object (Rochat 1989), and it is indirectly suggested by the marked delay in the use of the hands as exploratory tools observed in congenitally blind infants (Fraiberg 1977). The role of vision in the construction of reaching movements is even more straightforward. However, in the context of normal development, it is of interest how visual information can be gradually replaced with other sensory inputs, as shown, for example, by the successful reaching for sounding objects in the dark, already observed in normal 7-month-old infants (Clifton et al 1994). The same 'visual dominance' at the stage of motor learning has been described for head or trunk control in sitting and standing (Shumway-Cook and Woollacott 1985, Woollacott et al 1987, Sundermier and Woollacott 1998). Children have to rely more on visual information when they are at the stage of learning, but much less in the mature phase of postural control, when visual dominance disappears and children are able to accurately integrate multiple sensory inputs.

A few studies have tried to disentangle the specific role of vision in early development of manipulation and reaching by following their maturation in infants with congenital ocular abnormalities, such as cataract or retinal dystrophy (Fraiberg 1977, Warren 1984, Prechtl et al 2001, Fazzi et al 2002). A similar approach, however, cannot be easily used in children with neurological disorders, because of the concomitant general multisensory and motor impairment which generates a far more complex picture in terms of functional damage and reorganization processes. This is further complicated by the extreme inter-subject variability in neurological populations in terms of both structural and functional damage.

Some evidence of the crucial role of early visual development in hand function has been provided by longitudinal studies comparing early assessment of visual functions and later neurodevelopmental outcome in newborns with perinatal brain lesions. In term infants with hypoxic-ischaemic encephalopathy, visual function was found to be significantly correlated to outcome, and in particular to eye–hand coordination tasks (Mercuri et al 1999). A similar correlation was also found in preterm infants with periventricular brain damage in a study which also reported how, using multivariate analysis, visual impairment was more effective than motor disability score and extent of the lesion in determining the neurodevelopmental outcome (Cioni et al 2000). The strongest correlation coefficients were found with the eye–hand coordination subscores of the Griffiths scale, specifically assessing visually-guided hand tasks. More recently, eye–hand coordination skills have also been found to be very sensitive to transient disruption of brain function, as expressed by early-onset epileptic disorders (mainly West syndrome occurring in the first year), either in association or not with underlying brain lesions (Guzzetta et al 2002, Rando et al 2004).

Visual ventral/dorsal stream and motor action

The studies reported above have not only helped us to understand the extent to which visual impairment is associated with motor impairment in children with CP but have also indicated the role of different cortical and subcortical structures in various aspects of vision. The use of invasive electrophysiological studies in non-human primates and the improvements in functional neuroimaging in man have further increased our understanding of the anatomical structures and the mechanisms by which visual processing and action are interrelated. The transformation of visual information in a motor action requires not only the integrity of the 'classical' visual pathway and of the primary visual cortex but also that of an extended network involving other structures (Ungerleider and Mishkin 1982, Goodale and Milner 1992). In particular, the parietal cortex with its extensive connections to the visual cortex on the one side and to the premotor cortex on the other has been indicated to have a crucial role in the visual control of action (see Culham and Valyear 2006 for a review).

Experimental studies have shown that the parietal cortex is involved in the two basic motor processes that are responsible for the act of prehension under visual guidance: the reaching phase in which the arm moves towards the object (Connolly et al 2003), and the grasping phase in which the hand is adapted to the object to be grasped (Castiello 2005). The degree of segregation between the functions of reaching and grasping, however, is still only partially understood. Since the first description by Goodale and Milner (1992), who emphasized the pragmatic role in action control of the dorsal stream, i.e. the occipito-parieto visual pathway, several papers have tried to provide explanations of the role of the dorsal stream. In a recent review, on the basis of new anatomical data Rizzolatti and Matelli (2003) have suggested that the dorsal stream and its parietal areas form two distinct functional systems: the ventro-dorsal stream (v-d stream), responsible for space perception and action organization, and the dorso-dorsal stream (d-d stream), devoted to the 'on line' control of actions. The more dorsal parieto-frontal circuit, which involves the superior parietal lobule (SPL) and the dorsal premotor cortex (PMd), would be essential in controlling reaching movements; the ventral parieto-frontal circuit, involving the inferior parietal lobule (IPL) and the ventral premotor cortex (PMv), would be more involved in controlling grasping movements (Jeannerod et al 1995, Wise et al 1997). At this level, i.e. the IPL, and in par-ticular in the anterior intraparietal area (AIP), the computations of object properties for grasping and hand preshaping take place, independently from the ventral stream which is devoted to object recognition unrelated to motor action.

Despite having a certain degree of segregation, the two systems of grasping and reaching still show some overlap and interaction, both at the anatomical and at the functional level. Clear support for this view comes from neurological studies on individuals with posterior parietal lesions suffering from optic ataxia, a disorder of visually guided movements of the arms toward a goal, in which impairment of both reaching and grasping is usually observed (Perenin and Vighetto 1988).

It is therefore possible to formulate two statements: first, the ventral stream appears to be not essential in the act of prehension, even in the phase of grasping which requires a certain processing of the form of the object, as the dorsal stream (area AIP) is independently able to process the shape, size and orientation of three-dimensional objects (Culham et al

2003). Second, the functions of grasping and reaching show a partial degree of anatomical segregation within the dorsal stream, with a more dorsal parieto-frontal circuit primarily involved in reaching and a ventral parieto-frontal circuit mainly involved in grasping (Jeannerod et al 1995, Wise et al 1997).

Visual ventral/dorsal stream disorders in children

A further contribution to our understanding of the neurophysiological bases of prehension comes from the literature on individuals with brain lesions (Perenin and Vighetto 1988, Karnath and Perenin 2005). Most of the studies, however, have dealt with very localized lesions in adults, and much less has been reported on the possible effects of similar lesions of the dorsal stream in children in whom discrete and localized brain damage to the parietal cortex may be partly compensated for by reorganization of the immature nervous system. This is possibly the reason why, for instance, a clear picture of optic ataxia has never been reported following early brain damage. Furthermore, in children, even when more diffuse brain damage involving the occipito-parietal pathway is present, deficits in action control are usually attributed to impairment of the primary sensory-motor system, which cannot always be disentangled from possible deficits of visuo-motor transformation in the dorsal stream. Finally, assessment of extrastriatal visual functions requires a high degree of cooperation, which is not always easy to achieve in children, especially when they are suffering from developmental delay, often associated with learning disability or attentional deficits.

Because of these difficulties, a very limited number of studies have been performed so far exploring dorsal stream function in children with early brain damage, although there have been some attempts to assess dorsal stream-related functions in children with developmental disabilities. In particular, in three well-defined developmental disorders the dorsal stream has been extensively explored and found to be specifically impaired, i.e. Williams syndrome (Atkinson et al 1997, Nakamura et al 2001, Paul et al 2002, Atkinson et al 2003, Mendes et al 2005, Atkinson et al 2006), dyslexia (Felmingham and Jakobson 1995, Talcott et al 2000, Stein 2001) and autism (Spencer et al 2000, Bertone et al 2005, Pellicano et al 2005).

Our group has reported significant impairment of motion coherence thresholds, a dorsal stream-related function, in a group of children with congenital brain damage and hemiplegia, which was apparently unrelated to the site of damage (Gunn et al 2002), suggesting a more general vulnerability of the dorsal stream in these patients (Fig. 8.3). More recently, using a different type of coherent motion stimulus based on optic flow, we have also found a similar pattern of response in children with periventricular leukomalacia, a form of bilateral white matter damage typical of preterm infants (Morrone et al 2008). In cohorts with similar characteristics, vulnerability of the dorsal stream has also been suggested on the basis of visual perceptual tasks and brain MRI (Fazzi et al 2004, Jacobson et al 2006).

In the light of these studies, a series of possible dorsal stream-related dysfunctions in children with brain damage have been proposed, such as inaccurate visually guided reach (reaching beyond an object), or abnormal perception of the height of the ground ahead at floor boundaries, suggesting for each some possible therapeutic interventions (Dutton 2003). The possible correlation between dorsal stream function and constructive abilities was

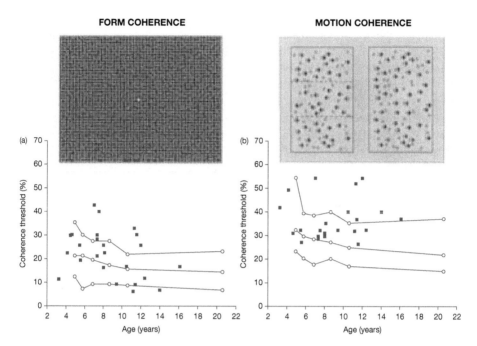

Fig. 8.3 Form and motion coherence thresholds in children with hemiplegia, plotted as a function of age. Individual children are represented by solid squares. Lines indicate performance of the 10th, 50th and 90th percentiles from the normal control groups

Source: Gunn et al 2002.

recently suggested by the observation, in a group of children with hemiplegia, of a significant correlation between motion thresholds and the block design test, in which children are required to put together red-and-white blocks according to a displayed model (Fig. 8.4).

These dysfunctions may in some cases be very subtle, only becoming apparent in particular conditions. This was, for instance, the case with GB, a young child affected with mild diplegia, with specific impairment of translational motion, who manifested some specific difficulties with a driving simulation video-game, which could be potentially harmful in the case of non-simulated driving. He showed very good ability in driving the car through the streets at various simulated car speeds, but he experienced difficulties with other driving actions, such as stopping the car before an obstacle crossing the street. This problem was not just a question of a delay in reaction times, as demonstrated by the fast arresting responses he presented in relation to non-moving stimuli (Morrone et al 2008).

In conclusion, the data presented in this chapter illustrate how a combined approach using new tools, including functional MRI, electrophysiology and specific psychophysical tests, has increased our knowledge on the specific contribution of visual disorders in the impairment of upper limb and hand function in children, and on the mechanisms underlying the tight link between these two functions. A number of questions still remain unanswered,

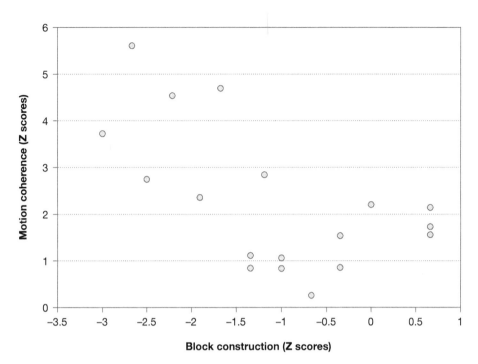

Fig. 8.4 Significant correlation (p < 0.05) between motion coherence thresholds and block construction task in a group of children with congenital hemiplegia and normal cognitive level.

and it is hoped that new research will contribute to clarify the mechanisms of compensation and reorganization of both visual and manual functions following early brain damage, and the best therapeutic windows for early intervention.

REFERENCES

Atkinson J (2000) *The Developing Visual Brain*. Oxford: Oxford University Press.

Atkinson J, King J, Braddick O, Nokes L, Anker S, Braddick F (1997) A specific deficit of dorsal stream function in Williams syndrome. *Neuroreport* 8: 1919–1922.

Atkinson J, Braddick O, Anker S, Curran W, Andrew R, Wattam-Bell J, Braddick F (2003) Neurobiological models of visuospatial cognition in children with Williams syndrome: measures of dorsal-stream and frontal function. *Dev Neuropsychol* 23: 139–172.

Atkinson J, Braddick O, Rose FE, Searcy YM, Wattam-Bell J, Bellugi U (2006) Dorsal-stream motion processing deficits persist into adulthood in Williams syndrome. *Neuropsychologia* 44: 828–833.

Bertone A, Mottron L, Jelenic P, Faubert J (2005) Enhanced and diminished visuo-spatial information processing in autism depends on stimulus complexity. *Brain* 128: 2430–2441.

Castiello U (2005) The neuroscience of grasping. *Nat Rev Neurosci* 6: 726–736.

Cioni G, Fazzi B, Coluccini M, Bartalena L, Boldrini A, van Hof-van Duin J (1997) Cerebral visual impairment in preterm infants with periventricular leukomalacia. *Pediatr Neurol* 17: 331–338.

Cioni G, Sales B, Paolicelli PB, Petacchi E, Scusa MF, Canapicchi R (1999) MRI and clinical characteristics of children with hemiplegic cerebral palsy. *Neuropediatrics* 30: 249–255.

Cioni G, Bertuccelli B, Boldrini A, Canapicchi R, Fazzi B, Guzzetta A, Mercuri E (2000) Correlation between visual function, neurodevelopmental outcome, and magnetic resonance imaging findings in infants with periventricular leucomalacia. *Arch Dis Child Fetal Neonatal Ed* 82: F134–F140.

131

Clifton RK, Rochat P, Robin DJ, Berthier NE (1994) Multimodal perception in the control of infant reaching. *J Exp Psychol Hum Percept Perform* 20: 876–886.

Connolly JD, Andersen RA, Goodale MA (2003) FMRI evidence for a 'parietal reach region' in the human brain. *Exp Brain Res* 153: 140–145.

Culham JC, Valyear KF (2006) Human parietal cortex in action. *Curr Opin Neurobiol* 16: 205–212.

Culham JC, Danckert SL, DeSouza JF, Gati JS, Menon RS, Goodale MA (2003) Visually guided grasping produces fMRI activation in dorsal but not ventral stream brain areas. *Exp Brain Res* 153: 180–189.

Dutton GN (2003) Cognitive vision, its disorders and differential diagnosis in adults and children: knowing where and what things are. *Eye* 17: 289–304.

Dutton GN, McKillop ECA, Saidkasimova S (2006) Visual problems as a result of brain damage in children. *Br J Ophthalmol* 90: 932–933.

Fazzi E, Lanners J, Ferrari-Ginevra O, Achille C, Luparia A, Signorini S, Lanzi G (2002) Gross motor development and reach on sound as critical tools for the development of the blind child. *Brain Dev* 24: 269–275.

Fazzi E, Bova SM, Uggetti C, Signorini SG, Bianchi PE, Maraucci I, Zoppello M, Lanzi G (2004) Visual-perceptual impairment in children with periventricular leukomalacia. *Brain Dev* 26: 506–512.

Fedrizzi E, Anderloni A, Bono R, Bova S, Farinotti M, Inverno M, Savoiardo S (1998) Eye-movement disorders and visual-perceptual impairment in diplegic children born preterm: a clinical evaluation. *Dev Med Child Neurol* 40: 682–688.

Felmingham KL, Jakobson LS (1995) Visual and visuomotor performance in dyslexic children. *Exp Brain Res* 106: 467–474.

Fraiberg S (1977) *Insights from the Blind*. New York: Basic Books.

Goodale MA, Milner AD (1992) Separate visual pathways for perception and action. *Trends Neurosci* 15: 20–25.

Gunn A, Cory E, Atkinson J, Braddick O, Wattam-Bell J, Guzzetta A, Cioni G (2002) Dorsal and ventral stream sensitivity in normal development and hemiplegia. *Neuroreport* 13: 843–847.

Guzzetta A, Cioni G, Cowan F, Mercuri E (2001a) Visual disorders in children with brain lesions: 1. Maturation of visual function in infants with neonatal brain lesions: correlation with neuroimaging. *Eur J Paediatr Neurol* 5: 107–114.

Guzzetta A, Fazzi B, Mercuri E, Bertuccelli B, Canapicchi R, van Hof-van Duin J, Cioni G (2001b) Visual function in children with hemiplegia in the first years of life. *Dev Med Child Neurol* 43: 321–329.

Guzzetta A, Mercuri E, Cioni G (2001c) Visual disorders in children with brain lesions: 2. Visual impairment associated with cerebral palsy. *Eur J Paediatr Neurol* 5: 115–119.

Guzzetta F, Frisone MF, Ricci D, Rando T, Guzzetta A (2002) Development of visual attention in West syndrome. *Epilepsia* 43: 757–763.

Henderson A, Pehoski C (2006) *Hand Function in the Child*. St Louis: Mosby.

Ipata AE, Cioni G, Bottai P, Fazzi B, Canapicchi R, van Hof-van Duin J (1994) Acuity card testing in children with cerebral palsy related to magnetic resonance images, mental levels and motor abilities. *Brain Dev* 16: 195–203.

Jacobson L, Flodmark O, Martin L (2006) Visual field defects in prematurely born patients with white matter damage of immaturity: a multiple-case study. *Acta Ophthalmol Scand* 84: 357–362.

Jeannerod M, Arbib MA, Rizzolatti G, Sakata H (1995) Grasping objects: the cortical mechanisms of visuomotor transformation. *Trends Neurosci* 18: 314–320.

Karnath HO, Perenin MT (2005) Cortical control of visually guided reaching: evidence from patients with optic ataxia. *Cereb Cortex* 15: 1561–1569.

Lanzi G, Fazzi E, Uggetti C, Cavallini A, Danova S, Egitto MG, Ginevra OF, Salati R, Bianchi PE (1998) Cerebral visual impairment in periventricular leukomalacia. *Neuropediatrics* 29: 145–150.

Mendes M, Silva F, Simoes L, Jorge M, Saraiva J, Castelo-Branco M (2005) Visual magnocellular and structure from motion perceptual deficits in a neurodevelopmental model of dorsal stream function. *Cogn Brain Res* 25: 788–798.

Mercuri E, Spano M, Bruccini G, Frisone MF, Trombetta JC, Blandino A, Longo M, Guzzetta F (1996) Visual outcome in children with congenital hemiplegia: correlation with MRI findings. *Neuropediatrics* 27: 184–188.

Mercuri E, Atkinson J, Braddick O, Anker S, Cowan F, Rutherford M, Pennock J, Dubowitz L (1997) Basal ganglia damage and impaired visual function in the newborn infant. *Arch Dis Child Fetal Neonatal Ed* 77: F111–F114.

Mercuri E, Haataja L, Guzzetta A, Anker S, Cowan F, Rutherford M, Andrew R, Braddick O, Cioni G, Dubowitz

L, Atkinson J (1999) Visual function in term infants with hypoxic-ischaemic insults: correlation with neurodevelopment at 2 years of age. *Arch Dis Child Fetal Neonatal Ed* 80: F99–F104.

Mercuri E, Anker S, Guzzetta A, Barnett A, Haataja L, Rutherford M, Cowan F, Dubowitz L, Braddick O, Atkinson J (2003) Neonatal cerebral infarction and visual function at school age. *Arch Dis Child Fetal Neonatal Ed* 88: F487–F491.

Mercuri E, Anker S, Guzzetta A, Barnett AL, Haataja L, Rutherford M, Cowan F, Dubowitz L, Braddick O, Atkinson J (2004) Visual function at school age in children with neonatal encephalopathy and low Apgar scores. *Arch Dis Child Fetal Neonatal Ed* 89: F258–F262.

Morrone MC, Guzzetta A, Tinelli F, Tosetti M, Del Viva M, Montanaro D, Burr D, Cioni G (2008) Inversion of perceived direction of motion caused by spatial undersampling in two children with periventricular leukomalacia. *J Cogn Neurosci* 20: 1094–1106.

Nakamura M, Watanabe K, Matsumoto A, Yamanaka T, Kumagai T, Miyazaki S, Matsushima M, Mita K (2001) Williams syndrome and deficiency in visuospatial recognition. *Dev Med Child Neurol* 43: 617–621.

Paul BM, Stiles J, Passarotti A, Bavar N, Bellugi U (2002) Face and place processing in Williams syndrome: evidence for a dorsal-ventral dissociation. *Neuroreport* 13: 1115–1119.

Pellicano E, Gibson L, Maybery M, Durkin K, Badcock DR (2005) Abnormal global processing along the dorsal visual pathway in autism: a possible mechanism for weak visuospatial coherence? *Neuropsychologia* 43: 1044–1053.

Perenin MT, Vighetto A (1988) Optic ataxia: a specific disruption in visuomotor mechanisms. I. Different aspects of the deficit in reaching for objects. *Brain* 111: 643–674.

Prechtl HF, Cioni G, Einspieler C, Bos AF, Ferrari F (2001) Role of vision on early motor development: lessons from the blind. *Dev Med Child Neurol* 43: 198–201.

Rando T, Bancale A, Baranello G, Bini M, De Belvis AG, Epifanio R, Frisone MF, Guzzetta A, La Torre G, Ricci D, Signorini S, Tinelli F, Biagioni E, Veggiotti P, Mercuri E, Fazzi E, Cioni G, Guzzetta F (2004) Visual function in infants with West syndrome: correlation with EEG patterns. *Epilepsia* 45: 781–786.

Rizzolatti G, Matelli M (2003) Two different streams form the dorsal visual system: anatomy and functions. *Exp Brain Res* 153: 146–157.

Rochat P (1989) Object manipulation and exploration in 2 to 5 month old infants. *Dev Psychol* 25: 871–874.

Shumway-Cook A, Woollacott MH (1985) The growth of stability: postural control from a development perspective. *J Mot Behav* 17: 131–147.

Spencer J, O'Brien J, Riggs K, Braddick O, Atkinson J, Wattam-Bell J (2000) Motion processing in autism: evidence for a dorsal stream deficiency. *Neuroreport* 11: 2765–2767.

Stein J (2001) The magnocellular theory of developmental dyslexia. *Dyslexia* 7: 12–36.

Steinlin M, Good M, Martin E, Banziger O, Largo RH, Boltshauser E (1993) Congenital hemiplegia: morphology of cerebral lesions and pathogenetic aspects from MRI. *Neuropediatrics* 24: 224–229.

Sundermier L, Woollacott MH (1998) The influence of vision on the automatic postural muscle responses of newly standing and newly walking infants. *Exp Brain Res* 120: 537–540.

Talcott JB, Hansen PC, Assoku EL, Stein JF (2000) Visual motion sensitivity in dyslexia: evidence for temporal and energy integration deficits. *Neuropsychologia* 38: 935–943.

Ungerleider L, Mishkin M (1982) Two cortical visual systems. In: Ingle DJ, GM, Mansfield RJW, editors. *Analysis of Visual Behaviour*. Cambridge, MA: MIT Press, pp. 549–586.

van Hof-van Duin J, Cioni G, Bertuccelli B, Fazzi B, Romano C, Boldrini A (1998) Visual outcome at 5 years of newborn infants at risk of cerebral visual impairment. *Dev Med Child Neurol* 40: 302–309.

Warren D (1984) *Blindness and Early Childhood Development*. New York: American Foundation for the Blind.

Wise SP, Boussaoud D, Johnson PB, Caminiti R (1997) Premotor and parietal cortex: corticocortical connectivity and combinatorial computations. *Annu Rev Neurosci* 20: 25–42.

Woollacott M, Debu B, Mowatt M (1987) Neuromuscular control of posture in the infant and child: is vision dominant? *J Mot Behav* 19: 167–186.

9

THE ROLE OF SENSATION FOR HAND FUNCTION IN CHILDREN WITH CEREBRAL PALSY

Annette Majnemer, Daniel Bourbonnais and Victor Frak

Importance of sensation for refined hand function

VISION AND HAND FUNCTION

One of the most important roles of the hand is prehension, that is, the ability to grasp, hold and manipulate objects. Vision is obviously critical to gathering information related to the potential intrinsic and extrinsic characteristics of the object (orientation of the object, size, distance from the body, estimation of the weight) (Hay and Beaubaton 1986). This visual information is then used to plan the reaching movement (Soechting and Flanders 1989, Crawford et al 2004) and postural adjustments underlying the prehensile act itself (Kaminski et al 1995). It is generally agreed that both vision and proprioception provide information on hand and body position, and that these inputs are contributing both before and during the reaching movements to enhance accuracy of reach of the target (Scheidt et al 2005, Bagesteiro et al 2006). Therefore, information on the internal status of the body (interoceptive) and on the relationship of the object to the body (exteroceptive) is necessary for planning and control of reaching movements.

It has been suggested that reaching to grasp an object can be divided into a transportation component, in which the arm brings the hand into the vicinity of the object to be grasped, and a manipulation component, in which final adjustments of the hand are made prior to grasp (Jeannerod 1984). During reaching, the grasp aperture increases throughout the transport phase, reaching a maximum before contact with the object, and is precisely adjusted when the hand is close to the object. Whether the onset of closing of the fingers is triggered by the decreased velocity of the forearm (Jeannerod 1984, Paulignan et al 1991) or by spatial information related to the distance of the hand from the target (Wang and Stelmach 2001) is still debated. Nonetheless, when under visual control, the distance between the thumb and index reflects the size of the object and the aperture is larger when vision is removed (Jeannerod 1981).

CUTANEOUS AFFERENTS AND MANIPULATION

When reaching an object, the ability to grasp it precisely between the thumb and index requires a close interplay between sensory inputs from the fingers and the mechanisms controlling the motor output of the hand and finger muscles. While holding an object between the index and thumb, the individual has to generate a shear force in order to overcome the weight of the object and prevent the object from slipping from the fingertips. The magnitude of the shear force is related to the friction coefficient of the object and the magnitude of the pinch force. Therefore, grip force can be modulated as a function of the friction between the fingertips and the object surface and, also, the weight of the object. Slippery and heavier objects will generally require larger grip forces. Usually the grip force is slightly larger than the minimal grip force mechanically required to hold the object, providing a security margin allowing small perturbations to be corrected without dropping the object. Many studies have demonstrated the precise coordination between the grip force and the shear force during the manipulation of an object (Johansson and Wesling 1984, Westling and Johansson 1984, Westling and Johansson 1987, Johansson and Wesling 1988a, Johansson and Cole 1992).

Recordings of the activity of individual afferent fibres in a human peripheral nerve have demonstrated the importance of the cutaneous receptors of the thumb and finger pads in controlling the opposing forces of a precision pinch grip while holding an object (Johansson and Westling 1984, 1987a). Different classes of cutaneous afferents encode various types of tactile stimuli applied to the skin of the digits. Slow and rapid receptors are respectively associated with dynamic and static indentations of the skin (Johansson and Westling 1987a) and are collectively implicated in the appreciation of texture and detection of slip. These mechanoreceptors provide information about changes in shear force or slip of the object on the skin (Johansson and Westling 1987a) which is used to adjust the safety margin required by the manipulation of the object. In addition, cutaneous afferents contribute to rapid and automatic grip force increases that are observed following unexpected restraint of the object (Johansson and Westling 1988b, Johansson et al 1992a, 1992b, 1992c). The grip force increases with a delay of approximately 70 ms, indicating a feedback mechanism probably involving a supra-spinal loop (Cole and Abbs 1988, Johansson and Westling 1988b, Macefield et al 1996). This evidence suggests an important role of cutaneous afferents for precise manipulation of a tool or an object.

PROPRIOCEPTIVE AFFERENTS
Afferent fibres from muscle receptors including muscle spindles and Golgi tendon organs and joint afferents have been recorded in humans during perturbation of an object gripped between the finger and the thumb (Macefield et al 1996). In contrast to tactile afferents, the activity of these afferents is not associated with the increased shearing force following perturbation, but rather, reflects the reactive forces generated by the muscles to restrain the object. Although this indicates a low contribution of muscle afferents to initiate an appro-priate change in grip force in response to an imposed change in shear force, this does not preclude the importance of muscle receptors in specifying the initial position and state of the hand effectors. This information is likely to be important for positioning the fingers in the correct biomechanical configuration to generate directionally-appropriate digital forces. Moreover, this proprioceptive information is probably important for establishing the spatial relationship of the hand with the environment when visual information is lacking. A series of studies were conducted in a patient with a loss of large myelinated fibres affecting all somatosensory modalities (kinaesthesia, tendon reflexes, touch, vibration). This patient

relied heavily on visual feedback of the limb to control arm movements (Teasdale et al 1993). Nonetheless, complex hand movements such as drawing ellipses on a sheet of paper, although slower, were still possible and the regularity and consistency of the drawings were comparable to those of healthy subjects. This regularity and consistency of the ellipses drawn was not affected by removal of vision; however, the position and orientation of the ellipses drifted with time. This suggests that proprioceptive information contributes in determining the positioning of the hand in the environment.

ROLE OF SENSATION IN ANTICIPATORY CONTROL OF GRIP FORCE

Skilled hand manipulation also requires a high level of motor control which relies mainly on prediction of the consequences of our own actions. Stopping or reversing a rapid movement of the arm while an object is held between finger and thumb of the hand requires an increase in shear force to counteract the inertia of the object. Considering the delays involved in cutaneous feedback loops (Cole and Abbs 1988, Johansson and Westling 1988b), this increase in grip force is produced by a predictive mechanism. This predictive behaviour of increasing grip force has been taken as evidence of the existence of an internal forward model of the limb and the object to be manipulated (Flanagan et al 1993). This model suggests that for self-produced movements, the central nervous system uses internal models of both the arm and the object to anticipate the resulting shear force and thereby adjust the grip force (Flanagan and Wing 1997).

It is probable that continuous sensory feedback is not necessary to perform a predictable task. Indeed, following digital anaesthesia, the pattern of force production is preserved during lifting and holding an object which has been previously manipulated (Johannson and Westling 1984). Only slight impairments of grip force regulation such as less precise adjustments to the skin and object friction characteristics and temporal delays between force adjustment phases for initiation of lifting (Johansson and Westling 1984) are observed. In contrast, digital anaesthesia of the fingers decreases or even abolishes grip force changes normally seen following a perturbation of the prehension (Johansson et al 1992c).

Inappropriate grip forces resulting from changing the weight of an object, which has been previously lifted by the subject, are re-scaled within a single trial (Johansson and Westling 1988a). This suggests that sensory feedback signals can effectively be used to recalibrate the grip force. However, it has been suggested that discrete sensory feedback provided primarily by cutaneous afferents is used to update anticipatory motor commands (Augurelle et al 2003).

SENSORY-MOTOR INTEGRATION

The relationship between sensory signals and motor commands has been extensively studied in neuroscience and recent advances in computational study of motor control have emphasized the importance of sensory feedback (Wolpert and Ghahramani 2000). This information is important not only for providing ongoing feedback control of prehension, but also for providing information to the nervous system on the status of the limb and hand in order to predict the effect of motor commands. Impairments of vision and somatosensory function

136

would impact specification of the initial state of the body, which is probably needed to determine with refinement the correct motor commands to be implemented.

Moreover, the integrity of sensory information is important for a sensory-driven control allowing the comparison of the actual somatosensory information and the expected somatosensory input. The sensory consequence of the movement would be predicted using an internal model in conjunction with a copy of the motor command generating the movement. Detection of a difference between predicted and observed sensory information would determine the corrective response as well as an updating of the motor command. Obviously, this sensory-driven control could be impaired in individuals with neurological impairments and associated deficits of somatosensory function such as cerebral palsy. Moreover, impairment in determining the intensity and timing of the motor command would also impair this sensory-driven control, since the sensory consequences would be incorrectly determined following an inappropriate estimation of the motor command. However, evidence suggests that individuals with neurological deficits can appropriately determine the intensity and timing of a motor command and use this information to define the intensity and timing of the anticipatory motor command. This could be illustrated by the observation that while both deafferented participants and participants with anaesthetized fingers generated elevated baseline grip forces on a held object while performing reversal of the arm movement, the precise temporal coupling between grip and load force profiles was maintained (Nowak et al 2001, Nowak and Hermsdorfer 2002). Interestingly, these individuals still modulated grip force even though the baseline levels were high enough, not justifying this modulation. This suggests that the intensity of the motor command required to maintain grip force during baseline force exertion is taken into account when determining the intensity of the predictive force counteracting the inertia of the object at movement reversal. This superimposition of predictive force on baseline force would probably not occur if the anticipatory force could not be scaled to baseline.

Recently, it has been shown that the sense of effort is preserved in individuals with neurological impairments, suggesting that force estimates may be preserved following brain damage. Indeed, force-matching tasks in which hemiparetic participants are required to produce equal sub-maximal grip forces in both hands have been studied (Bertrand and Mercier 2004). The results demonstrate that individuals with hemiparesis produce systematic errors in the force generated by the paretic hand, that is, the grip forces are lower on the paretic side, although they have sufficient strength to exert identical forces to those measured on the non-paretic side. The asymmetry between the two sides was found to be associated with the relative weakness on the paretic side (Fig. 9.1). These results suggest that individuals post-stroke rely on the perceived intensity of the effort (i.e. sense of effort) to scale the motor commands. For example, an individual scaling his motor commands to 65 per cent of the maximal voluntary force on each side (i.e. matching the intensity of the effort) would produce equal grip forces in both hands. Prior to the neurological insult, this strategy would produce comparable forces on both sides, but now results in asymmetrical forces because of the weakness affecting the upper limb contralateral to the cerebral lesion. Although these participants knew explicitly that they were weaker on the paretic side, they were totally unaware of the systematic errors they produced and all reported that they had succeeded in

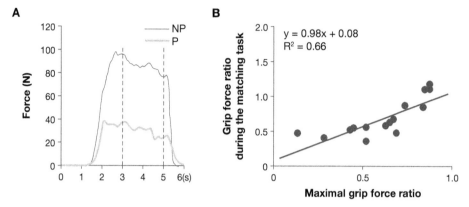

Fig. 9.1 The participant is asked to produce equal grip forces on both sides corresponding to 65 per cent of his maximal grip force on the paretic side. Although the force values clearly differ between sides (as shown in panel A: NP, non-paretic; P, paretic), the participant perceives that he is producing equal forces. The values included in the interval between the dotted lines were used to calculate the grip force ratio between the paretic and non-paretic sides, which is approximately 0.38 in this individual. These grip force ratios were calculated in 15 stroke patients and found to be significantly correlated to the maximal voluntary hand grip force ratios (as shown in panel B: regression equation and coefficient of determination (R^2)). This suggests that grip force matching is based on the perception of an identical scaled force production relative to maximal voluntary force. Source: Modified from Bertrand and Mercier 2004.

producing identical forces in both upper limbs. In the static tasks used, the absence of movement precluded the use of visual feedback and reduced the available proprioceptive feedback on the performance. It is still unknown how sensory feedback can be used to compensate for tasks undertaken in more natural conditions.

In summary, current evidence illustrates how sensory inputs such as visual, cutaneous and proprioceptive information are essential for the initiation and execution of refined hand movements. The essential role of sensory feedback following perturbation of a held object and for predictive control of hand movements has been emphasized. These principles should be considered when analysing results of clinical evaluation of sensation and hand function in children with cerebral palsy.

Relationship between sensation and hand function in children with cerebral palsy

Sensory Function in Children with Cerebral Palsy

Challenges of sensory assessment
Accurate measurement of cutaneous and proprioceptive sensation should be an important part of the rehabilitation management of children with neurological conditions such as cerebral palsy (CP). A comprehensive documentation of the extent and range of impairments and associated activity limitations is an essential component to programme planning and selection of therapeutic approaches to optimize function. Sensory impairments may

modulate motor performance, and therefore should be specifically evaluated in children with CP.

Quantitative sensory assessment should objectively ascertain the minimal energy or threshold required to reliably detect a particular sensory modality (Kahn 1992, Thibault et al 1994). Instructions should be simple and clear, and materials used need to be age-appropriate. For young children or those with developmental disabilities, the assessment should have minimum cognitive and language requirements. There should be minimal handling requirements if applied to children with physical limitations. Parameters for stimulus presentation should be standardized. Ideally, the assessment should be brief and easy to administer, to enhance feasibility of application in the clinical milieu. Accuracy of the results, including reliability and validity, should not be questioned (Kahn 1992, Cooper et al 1993).

It is therefore a challenge to evaluate sensation in children and youth with CP. There is a paucity of tools that may be applied to young children, particularly those with motor and other developmental deficits. Reliability estimates for sensory testing are often lacking, and informal approaches in the clinical setting may yield inconsistent results. Normative data for children of different ages are needed as there may be developmental changes expected with age. Adequate reliability across all modalities may not be feasible in infants and preschool children (Curry and Exner 1988). Although sections of standardized developmental assessments such as the Quick Neurologic Screening Test, the Miller Assessment for Preschoolers and the Sensory Integration and Praxis Tests may assess components of sensation, they were not designed for children with motor impairments. For example, adequate motor control is needed to test graphesthesia, stereognosis, kinesthesia and finger localization, as described in these tools. Furthermore, assessment of many modalities requires good attention and concentration skills (Cooper et al 1993, Yekutiel et al 1994, Clayton et al 2003).

There has been a recent interest in developing standardized measures of sensation appropriate for use in children with disabilities. In the Test of Sensory Functions in Infants (DeGangi et al 1988), sensory modulation is evaluated by therapists, but has limited reliability. The Sensory Profile (Dunn 1999) provides a parent report of their child's subjective experiences and responses to sensations within the natural environment. A number of investigators have applied sensory modalities commonly tested in adults with modifications to minimize language, motor and cognitive requirements, using materials that are familiar to children. Preliminary normative data are available for evaluation of the upper and lower extremities of children for modalities such as: pressure sensitivity using Semmes Weinstein monofilaments, two-point discrimination (using the Disk-criminator), directionality, proprioception, stereognosis, vibration, kinesthesia and thermal discrimination. Reliability estimates in studies to date show consistency between raters and on retest (Cooper et al 1993, Thibault et al 1994, Booth et al 1998). Further development on larger samples is necessary to determine thresholds by age.

Sensory findings in children with CP
As noted above, the feasibility of accurately assessing sensory abilities in children with CP is constrained by physical, cognitive and behavioural impairments which limit level of cooperation and ability to carry out procedures in a standardized fashion (Clayton et al 2003, McLaughlin et al 2005). Despite this, a number of studies have been conducted to evaluate the sensory abilities of children with CP (see Table 9.1), and there are a number of consistencies in the reported findings to date. A sizable proportion of children with CP will demonstrate sensory impairments, particularly with respect to stereognosis and two-point discrimination (Tizard et al 1954, Hohman et al 1958, Tachdjian and Minear 1958, Wigfield 1966, Wilson and Wilson 1967a, 1967b, Bolanos et al 1989, Lesny et al 1993, Van Heest et al 1993, Yekutiel et al 1994, Cooper et al 1995, Krumlinde-Sundholm and Eliasson 2002, McLaughlin et al 2005). Others have also reported deficits in other modalities, including kinesthesia, pressure sensitivity, proprioception, vibration sense and directionality (Opila-Lehman et al 1985, Van Heest et al 1993, Cooper et al 1995, McLaughlin et al 2005). Gender and age in this population do not appear to influence likelihood for impaired sensation (Wilson and Wilson 1967a, 1967b, Bolanos et al 1989, Cooper et al 1995). However, type of CP does appear to influence prevalence of sensory impairment. Specifically, children with spastic CP, especially those with a pattern of hemiplegia or diplegia, are much more likely to have sensory impairments (Hohman et al 1958, Tachdjian and Minear 1958, Monfraix et al 1961, Kenney 1966, Wigfield 1966, Bolanos et al 1989, Opila-Lehman et al 1985, Lesny et al 1993, Yekutiel et al 1994). There is stronger evidence supporting a high prevalence of sensory dysfunction in the upper extremity; however McLaughlin et al (2005) also found these deficits in the lower extremity. Abnormal somatosensory evoked potentials (absence of potentials or increased conduction time) lend further support to the high prevalence of sensory dysfunction in children with CP (Cooper et al 1995).

Impaired sensation is likely to be due to injury or malformation of cortical and subcortical structures such as the parietal lobe and thalamus (Clayton et al 2003). Furthermore, limited movement experiences which are important for motor control may also impede development of a sense of movement and position in space (Curry and Exner 1988). Decreased tactile exploration will limit sensory experiences which are important in early brain mapping of the somatosensory and associated brain structures (Clayton et al 2003). It has also been proposed that cutaneous and proprioceptive deficits may result in part secondary to selective dorsal rhizotomy (Thibault et al 1994); however, no evidence of a change in sensory status has been reported following this surgical intervention (McLaughlin et al 2005).

ASSOCIATION BETWEEN SENSATION AND HAND FUNCTION IN CHILDREN WITH CP

Theoretical rationale for this association
Upper extremity sensation is felt to be critical for the planning and execution of refined hand function including modulated grip force, in-hand manipulation, tool use and exploration with the hands (Clayton et al 2003). At the extreme, when there are severe sensory

TABLE 9.1
Summary of studies describing sensory abilities in children with CP

Authors/Year	Sample of children with CP	Sensory modalities affected
Bolanos et al 1989	51 CP, 170 controls 6–20 years	63% 2-point discrimination deficits, 9% astereognosis
Cooper et al 1995	9 CP (hemiplegia), 41 controls	89% sensory deficits bilaterally, stereognosis and proprioception most affected
Gordon & Duff 1999	15 CP (hemiplegia), 15 controls 4–18 years	Impaired 2-point discrimination, pressure sensitivity and stereognosis compared to controls
Hohman et al 1958	47 CP 6–16 years	72% deficits in form perception, 2-point discrimination, position sense; hemiplegia>quadriplegia>athetoid
Kenney 1966		73% sensory deficits, spastic>athetoid
Krumlinde-Sundholm & Eliasson 2002	25 CP (hemiplegia) 19 controls 5–18 years	Impairments in stereognosis and 2-point discrimination compared to controls
Lesny et al 1993	N = 220 7–14 years	Decreased 2-point discrimination compared to controls, especially for diplegia and hemiplegia
McLaughlin et al 2005	62 CP, 65 controls 3–18 years	Decreased toe position sense, direction of scratch and vibration sense when compared to controls
Monfraix et al 1961		Tactile agnosia 81% impaired if spastic, 43% impaired if athetoid
Opila-Lehman et al 1985	24 CP, 12 controls 8–15 years	Poor kinesthesia compared to controls, spastic form worse than athetoid
Tachdjian & Minear 1958	96 CP 6–19 years	42% sensory deficits; most common (>10%) modalities: stereognosis (42%), 2-point discrimination (32%), position sense (17%); spastic>athetoid
Tizard et al 1954	N = 106 (hemiplegia)	54% sensory deficits (stereognosis, 2-point discrimination and position sense most commonly affected)
Van Heest et al 1993	40 CP (hemiplegia)	97% astereognosis, 90% impaired 2-point discrimination, 46% proprioception deficit
Wigfield 1966	16–26 years	86% astereognosis for hemiplegic group, 1/11 for athetoid children
Wilson and Wilson 1967a	120 CP, 60 controls 7–21 years	48% impaired sensation: pressure sensitivity and/or 2-point discrimination; similar deficits in children with spasticity versus athetosis
Wilson and Wilson 1967b	120 CP, 60 controls 7–21 years	Haptic form discrimination deficit in 31% with spasticity versus 30% with athetosis; size discrimination deficit in 18% with spasticity versus 11% with athetosis
Yekutiel et al 1994	N = 55 6–17 years	51% deficits in stereognosis and/or 2-point discrimination

141

deficits, individuals tend to neglect the affected limb and a non-use phenomenon gradually emerges which can result in a progressive deterioration of limb functioning (Thibault et al 1994, McLaughlin et al 2005). In addition to neglect of the limb, decreased or absent afferent input to the brain appears to compromise motor learning and body image. This phenomenon has been demonstrated in both animal and human studies on congenital or acquired sensory deficits of central nervous system origin (Moberg 1976, McLaughlin et al 2005). The first section of this chapter provides a detailed overview of current evidence illustrating how sensory inputs are essential for refined motor control of the hand. Interpreting the temporal and spatial aspects of tactile input is felt to be critical for key everyday hand skills (Clayton et al 2003).

Therefore, it is critical that rehabilitation specialists objectively assess sensibility in children with CP, so as to appreciate how particular sensory deficits may undermine and limit hand function (Curry and Exner 1988). First, it is increasingly appreciated that move-ment experiences are important in the development of motor control; however, kinesthetic input may be limited or inadequate in children with CP. Therefore, as part of rehabilitation interventions, therapists should capitalize on more intact sensory systems (e.g. visual, auditory) to provide the needed feedback for accurate movement execution (Opila-Lehman et al 1985). Second, rehabilitation tends to focus predominantly on the motor disorder characteristic of CP; however, the impact of sensory deficits on motor performance cannot be overlooked. Sensory retraining approaches used successfully in adults following stroke to enhance sensibility are often applied, although rigorous studies to demonstrate effec-tiveness in children with CP are lacking (Yekutiel et al 1994). Finally, children can learn adaptive strategies which can enhance hand skill development over time. Hand function is dependent not only on physical (sensory and motor abilities) functioning, but also on cognitive (e.g. purposeful actions), behavioural (e.g. attention, concentration), social-emotional (e.g. motivation, self-efficacy, body image), and perceptual (e.g. integration of somatosensory information into motor actions) components. Therefore improvements can be optimized through training strategies that capitalize on strengths in these other component areas, in spite of sensory-motor deficits (Eliasson 2005).

Objective evidence for this association
There is a paucity of studies that have actually examined whether there is a relationship between sensation and hand function in children with CP. Tachdjian and Minear (1958) graded children based on hand use, and severity of sensory deficits was associated with severity of hand dysfunction. In those with no function, 88 per cent had sensory deficits; 69 per cent of those with poor hand function had sensory deficits; fair hand function was associated with deficits in 30 per cent; those with good hand function rarely had sensory deficits (7 per cent); and normal hand function was associated with normal sensation.

More recently, the impact of sensation on performance of precision grip was carefully evaluated in 15 children with CP compared to controls (Gordon and Duff 1999). The expectation was that sensory input would be critical for the adjustment of grip and scaling of forces. Indeed, stereognosis and two-point discrimination were highly correlated with pinch strength (dynamometer), grip force adaptation and grip force rate scaling (anticipatory control of force output). Pressure sensitivity also correlated with the preload-phase duration. These results provide objective evidence of the important relationship between tactile sensibility and fine motor control of fingertip force during precision grip. It is conceivable that sensory input provides children with the necessary information to adjust and adapt grip forces (anticipatory scaling of forces), and provides smoother transitions between phases of apprehension and release of small objects (Eliasson et al 1995, Gordon and Duff 1999).

As described above, in addition to providing input to initiate movements, sensory inputs also provide feedback to modify forces. It appears that children with CP may have excessive grip force so as to compensate for decreased sensory input, as is noted in adults with cutaneous anaesthesia. Indeed, Curry and Exner (1988) demonstrated that preschool children with CP had a preference for hard textures and avoided softer objects, in contrast to typically developing preschool children. These children may also be less likely to use reflex mechanisms to prevent slipping, and are less able to adapt their grip to different textures (Eliasson et al 1995). Because of poor awareness of position in space and decreased tactile sensibility, these children may rely on other sensory systems to optimize motor performance. In a study by Cherng et al (1999), there were the greatest differences in static standing balance in children with spastic diplegia compared to matched non-disabled children when vision was either occluded or unreliable (i.e. sensory conflict conditions). Various measures of tactile sensibility (two-point discrimination, stereognosis, light touch) significantly correlated with hand function in terms of dexterity (pick-up test) in children with hemiplegia (Krumlinde-Sundholm and Eliasson 2002). However, correlations between sensibility and performance on bimanual tasks were weak. It should be noted that severity of sensory impairment does not necessarily correlate with severity of motor function or activity limitations; but, rather, sensibility across modalities influences hand function, contributing to the variance (Wigfield 1966, Cooper et al 1995).

The clinical implications with respect to the best intervention strategies to optimize hand function remain unclear. There is a lack of evidence demonstrating the effectiveness of particular treatment approaches such as sensory retraining and repetitive sensory stimulation, or more adaptive motor learning strategies that are specifically targeted at children with CP who have sensory deficits. A repetitive multi-sensory training programme using a sensory story with contrasting sensory words (e.g. soft/stiff, smooth/sharp, hot/cold) was conducted with six children with hemiplegia. An increased awareness and a greater frequency of use of the affected limb were noted in this observational study, with apparent carryover to play activities (Barrett and Jones 1967). Another study compared a group of children with CP who received sensory-perceptual-motor training over a three-month period with a reference sample who received home programmes only. Of those receiving sensory-perceptual-motor treatment, one sample had individual treatment, and another sample had group treatments. Both experimental groups improved from baseline on a variety of sensory integration subtests when compared to the reference group who did not receive the direct treatment. The authors propose that this approach may increase sensory experiences and assist in the assimilation of sensory information, with the expectation of enhancing motor function (Bumin and Kayihan 2001). Clearly, future studies are needed to address whether particular sensory treatment approaches, whether emphasizing remediation or adaptation, can enhance upper extremity function in this population of interest.

Conclusions

This chapter reviews the importance of sensations such as vision, as well as cutaneous sensibility and proprioception, for the refined motor control of the hand. Intact sensory receptors provide the input needed for modulation and adjustment of movements to ensure that they are accurate and smooth. Cerebral palsy is a non-progressive disorder of movement and posture, often accompanied by disturbances of sensation. For rehabilitation specialists evaluating children with CP in the clinical setting, it is essential that the potential influence of sensory impairments be considered, as it may impact on sensory-motor integration needed for refined hand movements to execute everyday tasks and activities. Therapeutic interventions may focus on maximizing tactile sensibility using sensory retraining and stimulation approaches, with the expectation that sensory input will improve and prehension patterns will become more precise. Conversely, capitalizing on more intact sensory modalities and use of adaptive strategies may be employed to enhance learning of functional hand skills, in spite of sensory-motor deficits. Evidence to support the effectiveness of either remediation or compensatory approaches is lacking, and needs to be addressed in future studies, so as to promote hand function needed to independently execute everyday self-care, school and leisure activities in children and young people with CP.

REFERENCES

Augurelle AS, Smith AM, Lejeune T, Thonnard JL (2003) Importance of cutaneous feedback in maintaining a secure grip during manipulation of hand-held objects. *J Neurophys* 89: 665–671.
Bagesteiro LB, Sarlegna FR, Sainburg RL (2006) Differential influence of vision and proprioception on control of movement distance. *Exp Brain Res* 171: 1–13.
Barrett ML, Jones MH (1967) The 'sensory story': a multi-sensory training procedure for toddlers. 1. Effect on motor function of hemiplegic hand in cerebral palsied children. *Dev Med Child Neurol* 9: 448–456.
Bertrand AM, Mercier C (2004) Effects of weakness on symmetrical bilateral grip force exertion in subjects with hemiparesis. *J Neurophys* 91: 1579–1585.
Bolanos AA, Bleck EE, Firestone P, Young L (1989) Comparison of stereognosis and two-point discrimination testing of the hands of children with cerebral palsy. *Dev Med Child Neurol* 31: 371–376.
Booth S, Estevez W, Cooper J, Majnemer A (1998) A standardized paediatric sensory assessment for the lower extremity: preliminary results of a reliability study in normal school-aged children. *Can J Occup Ther* 65: 92–103.
Bumin G, Kayihan H (2001) Effectiveness of two different sensory-integration programmes for children with spastic diplegic cerebral palsy. *Dis Rehabil* 23: 394–399.
Cherng R-J, Su F-C, Chen J-J, Kuan T-S (1999) Performance of static standing balance in children with spastic diplegic cerebral palsy under altered sensory environments. *Phys Med Rehabil* 78: 336–343.
Clayton K, Fleming JM, Copley J (2003) Behavioral responses to tactile stimuli in children with cerebral palsy. *Phys Occup Ther Pediatr* 23: 43–62.
Cole KJ, Abbs JH (1988) Grip force adjustments evoked by load force perturbations of a grasped object. *J Neurophys* 60: 1513–1522.
Cooper J, Majnemer A, Rosenblatt B, Birnbaum R (1993) A standardized sensory assessment for children of school-age. *Phys Occup Ther Pediatr* 13: 61–80.
Cooper J, Majnemer A, Rosenblatt B, Birnbaum R (1995) The determination of sensory deficits in children with hemiplegic cerebral palsy. *J Child Neurol* 10: 300–309.
Crawford JD, Medendorp WP, Marotta JJ (2004) Spatial transformations for eye–hand coordination. *J Neurophys* 92: 10–19.

Curry J, Exner C (1988) Comparison of tactile preferences in children with and without cerebral palsy. *Am J Occup Ther* 42: 371–377.

DeGangi GA, Berk RA, Greenspan SI (1988) The clinical measurement of sensory functioning in infants: a preliminary study. *Phys Occup Ther Pediatr* 8: 1–23.

Dellon AL (1984) Touch sensibility in the hand. *J Hand Surg* 9B: 11–13.

Dunn W (1999) *Sensory Profile*. San Antonio, TX: Psychological Corporation.

Eliasson A-C (2005) Improving the use of hands in daily activities: aspects of the treatment of children with cerebral palsy. *Phys Occup Ther Pediatr* 25: 37–60.

Eliasson A-C, Gordon AM, Forssberg H (1995) Tactile control of isometric fingertip forces during grasping in children with cerebral palsy. *Dev Med Child Neurol* 37: 72–84.

Flanagan JR, Wing AM (1997) The role of internal models in motion planning and control: evidence from grip force adjustments during movements of hand-held loads. *J Neurosci* 17: 1519–1528.

Flanagan JR, Tresilian J, Wing AM (1993) Coupling of grip force and load force during arm movements with grasped objects. *Neurosci Lett* 152: 53–56.

Gordon AM, Duff SV (1999) Relation between clinical measures and fine manipulative control in children with hemiplegic cerebral palsy. *Dev Med Child Neurol* 41: 586–591.

Hay L, Beaubaton D (1986) Visual correction of a rapid goal-directed response. *Percept Mot Skills* 62: 51–57.

Hohman LB, Baker L, Reed R (1958) Sensory disturbances in children with infantile hemiplegia, triplegia, and quadriplegia. *Am J Phys Med* 37: 1–6.

Jeannerod M (1981) Intersegmental coordination during reaching at natural visual objects. In: Long J, Baddeley A, editors. *Attention and Performance*, Vol 9, Hillsdale, NJ: Erlbaum, pp 153–168.

Jeannerod M (1984) The timing of natural prehension movements. *J Mot Behav* 16: 235–254.

Johansson RS, Cole KJ (1992) Sensory-motor coordination during grasping and manipulative actions. *Curr Opin Neurobiol* 2: 815–823.

Johansson RS, Westling G (1984) Roles of glabrous skin receptors and sensorimotor memory in automatic control of precision grip when lifting rougher or more slippery objects. *Exp Brain Res* 56: 550–564.

Johansson RS, Westling G (1987a) Signals in tactile afferents from the fingers eliciting adaptive motor responses during precision grip. *Exp Brain Res* 66: 141–154.

Johansson RS, Westling G (1987b) Significance of cutaneous input for precise hand movements. *Electroenceph Clin Neurophys* Suppl 39: 53–57.

Johansson RS, Westling G (1988a) Coordinated isometric muscle commands adequately and erroneously programmed for the weight during lifting task with precision grip. *Exp Brain Res* 71: 59–71.

Johansson RS, Westling G (1988b) Programmed and triggered actions to rapid load changes during precision grip. *Exp Brain Res* 71: 72–86.

Johansson RS, Riso R, Hager C, Backstrom L (1992a) Somatosensory control of precision grip during unpredictable pulling loads. I. Changes in load force amplitude. *Exp Brain Res* 89: 181–191.

Johansson RS, Hager C, Riso R (1992b) Somatosensory control of precision grip during unpredictable pulling loads. II. Changes in load force rate. *Exp Brain Res* 89: 192–203.

Johansson RS, Hager C, Backstrom L (1992c) Somatosensory control of precision grip during unpredictable pulling loads. III. Impairments during digital anesthesia. *Exp Brain Res* 89: 204–213.

Kahn R (1992) Quantitative sensory testing. *Muscle Nerve* 15: 1155–1157.

Kaminski TR, Bock C, Gentile AM (1995) The coordination between trunk and arm motion during pointing movements. *Exp Brain Res* 106: 457–466.

Kenney WE (1966) The importance of sensori-perceptu-gnosia in the examination, the understanding and the management of cerebral palsy. *Clin Orthop Relat Res* 46: 45–52.

Kerem M, Livanelioglu A, Topcu M (2001) Effects of Johnstone pressure splints combined with neurodevelopmental therapy on spasticity and cutaneous sensory inputs in spastic cerebral palsy. *Dev Med Child Neurol* 43: 307–313.

Krumlinde-Sundholm L, Eliasson A-C (2002) Comparing tests of tactile sensibility: aspects relevant to testing children with spastic hemiplegia. *Dev Med Child Neurol* 44: 604–612.

Lesny I, Stehlik KA, Tomasek J, Tomankova A, Havlicek I (1993) Sensory disorders in cerebral palsy: two-point discrimination. *Dev Med Child Neurol* 35: 402–405.

Levin S, Pearsall G, Ruderman RJ (1978) Von Frey's method of measuring pressure sensibility in the hand: an engineering analysis of the Weinstein-Semmes pressure aesthesiometer. *J Hand Surg* 3: 211–216.

Macefield VG, Johansson S (1996) Control of grip force during restraint of an object held between finger and thumb: responses of muscle and joint afferents from the digits. *Exp Brain Res* 108: 172–184.

145

Macefield VG, Rothwell JC, Day BL (1996) The contribution of transcortical pathways to long-latency stretch and tactile reflexes in human hand muscles. *Exp Brain Res* 108: 147–154.

McLaughlin JF, Felix SD, Nowbar S, Ferrel A, Bjornson K, Hays RM (2005) Lower extremity sensory function in children with cerebral palsy. *Pediatr Rehabil* 8: 45–52.

Moberg E (1976) Reconstructive hand surgery in tetraplegia, stroke, and cerebral palsy: some basic concepts in physiology and neurology. *J Hand Surg* 1: 29–34.

Monfraix C, Tardieu G, Tardieu C (1961) Disturbances of manual perception in children with cerebral palsy. *Cereb Palsy Bull* 3: 544–552.

Nowak DA, Hermsdorfer J (2002) Coordination of grip and load forces during vertical point-to-point movements with a grasped object in Parkinson's disease. *Behav Neurosci* 116: 837–850.

Nowak DA, Hermsdorfer J, Glasauer S, Philipp J, Meyer L, Mai N (2001) The effects of digital anaesthesia on predictive grip force adjustments during vertical movements of a grasped object. *Eur J Neurosci* 14: 756–762.

Opila-Lehman J, Short MA Trombly CA (1985) Kinesthetic recall of children with athetoid and spastic cerebral palsy and of non-handicapped children. *Dev Med Child Neurol* 27: 223–230.

Paulignan Y, MacKenzie C, Marteniuk R, Jeannerod M (1991) Selective perturbation of visual input during prehension movements, 1. The effects of changing object position. *Exp Brain Res* 83: 502–512.

Scheidt RA, Conditt MA, Secco EL, Mussa-Ivaldi FA (2005) Interaction of visual and proprioceptive feedback during adaptation of human reaching movements. *J Neurophys* 93: 3200–3213.

Soechting JF, Flanders M (1989) Sensorimotor representations for pointing to targets in three-dimensional space. *J Neurophys* 62: 582–594.

Tachdjian MO, Minear WL (1958) Sensory disturbances in the hands of children with cerebral palsy. *J Bone Joint Surg* 40A: 85–90.

Teasdale NR, Forget R, Bard C, Paillard J (1993) The role of proprioceptive information for the production of isometric forces and for handwriting tasks. *Acta Psychol* 82: 179–191.

Thibault A, Forget R, Lambert J (1994) Evaluation of cutaneous and proprioceptive sensation in children: a reliability study. *Dev Med Child Neurol* 36: 796–812.

Tizard JPM, Paine RS, Crothers B (1954) Disturbances of sensation in children with hemiplegia. *JAMA* 155: 628–632.

Van Heest AE, House J, Putnam M (1993) Sensibility deficiencies in the hands of children with spastic hemiplegia. *J Hand Surg* 18A: 278–281.

Wang J, Stelmach E (2001) Spatial and temporal control of trunk-assisted prehensile actions. *Exp Brain Res* 136: 231–240.

Westling G, Johansson RS (1984) Factors influencing the force control during precision grip. *Exp Brain Res* 53: 277–284.

Westling G, Johansson RS (1987) Responses in glabrous skin mechanoreceptors during precision grip in humans. *Exp Brain Res* 66: 128–140.

Wigfield ME (1966) Cerebral palsy: altered sensation, astereognosis and sensory perception in relation to vocational training and job performance. *Clin Orthop Relat Res* 46: 93–108.

Wilson BC, Wilson JJ (1967a) Sensory and perceptual functions in the cerebral palsied: I. Pressure thresholds and two-point discrimination. *J Nerv Ment Dis* 145: 61–68.

Wilson BC, Wilson JJ (1967b) Sensory and perceptual functions in the cerebral palsied: II. Stereognosis. *J Nerv Ment Dis* 145: 53–60.

Witney AG, Wing A, Thonnard JL, Smith AM (2004) The cutaneous contribution to adaptive precision grip. *Trends Neurosci* 27: 637–643.

Wolpert DM, Ghahramani Z (2000) Computational principles of movement neuroscience. *Nat Neurosci* 3(Suppl): 1212–1217.

Yekutiel M, Jariwala M, Stretch P (1994) Sensory deficit in the hands of children with cerebral palsy: a new look at assessment and prevalence. *Dev Med Child Neurol* 36: 619–624.

10
TYPICAL AND ATYPICAL DEVELOPMENT OF THE UPPER LIMB IN CHILDREN

Jeanne R. Charles

Introduction

The ability to reach and grasp an object includes actions that allow one to actively explore and interact with the environment. Goal-directed reaching and prehension are described as grasp, manipulation and release (Duff and Charles 2004). The skills of reach and prehension develop throughout early childhood and involve integration of the sensorimotor, visual and cognitive systems. From a fine motor perspective it requires recognition of an object, accurate reach toward the object, correct hand orientation, pre-shaping of the hand aperture as it approaches the object, and finally grasping the object. Task completion involves timing and coordination of all these systems. Skilful actions are also possible due to the many degrees of freedom of the upper extremities in joint and muscle space (Newell and McDonald 1997). This flexibility contributes to adaptability within one's environmental context and is crucial for the development of functional skills such as dressing, writing, eating, and engaging in sports activities. Mature reach and grasp use a feed-forward mechanism (anticipatory control) which develops during childhood. Prior to the development of feed-forward control, the young child uses a feedback mechanism whereby information about the task being performed is processed 'online' as the task is performed (Forssberg et al 1991). For developing skills, the challenge is to learn to overcome constraints within themselves and their environment (Thelen and Spencer 1998, Eliasson 2005). The purpose of this chapter is to discuss the development of motor control for reach and prehension in typically developing children and children with movement disorders due to central nervous system (CNS) damage.

Systems influencing functional development of the upper extremity

Both the environmental context and the postural context affect the nature and success of movements (Thelen and Spencer 1998, cf. Reed 1989). No functional movement, such as reaching, exists in isolation but rather is embedded in complex situations and nested into a given postural setting. In typical reaching movements the eyes, head and upper extremity can move sequentially or in conjunction depending on the constraints of the task. Thus, the development of reaching and prehension relies on control and coordination of a number of systems: sensorimotor, visual/spatial, postural and cognitive. The dynamics of reaching and grasping an object involve: transformation of visual space to a body-centred coordinate system and generation of a smooth, straight pathway from an initial starting position to the object with acceleration, followed by deceleration as the hand approaches the object. In addition, the arm must be supported against gravity and at the same time generate forces that are appropriate to move the hand to the object and generate coordinated forces to shape the hand and pick up an object without crushing or dropping it. Finally, the neuromotor system must account for passive and elastic forces that are generated by the movement (Thelen and Spencer 1998). Therefore, it is important to understand the contribution of a number of systems in order to have a comprehensive understanding of how they interact in the motor control of the upper extremity.

Postural control is important in the development of reach as well as manipulation (prehension). It is the ability to control the body in space for purposes of stability and spatial orientation (Shumway-Cook and Woollacott 2001). Maintaining balance through body stability and appropriate spatial orientation is a means of offsetting gravitational forces acting on the body without interfering with manipulative activity (Bertenthal and von Hofsten 1998). It also serves as a reference for movement organization. For example, in reaching toward an object, the organization of the head, neck and trunk in space serves as a frame of reference in planning the appropriate hand and arm trajectory (Massion 1998, Fallang et al 2000). Thus, understanding postural control is important in understanding development of reaching and prehension (Shumway-Cook and Woollacott 2001). (See Chapter 5 for more detailed discussion on postural contributions to reach and grasp.)

EARLY SENSORIMOTOR DEVELOPMENT
Movement of the upper extremities is detected *in utero*. By 15 weeks gestation, for example, the fetus will rotate the head and bring the hand to the mouth (Sparling et al 1999, D'Elia et al 2001). While this movement has been interpreted as generalized and non-specific, studies have related this movement to the *in utero* maturation of the nervous system (D'Elia et al 2001). Thus, direct connections from the pyramidal tract to motor neurons are established before birth (Eyre et al 2001).

Recent research has expanded our view of the development of reaching and hand development. Von Hofsten (1980) examined visual tracking and generalized reaching behaviours in infants from birth to 3 months of age and found that if the postural requirements are eliminated with the trunk supported, newborn infants will track a moving object and make generalized reaching movements toward it. Van der Meer et al (1995) documented that newborns generate force in the upper extremities when stimulated. One study (Wallace and Whishaw 2003) classified spontaneous hand and digit movements in infants ranging in age from 1 to 5 months. Four grasping patterns were observed (fist, pre-precision grip, precision grip, and self-directed grasp) which developed from 'vacuous' to more self-directed over time. The authors compared these movements to babbling behaviour as a precursor to speech, describing them as precursors to visually directed movement, and hypothesized that their progression is correlated to development of the pyramidal tracts.

Finally, newborn infants were found to purposefully imitate index finger movement (Nagy et al 2005). Index finger protrusion as an indicator of imitation of fine motor development was examined in 39 neonates ranging from 3 to 96 hours old. Through videotape analysis of the frequency and duration of hand movements, the authors found that neonates immediately after birth were capable of imitating finger extension movements which were differentiated from general hand movements. The authors concluded that corticospinal connections that are known to be established as early as the 24th week post-conception coupled with the extensive spinal nerve growth before birth allow for these types of movements.

DEVELOPMENT OF GRASP AND OBJECT MANIPULATION

Use of the hand for object manipulation involves grasp, release, and the ability to transfer objects from one hand to the other. Stereotyped reflex patterns are often described in newborn infants. However, as mentioned previously, studies have indicated that these early movements can be considered less reflexive and more voluntary. The appearance of precision grasp (pad of radial fingers to pad of thumb) which emerges at around 10–12 months can be considered a developmental marker for advanced hand skills (Pehoski 2006). The actual development of object manipulation, however, occurs over a fairly long period of time.

The development of functional grasp occurs later and is usually seen in rudimentary form by 4–5 months of age. Previously it was thought that ulnar grasp develops first at around 3–4 months (Case-Smith 2006). However, more recent work suggests that isolated forefinger movement may be used earlier in grasp development as a means to contact and explore objects (Berthier and Keen 2006). By 6 months of age the infant has developed the skill of adjusting the hand to an object, orienting and adjusting the grip based on visual and tactile clues. As both upper extremities are brought together consistently, bimanual manipulation of objects is observed (about 8 months); exploration of an object with the fingers can begin with one hand while the other stabilizes the object. Thumb opposition and beginning finger individuation develop at 10–12 months, which allows for greater flexibility and leads to the development of a range of grasp patterns (Newell and McDonald 1997) (Figs 10.1 and 10.2).

To summarize, basic skills of reaching and grasping are demonstrated early in development. More precise reaching and grasping skills are seen by 4–5 months of age, with adult grasping patterns observed by 9 months of age (von Hofsten 1991) and precision grasping demonstrated by 12–18 months of age (von Hofsten and Fazel-Zandy 1984).

Less studied is the development of object release; however, controlled release generally develops after grasp (Pehoski 2006). At around 5–6 months, infants start the release of an object in a more purposeful way. Later (10–11 months) children generally reinforce purposeful object release through play by flinging items in a ballistic extension synergistic movement pattern (elbow, wrist and finger extension). By 1 year of age children have acquired graded object release (Pehoski 2006).

Development of functional hand skills and object manipulation continues to be refined over an extended period of time (Newell and McDonald 1997) with complex in-hand manipulation skills not mastered until 7 years of age (Exner 1990, Pehoski et al 1997 a, 1997b). In-hand manipulation skills have also been referred to as: the adjustment of an object in the hand after grasp (Pehoski 2006; see Exner 1990, 1992). These skills are necessary for such functional skills as handwriting and buttoning because they enable an object

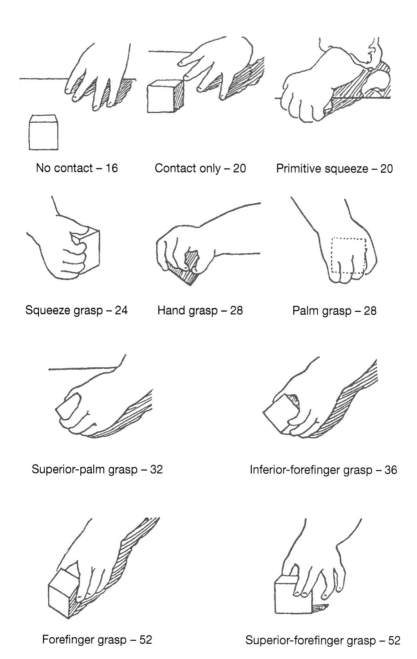

No contact – 16   Contact only – 20   Primitive squeeze – 20

Squeeze grasp – 24   Hand grasp – 28   Palm grasp – 28

Superior-palm grasp – 32   Inferior-forefinger grasp – 36

Forefinger grasp – 52   Superior-forefinger grasp – 52

Fig. 10.1 Grasping patterns.

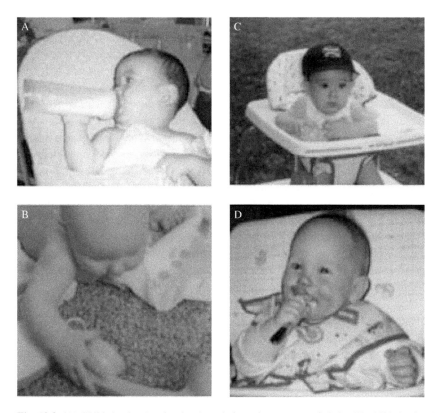

Fig. 10.2 (A) Child shaping hand to bottle and also using support of chair; (B) child shaping hand to phone; (C) child shaping hand to large object; (D) child using palmer grasp for self-feeding.

to be more efficiently positioned in the hand. In hand manipulation, actions can be defined as follows: the ability to move an object from the fingers to the palm and from the palm to the fingers (translation), the ability to rotate an object in the fingers (rotation), and the ability to move an object in a linear direction on the finger surface (shift). Rotation skills can be simple, such as rolling or turning an object in the fingers, or complex, such as rotating the object 180 degrees. Examples of these types of manipulation in functional skills include: moving a coin from the palm to the fingers to place in a vending machine (translation), rotating a pen through the fingers (rotation), and moving a pencil that is in the hand so the fingers are closer to the point (shift) (Exner 1990, 1992).

DEVELOPMENT OF REACH
The development of reaching has been defined as a search of task space for movement by von Hofsten and Rönnqvist (1993), and movement toward an object that takes the hand to an object quickly, accurately and efficiently by Berthier and Keen (2006). Reaching consists of two phases: transporting the hand to the object, and shaping the hand to the object. Within the constraints of this task, the infant learns to coordinate a relatively

immature neuromuscular system while controlling many degrees of freedom of movement in the arm and shoulder. Successful reaching and grasping objects is consistently demonstrated by infants by 4 months of age. At this early stage of reaching, infants try to reach for objects in the minimal amount of time (Berthier et al 1999).

Studies examining the development of a mature less variant reach in older infants and young children provide some insight into reach development. Thelen and Konczak conducted studies to measure the inverse dynamics associated with reaching in infants, and found that the path of an infant's reaching is curvilinear initially and becomes straighter at 6 months of age, indicating that hand paths and joint torques become smoother with development (Thelen et al 1993, Konczak et al 1995, Konczak and Dichgans 1997, Konczak et al 1997) (see Fig. 10.3). During the onset of reaching at 11 weeks, infants use primarily the proximal muscles of the arm and torso for reaching and tend to keep the elbow extended (Konczak et al 1995, 1997, Berthier et al 1999). Berthier et al (1999) propose that this strategy controls for degrees of freedom by limiting the reach within a small spatial plane, and may also increase the utility of feedback information obtained by these exploratory movements by stiffening the distal muscles. By using proximal muscles and making repeated similar movements, the infant's learning is thought to occur more rapidly.

DEVELOPMENT OF PRECISION GRIP
Coordination of precision grip develops rapidly during the first years of life. The refinement continues for many years and adult-like sensorimotor control is not attained until the early teenage years (Forssberg at al 1991, 1992, 1995). Precise grasping relies on the perceptual system which provides information about the position of the hand in space as well as the position of the target. This information is used to accommodate the size of the hand aperture to the size of the object for a smooth and precise grip (Jeannerod 1984). The pre-shaping activity of the digits develops from 8 months with rapid development during the following months (von Hofsten and Rönnqvist 1988). Yet, younger children (age 4 years) open their hands wider than older children (12 years). In addition, older children demonstrate a tighter coupling of maximum grip aperture to reach deceleration than younger children (Kuhtz-Buschbeck et al 1999).

Force control is another crucial factor for smooth and precise grasping. The invariant coordination pattern of the load (tangential to the grip surface) and grip forces (normal force) develops normally during the first years and continues gradually until teenage years when the lifts are completely adult-like (Forssberg et al 1991). The early pattern is characterized by a delay between movement phases and a sequential onset of the grip and load forces, as well as large intra-individual variability, resulting in immature and dyscoordinated movements (Fig. 10.4).

The amount of force generated during grasp depends on the size, friction and weight of the object and is built up by previous practice (Gordon et al 1991, Forssberg et al 1992, 1995). This internal representation of objects' properties is necessary to produce rapid and well-coordinated transitions between the various movement phases due to a long delay between motor command and sensory feedback (Johansson and Westling 1990, Gordon et al 1991). Uni-peaked force rate profiles are considered to be a result of an internal model.

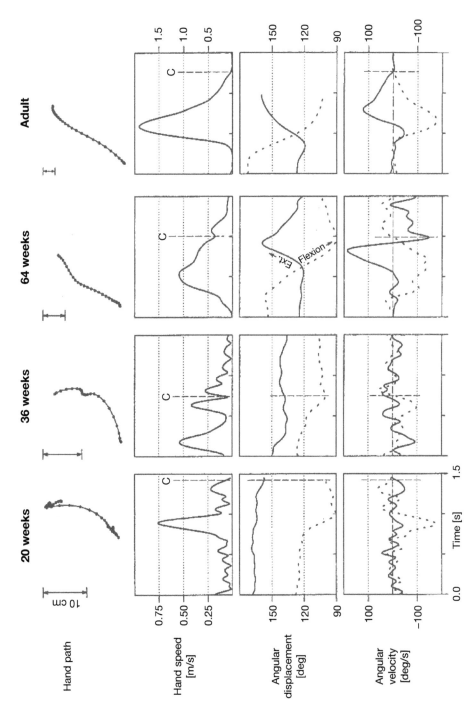

Fig. 10.3 Angular and endpoint kinematics of four individual infant reaches.

153

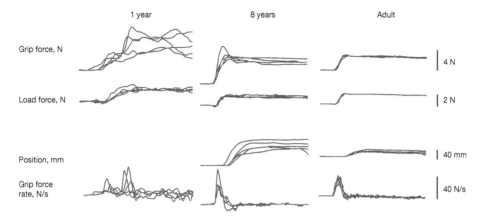

Fig. 10.4 Superimposed traces of representative lifts performed at different ages in three children with cerebral palsy with various degrees of severity. Grip force, load force, position, and grip force rate are shown as functions of time. When lifting the object, the grip force starts to increase; then the grip force and load force increase until the object starts to move. When the forces overcome gravity, the signal measuring position increases, followed by a static phase when the object is held in the air.

Source: Modified from Forssberg et al 1991.

In early age the force rates profiles are multi-peaked, indicating that children have to rely on sensory feedback mechanisms to control the force output. With continued development, these transform toward more uni-peaked force rates profiles (Forssberg et al 1992, Gordon et al 1992, Duque et al 2003).

These mechanisms can be seen in daily activities – for example, a 1-year-old usually crushes an ice-cream cone, whereas a 2-year-old can manage it quite well. At this age, they start to generate grip and load forces in parallel and scale the forces toward the object's different weight and friction. In 4-year-old children the motor output is less varied and more coordinated. The children have more coordinated and reliable movements and are able to, for example, carry a puppy and handle fragile objects. However, the appropriate anticipatory scaling with acceleration of the lift to harmonize with the weight of the object is not developed until 6 to 8 years of age. Even so, there are still large variations in the ability to properly scale the forces according to frictional demands. It is not until ages 10 to 12 that scaling approaches adult levels. Efficient control of finger movements continues to develop until adolescence, when children can learn to play musical instruments and develop good handwriting with accurate speed.

Atypical development due to prenatal/perinatal CNS damage

Reach Differences in Children with Cerebral Palsy
Reach to grasp movements in children with atypical sensorimotor development due to prenatal/perinatal CNS damage are typically clumsy to a variant extent. The movements are characterized in experimental studies by decreases in speed and velocity profiles with

proportionately longer deceleration phases, as well as a lack of movement smoothness which is denoted by a greater number of sub-movements (Trombly 1992, 1993). Disrupted inter-segmental relationships in reaching and grasping are found in children with hemiplegic cerebral palsy (CP). In a study by Steenbergen et al (2000a), results showed that the reaching task is initiated with movement largely at the shoulder with less elbow extension followed by a decrease in shoulder involvement. The children also completed the reaching with increased trunk movement. Deviant sitting posture during reaching is also described for children with hemiplegia; they tend to sit with their trunks more flexed and with the pelvis rotated posteriorly compared to typically developing children. In another study, children with bilateral CP were noted to have increased shoulder retraction and elbow flexion (van der Heide et al 2005). The quality of reaching depended on the adequacy of postural control. Children with hemiplegic (unilateral) CP also had limited ability to modulate postural muscles in relation to a specific reaching task: however, it appeared they could 'learn' to use trunk displacement in order to establish a better quality reach; while this was more difficult for the group of children with bilateral CP (van der Heide et al 2004).

There have been fewer studies examining upper extremity movement in children with more severe CP, i.e. children with spastic quadriplegia. In one study examining trunk recruitment during a reaching task, young adults with quadriplegia and a healthy control group transported either water or sugar by spoon and deposited each in a bowl that was either large or small (van Roon et al 2004). The results demonstrated that all participants used a similar type of grasp, and both groups transported similar amounts of substance to the bowl. However the adults with spastic quadriplegia were moving more slowly in the transport phase of the task and had larger trunk displacement during the task. Both groups could grade the amount of trunk displacement to variations in the accuracy demands of the task.

Grasp Differences in Children with Cerebral Palsy
Children with CP demonstrate differences in the development of grasping when compared to typically developing children. The parallel grip and load force typical of normal development is rarely seen. Instead, the forces increase sequentially, with the grip force increasing before the load force (Fig. 10.5). Consequently, children with CP do not produce force rates in mainly bell-shaped profiles, but in stepwise, irregular, and extremely variable profiles (Eliasson et al 1991, Forssberg et al 1999). However, this slow, sequential initiation of movements is an adequate strategy providing security in a manipulative task where the coordination of force generation is not fully functional. The same pattern with prolonged and uncoordinated movement phases is seen when the children have to replace and release objects (Eliasson and Gordon 2000). The question is to what extent this pattern is rigid or possible to influence by training. A study using constraint-induced movement therapy showed that extensive training may improve the grip–lift force synergy (Charles et al 2001). Follow-up over a long period reveals that improvement continues to take place, supporting a dynamic view of the nervous system (Eliasson et al 2006).

Other studies (Eliasson et al 1992, 1995, Forssberg et al 1999) further delineated problems of children with CP and their poor coordination of precision grip forces as:

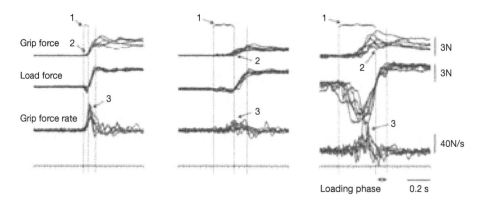

Fig. 10.5 Superimposed trajectories for children with normally developed grip–lift synergy, characterized by a short preload phase (1), low grip force at load force onset (2), followed by a parallel increase of the grip and load forces until the load force overcomes gravity with the peak grip force rate occurring in about the middle of the loading phase (3). The second child has an immature grip–lift synergy where the preload phase is prolonged (1), the grip forces at load force onset are higher (2), and the peak grip force rate occurs at different times (3), sometimes during the preload phase. The third child has no grip–lift synergy, with the preload phase being dramatically prolonged (1), and there being a sequential onset of grip and load forces (2), resulting in a very early peak grip force rate (3). The vertical dotted lines indicate the shift between the preload and loading phases.

Source: Adapted from Forssberg et al 1999.

inappropriate scaling of forces to an object's weight, with a stepwise increase in force as they picked up an object (lack of anticipatory control); needing successive lifts of an object to build up internal representations from weight and tactile information about an object. Later studies investigating grasp control in children with hemiplegic CP demonstrated that these children did learn some anticipatory control with continued practice lifting an object with the same properties (Gordon and Duff 1999, Duff and Gordon 2003). The same learning ability was seen when investigating reach and grasping (Steenbergen et al 1998). Typically, children with CP spent more time in contact with an object to be lifted, in contrast to the time they took to reach the object. Again, after several lifts of the object, time in contact with the object decreased, suggesting that children with CP are able to control and modify fingertip forces in advance with practice (Steenbergen et al 1998).

Later studies have examined movement planning and tested the minimization of movement costs and postural discomfort as constraints on grip selection (Steenbergen et al 2000b). Unlike control participants whose grip selection was driven by minimal postural discomfort and movement costs, participants with hemiplegia imposed different constraints on grip selection. If movements were difficult with the impaired hand, grip selection and planning to minimize movement costs resulted in reduced joint rotation.

Weakness is another problem in children with CP. Isometric force generation in typically developing children increased as a function of maturation (Smits-Engelsman et al 2003). However, in children with CP, the older children (over 10 years) demonstrated decreased force generation in the involved hand. In younger children with CP, the

156

non-involved hand showed peak values and frequency spectra that were commensurate with chronological age, while in older children with CP the non-involved hand was weaker than in control participants of the same age (Smits-Engelsman et al 2004).

Conclusion

Functional use of the upper extremity is a process that involves integration of several systems, maturation of the CNS, the constraints of the task, and the environment. There are dramatic observable changes during the first year but development of the child's upper limb control continues throughout childhood into the adolescent period. While damage to the CNS may result in atypical development of the various systems, there is a large variation in skills among children with CP: some exhibit only minor abnormalities while others experience significant impairment of reach, grasp and manual ability. When compared to typically developing children, the grip patterns of children with CP are invariant, and prolonged movement phases, as well as uncoordinated movements, are a typical sign related to their disability.

REFERENCES

Bertenthal B, von Hofsten C (1998) Eye, head and trunk control: the foundation for manual development. *Neurosci Biobehav Rev* 22: 515–520.
Berthier NE, Keen R (2006) Development of reaching in infancy. *Exp Brain Res* 169: 507–518.
Berthier NE, Clifton RK, McCall DD, Robin DJ (1999) Proximodistal structure of early reaching in human infants. *Exp Brain Res* 127: 259–269.
Case-Smith J (2006) Hand skill development in the context of infants' play: birth to 2 years. In: Henderson A, Pehoski C, editors. *Hand Function in the Child: Foundations for Remediation.* St Louis, MO: Mosby, pp. 128–141.
Charles J, Lavinder G, Gordon AM (2001) Effects of constraint-induced therapy on hand function in children with hemiplegic cerebral palsy. *Pediatr Phys Ther* 13: 68–76.
D'Elia A, Pighetti M, Moccia G, Santangelo N (2001) Spontaneous activity in normal fetuses. *Early Hum Dev* 65: 139–147.
Duff SV, Charles J (2004) Enhancing prehension in infants and children: fostering neuromotor strategies. *Phys and Occ Ther Ped* 24: 129–172.
Duff SV, Gordon AM (2003) Learning of grasp control in children with hemiplegic cerebral palsy. *Dev Med Child Neurol* 45: 746–757.
Duque J, Thonnard JL, Vandermeeren Y, Sebire G, Cosnard G, Olivier E (2003) Correlation between impaired dexterity and corticospinal tract dysgenesis in congenital hemiplegia. *Brain* 126: 732–747.
Eliasson AC (2005) Improving the use of hands in daily activities: aspects of the treatment of children with cerebral palsy. *Phys Occup Ther Ped* 25: 37–60.
Eliasson AC, Gordon AM (2000) Impaired force coordination during object release in children with hemiplegic cerebral palsy. *Dev Med Child Neurol* 42: 228–234.
Eliasson AC, Gordon AM, Forssberg H (1991) Basic co-ordination of manipulative forces of children with cerebral palsy. *Dev Med Child Neurol* 33: 661–670.
Eliasson AC, Gordon AM, Forssberg H (1992) Impaired anticipatory control of isometric forces during grasping by children with cerebral palsy. *Dev Med Child Neurol* 34: 216–225.
Eliasson AC, Gordon AM, Forssberg H (1995) Tactile control of isometric fingertip forces during grasping in children with cerebral palsy. *Dev Med Child Neurol* 37: 72–84.
Eliasson AC, Forssberg H, Ya-Ching Hung, Gordon AM (2006) Development of hand function and precision grip control in individuals with cerebral palsy: a 13 year follow up. *Pediatrics* 118: 1226–1236.
Exner CE (1990) The zone of proximal development in in-hand manipulation skills of nondysfunctional 3- to 4-year-old children. *Am J Occup Ther* 44: 884–891.

Exner CE (1992) In-hand manipulation skills. In: Case-Smith J, Pehoski C, editors. *Development of Hand Skills*. Rockville, MD: American Occupational Therapy Association.

Eyre JA, Taylor JP, Villagra F, Smith M, Miller S (2001) Evidence of activity-dependent withdrawal of corticospinal projections during human development. *Neurology* 57: 1543–1554.

Fallang B, Saugstad OD, Hadders-Algra M (2000) Goal directed reaching and postural control in supine healthy infants. *Behav Brain Res* 115: 9–18.

Forssberg H, Eliasson AC, Kinoshita H, Johansson RS, Westling G (1991) Development of human precision grip I: Basic coordination of forces. *Exp Brain Res* 85: 451–457.

Forssberg H, Kinoshita H, Eliasson AC, Johansson RS, Westling G, Gordon AM (1992) Development of human precision grip II: Anticipatory control of isometric forces targeted for object's weight. *Exp Brain Res* 90: 393–398.

Forssberg H, Kinoshita H, Eliasson AC, Johansson RS, Westling G (1995) Development of human precision grip IV: Tactile adaptation of isometric finger forces to the frictional condition. *Exp Brain Res* 104: 323–330.

Forssberg H, Eliasson AC, Redon-Zouitenn C, Mercuri E, Dubowitz L (1999) Impaired grip-lift synergy in children with unilateral brain lesions. *Brain* 122: 1157–1168.

Gesell A, Amatruda CS (1947) *Developmental Diagnosis, 2nd edn.* New York: Paul B. Hoeber.

Gordon AM, Duff SV (1999) Fingertip forces during object manipulation in children with hemiplegic cerebral palsy. I: Anticipatory scaling. *Dev Med Child Neurol* 41: 166–175.

Gordon AM, Forssberg H, Johansson RS, Westling G (1991) Integration of sensory information during the programming of precision grip: comments on the contributions of size cues. *Exp Brain Res* 85: 226–229.

Gordon AM, Forssberg H, Johansson RS, Eliasson AC, Westling G (1992) Development of human precision grip III: Integration of visual size cues during programming of isometric forces. *Exp Brain Res* 90: 399–403.

Hadders-Algra M (2000) The neuronal group selection theory: a framework to explain variation in normal motor development. *Dev Med Child Neurol* 42: 566–572.

Heriza CB (1991) Implications of a dynamical systems approach to understanding infant kicking behavior. *Phys Ther* 71: 222–235.

Jeannerod M (1984) The timing of natural prehension movements. *J Mot Behav* 16: 235–254.

Johansson RS, Westling G (1990) Tactile afferent signals in the control of precision grip. In: Jeannerod M, editor. *Attention and Performance*. Hillsdale, NJ: Erlbaum.

Konczak J, Dichgans J (1997) The development toward stereotypic arm kinematics during reaching in the first 3 years of life. *Exp Brain Res* 117: 346–354.

Konczak J, Borutta M, Topka H, Dichgans J (1995) The development of goal-directed reaching in infants: hand trajectory formation and joint torque control. *Exp Brain Res* 106: 156–168.

Konczak J, Borutta M, Dichgans J (1997) The development of goal-directed reaching in infants. II. Learning to produce task-adequate patterns of joint torque. *Exp Brain Res* 113: 465–474.

Kuhtz-Buschbeck J, Boczek-Funcke A, Illert M, Joehnk K, Stolze H (1999) Prehension movements and motor development in children. *Exp Brain Res* 128: 65–68.

Massion J (1998) Postural control systems in developmental perspective. *Neurosci Biobehav Rev* 22: 465–472.

Nagy E, Compagne H, Orvos, H, Pal A, Molnar P, Jansky I, Loveland KA, Bardos G (2005) Index finger movement imitation by human neonates: motivation, learning, and left hand preference. *Pediatr Res* 58: 749–775.

Newell K, McDonald PV (1997) The development of grasp patterns in infancy. In: Connolly K, Forssberg H, editors. *Neurophysiology and Neuropsychology of Motor Development*. London: Mac Keith Press, pp. 232–256.

Pehoski C (2006) Object manipulation in infants and children. In: Henderson A, Pehoski C, editors. *Hand Function in the Child: Foundations for Remediation*. St Louis, MO: Mosby, pp.143–160.

Pehoski C, Henderson A, Tickle-Degnan L (1997a) In-hand manipulation in young children: rotation of an object in fingers. *Am J Occup Ther* 51: 544–552.

Pehoski C, Henderson A, Tickle-Degnan L (1997b) In-hand manipulation in young children: translation movements. *Am J Occup Ther* 51: 719–728.

Reed ES (1989) Changing theories of postural development. In: Woollacott MH, Shumway-Cook A, editors. *Development of Posture and Gait across the Life Span*. Columbia, SC: University of South Carolina Press, pp. 1–24.

Shumway-Cook A, Woollacott MH (2001) Development of postural control. In: *Motor Control: Theory and Practical Applications, 2nd edn.* Philadelphia: Lippincott Williams & Wilkins, pp. 192–221.

Smits-Engelsman B, Westenberg Y, Duysens J (2003) Development of isometric force and force control in children. *Cogn Brain Res* 17: 68–74.

Smits-Engelsman B, Rameckers EA, Duysens J (2004) Late development deficits in force control in children with hemiplegia. *Neuroreport* 15: 1931–1935.

Sparling JW, Van Tol J, Chesheir NC (1999) Fetal and neonatal hand movement. *Phys Ther* 79: 24–39.

Steenbergen B, Hulstijn W, Lemmens IHL, Meulenbroek RGJ (1998) The timing of prehensile movements in subjects with cerebral palsy. *Dev Med Child Neurol* 40: 108–114.

Steenbergen B, van Thiel E, Hulstijn W, Meulenbroek R (2000a) The coordination of reaching and grasping in spastic hemiparesis. *Hum Mov Sci* 19: 75–105.

Steenbergen B, Hulstijn W, Dortman S (2000b) Constraints on grip selection in cerebral palsy. Minimizing discomfort. *Exp Brain Res* 134: 385–397.

Thelen E, Spencer JP (1998) Postural control during reaching in young infants: a dynamic systems approach. *Dev Psychobiol* 30: 89–102.

Thelen E, Corbetta D, Kamm K, Spencer JP, Schneider K, Zernicke RF (1993) The transition to reaching; mapping intention and intrinsic dynamics. *Child Dev* 64: 1058–1098.

Trombly CA (1992) Deficits of reaching in subjects with left hemiparesis: a pilot study. *Am J Occup Ther* 46: 887–897.

Trombly CA (1993) Observations of improvement in reaching in five subjects with left hemiparesis. *J Neurol Neurosurg Psychiatry* 56: 40–45.

van der Heide JC, Begeer C, Fock JM, Otten B, Stremmelaar E, van Eykern LA, Hadders-Algra M (2004) Postural control during reaching in preterm children with cerebral palsy. *Dev Med Child Neurol* 46: 253–266.

van der Heide JC, Fock JM, Otten B Stremmelaar E, Hadders-Algra M (2005) Kinematic characteristics of postural control during reaching in preterm children with cerebral palsy. *Pediatr Res* 58: 586–593.

van der Meer AL, van der Weel FR, Lee DN (1995) The functional significance of arm movements in neonates. *Science* 267: 693–695.

van Roon D, Steenbergen B, Meulenbrock RGJ (2004) Trunk recruitment during spoon use in tetraparetic cerebral palsy. *Exp Brain Res* 155: 186–195.

von Hofsten C (1980) Predictive reaching for moving objects by human infants. *J Exp Child Psychol* 30: 369–382.

von Hofsten C (1991) Structuring of early reaching movements: a longitudinal study. *J Mot Behav* 23: 280–292.

von Hofsten C, Fazel-Zandy S (1984) Development of visually guided hand orientation in reaching. *J Exp Child Psychol* 38: 208–219.

von Hofsten C, Rönnqvist L (1988) Preparation for grasping an object: a developmental study. *J Exp Psychol Hum Percept Perform* 14: 610–621.

von Hofsten C, Rönnqvist L (1993) The structuring of neonatal arm movements. *Child Dev* 64: 1046–1057.

Wallace PS, Whishaw IQ (2003) Independent digit movements and precision grip patterns in 1–5-month-old infants: hand babbling, including vacuous then self-directed hand and digit movements, precedes targeted reaching. *Neuropsychologia* 41:1912–1918.

159

11
BIMANUAL COORDINATION IN CHILDREN WITH HEMIPLEGIC CEREBRAL PALSY

Andrew M. Gordon and Bert Steenbergen

Children with hemiplegic cerebral palsy (CP) have largely unilateral impairments in upper extremity movement (see Chapters 1, 4 and 10 for details). These impairments do not have much impact on unimanual activities of daily living (e.g. combing hair, brushing teeth, drinking, etc.) since these tasks may be performed effectively with their non-involved extremity. Furthermore, children with hemiplegic CP are remarkably adept at reaching with the non-involved extremity toward objects that are located in the contralateral hemispace. Similarly, they may use the non-involved extremity alone in a compensatory manner during tasks that typically developing children/adults would normally perform bimanually. For example, to place a milk container in the refrigerator, children with hemiplegia may perform the task exclusively with their non-involved extremity, by setting the container down on the counter with the non-involved hand in order to open the refrigerator with that hand, maintaining the door open with their body and then grasping, transporting and releasing the container on the shelf. The consequence of such sequential behaviour is that the children are clumsy and take time to perform tasks.

In addition to severe impairments, children with hemiplegia often have 'developmental disuse' whereby they may never have learned to use their involved extremity effectively for many motor tasks, or may only use it in the simplest manner, for example as a passive stabilizer (e.g. placing the involved extremity passively on a book page or piece of paper while reading or writing). When asked to perform bimanual tasks with specific spatio-temporal demands, they either fail to complete the task or exhibit poor coordination between the two extremities.

In this chapter we will briefly describe the development of bimanual coordination and the inherent constraints of such tasks. Next, we provide an overview of experimental studies on bimanual control in children with hemiplegic CP. Finally, we will discuss recent advances in rehabilitation which aim to improve bimanual coordination and thereby facilitate activities of daily living. These advances are exemplified by preliminary findings of a new intervention for children that specifically focuses on coordination of both hands together.

Neural control and development of bimanual coordination in typically developing children

Bimanual coordination involves a large number of neural structures, including the cerebellum, premotor cortex, supplementary motor cortex, parietal cortex and corpus callosum (see Swinnen and Wenderoth 2004). A number of studies suggest that development of bimanual coordination (especially for asymmetrical tasks) in typically developing individuals is related to maturation and myelination of the corpus callosum, connecting the two hemispheres. These connections are incomplete at birth and myelination may continue over the first decade of life (Yakovlev and Lecours 1967, LaMantia and Rakic 1990). This development corresponds with the ontology of spatial and temporal features of bimanual coordination (e.g. Fagard et al 1985, Njiokiktjien et al 1986, Jeeves et al 1988, Fagard et al 2001). Specifically, the contrast between the ease of performing symmetrical bimanual movements and the greater difficulty involved in performing asymmetrical movements, which is particularly strong in children, diminishes during the first decade of development, thus parallelling the process of myelinization of the corpus callosum (Abercrombie 1970, Njiokiktjien et al 1986, Fagard 1987, Fagard et al 2001, Fagard and Corroyer 2003). Bimanual performance measured by a computerized bimanual performance test has been found to involve interhemispheric interactions as well (Marion et al 2003).

Although preferences in bimanual control change during development, research has revealed several spatial and temporal motor constraints in adults that may inform us on the preferences of the central nervous system when controlling bimanual actions (e.g. Steenbergen et al 2003). For example, movements involving homologous (same) muscle groups in each limb appear to be easier to perform than movements involving non-homologous muscle groups (Cohen 1970, Annett and Sheridan 1973, Kelso et al 1983). In addition, spatial and temporal interference have been abundantly shown during bimanual movement performance. Kelso and coworkers were among the first to show tight temporal coupling between limbs when the task requirements of each limb (with respect to movement accuracy and amplitude) were different (Kelso et al 1979, 1983). Spatial interference effects were shown by having both hands draw figures that differed in shape. Franz et al showed spatial interference effects when one hand had to draw circles, while the other drew lines (Franz et al 1991): circles became ellipsoid and lines became circle-like. Evidence for the role of the corpus callosum in spatial interference was found in patients who had a 'split-brain' following callostomy, as these patients did not demonstrate these spatial interference effects (Franz et al 1996). Finally, coordination of the two hands together has been shown to require appropriate control of the trunk in an anticipatory manner (e.g. Schmitz and Assaiante 2002, Roncesvalles et al 2005). Together, these studies suggest that the ability to coordinate both hands develops over the first decade and is related to maturation of the corpus callosum. In adults, complex interactions exist between the hands which pertain to spatial and temporal coupling or uncoupling.

Coordination of bimanual movements in children with hemiplegic CP

Early damage to the developing brain may inhibit the development of skilled bimanual interactions, or the developing child may fail to engage in sufficient practice to develop these skills. The latter is specifically prominent in children with hemiplegic cerebral palsy. Hemiplegic cerebral palsy is usually the result of middle cerebral artery infarct, hemi-brain atrophy, periventricular white matter damage, brain malformation or posthaemorrhagic porencephaly (Uvebrant 1988, Bouza et al 1994, Okumura et al 1997, Cioni et al 1999), which may result in damage to areas involved in bimanual coordination, including the motor cortex, premotor cortex, supplementary motor area (SMA) and parietal cortex (Toyokura et al 1999, Debaere et al 2001, Immisch et al 2001, Gribova et al 2002). Damage to areas such as the SMA and the parietal lobe has been shown to result in bimanual coordination impairments (Serrien et al 2001, Serrien et al 2002, Steyvers et al 2003). The timing of the brain damage may also impact the severity of motor impairment (see Chapter 4).

Most evident in hemiplegic cerebral palsy are movement deviations contralateral to the brain damage, and most studies of hand function in children with hemiplegia have indeed focused on unimanual coordination (see Chapter 26). However, the majority of manual activities of daily living require that the two hands work together (see Chapters 21 and 25). In light of the recent modification of the definition of CP that it is a 'disorder of movement and posture causing activity limitation' (Rosenbaum et al 2007), this dearth of information on bimanual coordination in CP is problematic in understanding the motor impairments underlying the disease. One recent qualitative study of bimanual control in adolescents with hemiplegic CP found that the planning of bimanual activities involved a complex process that was influenced not only by motor factors, but also by a range of other internal and external factors (Skold et al 2004). In particular, factors such as feasibility of success, social aspects and personal aspects, as well as tolerating some negative consequences of the action, came into play when choosing movement strategies.

Most research has focused on how the two hands interact, and has examined whether one hand facilitates or interferes with movement of the other hand. Although the non-involved extremity had previously been clinically described to have a beneficial effect on the involved extremity (Brown et al 1987), most work on bimanual coordination in this population has been performed in the last decade (Utley and Steenbergen 2006). In one of the pioneering experimental studies, Sugden and Utley (1995) examined the mutual influence of one hand on the other by asking participants to reach at preferred speed either unimanually or bimanually. Temporal synchronization between the two hands was found under bimanual responding, but the way in which this was achieved differed between and within participants. Either one of the two hands or both adapted during the bimanual movements as compared to moving unimanually. Utley and Sugden (1998) showed a speeding up of the involved hand during bimanual reach and grasp and reach, touch and grasp. In Fig. 11.1, an example is shown of the involved hand moving faster (compared to unimanual movement) and being coupled to the movement of the non-involved hand when the movements are produced bimanually as participants reach toward a cube to grasp it (not shown).

In a separate series of studies by Steenbergen and colleagues, similar temporal synchrony in bimanual conditions was found when participants were asked to respond as quickly as possible (Steenbergen et al 1996). In contrast to Sugden and Utley's (1995) study, they showed that temporal coupling was established in a uniform manner. For all participants, the non-involved hand slowed down under bimanual responding. Performance of the involved hand was relatively unaffected by the movement condition. The greater effect on the involved hand's speed in Sugden and Utley's (1995) study than in Steenbergen and colleagues' (1996, 2000) studies may be explained by the task instructions. The speeding

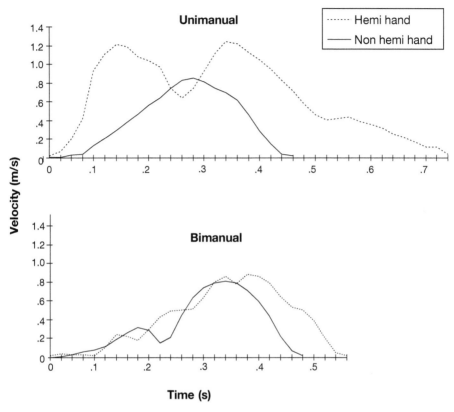

Fig. 11.1 Superimposed velocity profiles for each hand when a 10-year-old child with severe hemiplegia reaches either unimanually (top) or bimanually (bottom).

Source: Adapted from Utley et al 2004.

up of the involved extremity in the former study may have been possible because the tasks were performed at self-pace. In contrast, the latter studies required participants to perform the task as fast as possible. Thus, unlike under self-paced conditions, there may not have been room for the involved extremity to move any faster (i.e. a ceiling effect).

As well as temporal synchrony of the end effectors, the studies cited above also examined coupling at the level of joint angle displacements of the elbow and shoulder (Steenbergen et al 2000) and postural and spatial coupling (Sugden and Utley 1995). Coupling between shoulder and elbow angular displacement was found under bimanual responding (Steenbergen et al 2000), but Sugden and Utley (1995) showed that spatial (hand trajectory) and postural (hand posture) coupling were not always found.

Taken together, the results of these studies suggest that during symmetrical movements there is a coupling of movements of the two extremities, with one or both of the movements being affected. It is also evident that the influence of the other hand is not always beneficial. This may be illustrated by a recent study (Steenbergen et al 2008) in which we asked children with hemiplegic CP to grasp, pick up, transport and release either one object unimanually with the involved hand or two objects simultaneously with both hands. Fig. 11.2 shows the total movement time of the involved hand when transporting one or two objects. Overall, bimanual movements were 13 per cent slower compared to unimanual movements, which may be due to the increased attention required to manipulate two objects. Thus, the extent to which bimanual movement benefits or interferes with unimanual function appears to be task-dependent.

Importantly, unlike the above studies, most bimanual activities involve a decoupling of movement of the two extremities such that the movements must be performed in an asymmetrical manner (e.g. typing, buttoning, shoelace tying). Many children with hemiplegia demonstrate the presence of mirror movements (Kuhtz-Buschbeck et al 2000), particularly those with greater severity. During asymmetrical movements, however, the non-involved hand cannot serve as a template for the involved hand, and instead the two limbs must be decoupled to act independently. The distinction is important given recent findings by Volman and colleagues (2002). These investigators asked children with hemiplegia to draw circles with their two hands, using either homologous or non-homologous muscles of the two extremities. During homologous task performance, there was reduced temporal variability and increased smoothness of the non-involved hand. Conversely, when non-homologous muscles were employed across the two limbs, the non-involved extremity had to adapt to the performance of the involved limb. In a follow-up study, it was shown that amplitude and form incongruence resulted in differential effects (Volman 2005). As seen in Fig. 11.3, when children with hemiplegic CP were asked to draw a circle with one hand and a line with the other, the circles became more linear and

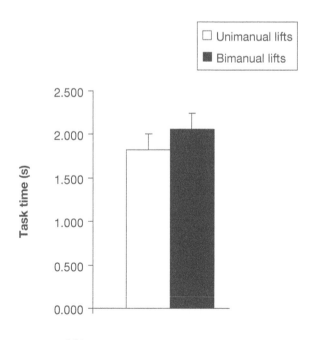

Fig. 11.2 Total task time as children with hemiplegic CP grasp, pick up, transport and release either one object unimanually (unfilled bars) or two objects (filled bars) simultaneously with both hands.
Source: Steenbergen et al 2008.

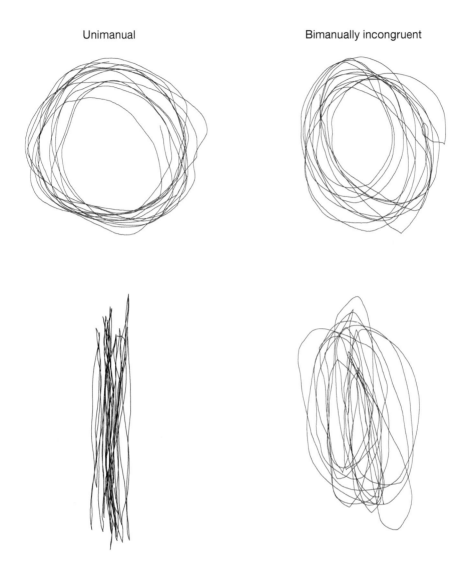

Fig. 11.3 Examples of circle drawing (top) and line drawing (bottom) for the involved right hand of a 10-year-old boy with hemiplegia when asked to draw these shapes either unimanually (left panels) or during a bimanual incongruent situation where the non-involved hand simultaneously draws the opposite (right panels). Note the spatial interference whereby the incongruent task of one hand is detrimental to the other hand.

Source: Adapted from Volman 2005.

the lines more ellipsoid compared to when either was drawn individually, regardless of the hand performing each task. When asked to draw circles of differing sizes with the two hands (not shown), each hand influenced the other, but the direction of influence depended on which hand drew a given-size circle. Thus, in addition to being dependent on speed-related task constraints, the influence of each hand on the other may be dependent on task constraints related to spatial characteristics of the objects. For example, Utley et al (2004) found that asking participants to grasp larger objects with their involved extremity improved performance compared to their non-involved extremity.

A final consideration concerns the type of tasks that were studied. In order to determine how the two hands interact during a common functional task, we recently examined bimanual coordination requiring asymmetrical control using a drawer-opening task (Hung et al 2004). Children were asked to reach forward and open a drawer with one hand and activate a light switch inside the drawer with the contralateral hand. This task involves a variety of neural structures (Wiesendanger and Serrien 2004) as well as integration of proprioception from both limbs (Kazennikov and Wiesendanger 2005). Fig. 11.4 shows an example of kinematic traces of both hands for a typically developing child performing the task at self-paced speed (A), and for a child with hemiplegia performing the task at self-paced speed (B) and as fast as possible (C). The control child (A) began moving the task hand (b) shortly after initiating the drawer-opening hand movement (a) and thus had considerable movement overlap time of the two hands (b–e) and a short goal synchronization duration whereby both hands complete their tasks (e–f). In contrast, the child with hemiplegic CP (B) was much slower and their movements were more sequential, with the task hand initiating movement well after the drawer hand reached the drawer and began pulling it open (minima in drawer-opening hand trace). Thus, there was less movement overlap (b–e) and a longer goal synchronization time (e–f) when moving at self-pace. However, when moving as fast as possible, the task was completed much more quickly, and the coordination begins to approximate that of the typically developing child (C). The results further highlight the importance of movement constraints on task performance and suggest that movement speed may facilitate better bimanual coordination under asymmetric task conditions.

The overlap of movement was influenced by the hand used for each task for the hemiplegic CP group. When the involved hand served as the drawer hand, the non-involved hand waited for the involved hand to open the drawer (i.e. minimizing movement overlap) before initiating its movement. However, the non-involved hand compensated by increasing its velocity at the end of the task.

In a subsequent study we manipulated the task constraints by varying the difficulty of grasping the drawer handle (Gordon, Charles and Hung, unpublished data). The drawer handle was varied to be either a 3.5 cm knob that required precision grasp, or a loop handle that simply required curling the fingers around it. The results indicated that making the handle easier to grasp (i.e. by using the loop) improved movement overlap. This can be seen in Fig. 11.5, which plots the movement times of the drawer-reaching hand and the task hand, with the relative delay of onset indicated by the difference in onset times. Regardless of which hand was used to open the drawer, the task time (denoted by end of task hand movement) was shorter when the handle was easier to grasp and the button to manipulate was larger.

To summarize, performance of bimanual tasks in children with hemiplegic CP may be dependent on a number of factors, such as the speed of the movements, the extent to which

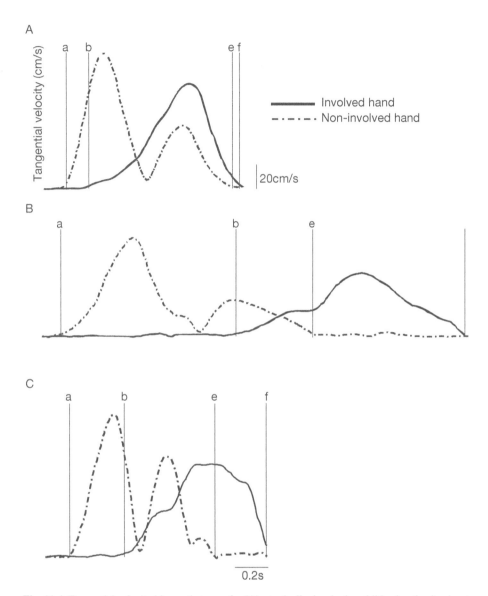

Fig. 11.4 Tangential velocity kinematic traces for (A) a typically developing child using the dominant hand to open the drawer at self-pace, (B) a child with hemiplegic CP using the non-involved hand to open the drawer at self-pace, (C) the same child using the non-involved hand to open the drawer as fast as possible. Note that the velocity traces of the task hand terminate above zero if the hand does not decelerate before contacting the switch. (a) Movement onset of the drawer hand. (b) Movement onset of the task hand. (e) Movement offset of the drawer hand when the drawer is completely opened. (f) Movement offset of the task hand. (b–e) Movement overlap time for the two hands. (e–f) Goal synchronization duration.

Source: Adapted from Hung et al 2004.

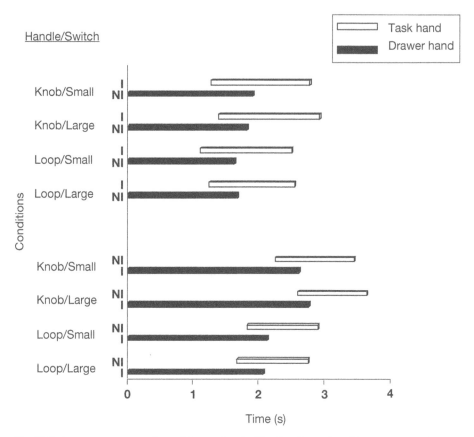

Fig. 11.5 Average movement time of the two hands. The first four pairs of bars represent the non-involved (NI) hand as the drawer hand, and involved (I) hand as the task hand condition. The lower four pairs of bars represent the reverse. The total distance on the x-y axis represents task time, and the onset of the task hand relative to the drawer hand shows movement overlap.

Source: Gordon, Hung and Charles, unpublished data.

the hands produce similar or different movements, whether the task requires symmetric or asymmetric control, and the accuracy requirements for each hand. These results, as well as findings from typically developing children and adults, suggest that the non-involved extremity may be useful in providing a template for the involved extremity to improve performance (see also Steenbergen et al 2003). These findings may have implications for rehabilitation, which will be outlined below. However, one major limitation in our understanding of both the mechanisms of bimanual coordination impairments and the potential for rehabilitation is that most studies to date have focused on moderately impaired individuals. Little is known about impairments in mildly or severely afflicted individuals.

Rehabilitation of bimanual coordination

Performance of a movement with one hand may provide a template for performing the task with the contralateral hand (Gordon et al 1994, 1999, 2006a). Such findings provide the rationale for using mirroring, where a task is first performed with the non-involved extremity to provide an understanding of task constraints during intensive unimanual training (e.g. constraint-induced therapy; Gordon et al 2005).

There is some evidence suggesting that extensive unimanual practice associated with constraint-induced therapy can transfer to improvements in bimanual coordination (Eliasson et al 2005; see also Charles and Gordon 2005, and Chapter 20). Principles of motor learning emphasize the importance of task specificity in practice in order to maximize learning (see Schmidt and Lee 2005). Thus, if the goal is to improve bimanual coordination, but also to increase use of the involved hand, intensive unimanual training (which focuses on unimanual tasks, which are unlikely to be performed with the involved extremity following removal of the constraint) would be less efficient than bimanual training. Since ipsilateral pathways are thought to be implicated in the recovery of function after stroke (Marshall et al 2000), tasks recruiting these pathways, such as symmetrical bilateral movements (Hallett 2001, Stinear and Byblow 2004), may be beneficial. Bilateral practice may result in changes in plasticity (Cauraugh and Summers 2005) and cortical excitability in the undamaged hemisphere (Stinear and Byblow 2004) in stroke patients, providing a rationale for bimanual therapy at the neural level. This rationale has driven the development of bimanual interventions in adults with stroke (for a review see Rose and Winstein 2004, Cauraugh and Summers 2005). Most of these studies reported functional improvements of the involved upper extremity with bimanual training. However, these studies have largely used repetitive non-functional tasks (e.g. repetitive cycling with the two hands) or cyclical tasks. More functional training may be of benefit in children with CP (Ketelaar et al 2001, Ahl et al 2005).

Recently, we have developed (Gordon et al 2007) a new structured intervention for children with hemiplegia which provides the intensity of practice of constraint-induced (CI) therapy, but which focuses on coordination of both hands together: Hand-Arm Bimanual Intensive Training (HABIT). HABIT was developed based on: (1) our experience with CI therapy in children with CP; (2) the results of bimanual coordination studies described above; (3) principles of motor learning (specificity of practice, types of practice, feedback); and (4) principles of neuroplasticity (practice-induced brain changes arising from repetition, increasing movement complexity, motivation, and reward) (e.g. Nudo 2003, Kleim et al 2004).

HABIT retains the two major elements of paediatric CI therapy (intensive structured practice and child-friendliness) and engages the child in bimanual activities 6 hours/day for 10 days (60 hours). However, it differs from 'traditional' CI therapy in that there is an absence of physical restraint, and activities that necessitate bimanual hand use rather than unimanual performance are employed. HABIT also differs from conventional physical and occupational therapy in several ways. The intensity of HABIT is far greater than that of conventional therapies, providing sufficient opportunity for practice using principles of motor learning. It is far more structured than conventional therapy, as described below.

Finally, rather than encouraging use of the involved hand in any manner (e.g. as a passive assist), we ask children to use it as a typically developing child uses their non-dominant hand. Specifically, we ask them to focus on how the hand and arm are performing at the end-point of the movement.

To conduct HABIT, specific bimanual activities involving performance of play or functional activities are selected by considering joint movements with pronounced deficits, improvement of which interventionists believe have greatest potential. The age-appropriate fine motor and manipulative gross activities (see Table 11.1) are chosen to elicit whole or part practice, and these activities determine how the involved hand and arm are used. Specific activities are selected by considering the role of the involved limb in the activity. While task demands are graded to allow for success, children are asked to use the involved limb in the same manner as that of the non-dominant limb of a typically developing child.

TABLE 11.1
HABIT activities

Activity category	Repetitive task practice	Whole task practice	Role of involved hand	Graded constraints
Manipulative games and tasks	Precision grasp in symmetrical bimanual tasks	Precision grasp, wrist extension and supination	Stabilizer, manipulator, active/passive assist, symmetrical and asymmetrical movements	Changing spatial and temporal constraints of the task, for symmetrical tasks increasing frequency task is completed within a fixed time period
Card games	Active wrist supination in symmetrical bimanual tasks	Grasp, wrist stabilization and supination	Stabilizer, manipulator, active/passive assist, symmetrical and asymmetrical movements	Changing spatial and temporal constraints of the task, for symmetrical tasks increasing frequency task is completed within a fixed time period
Video games	Finger individuation	Finger individuation	Manipulator, active assist, symmetrical movements	Changing temporal constraints of task
Functional tasks	All movements	Precision grasp, wrist extension and supination	Stabilizer, manipulator, active/passive assist, symmetrical and asymmetrical movements	Stabilizer, manipulator, active/passive assist, symmetrical and asymmetrical movements
Gross motor	Shoulder, upper extremity movement, shoulder flexion, abduction and elbow, wrist extension	Shoulder, upper extremity movement, shoulder flexion, abduction and elbow, wrist extension	Stabilizer, manipulator, active/passive assist, symmetrical and asymmetrical movements	Stabilizer, manipulator, active/passive assist, symmetrical and asymmetrical movements
Arts and crafts	Wrist and finger extension in symmetrical bimanual tasks	Precision grasp, wrist extension and supination	Stabilizer, manipulator, active/passive assist, symmetrical and asymmetrical movements	Stabilizer, manipulator, active/passive assist, symmetrical and asymmetrical movements

During these activities the children receive instructions from the interventionist but also have to engage in their own active problem solving. Task performance is recorded and both positive reinforcement and knowledge of performance are used to motivate performance and to reinforce target movements.

HABIT is conducted in groups of two to four children, to provide social interaction, modelling, and encouragement. The choice of specific activities is not as important as the movements they elicit. Movement deficits of the involved extremity and bimanual coordination deficits are determined during the pre-intervention evaluation. Bimanual activities are then selected that will improve these movement deficits and engage the child in activities of increasingly complex coordination. Directions specifying how each hand will be used during the activity are given to the child before the start of each task in order to avoid use of compensatory strategies (performing the task unimanually with the non-involved extremity). Two types of practice are employed. During performance of **whole task practice**, activities are performed continuously for at least 15–20 minutes in the context of playing a game or performing functional activities. Targeted movements and spatial and temporal coordination are practised within the context of completing the task. **Part task practice** involves practising a targeted movement exclusive of other movements. Specifically, we used symmetrical bimanual movements such as putting game pieces away with both hands simultaneously. The task difficulty is graded as the child's performance improves by requiring greater speed or accuracy, or by providing tasks that require more skilled use of the involved hand and arm (for example, moving from activities in which the involved limb is used as a stabilizer to activities where it is used as a manipulator; see Krumlinde-Sundholm and Eliasson 2003, and Chapter 10).

We recently conducted a preliminary randomized control trial of HABIT (Gordon et al 2007) with 20 children with hemiplegic CP between the ages of 3.5 and 14 years. All children demonstrated moderate hand involvement (Type IIa; Zancolli and Zancolli 1981). The inclusion criteria for children with hemiplegic cerebral palsy were identical to those used in the paediatric constraint-induced therapy studies (Charles et al 2006, Gordon et al 2006b).

The results indicate significant ($p < 0.05$) improvement in the scores on the Assisting Hand Assessment and bimanual items of the Bruininks-Oseretsky Test of Motor Proficiency (Gordon et al 2007). The children also showed improvement on performance of the drawer task described above (Hung et al 2004). This can be seen in Fig. 11.6, which shows that the time between opening the drawer and pressing the light switch (goal-synchronization) averaged more than a second during the pretest, but decreased substantially following participation in the study for all eight participants who performed the task following treatment.

Collectively, these results suggest that improvement in coordination can be elicited without a physical restraint, and that bimanual coordination can be improved with intensive bimanual practice.

Despite our successful application of HABIT with children with hemiplegia, this is only preliminary evidence of its efficacy, and considerable work needs to be performed to ensure that it complies with the rigour of evidence-based medicine. Whether HABIT is as efficacious as CI therapy, or whether children would benefit by first 'jump-starting' the

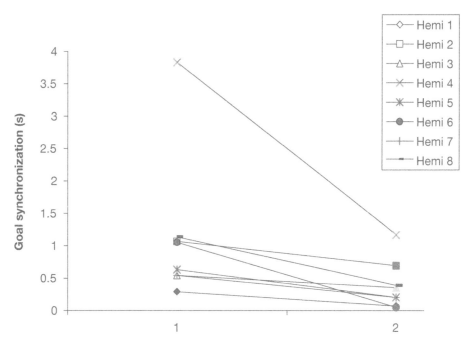

Fig. 11.6 Goal synchronization time (e–f, Fig. 11.4) of the eight participants receiving the HABIT treatment.

Source: Adapted from Gordon et al 2007.

involved extremity by using CI therapy followed subsequently by HABIT training, remains to be determined.

ACKNOWLEDGEMENTS

This work was supported by a grant from the United Cerebral Palsy Research and Education Foundation awarded to the first author. The second author was supported by a grant awarded by The Netherlands Organization for Scientific Research (NWO) for the research project 'Adaptation in movement disorder'. We would like to thank Andrea Utley for assistance with graphics and helpful discussions of this work.

REFERENCES

Abercrombie MLJ (1970) Learning to draw. In: Connolly K, editor. *Mechanisms of Motor Skill Development.* London: Academic Press, pp. 307–324.
Ahl LE, Johansson E, Granat T, Carlberg EB (2005) Functional therapy for children with cerebral palsy: an ecological approach. *Dev Med Child Neurol* 47: 613–619.
Annett J, Sheridan MR (1973) Effects of S–R and R–R compatibility on bimanual movement time. *Q J Exp Psychol* 25: 247–252.
Bouza H, Dubowitz L, Rutherford M, Cowan F, Pennock JM (1994) Late magnetic resonance imaging and clinical findings in neonates with unilateral lesions on cranial ultrasound. *Dev Med Child Neurol* 36: 951–964.

Brown JK, Rensburg van E, Walsh G, Lakie M, Wright GW (1987) A neurological study of hand function of hemiplegic children. *Dev Med Child Neurol* 29: 287–304.

Cauraugh JH, Summers JJ (2005) Neural plasticity and bilateral movements: a rehabilitation approach for chronic stroke. *Prog Neurobiol* 75: 309–320.

Charles J, Gordon AM (2005) A critical review of constraint-induced movement therapy and forced-use in children with hemiplegia. *Neural Plast* 12: 245–262.

Charles J, Wolf S, Schneider JA, Gordon AM (2006) Efficacy of a child-friendly form of constraint-induced movement therapy in hemiplegic cerebral palsy: a randomized control trial. *Dev Med Child Neurol* 48: 635–642.

Cioni G, Sales B, Paolicelli PB, Petacchi E, Scusa MF, Canapicchi R (1999) MRI and clinical characteristics of children with hemiplegic cerebral palsy. *Neuropediatrics* 30: 249–255.

Cohen L (1970) Interaction between limbs during bimanual voluntary activity. *Brain* 93: 259–272.

Debaere F, Swinnen SP, Beatse E, Sunaert S, Van Hecke P, Duysens J (2001) Brain areas involved in interlimb coordination: a distributed network. *Neuroimage* 14: 947–958.

Eliasson AC, Krumlinde-Sundholm L, Shaw K, Wang C (2005) Effects of constraint-induced movement therapy in young children with hemiplegic cerebral palsy: an adapted model. *Dev Med Child Neurol* 47: 266–275.

Fagard J (1987) Bimanual stereotypes: bimanual coordination in children as a function of movements and relative velocity. *J Mot Behav* 19: 355–366.

Fagard J, Corroyer D (2003) Using a continuous index of laterality to determine how laterality is related to interhemispheric transfer and bimanual coordination in children. *Dev Psychobiol* 43: 44–56.

Fagard J, Morioka M, Wolff PH (1985) Early stages in the acquisition of a bimanual motor skill. *Neuropsychologia* 23: 535–543.

Fagard J, Hardy-Leger I, Kervella C, Marks A (2001) Changes in interhemispheric transfer rate and the development of bimanual coordination during childhood. *J Exp Child Psychol* 80: 1–22.

Franz EA, Zelaznik HN, McGabe G (1991) Spatial topological constraints in a bimanual task. *Acta Psychol* 77: 137–151.

Franz EA, Eliassen J, Ivry RB, Gazzaniga M (1996) Dissociation of spatial and temporal coupling in the bimanual movements of callotosomy patients. *Psychol Sci* 7: 306–310.

Gordon AM, Forssberg H, Iwasaki N (1994) Formation and lateralization of internal representations underlying motor commands during precision grip. *Neuropsychologia* 32: 555–568.

Gordon AM, Charles J, Duff SV (1999) Fingertip forces during object manipulation in children with hemiplegic cerebral palsy. II: bilateral coordination. *Dev Med Child Neurol* 41: 176–185.

Gordon AM, Charles J, Wolf SL (2005) Methods of constraint-induced movement therapy for children with hemiplegic cerebral palsy: development of a child-friendly intervention for improving upper-extremity function. *Arch Phys Med Rehabil* 86: 837–844.

Gordon AM, Charles J, Steenbergen B (2006a) Fingertip force planning during grasp is disrupted by impaired sensorimotor integration in children with hemiplegic cerebral palsy. *Pediatr Res* 60: 587–591.

Gordon AM, Charles J, Wolf SL (2006b) Efficacy of constraint-induced movement therapy on involved upper-extremity use in children with hemiplegic cerebral palsy is not age-dependent. *Pediatrics* 117: e363–e373.

Gordon AM, Charles J, Schneider JA, Chinnan A (2007) Efficacy of a Hand-Arm Bimanual Intensive Therapy (HABIT) for children with hemiplegic cerebral palsy: a randomized control trial. *Dev Med Child Neurol* 49: 830–838.

Gribova A, Donchin O, Bergman H, Vaadia E, Cardoso De Oliveira S (2002) Timing of bimanual movements in human and non-human primates in relation to neuronal activity in primary motor cortex and supplementary motor area. *Exp Brain Res* 146: 322–335.

Hallett M (2001) Plasticity of the human motor cortex and recovery from stroke. *Brain Res Rev* 36: 169–174.

Hung YC, Charles J, Gordon AM (2004) Bimanual coordination during a goal-directed task in children with hemiplegic cerebral palsy. *Dev Med Child Neurol* 46: 746–753.

Immisch I, Waldvogel D, van Gelderen P, Hallett M (2001) The role of the medial wall and its anatomical variations for bimanual antiphase and in-phase movements. *Neuroimage* 14: 674–684.

Jeeves MA, Silver PH, Jacobson I (1988) Bimanual co-ordination in callosal agenesis and partial commissurotomy. *Neuropsychologia* 26: 833–850.

Kazennikov OV, Wiesendanger M (2005) Goal synchronization of bimanual skills depends on proprioception. *Neurosci Lett* 388: 153–156.

Kelso JAS, Southard DL, Goodman D (1979) On the nature of human interlimb coordination. *Science* 203: 1029–1031.

Kelso JAS, Putnam CA, Goodman D (1983) On the space-time structure of human interlimb co-ordination. *Q J Exp Psychol* 35: 347–375.

Ketelaar M, Vermeer A, Hart H, van Petegem-van Beek E, Helders PJ (2001) Effects of a functional therapy program on motor abilities of children with cerebral palsy. *Phys Ther* 81: 1534–1545.

Kleim JA, Hogg TM, VandenBerg PM, Cooper NR, Bruneau R, Remple M (2004) Cortical synaptogenesis and motor map reorganization occur during late, but not early, phase of motor skill learning. *J Neurosci* 24: 628–633.

Krumlinde-Sundholm L, Eliasson AC (2003) Development of the assisting hand assessment: a Rasch-built measure intended for children with unilateral upper limb impairments. *Scand J Occup Ther* 10: 16–26.

Kuhtz-Buschbeck JP, Sundholm LK, Eliasson AC, Forssberg H (2000) Quantitative assessment of mirror movements in children and adolescents with hemiplegic cerebral palsy. *Dev Med Child Neurol* 42: 728–736.

LaMantia AS, Rakic P (1990) Axon overproduction and elimination in the corpus callosum of the developing rhesus monkey. *J Neurosci* 10: 2156–2175.

Marion SD, Kilian SC, Naramor TL, Brown WS (2003) Normal development of bimanual coordination: visuomotor and interhemispheric contributions. *Dev Neuropsychol* 23: 399–421.

Marshall RS, Perera GM, Lazar RM, Krakauer JW, Constantine RC, DeLaPaz RL (2000) Evolution of cortical activation during recovery from corticospinal tract infarction. *Stroke* 31: 656–661.

Njiokiktjien C, Driessen M, Habraken L (1986) Development of supination-pronation movements in normal children. *Hum Neurobiol* 5: 199–203.

Nudo RJ (2003) Adaptive plasticity in motor cortex: implications for rehabilitation after brain injury. *J Rehabil Med* (41 Suppl): 7–10.

Okumura A, Kato T, Kuno K, Hayakawa F, Watanabe K (1997) MRI findings in patients with spastic cerebral palsy. II: correlation with type of cerebral palsy. *Dev Med Child Neurol* 39: 369–372.

Roncesvalles MN, Schmitz C, Zedka M, Assaiante C, Woollacott M (2005) From egocentric to exocentric spatial orientation: development of posture control in bimanual and trunk inclination tasks. *J Mot Behav* 37: 404–416.

Rose DK, Winstein CJ (2004) Bimanual training after stroke: are two hands better than one? *Top Stroke Rehabil* 11: 20–30.

Rosenbaum P, Paneth N, Leviton A, Goldstein M, Bax M, Damiano D, Dan B, Jacobsson B (2007) A report: the definition and classification of cerebral palsy. April 2006. *Dev Med Child Neurol* 109(Suppl): 8–14.

Schmidt RA, Lee TD (2005) *Motor Control and Learning: A Behavioral Emphasis.* Champaign, IL: Human Kinetics.

Schmitz C, Assaiante C (2002) Developmental sequence in the acquisition of anticipation during a new co-ordination in a bimanual load-lifting task in children. *Neurosci Lett* 330: 215–218.

Serrien DJ, Nirkko AC, Lovblad KO, Wiesendanger M (2001) Damage to the parietal lobe impairs bimanual coordination. *Neuroreport* 12: 2721–2724.

Serrien DJ, Strens LH, Oliviero A, Brown P (2002) Repetitive transcranial magnetic stimulation of the supplementary motor area (SMA) degrades bimanual movement control in humans. *Neurosci Lett* 328: 89–92.

Skold A, Josephsson S, Eliasson AC (2004) Performing bimanual activities: the experiences of young persons with hemiplegic cerebral palsy. *Am J Occup Ther* 58: 416–425.

Steenbergen B, Hulstijn W, de Vries A, Berger M (1996) Bimanual movement coordination in spastic hemiparesis. *Exp Brain Res* 110: 91–98.

Steenbergen B, Van Thiel E, Hulstijn W, Meulenbroek RG (2000) The coordination of reaching and grasping in spastic hemiparesis. *Hum Mov Sci* 19: 75–105.

Steenbergen B, Utley A, Sugden DA, Thiemann P (2003). Discrete bimanual movement coordination in adults, during development, and in hemiparetic cerebral palsy: review and preliminary results of an experiment. In: Savelsbergh G, Davids K, Van der Kamp J, Bennett SJ, editors. *Development of Movement Co-ordination in Children: Applications in the Fields of Ergonomics, Health Sciences and Sport.* London: Routledge, pp. 156–176.

Steenbergen B, Charles J, Gordon AM (2008) Fingertip force control during bimanual object lifting in hemiplegic cerebral palsy. *Exp Brain Res* 186: 191–201.

Steyvers M, Etoh S, Sauner D, Levin O, Siebner HR, Swinnen SP, Rothwell JC (2003) High-frequency transcranial magnetic stimulation of the supplementary motor area reduces bimanual coupling during anti-phase but not in-phase movements. *Exp Brain Res* 151: 309–317.

Stinear JW, Byblow WD (2004) Rhythmic bilateral movement training modulates corticomotor excitability and enhances upper limb motricity poststroke: a pilot study. *J Clin Neurophysiol* 21: 124–131.

Sugden D, Utley A (1995) Interlimb coupling in children with hemiplegic cerebral palsy. *Dev Med Child Neurol* 37: 293–309.

Swinnen SP, Wenderoth N (2004) Two hands, one brain: cognitive neuroscience of bimanual skill. *Trends Cogn Sci* 8: 18–25.

Toyokura M, Muro I, Komiya T, Obara M (1999) Relation of bimanual coordination to activation in the sensorimotor cortex and supplementary motor area: analysis using functional magnetic resonance imaging. *Brain Res Bull* 48: 211–217.

Utley A, Steenbergen B (2006) Discrete bimanual co-ordination in children and young adolescents with hemiparetic cerebral palsy: recent findings, implications and future research directions. *Pediatr Rehabil* 9: 127–136.

Utley A, Sugden D (1998) Interlimb coupling in children with hemiplegic cerebral palsy during reaching and grasping at speed. *Dev Med Child Neurol* 40: 396–404.

Utley A, Steenbergen B, Sugden DA (2004) The influence of object size on discrete bimanual co-ordination in children with hemiplegic cerebral palsy. *Disabil Rehabil* 26: 603–613.

Uvebrant P (1988) Hemiplegic cerebral palsy aetiology and outcome. *Acta Paediatr Scand* 345(Suppl).

Volman MJ (2005) Spatial coupling in children with hemiplegic cerebral palsy during bimanual circle and line drawing. *Motor Control* 9: 395–416.

Volman MJ, Wijnroks A, Vermeer A (2002) Bimanual circle drawing in children with spastic hemiparesis: effect of coupling modes on the performance of the impaired and unimpaired arms. *Acta Psychol* 110: 339–356.

Wiesendanger M, Serrien DJ (2004) The quest to understand bimanual coordination. *Prog Brain Res* 143: 491–505.

Yakovlev PI, Lecours AR (1967) The myelogenetic cycle of regional maturation of the brain. In: Minkowski A, editor. *Regional Development of the Brain in Early Life*. Philadelphia: Davis, pp. 3–65.

Zancolli EA, Zancolli ER, Jr (1981) Surgical management of the hemiplegic spastic hand in cerebral palsy. *Surg Clin North Am* 61: 395–406.

175

12
CHOOSING AND USING ASSESSMENTS OF HAND FUNCTION

Lena Krumlinde-Sundholm

The hand function of children with cerebral palsy can be approached and understood from a variety of angles, and there are many different components affecting skilled use of the hands. The methods used to assess hand function are also multifaceted. However, little has been written about what the commonly used hand function instruments really measure and the rationale behind choosing a particular test.

> We sometimes measure what we measure because we can measure it. . . . We do not measure what we should measure because it is more difficult and more complex. We then use the easy measure to infer things about the difficult measure.
>
> (Simmonds 1997)

This quotation pinpoints the dilemma in the choice of assessment tools. Which tools are available? Do we perhaps pick a test just because we have it, and because it measures 'hand function'? What does it really measure? What do we want to know and what do we want to use the information for? Does the assessment used reflect the same qualities of hand function that are targeted in the intervention and the qualities we wish to evaluate? The reason for doing the assessment must guide the choice of instruments, not just the fact that a particular instrument is available. The purpose of this chapter is to draw attention to different conceptual factors that should be considered when choosing and using standardized test instruments, and to discuss the significance of each instrument's different psychometric properties.

The use of standardized assessments requires knowledge of test administration, scoring and interpreting results for the measures to be valid and reliable. Awareness among clinicians about the importance of using standardized assessment tools has grown in recent years, and the inadequacy of the 'cafeteria approach' – collecting different test items from different protocols – is recognized, but this approach is still sometimes used. In a recent study about measurement practice in paediatric rehabilitation, Hanna and collaborators (2007) reported that about 50 per cent of clinicians surveyed stated that they sometimes modified test procedures or used only selected items from the standardized test procedures. There is increasing pressure on clinicians to evaluate their interventions for cost effectiveness in times of restrictive budgets as well as to prove their effectiveness in terms of client outcomes.

It is also widely acknowledged that the systematic use of standardized clinical assessments is a basic requirement for collecting evidence about treatment effects. The most prominent barrier to clinicians' regular use of standardized tests is the time required to administer them, as well as a perceived lack of knowledge about measures (Law et al 1999, Hanna et al 2007). It can also be a challenge to find the right tools which are useful, i.e. that meet the needs of the clients while also being valid, reliable measures that are sensitive to change.

Hand function is complex, and indeed influenced by many intra-personal components as well as environmental issues already highlighted in this book. Development of hand function and skilled use of the hands is influenced, for example, by visual and perceptual skills, age, cognition, social and cultural factors, the task *per se*, and environmental factors. How should the complex concept 'hand function' best be assessed, and which assessments are appropriate to use for children, at different ages and developmental stages, and in particular for the heterogeneous group of children with cerebral palsy? It would be terrific to have one universal tool, something corresponding to a Swiss army knife, which could be used for all needs and which would simply assess 'hand function'. Even though hand function as such is a very small part of a person's overall functional ability, the use of one's hands is essential for completion of most daily activities, and for infants for moving and exploring their environment. Unfortunately, a single universal instrument does not exist. Instead we need to carefully select the right tool for the task we wish to evaluate and address in intervention. In order to choose from the different instruments available, it may be helpful to use some frames of reference and basic concepts concerning test features as a starting point.

What can tests do?

> Measures are tools used to perform specific tasks. . . . It is therefore essential that we be clear about what we wish to accomplish before beginning to measure and then seek the tools that will enable us to do that task.
>
> (Rosenbaum 1998)

TESTS VERSUS CLASSIFICATIONS

The label *test* is usually reserved for instruments that use a standardized procedure and are evaluated for their measurement accuracy of behavioural parameters within a specific population. Special test materials, score forms and a detailed manual are typically provided. The test comprises a number of items that are typically selected through an item analysis. These items are administered in a standardized manner and are scored, often using a rating scale or a timed performance. Within a test a description of a number of observations is obtained. Test results are often reported as the sum of scores, expressed as a raw score that commonly is converted to different scales such as z-values, percentiles or age-equivalence. In order to be sensitive enough to detect differences between individuals, the test needs to include a number of items which range over a wide span of difficulty suitable for the target group. That is, persons with a low ability level can pass the more easy items and persons with a higher ability can pass the more difficult items as well as the easy ones. A test's ability to effectively discriminate differences in a variety of persons at different ability levels is important and demands a number of test items that are well targeted for the intended population.

The purpose of classifications is to group data, persons or objects into classes and/or categories according to common characteristics. A classification can be seen as a one-item test. For example, in the Manual Ability Classification System (MACS; Eliasson et al 2006), children's ability to handle objects in daily activities (the one item) is classified using five levels (categories). Classifications are useful to describe and to group people who have similar characteristics. Because classifications do not include detailed descriptions, they are not intended to measure or detect change, especially when the behaviours classified are complex. The purpose of classification systems is simply to describe common characteristics in groups that are thought to have meaning (validity). Use of classification systems can increase communication between professionals, as well as assist in understanding and identifying the best practice for children who perform at different levels.

As an example, in the MACS the five levels are used to describe manual abilities in children within the whole wide severity spectrum of CP, from very mild to very severe disability. The five levels each include children with a range of manual abilities but grouped together by the common characteristics as defined in the classification. Since classes are crude, the MACS is not likely to detect change. Of course, an individual whose ability is close to the border between two classes might change level, e.g. after intervention or with growth, but most persons are likely to stay in the same level over time. This has been shown for the Gross Motor Function Classification System (GMFCS) (Palisano et al 1997), and stability over time is a feature which makes a classification useful as a predictor for the future, as well as assisting clinicians in making relevant intervention plans (Palisano et al 2006). Thus, the usefulness of a classification is generally to describe common characteristics of individuals, not necessarily to measure change.

TYPES OF TESTS

There are two main types of standardized tests: norm-referenced and criterion-referenced. In a *norm-referenced test* the child's performance is compared to the average performance of a normative sample of typically developed age-matched peers. The results determine how far from the mean score of the normative sample of peers the child's performance is deviating, this being commonly given as standard deviation-based scores (standard scores, t-scores, z-scores, percentiles) or as age-equivalent scores. Norm-referenced tests often have a general content covering a variety of skills. Since they are intended to reflect typical performance in non-disabled individuals, the test items can be clinically irrelevant and far too advanced for a child with an identified disability such as cerebral palsy. Furthermore, the framework of norm-referenced tests does not account for the fact that children with disabilities do not always follow typical developmental patterns. The use of a developmental framework for measurement of outcomes can lead to a focus on normalization, in which children with disabilities are evaluated according to 'normal' patterns (Haley et al 1991). The most important contribution of norm-referenced tests for children with disabilities is their use in identifying a child's need and eligibility for therapy services by determining the extent of the child's delay or dysfunction.

Criterion-referenced tests provide information about how a child performs on specific tasks, i.e. whether the child's performance meets the criteria stipulated for successful performance rather than whether his or her performance is age-appropriate. Thus, the child's performance is compared to a defined list of tasks or skills. Typically a rating system is used, scoring a progression of skills *per se*, as opposed to relating skills to age levels. Interpretation is based on raw scores, sometimes expressed as the percentage of the total sum or as a scaled score. If Rasch analysis or Item Response Theory was used to develop the scale, the child's raw scores are converted to equal interval scaled scores. Criterion-referenced tests often measure functional skills and can be used to identify change since the score is based on number of tasks passed according to the criteria, not taking into account the age of the child.

THE PURPOSE OF A TEST

There are three main purposes for which measures or standardized tests in general are constructed (Boyce et al 1991, Rosenbaum 1998):

1   *Discriminative/descriptive tests* are measures intended to answer questions like 'does this individual at this specific time differ in the feature of interest from others, and if so, how much?' Discriminative tests are often age norm-referenced and they provide information about a child's development compared to typical development.
2   *Screening/predictive measures* are used to separate populations – to separate those children who are suspected of having developmental differences from those who score within age expectations. Screening measures are not meant to evaluate a functional status in detail; they identify children who will require additional in-depth testing.
3   *Evaluative measures* have to be capable of detecting change over time. These tests are often criterion-referenced, meaning that they are scored on preset criteria for performance related to ability to accomplish a number of specific skills, rather than comparing the performance with a normative sample.

When choosing a test, it is important not to use an instrument for purposes other than those with supporting evidence of a specific use (descriptive, screening or evaluative). This information should be available in the test manual.

USE OF SCORES

Davies and Gavin (1998) emphasize another important point to consider when choosing the method of assessment: the application of the results. Do the measurement data have limitations in how they may apply to an individual child's performance profile or to outcomes on a group level? First, the type of measurement decides how the results can be used. Most assessments of human abilities are constructed using ordinal level scores. Ordinal scales collect data describing a category as 'less than' or 'more than' with an assigned number. These categories that are rated provide raw scores. However, since these numbers do not represent equal intervals on a continuum of performance levels, the scores merely reflect a change of ability as greater or lesser – that is, without assigning a value to the degree of this change. The information about a child is then limited, and no comparisons can be drawn as to whether one individual has gained more than another. When analysing ordinal level data, non-parametric statistics are appropriate for use. However, equal-interval ability scores can be produced from ordinal level raw scores by using a Rasch measurement analysis (Wright and Stone 1979, Wright and Linacre 1989, Bond and Fox 2007).

How different types of test scores can be understood and used is described by Davies and Gavin (1998):

- *Raw scores* are mostly ordinal level data and should, as mentioned above, be interpreted with caution. An increase in a sum of raw scores may not indicate an increase in ability; rather, it might just reflect more items (though not necessarily more difficult items) being passed.
- *Age-equivalent scores* are most commonly based on the matching of the raw scores of the child being tested with the standardized sample data. Age-equivalent scores are ordinal and the authors recommend that they should not be used in studies evaluating treatment outcome.
- *Percentile scores* are generated from the distribution of the raw scores in the standard-ization sample. They represent the percentage of persons from the standardization sample whose raw scores are at the same or a lower level than the tested person's raw scores. One disadvantage of percentile scores is that those persons who score at the extreme ends of the scale need a bigger absolute difference in raw scores for a change to be noted in their percentile scores than those whose scores lie in the middle of the scale. Since standardization samples are usually from normal non-disabled populations and children tested most often have disabilities and perform at the extreme lower end, changes in their abilities would have to be quite large to be apparent with percentile scores. Percentile scores are also ordinal data and should be analysed with non-parametric procedures.
- *Standard scores* or *z-scores* are expressed as the standard deviation of the individual's raw score compared to the mean of raw score of the standardization sample. The mean is commonly 0 with a standard deviation of 1. Standard scores can be changed to any other convenient scale – often a 0–100 scale, with a mean of 50 where 1 standard deviation is 10 – and are referred to as T-scores. Standard scores reflect an individual's performance in comparison to the standardization sample and are most useful if the standardization group is directly relevant to the person being tested. Fig. 12.1 illustrates some commonly used scores and their relation to the curve of normal distribution (Richardson 2005).

IMPLICATIONS FOR USE

To better understand the results from different types of standardized tests of hand function which may be used with children who have a disability, we may take the example of a preschool-aged child with spastic bilateral cerebral palsy (diplegia), on MACS level 3 and GMFCS level 3.

A descriptive norm-referenced test may be suitable to describe aspects of age-related hand function such as precision in stacking blocks, speed-related dexterity or skills in use of pen or scissors. Such a test will provide information about how far this child's

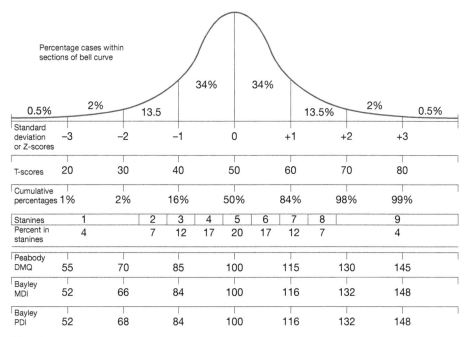

Fig. 12.1 The curve of normal distribution and associated standard scores.

Source: Richardson 2005, p. 255 (© Elsevier 2005).

performance deviates from the performance of other children of his or her age. It will show that this child is eligible for rehabilitation services because he or she has pronounced difficulties. This could also be shown with a screening test or maybe also from a classification, providing that there was evidence supporting their validity and reliability for children with cerebral palsy. In contrast, a criterion-referenced test will show what manual tasks the child is able to do and what he/she cannot do, expressed as a higher or lower ability score. The test may also provide information about what skills the child needs to practise.

Furthermore, the norm-referenced test results will not be useful for detecting change over time. Results based on standard scores (T-scores, z-scores, percentiles or age-equivalent scores) from repeated testing will probably show lower results over time in individuals who have pronounced difficulties as compared to norms. A person like the child in our example, who obtains low scores on a norm-referenced test at an early age, where typically developed children also accomplish few items, will with time be placed further away from the expected age-related norm even though his or her skills have in fact improved. This is because the child must not only gain in skills at his current age level but also show gains reaching the next age level of development to achieve scores appropriate to age. Thus, a person with, for example, CP may never 'catch up' with the increasing demands on the age norm-referenced score levels, and although he or she may have achieved improvement in skills, the distance to the normal performance increases with each 6- or 12-month increment. By using a criterion-referenced test the improved skills may be captured and credited and the child's change over time will be measured in relation to himself and not compared to able-bodied peers.

Psychometric properties

Outcome measures need to fulfil some basic criteria concerning psychometric properties in order to be useful. In addition to being standardized, having a stated purpose and being clinically applicable, tests used to evaluate outcomes need to produce valid and reliable measures (American Educational Research Association 1999, Streiner and Norman 2003). However, an assessment instrument, as such, does not possess a general attribute of being valid and reliable in the sense that it is valid and reliable for any population. Rather, there may be evidence supporting the fact that a specific test will produce valid and reliable measures for a proposed target group. This means that the psychometric properties are only applicable when the assessment is used with persons within the age and diagnoses that it is intended for and when it is used as stated in the manual, e.g. using all test items in the stipulated context. If the assessment is applied differently, for example to a different population, the user needs to show that the psychometric properties are re-evaluated for that purpose (Streiner and Norman 2003).

VALIDITY AND RELIABILITY

Validity refers to the extent to which an instrument actually measures what it is supposed to measure (Streiner and Norman 2003). Given this definition, validity is influenced by the purpose and the construct of a measure, the item content and the rationale for the item selection. The validity may be the most important aspect of an instrument (American Educational Research Association 1999) and yet it is a property not always thoroughly evaluated and described. The concept of the test should be created from theory, and the methods used for item selection and reduction, the relation to other instruments and consistency with theoretically derived hypotheses must be reported and evaluated in establishing validity. A current often recommended method to create or revise instruments is to use modern test theory, e.g. the Rasch measurement model, to establish evidence of internal scale validity and sound psychometric properties. Traditionally, three different types of validity have mainly been spoken of: construct-, content- and criterion-related validity. Since the revision from 1999 of the 'Standards for Education and Psychological Testing' (American Educational Research Association 1999) the terminology has changed towards a less strict use of these 'labels', the recommendation being instead to focus more on 'types of evidence' supporting the interpretations that can be made from the test's scores. Thus, one cannot say that a test is valid in itself, but rather that there are valid uses of the test.

Reliability refers to the trustworthiness or the reproducibility of the measure: can the same results be obtained from the same rater (intrarater reliability) or from different raters (interrater reliability) and for repeated test occasions (test-retest reliability)? Reliability is most often expressed by a correlation coefficient. Many different methods for reliability evaluation are used, but the discussion by Streiner and Norman (2003: 151) about which method is best practice for reliability calculations suggests that Pearson correlation co-efficients are theoretically incorrect, and that the method of Altman and Bland is equivalent to the results of error variance in intraclass correlation coefficients (ICC). Their recommendation is to use kappa or intraclass correlation coefficients, which in the end yield identical results. According to Polit and Hungler (1999) a general guideline for interpreting the meaning of a reliability coefficient is that for group level comparisons 0.70–0.80 is sufficient, and for making decisions for individuals a coefficient of 0.90 or more is required. Accordingly, and contrary to what is commonly believed, for measuring individuals a rather precise measure with a small measurement error is needed. When the measure is applied to a group of individuals less precision is required since taking the average of observations reduces the error of measurement (Dekker et al 2005).

Reliability and validity are in some respects closely related. If results from a test are not reliable they likewise cannot be valid. However, test results may show evidence of reliability, yet still not be valid for the task to be measured. For example, standing a person on a scale to measure weight may show excellent agreement between occasions, but if the intention was to know how tall a person is the scale was not a valid tool for that purpose. Even though the relationship between height and weight often is fairly strong, the scale does not measure what was intended to be measured. Although this concept may appear to be too obvious to need mentioning, quite often, even in measures of hand function, it may be violated. Hand function tests that are available for use are not always developed from a clear rationale and these tests are often interpreted to cover a wider range of aspects than intended.

For example, improved functional manual ability is the aim for an intervention and measures of grip strength and speed of dexterity are applied before and after the intervention. However, improved grip strength may not lead to better functional ability, e.g. fastening buttons or making a sandwich. Likewise improved speed may not imply better handwriting. Tests of grip strength and dexterity may not necessarily reflect changes in performing functional manual tasks. Consequently, the aims of an intervention need to be carefully expressed and analysed in terms of their components and then matched with instruments which are also analysed concerning their content and construct. As a minimum requirement, outcome measures must specifically address the aims of the interventions (Cieza et al 2005).

RESPONSIVENESS TO CHANGE
If a test is used with the intention to measure change, it must have been demonstrated to be sensitive to change (to be able to measure any degree of change), and to be able to detect clinically meaningful changes (to be responsive to change). Streiner and Norman (2003) provide an overview of the different approaches to, and diverse opinions about, this essential topic. They advocate that the sensitivity of an instrument to detect change should be viewed as a form of construct validity, and not as a psychometric property *per se*. Regardless of terminology, this feature of an instrument is most important for its usefulness in rehabilitation.

STANDARD ERRORS OF MEASUREMENT
The child's result on a test administered is never 100 per cent accurate, a 'true score'; we can only obtain an estimate of a child's behaviour within a specific confidence interval. All test outcomes have a certain amount of measurement error, a variance of the outcome depending on rater error/variability or individual variation of performance from time

to time. The size of this error can be calculated from the reliability coefficient, preferably from a test-retest situation. Rater reliability is most commonly reported with a reliability coefficient, which is an expression of the extent to which raters can distinguish between individuals on different levels of the measured trait. However, the reliability coefficient does not indicate how in practice to estimate measurement error for the score of an individual. The Standard Error of Measurement (SEM) is more useful for this as it is given in the same unit of measurement as the actual scores in the test. The SEM can be used to calculate a confidence interval with 95 per cent probability around an observed score within which the true score of the child would lie (American Educational Research Association 1999). To establish that a change has really occurred for an individual, and that the changed score is not merely an expression of rater error, the difference between the first score and the second score must exceed ±2 SEM for both occasions, that is, there should be no overlap of the intervals. Hanna and collaborators (2007) state that therapists, in their opinion, have little understanding of the meaning of SEM and how to use this information to interpret change for their clients. Since knowledge about this construct, as well as of other psychometric properties of instruments, is important, the authors have created 'Clinical Measurement Practical Guidelines for Service Providers', available on the CanChild Centre for Childhood Disability Research website (Hanna et al 2005; http://www.canchild.ca/Default.aspx?tabid=1136). In this article clinicians can find readable information about clinical measures and what may happen if one modifies measures.

We may use an example to illustrate the use of SEM to interpret change: a child obtains 56 points on the Assisting Hand Assessment (Krumlinde-Sundholm et al 2007) at baseline, and after a treatment period the score is now 60 points. Is this a 'true' improvement? The SEM for the subtest is given in the manual as 1.2 points for an intrarater condition. To get a confidence interval of 95 per cent, ±2 SEM should be calculated. In the example, +2.4 points should be added to the first score (56) and –2.4 points deducted from the second score (60). Since the scores then overlap this suggests that the apparent change may be due to chance variation and not be a 'true' change (Fig. 12.2, example 1). If the second assessment had given a score of 61 points there would be no overlap, indicating that we can be 95 per cent certain that a real change occurred (Fig. 12.2, example 2).

However, Eliasziw and coworkers (1994) argue that using ±2 SEM is somewhat too severe, since the risk of the true score falling exactly within the small overlapping area is really very small, and they propose that a significant clinical difference can rather be calculated by use of the formula:

$$Z_{\text{intra or inter}} = \frac{\text{assessment 1} - \text{assessment 2}}{\sqrt{2}\ \text{SEM intra or inter}}$$

Using the AHA-example above, with this formula a change of 4 points would indicate a significant change ($p < 0.005$), so that the change seen in example 1 would be regarded as significant.

A third way of evaluating 'real' change sometimes seen in the literature is suggested by Schreuders and coworkers (2003): calculation of the Smallest Detectable Difference (SDD), using the following formula:

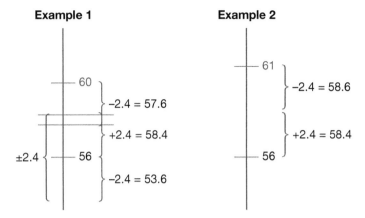

Fig. 12.2 Illustration of the use of the Standard Error of Measurement (SEM) to interpret change. In example 1, the interval of ±2 SEM is overlapping, indicating that the difference in the scores may be due to measurement error. In example 2, there is no overlap, indicating that a change has occurred.

$$SDD = SEM \times 1.96 \times \sqrt{2}$$

For the AHA-example above, this results in SDD = 3.32.

IMPLICATIONS FOR USE

Different psychometric properties are important for specific areas of use. For example, if the question asked is whether a child's hand function is normally developed, a descriptive test with good internal consistency, content and construct validity and well researched norms is important. However, if the question to be answered is whether or not change has occurred after a treatment period, the test chosen must be evaluative, and it must have good intra- or interrater reliability, content and construct validity and sensitivity to change. Furthermore, information about the size of the measurement error in terms of SEM or the smallest detectable difference is important for interpreting change in individuals.

Test manuals must include information concerning the test's specific purpose, and evidence of whether the test fulfils this purpose should be reported in the manual and in referee-reviewed journals. Selecting an instrument with overall 'good' psychometric properties is not always the best solution; instead, in the perspective of a specific clinical or research context, an instrument best suited for a particular task and purpose should be chosen. The starting point is to specify the particular purpose of measurement. Rudman and Hannah (1998) presented an Instrument Evaluation Framework which can be very useful for clinicians as well as researchers. The model can help therapists decide what properties are the most important for the task they need or want to measure (Fig. 12.3).

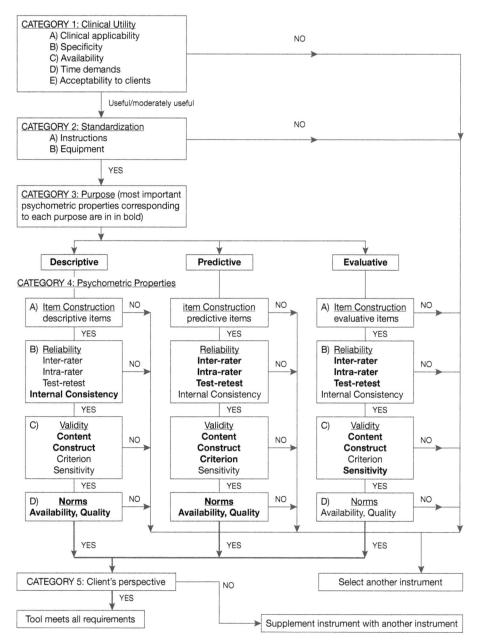

Fig. 12.3 The instrument evaluating framework for selecting instruments in hand therapy. Before initiating the evaluation process, the user must determine what is to be measured (outcome) and why it is to be measured (purpose). Note: most important psychometric properties corresponding to each purpose are in bold type.

Source: Rudman and Hannah 1998, p. 267 (© Elsevier 1998).

Organizing frameworks

When making the decision about which assessment instrument to use, an organizing framework may be useful to guide the process. First, the purpose of conducting an assessment must be clearly expressed. What is it you want to measure and why? If intervention outcome is what you are interested in, the content and target area of the intervention as well as the goals for the intervention must correspond to the outcome measures chosen. If you expect transition effects on other domains of functioning, these domains need to be measured as well. When choosing an assessment instrument, different frameworks can be used.

INTERNATIONAL CLASSIFICATION OF FUNCTIONING, DISABILITY AND
HEALTH (ICF)

The framework outlined in the international model for classification of functioning, disability and health (ICF; WHO 2001) can be used to clarify focuses of measurements. The process of linking standardized assessments to the ICF classification has started (e.g. Granlund et al 2004, Stucki 2005, Østensjø et al 2006, Schepers et al 2007) but has not yet included measures of hand function for children with cerebral palsy. Specific rules for linking health status measures to the ICF have been proposed (Cieza et al 2005), whereby 'what to measure' for a specific diagnostic group is first defined and then 'how to measure' is suggested by careful analyses and coding of each item in the assessments. This makes it possible to link assessments to aims of intervention with the framework of the ICF. Such information would be most useful, but is still lacking for the area of hand function and cerebral palsy. What is presented below is only a rough attempt to organize different features of assessments to the ICF domains.

In the ICF, *body functions* are defined as the physiological functions of body systems, and body structures refer to the anatomical construct of the body. Problems in this domain are referred to as impairments. *Activity* is defined as the execution of tasks by or actions of an individual, and *participation* refers to involvement in life situations. Difficulties in these areas are denoted as activity limitations and participation restrictions. Accordingly, basic components of motor and sensory functions, e.g. range of motion, grip strength, spasticity and tactile sensibility, are regarded as aspects of body functions (chapters b2 and b7). Skills such as grasping, picking up, manipulating, reaching, turning and releasing objects are listed under the activity and participation domain in the ICF (chapter d4, Mobility d430–d449). This domain also incorporates more complex, hand-related activities such as eating and grooming (chapter d5, Self care d510–570), cooking or cleaning (chapter d6, Household tasks d630–649). Thus, assessment instruments regarded as 'measures of hand function' are found in all the functioning domains: the body function/structure domain or the activity and participation domain. However, this latter domain covers a wide range of hand-related behaviour, from simple actions such as grasping, to complex tasks such as cutting food or cleaning. This wide definition of activity and participation makes the ICF less useful or at least more complex for the purpose of clarifying differences of focus in assessments.

One interesting aspect expressed in the ICF is the differentiation between the qualifiers *capacity* and *performance*. Capacity is referred to as the person's ability to execute a task or an action on the highest probable level of functioning that a person may reach in a standardized environment, e.g. in a typical clinical test setting. Transferred to a hand function test situation, *capacity* is examined in any test where the person is asked to grasp, press, lift or transport objects by using the hands, to show what they *can do*. This concept is quite straightforward. However, when it comes to the performance qualifier, the ICF leaves room for different interpretations and also encourages a debate, especially concerning the concept of participation. *Activity performance* is used to reflect participation in life situations. This use of 'participation' has been debated and it has been described by many as a simplification (Hemmingson and Jonsson 2005). The ICF suggests different ways of using the terms activity and participation, and the actual use of these terms will from here on determine their definitions. The concept of *performance* incorporates the real-life environment and thus social and environmental aspects of completion of activities. In relation to hand function assessments the real-life environment is rarely utilized. Hand function assessments are not usually executed in a person's normal environment with the use of objects in that particular environment. Most tests use standardized blocks, pegs and specially manufactured objects, though some tests do include handling of ordinary common objects. Questionnaires describing hand use in daily life may be viewed as representing the performance/participation aspect.

In another sense, beyond distinguishing between activity and participation, the general meaning of capacity and performance could be a useful concept to describe two importantly different aspects of activity. Capacity can be used for describing actions and activities performed with the best possible ability upon request, and performance to describe how actions and activities are usually performed, i.e. the typical performance. This distinction is clinically very meaningful. The concepts of 'can do' and 'does do' are not always equivalent, a fact well recognized by clinicians. By making a distinction between these two concepts, in relation to hand function, we can gain a broadened view of a child's abilities. For example, even if a child with hemiplegic cerebral palsy can pick up objects from the table with the affected hand when asked to (the capacity), he might not normally use this capacity, using instead the better hand for grasping objects, thereafter placing them in the hemiplegic hand (the performance). So, from a hand function test point of view, we should specify what we want to know and measure: the child's best capacity or his typical performance? These two aspects are different and it is important to pay attention to both. If the difference between capacity and actual performance is large, the child may have potential for a more effective performance, so that intervention can focus on establishing a useful habitual behaviour and helping the child to learn to use a specific capacity. If the child is already fully using the capacities he has in daily typical performance but still perceives a poor result or a great effort, intervention needs to focus on improving the capacity (or on finding compensations). In the first scenario, the intervention recommendation may be intensive occupational therapy; the second scenario may lead to a surgical procedure aiming to obtain a more advantageous biomechanical prerequisite for handling objects. Consequently, we need measures of hand function for both of these concepts, to allow outcome differentiation and to guide treatment.

Most hand function tests measure capacity with standardized items based on speed or accuracy or test situations where children show what they *can* do when asked to. This applies

TABLE 12.1

Examples of instruments used to evaluate aspects of hand function and their characteristics concerning (i) domain in the International Classification of Functioning and Health (ICF), (ii) whether their focus is on unimanual, bimanual or evaluation of task outcome, (iii) the type of measure

	ICF domain			Performance perspective			Type of measure	
	BF BS	A & P *capacity*	A & P *performance*	Unimanual	Bimanual	Result of tasks	Norm-referenced	Criterion-referenced
Range of motion, goniometry	✓			✓			✓	
Grip strength, dynamometry	✓			✓			✓	
Tactile sensibility, e.g. 2PD, stereognosis	✓			✓			✓	
Muscle tone, e.g. MAS	✓							✓
PDMS-2		✓		✓			✓	
Jebsen-Taylor test of hand function		✓		✓			✓	
QUEST	✓	✓		✓				✓
Melbourne Assessment		✓		✓				✓
AHA			✓		✓			✓
SHUEE	✓	✓		✓				✓
ABILHAND-Kids			✓			✓		✓

BF = body function, BS = body structure, A & P = activity and participation, 2PD = two-point discrimination, MAS = Modified Ashworth Scale, PDMS-2 = Peabody Developmental Motor Scale-2, QUEST = Quality of Upper Extremity Skills Test, AHA = Assisting Hand Assessment, SHUEE = Shriners Hospital for Children Upper Extremity Evaluation.

to tests such as the Jebsen and Taylor test of hand function (Jebsen et al 1969, Taylor et al 1973), the Melbourne Assessment of Unilateral Upper Limb Function (Johnson et al 1994, Randall et al 2001), the Quality of Upper Extremity Skills Test (QUEST; DeMatteo et al 1992) or the Movement Assessment Battery for Children (Movement ABC; Henderson and Sugden 1992). Assessments involving what children *do* in fact do are often in the form of questionnaires, commonly asking about accomplishment of certain activities (e.g. can, with difficulty or cannot), rather than how the hands are used to execute the activities. An example of this is the ABILHAND-Kids (Arnould et al 2004). Although the overall aim for most hand-function-directed interventions is to improve performance, i.e. the functional use of the hands, there is a lack of observation-based instruments using this perspective. The Assisting Hand Assessment is a newly developed test which measures how effectively children with a unilateral disability actually use the affected hand in bimanual play (Krumlinde-Sundholm and Eliasson 2003, Holmefur et al 2007, Krumlinde-Sundholm et al 2007).

THE FUNCTIONAL REPERTOIRE OF THE HAND MODEL
Another approach to guide assessments and therapy, directed specifically towards hand function, is proposed by Kimmerle and coworkers (2003) in their Functional Repertoire of the Hand Model (FRH model). This model consists of four key components which can be used to delineate theoretically different aspects of hand function.

The first component of the FRH model, *Personal constraints*, includes physical and psychological impairment-based limitations such as range of motion, sensibility, muscle control, socio-cultural framework and self-perception of hand function. Kimmerle and coworkers point out that these components *per se* do not define a person's ability to function, but may be the underlying reason for limitations, and as such are important targets for intervention and assessment. In the second key component, *Hand roles*, the different roles the two hands play are recognized. The importance of bimanual handling of objects, i.e. how the two hands are used simultaneously and jointly, has not previously received much attention in hand function interventions and assessments but may well be the most important aspect of the functional use of the hands in daily life activities.

The third key component of the FRH model concerns *Hand actions*, which are divided into *Gestures* and *Object-related Hand Actions*. The hand action capabilities are expressed in the categories of reaching, grasping and manipulating objects and are defined by reference to fundamental actions needed in a variety of tasks. The last key component of the FRH model is called *Task Parameters*. In this component it is recognized that different tasks place different demands on the hand function and that handling of objects involves different challenges regarding the object's size and shape, the movement patterns involved (e.g. single, discrete, repeated, continuous, or sequences of actions), performance demands, and spatial, temporal and force demands. The task itself is crucial, and for individuals their hand function may be quite sufficient for performing some tasks but not for others.

The FRH model may provide therapists with a structure for decisions about assessments and therapies, a framework for analysis of hand function.

A topic far too little discussed but of considerable importance concerns what assessments to choose to evaluate different interventions. Which tools will reflect changes and assist in understanding and interpreting the results? Interventions need to be evaluated from a broad perspective but it is even more important that the components measured are the same components that are expected to be changed (Majnemer and Mazer 2004). Considering this, therapists and physicians need to express in more detail what components of hand function they anticipate or hypothesize the treatment will influence, and what the goal for the intervention is, in more specific terms than 'improved hand function'. At a basic level, the assessment of choice must reflect the component directly targeted in the intervention, in order to evaluate the treatment effect. If an extended or transfer effect to other areas is hoped for, these areas must also be measured. Even though we seemingly have many assessment tools to measure hand function, there are few that have proved to be valid for use with individuals with CP as well as being reliable and responsive to change. The wide variation of assessment used in intervention studies is probably a consequence of the lack of suitable 'criterion standard' assessments. It would also be useful to find a consensus about matching certain assessments to different types of interventions so as to be able to compare results from different studies and to conduct meta-analyses.

What to assess?

Since no general universal measure of 'hand function' exists, clinicians and researchers need to clearly formulate what components or qualities of hand function may be important to measure from the perspective of why they should be measured. Is the purpose to establish eligibility for therapy services, to take decisions on type of intervention, to plan and guide intervention, or to evaluate outcomes? Choosing the instrument must be guided by an explicit purpose. What elements are, then, of importance?

PERCEPTIONS AND EXPECTATIONS

First, what are the client's perceptions and expectations about their hand function? Formulating these is of great importance, and it is also highly important to have clients and service providers match their perceptions about the hand functioning, goals and possible outcome, i.e. for them to 'speak the same language'. Are the expectations realistic? Are they measurable? Will both clinicians and clients have the same frame of reference and perception about the meaning of a 'good' outcome? One further aspect, very central to clients but difficult to evaluate, is the perception of the *cosmetic appearance* of the hand and the experience of relaxation and *well-being*.

FUNCTIONAL ACTIVITY PERFORMANCE

Improved functional performance is probably the ultimate and hoped-for outcome of all kinds of interventions, and it is therefore of interest to measure. Individualized measures offer support in defining the nature of functional performance problems. The Goal Attainment Scale (GAS; Kiresuk and Sherman 1968, Ottenbacher and Cusick 1990) and the Canadian Occupational Performance Measure (COPM; Law et al 2000) have been found to be useful, also for hand-related goals (Cusick et al 2006, Wallen et al 2007). Undoubtedly, a collaborative client–therapist approach to identifying problem areas and to setting goals for interventions is an excellent way of identifying important functional goals. This in turn helps to sharpen the focus, and to strengthen the motivation for carrying through task-specific practice, one important agent for motor learning (Smith and Wrisberg 2000). Whether functional goals can be achieved simply by transfer effects from interventions on body function level without task-specific training remains to be proven, and deviating results concerning stability of goal areas and ability ratings for test-retest conditions (Eyssen et al 2005) are of concern and call for further investigation.

Another option for measuring functional performance is to use questionnaires measuring ability in task performance. Few such instruments, however, focus on manual abilities. The ABILHAND-Kids (Arnould et al 2004) is one such measure, which has proved useful in identifying individuals of different ability levels. ABILHAND-Kids has been thoroughly evaluated for validity and reliability by use of the Rasch measurement model, which makes it unique among manual ability-related questionnaires used for children with cerebral palsy. Whether effects of treatment can be captured with this instrument is still unknown.

The level of functional performance and the relevance to performing various daily life tasks differ considerably within the heterogeneous group of individuals with cerebral palsy, as well as between different age groups. For example, handwriting is not relevant for a child on MACS level V, but the ability to push a button or to point accurately on a communication device is highly relevant. It is likely that development of subgroup-specific and activity-based measures would provide new opportunities to actually evaluate hand function-related activity performance.

SKILFULNESS IN OBJECT MANIPULATION
Typically there is a relation between skilful hand use and speed of performance where components such as force control, coordination and dexterity are blended. An example of a timed test is the classic Box and Block test (Mathiowetz et al 1985a, 1985b), in which cubes that are fairly easy to grasp are moved between two containers; or the Nine-Hole Peg test, in which small pegs, more difficult to grasp, are inserted and removed from a peg board (Kellor et al 1971, Poole et al 2005). Another example is the Jebsen and Taylor test of hand function (Jebsen et al 1969, Taylor et al 1973), which uses objects of different sizes, shapes and weights, selected with the intent that they should represent different fine motor demands in daily life. Timed tests reflect capacity and commonly test one hand at a time. There is an age-related component of speed and dexterity; thus these tests have age norms. There is also possibly a training effect from repeatedly carrying out speed-related tests. Whether timed performance is stable for test-retest conditions in individuals with fluctuating muscle tone and motor control difficulties has not been well investigated. Demonstration of stable repeated baseline measures is needed for both research and clinical use of timed tests for children with cerebral palsy, and it may be debated whether speed is an important feature of hand function in individuals with cerebral palsy.

Another characteristic of hand function anticipated to have importance for skilful handling of objects is the *quality of movements*. Two examples of standardized tests measuring quality of movement are the Melbourne Assessment of Unilateral Upper Limb Function (Randall et al 1999, 2001) and the Quality of Upper Extremity Skills Test (QUEST; DeMatteo et al 1992, 1993). The Melbourne Assessment is valid for use with children with cerebral palsy aged 5–15. It evaluates quality of movements in functional tasks such as pointing, grasping and reaching. The movements are scored for accuracy, joint position, differentiation and fluency of movement for each hand and arm separately. QUEST was developed for the purpose of measuring components of movements focused on in neurodevelopmental treatment (NDT) such as dissociated movements, grasp patterns, weight bearing and protective extension. It is valid for use with children with cerebral palsy from 18 months to 8 years of age. Capacity is observed and scored on items for each hand separately but the total score includes measures of both hands. For both tests a major part of the total score concerns arm-related movements and a smaller part concerns hand manipulative skills.

A third aspect of object manipulation is measured with the Assisting Hand Assessment (AHA; Krumlinde-Sundholm and Eliasson 2003, Holmefur et al 2007, Krumlinde-Sundholm et al 2007). The AHA measures how effectively children with a unilateral disability spontaneously use the affected hand in *bimanual performance* (play). The AHA is valid for children with hemiplegic cerebral palsy or brachial plexus palsy from 18 months to 12 years of age. In the AHA it is the collaborative use of both hands that is the focus, and the test measures performance as opposed to capacity, since the children are not specifically asked to use their affected hand but encouraged to play with selected toys where bimanual use is required. Items in the AHA measure, for example, effectiveness in terms of initiation of use, stabilization and manipulation of objects, and flow of performance.

BIOMECHANICAL PREREQUISITES OF FUNCTIONING
Biomechanical prerequisites are perceived to be important for effective use of the hands and several interventions aim to improve biomechanical features of the hand and arm by, for example, surgery, tone reduction, splinting or casting. Standard body function-directed measures are needed to evaluate whether the desired effect was accomplished: range of motion, joint alignment, muscle strength and muscle tone. Other assessments that focus on movement are the House Thumb position classification (House et al 1981) and the Zancolli scale for simultaneous wrist and finger extension (Zancolli and Zancolli 1981). If a transfer effect to activity level components is anticipated in terms of improved dexterity, quality of movements in task performance or bimanual performance, this has to be evaluated separately. For this purpose other tests such as those previously mentioned are needed.

The Shriners Hospital Upper Extremity Evaluation (SHUEE; Davids et al 2006) is a new assessment which incorporates different subscales of traditional measures of range of motion and muscle tone, dynamic position analysis and spontaneous functional analysis; a grasp-release analysis is also performed. SHUEE is intended for use with clients with hemiplegia aged 3–18 to guide and evaluate surgical and tone-reduction interventions.

AN EXAMPLE

As an example, consider a situation where the effects of injections of botulinum A toxin in the upper limb of a child with hemiplegia are to be evaluated. The hypothesis is that apart from reducing tone this treatment will also improve alignment or position of the wrist and fingers, with a resultant increase in speed and dexterity. Another hoped-for outcome is that spontaneous use of the affected hand will increase and that bimanual and functional task performance will improve both in an overall manner and for specific goals. One possible undesirable effect is weakened grip. Consequently, all these elements should be evaluated, and this requires use of many of the instruments mentioned above. However, a balance must be struck so as to ensure a reasonable number of hours for both clients and therapists to administer these instruments. Careful analysis of anticipated effects, as well as a critical analysis of the assessment instruments available, should help to clarify the intentions of interventions and guide the choice of instruments. The framework of the ICF and/or the FRH model may serve to help specify aims of interventions and choices of assessments. Careful analysis of the potential assessment tool is needed: the type of standardization and reference frame, the properties concerning content and construct validity, and reliability of measures for the target group of clients in relation to the purpose of the evaluation. Clinical utility, client compliance and time demands are likewise important aspects. In the future it is hoped that the tendency to use a test simply because it is available will become less common, and instead tests will be carefully chosen after analysis of what needs to be measured.

WHERE TO GO

Even though a lot of measures exist, both clinicians and researchers find it hard to select instruments suitable for individuals within the heterogeneous group of cerebral palsy. The norm-referenced tests are probably only relevant for individuals on MACS level I and possibly level II, and not as relevant for unilaterally involved persons. It is not possible to find one assessment that can measure clinically relevant aspects of hand function for all persons with cerebral palsy. It would be very helpful to have information about relevant subgroups for the tests reported in the manuals, and the MACS may prove to be a useful classification system for this.

Most of the assessments mentioned in this chapter require relatively good hand function and are not applicable for individuals on MACS level IV or V. There is a lack of standardized instruments to assist in making decisions about preferable placing of joysticks or switches, or evaluating whether a seating position facilitates accuracy of arm and hand use. This makes it difficult to measure effects of intervention with aims of this type, and for evidence-based interventions to be made.

Finally, it appears that we still need additional instruments, but with a reconsidered perspective. We definitely need instruments that have a functional and bimanual perspective, since using our two hands together is what we commonly need for performing daily life tasks. Many tests, perhaps in an attempt to be objective, have become very technical or contrived and therefore the test items may be experienced as irrelevant for the daily functions a child experiences. Thus, we need tests where real-life objects are handled in relevant situations. The concept of such a test must be created from theory and the constructs included in the test solidly built with careful item selection, preferably modelled on modern test theory, such as the Rasch measurement model, to establish evidence of internal scale validity and sound psychometric properties. The wished-for instrument would also be useful for guiding interventional planning. Lastly, of course, instruments need to be responsive to clinically meaningful change in order to make it possible to determine successful intervention strategies.

Considerations

What does it mean for parents and children to be subjected to assessments? Therapists have an ethical responsibility not only to take into account aspects of choosing the correct test, using it according to the standardized protocol and for the correct purpose, but also to anticipate how the test situation may affect the child and parents, as well as how the test results will be used. Critical decisions about intervention services or programmes are often based on the test results. Moreover, some parents, and possibly also some children, experience clinical tests as stressful because the test situation itself puts in question the child's abilities and perhaps places difficult demands on the child, all of which often makes the child's shortcomings visible and evident. Most therapists, however, have experienced that children do like performing clinical tests, seeing them as a game or a competition for setting records. Thus, the presentation of the assessment by the therapist to the family is of key importance. It must also be stressed that in family-centred clinical practice, establishing rapport and finding out family priorities/concerns must precede and be in line with any assessment procedure. Similarly, the test results must be reported in an understandable way and interpretation of results must include information about how accurate the results are, i.e. how confident the therapist is that the results are accurate in terms of test procedure and reliability. Clinical measures are important for a number of reasons, but should not be applied routinely without a specific purpose being stated.

REFERENCES

American Educational Research Association (1999) *Standards for Educational and Psychological Testing.* Washington, DC: American Educational Research Association.
Arnould C, Penta M, Renders A, Thonnard J-L (2004) ABILHAND-Kids: a measure of manual ability in children with cerebral palsy. *Neurology* 63: 1045–1052.
Bond TG, Fox CM (2007) *Applying the Rasch model. Fundamental Measurement in the Human Sciences, 2nd edn.* Mahawa, NJ: Lawrence Erlbaum.
Boyce WF, Gowland C, Rosenbaum PL (1991). Measuring quality of movement in cerebral palsy: a review of instruments. *Phys Ther* 71: 813–819.
Cieza A, Geyh S, Chatterji S, Kostanjsek N, Üstünd B, Stucki G (2005) ICF linking rules: an update based on lessons learned. *J Rehabil Med* 37: 212–218.
Cusick A, McIntyre S, Novak I, Lannin N, Lowe K (2006) A comparison of goal attainment scaling and the Canadian occupational performance measure for paediatric rehabilitation research. *Pediatr Rehabil* 9: 149–157.
Davids JR, Peace LC, Wagner LV, Gidewall MA, Blackhurst DW, Roberson WM (2006) Validation of the Shriners Hospital for Children Upper Extremity Evaluation (SHUEE) for children with hemiplegic cerebral palsy. *J Bone Joint Surg Am* 88: 326–333.
Davies PL, Gavin WJ (1998) Measurement issues in treatment effectiveness studies. *Am J Occup Ther* 53: 363–372.

195

Dekker J, Dallmeijer AJ, Lankhorst G (2005) Clinimetrics in rehabilitation medicine: current issues in developing and applying measurement instruments. *J Rehabil Med* 37: 193–201.

DeMatteo C, Law M, Russel DJ, Pollock N, Rosenbaum P, Walter S (1992) *Quality of Upper Extremity Skills Test Manual*. Hamilton, Ontario: Canchild, McMasters University.

DeMatteo C, Law M, Russell D, Pollock N, Rosenbaum P, Walter S (1993) The reliability and validity of the Quality of Upper Extremity Skills Test. *Phys Occup Ther Pediatr* 13: 1–18.

Eliasson AC, Krumlinde-Sundholm L, Rösblad B, Beckung E, Arner M, Öhrvall AM, Rosenbaum P (2006) The Manual Ability Classification System (MACS) for children with cerebral palsy: scale development and evidence of validity and reliability. *Dev Med Child Neurol* 48: 549–554.

Eliasziw M, Young M, Woodbury G, Fryday-Field K (1994) Statistical methodology for the concurrent assessment of interrater and intrarater reliability: using goniometric measurements as an example. *Phys Ther* 74: 777–788.

Eyssen IC, Beelen A, Dedding C, Cardol M, Dekker J (2005) The reproducibility of the Canadian Occupational Performance Measure. *Clin Rehabil* 19: 888–894.

Granlund M, Eriksson L, Ylvén R (2004) Utility of International Classification of Functioning, Disability and Health's participation dimension in assigning ICF codes to items from extant rating instruments. *J Rehabil Med* 36: 130–137.

Haley SM, Coster WJ, Ludlow LH (1991) Pediatric functional outcome measures. *Phys Med Rehabil Clin North Am* 4: 689–723.

Hanna SE, Russell D, Bartlett D, Kertoy M, Rosenbaum P, Swinton M (2005) Clinical measurement: practical guidelines for service providers. CanChild Centre for Childhood Disability Research. www.fhs.mcmaster.ca/canchild

Hanna SE, Russell DJ, Bartlett DJ, Kertoy M, Rosenbaum PL, Wynn K (2007) Measurement practices in pediatric rehabilitation: a survey of physical therapists, occupational therapists, and speech-language pathologists in Ontario. *Phys Occup Ther Pediatr* 27: 25–42.

Hemmingson H, Jonsson H (2005) An occupational perspective on the concept of participation in the international classification of functioning, disability and health – some critical remarks. *Am J Occup Ther* 59: 569–576.

Henderson SE, Sugden DA (1992) *Manual for the Movement Assessment Battery for Children*. Sidcup, Kent: Psychological Corporation.

Holmefur M, Krumlinde-Sundholm L, Eliasson AC (2007) Interrater and intrarater reliability of the Assisting Hand Assessment. *Am J Occup Ther* 61: 79–84.

House JH, Gwathmey FW, Fidler MO (1981) A dynamic approach to the thumb-in-palm deformity in cerebral palsy. *J Bone Joint Surg* 63: 216–225.

Jebsen RH, Taylor N, Trieschmann RB, Trotter MJ, Howard LA (1969) An objective and standardized test of hand function. *Arch Phys Med Rehabil* 50: 311–319.

Johnson LM, Randall MJ, Reddihough DS, Oke LE, Byrt TA, Bach TM (1994) Development of a clinical assessment of quality of movement for unilateral upper-limb function. *Dev Med Child Neurol* 36: 965–973.

Kellor M, Frost J, Silberberg N, Iversen I, Cummings R (1971) Hand strength and dexterity. *Am J Occup Ther* 25: 77–83.

Kimmerle M, Mainwaring L, Borenstein M (2003) The functional repertoire of the hand and its application to assessment. *Am J Occup Ther* 57: 489–498.

Kiresuk TJ, Sherman RE (1968) Goal attainment scaling: a general method for evaluating community mental health programs. *Community Ment Health J* 4: 442–453.

Krumlinde-Sundholm L, Eliasson A (2003) Development of the Assisting Hand Assessment, a Rasch built measure intended for children with unilateral upper limb impairments. *Scand J Occup Ther* 10: 16–26.

Krumlinde-Sundholm L, Holmefur M, Kottorp A, Eliasson AC (2007) The Assisting Hand Assessment: current evidence of validity, reliability and responsiveness to change. *Dev Med Child Neurol* 49: 259–264.

Law M, King G, Russell D, MacKinnon E, Hurley P, Murphy C (1999). Measuring outcomes in children's rehabilitation: a decision protocol. *Arch Phys Med Rehabil* 80: 629–636.

Law M, Baptiste S, Carswell A, McColl MA, Polatajko H, Pollock N (2000) *Canadian Occupational Performance Measure*. Toronto: CAOT Publications, ACE.

Majnemer A, Mazer B (2004) New directions in the outcome evaluation of children with cerebral palsy. *Semin Pediatr Neurol* 11: 11–17.

Mathiowetz V, Volland G, Kashman N, Weber K (1985a) Adult norms for the Box and Block test of manual dexterity. *Am J Occup Ther* 39: 386–391.

Mathiowetz V, Federman S, Wiemer D (1985b) Box and Block test of manual dexterity: norms for 6–19 year olds. *Can J Occup Ther* 55: 241–245.

Østensjø S, Bjørbäkmo W, Carlberg EB, Vollestad NK (2006) Assessment of everyday functioning in young children with disabilities: an ICF-based analysis of concepts and content of the Pediatric Evaluation of Disability Inventory (PEDI). *Disabil Rehabil* 28: 489–504.

Ottenbacher KJ, Cusick A (1990) Goal attainment scaling as a measure of clinical service evaluation. *Am J Occup Ther* 44: 519–525.

Palisano R, Rosenbaum P, Walter S, Russell DJ, Wood EP, Galuppi B (1997) Development and reliability of a system to classify gross motor function in children with cerebral palsy. *Dev Med Child Neurol* 39: 213–223.

Palisano RJ, Cameron D, Rosenbaum PL, Walter SD, Russell D (2006) Stability of the Gross Motor Function Classification System. *Dev Med Child Neurol* 48: 424–428.

Polit DF, Hungler BP (1999) *Nursing Research*. Philadelphia: Lippincott Williams & Wilkins.

Poole JL, Burtner PA, Torres TA, McMullen CK, Markham A, Marcum ML, Anderson JB, Qualls C (2005) Measuring dexterity in children using the nine-hole peg test. *J Hand Ther* 18: 348–351.

Randall MJ, Johnson LM, Reddihough DS (1999) *The Melbourne Assessment of Unilateral Upper Limb Function*. Melbourne: Royal Children's Hospital.

Randall M, Carlin JB, Chondros P, Reddihough D (2001) Reliability of the Melbourne assessment of unilateral upper limb function. *Dev Med Child Neurol* 43: 761–767.

Richardson PK (2005) Use of standardized tests in pediatric practice. In: Case-Smith J, editor. *Occupational Therapy for Children*. St Louis, MO: Mosby, pp. 217–245.

Rosenbaum P (1998) Screening tests and standardized assessments used to identify and characterize developmental delays. *Semin Pediatr Neurol* 5: 27–32.

Rudman D, Hannah S (1998) An instrument evaluation framework: description and application to assessments of hand function. *J Hand Ther* 11: 266–277.

Schepers VP, Ketelaar M, van de Port IG, Visser-Meily JM, Lindeman E (2007) Comparing contents of functional outcome measures in stroke rehabilitation using the International Classification of Functioning, Disability and Health. *Disabil Rehabil* 29: 221–230.

Schreuders TA, Roebroeck ME, Goumans J, van Nieuwenhuijzen JF, Stijnen TH, Stam HJ (2003) Measurement error in grip and pinch force measurements in patients with hand injuries. *Phys Ther* 83: 806–815.

Simmonds MJ (1997). Muscle strength. In: Van Deusen J, Brunt D, editors. *Assessment in Occupational Therapy and Physical Therapy*. Philadelphia: W.B. Saunders, pp. 27–48.

Smith RA, Wrisberg CA (2000) *Motor Learning and Performance. A Problem-Based Learning Approach, 2nd edn*. Champaign, IL: Human Kinetics.

Streiner DL, Norman GR (2003) *Health Measurement Scales: A Practical Guide to their Development and Use, 3rd edn*. Oxford: Oxford University Press.

Stucki G (2005) International Classification of Functioning, Disability, and Health (ICF): a promising framework and classification for rehabilitation medicine. *Am J Phys Med Rehabil* 84: 733–740.

Taylor N, Sand PL, Jebsen RH (1973). Evaluation of hand function in children. *Arch Phys Med Rehabil* 54: 129–135.

Wallen M, O'Flaherty SJ, Waugh M-C (2007) Functional outcomes of intramuscular botulinum toxin type A and occupational therapy in the upper limbs of children with cerebral palsy: a randomized controlled trial. *Arch Phys Med Rehabil* 88: 1–10.

World Health Organization (2001) *International Classification of Functioning, Disability and Health*. Geneva: World Health Organization.

Wright BD, Linacre JM (1989) Observations are always ordinal; measurements, however, must be interval. *Arch Phys Med Rehabil* 70: 857–860.

Wright B, Stone M (1979) *Best Test Design, Rasch Measurement*. Chicago: Mesa Press.

Zancolli EA, Zancolli ER (1981) Surgical management of the hemiplegic spastic hand in cerebral palsy. *Surg Clin North Am* 61: 395–406.

13
ORTHOPAEDIC INTERVENTION IN THE UPPER EXTREMITY IN THE CHILD WITH CEREBRAL PALSY: MUSCULOSKELETAL SURGERY

L. Andrew Koman, Zhongyu Li and Beth Paterson Smith

Introduction

Significant functional limitations of the upper limbs are observed in 80 per cent of individuals with cerebral palsy having hemiparesis or quadriparesis. This limb involvement negatively impacts self-esteem, interferes with functional activities, impairs caregiving activities, and/or produces pain. Historically, less than 20 per cent of paediatric patients with cerebral palsy with affected limbs are candidates for effective surgical intervention (Carroll and Craig 1951, Green and Banks 1962, Goldner 1974, Goldner et al 1990, Koman et al 1990, Koman et al 2002). In addition to improving function, surgery may be employed to diminish pain, to decrease or prevent deformity, and to improve self-esteem and appearance. This is in marked contrast to the lower extremity in which surgery is more frequently indicated. Interventions (e.g. therapy, splinting, electrical stimulation, constraint-induced therapy, oral antispasticity medications, parenteral chemodenervation/neuromuscular blocking agents, and intrathecal baclofen) are used to maintain upper extremity range of motion, prevent osseous deformity and delay or diminish joint contracture. Therefore, their successful use may increase the number of eligible candidates for upper extremity surgical procedures.

This chapter is designed as an overview of the complex topic of orthopaedic upper extremity surgical interventions. The chapter will discuss the evaluation of the spastic limb; diagnostic testing techniques; indications for surgery; surgical options for specific deformity(ies); and post-operative care protocols. Optimal orthopaedic management of the upper limb in children with cerebral palsy requires careful patient assessment, a patient-oriented, outcome-driven treatment approach, and consistent and long-term post-operative care.

Evaluation

HISTORY AND PHYSICAL EXAMINATION
A complete history and physical examination is crucial and should include input from the patient, caregiver(s), therapists, teachers, social workers, and other health-care providers. Evaluations performed within the World Health Organization's Classification of Function, Disability and Health domains are helpful (WHO 2001). Patient evaluations using functional

classifications (e.g. House Scale; House et al 1981) and standardized testing regimens (e.g. Melbourne Assessment of Unilateral Limb Function (Johnson et al 1994, Randall et al 2001) provide valuable objective information. For patients with mild to moderate involvement, a complete Melbourne Assessment is obtained. Active and passive range of motion are recorded in a standardized manner – we utilize the upper extremity rating scale (UERS). The Jebsen Hand Function Test is helpful in mild to moderately involved patients. Degree of spasticity, absence or presence and magnitude of involuntary movement disorders (dystonia) and effectiveness of upper limb motor control are assessed, quantified, and recorded. Muscles that are being considered for transfer are assessed to determine phasic and nonphasic control. If there is a clinical concern, electromyography is requested. A global instrument such as the WeeFim (see Appendix) is available to measure self-care and functional skills (ICF Activities level). The patient should be observed – if appropriate – during ambulation and while standing, sitting and recumbent in order to observe possible posturing and motion patterns. Because the time of day, degree of anxiety, and level of fatigue may influence clinical findings, serial evaluations are helpful to fully assess patients. Sensibility testing includes evaluations of proprioception, stereognosis, and two-point discrimination. Limited sensory capability is a relative contraindication for sophisticated surgical techniques (Van Heest et al 1999). These tests are helpful in identifying patients who are suitable candidates for complex reconstruction procedures.

If the surgical recommendations are not consistent, caution is urged and further consideration is important. Proactive planning with multiple team members is key to the success of the surgical intervention. This includes formalizing the surgical plan, outlining the immediate post-operative regime – e.g. period and type of immobilization – and designing a rehabilitation programme.

DIAGNOSTIC EVALUATION
Evaluations using radiology, electromyography, motion analysis, and diagnostic muscle blockade can provide valuable diagnostic information to individualize the surgery to a particular child. Joint and osseous deformities may be evaluated using plain roentgenograms, computerized tomography (CT), and magnetic resonance imaging. Three-dimensional reconstructions of CT images are helpful in assessing joint congruity before performing soft tissue or bony interventions. Both surface and needle electromyography provide a qualitative and quantitative assessment of voluntary motor recruitment and the appropriateness of motor activations (Hoffer et al 1979, Mowery et al 1985, Hoffer et al 1986). Three-dimensional upper extremity motion analysis provides a quantitative measure of a patient's motor performance and functional capacity, but is rarely used. Diagnostic motor blockade produced by injecting bupivacaine or botulinum A toxin may be used to predict post-surgical outcomes and the appropriateness of surgical interventions in the muscles identified for surgery (Autti-Ramo et al 2000, Koman et al 2002). All these diagnostic tools assist the surgeon and family in their decision making.

Global surgical goals for best outcomes include: (1) improved function, (2) facilitation of care, (3) pain reduction, and (4) enhancement of self-esteem. Specific surgical interventions performed at one or more levels (i.e. shoulder, elbow, wrist, hand) are necessary to reduce spasticity and/or pain, to balance or stabilize joint movements, to improve selective motor control, and/or to augment or diminish uncontrollable motor power in order to achieve each patient's specific goals. Surgical interventions may be reduced to a checklist of options (Table 13.1). The presence of involuntary movement disorders is a relative contraindication for tendon transfers. The art and science of surgery depends on the selection of the appropriate procedure(s) required to achieve both specific and global outcomes individualized for each patient.

Operative procedures

SHOULDER

Adduction and internal rotation shoulder deformities are common in individuals with cerebral palsy, and these deformities may be dynamic or static in nature. The shoulder joint may be dislocated, subluxed, or contracted in one or more planes. Furthermore, the glenoid or humeral head may be deformed, dysplastic, and/or arthritic. In dynamic deformities, glenohumeral articulation is often congruous and stable with satisfactory articular surfaces. Treatment options for shoulder deformities include muscle lengthening and muscle/tendon transfer, though these procedures are rarely performed. For shoulder internal rotation deformity, release of the pectoralis major and subscapularis by Z-lengthening may be effective, although capsular release is often required. External rotation power may be augmented by transfer of the latissimus dorsi and teres major (Fig.13.1). For patients with significant adduction and internal rotation shoulder contractures, release of the latissimus and teres major in conjunction with the procedures described above may be required. Alternatively, a proximal or distal osteotomy of the humerus is a possible option to improve either external rotation or internal rotation. However, osteotomy is reserved for arthritic or dysplastic/subluxed joints or for patients who have failed previous tendon transfers. In patients without arthritis or significant humeral head or glenoid deformity, subluxation and dislocation may require open reduction, capsular release and/or capsulodesis, and/or humeral or glenoid osteotomy. Shoulder fusion has been reported to manage refractory pain secondary to arthritis, but we have no experience with this procedure in patients with cerebral palsy (Landi et al 2004).

ELBOW

Elbow flexion deformity – except in essentially normal children – does not require treatment until the flexion deformity exceeds 30 degrees (Manske et al 2001). Unbalanced spasticity of the biceps brachii, brachialis, brachioradialis, and/or flexor/pronator muscles may result in joint contracture and shortening of musculotendinous units. Deformities are usually a combination of fixed contracture of the capsule and muscles and dynamic motor imbalance. Associated hyperpronation may result in dysplasia and subluxation of the radial head,

TABLE 13.1
Specific interventions (common choices)

Joint area	Need	Options
Shoulder	Joint stabilization Increase external rotation Increase internal rotation	Fusion, capsular reconstructions Lengthen pectoralis major/ subscapularis; transfer LD and/or teres major Lengthen/release infraspinatus/teres minor
Elbow	Stabilization Increase extension	Fusion Lengthen or release biceps brachii; brachialis brachioradialis release (slide); flexor-pronator mass release; joint capsule release; humeral osteotomy; excise radial head
Forearm	Improve supination	Reroute, lengthen, or release PT; osteotomy radius ulna; release flexor-pronator muscle, excise radial head
Wrist	Stabilize Increase range of motion Extension	Fusion; (tendon transfer; release; proximal row) carpectomy Transfers of FCU, ECU, FCR, BR, FDS, FDP
Thumb	Stabilization Increase extension Improve power Improve abduction	Volar plate arthroplasty, fusion MCP joint Plication/transfer, EPL, APB, EPB; release/lengthen FPL Reinforce EPL, reinforce FPL Release adductor, abduction transfer, osteotomy metacarpal
Fingers	Flexion Swan neck	FDS to FDP transfer; flexor/ pronator release (slide), lengthen FDS, lengthen FDP EDC FDS tenotomy; fusion PIP joint; tenodesis FDS

Abbreviations
APB   abductor pollicis brevis
APL   abductor pollicis longus
BR   brachioradialis
ECU   extensor carpi ulnaris
EPB   extensor pollicis brevis
EPL   extensor pollicis longus
FCU   flexor carpal ulnar
FDS   flexor digitorum superficialis/profundus
FCR   flexor carpi radialis
LD   latissimus dorsi
MCP   metacarpophalangeal
PIP   proximal interphalangeal joint
PM   pectoralis major
PT   pronator teres

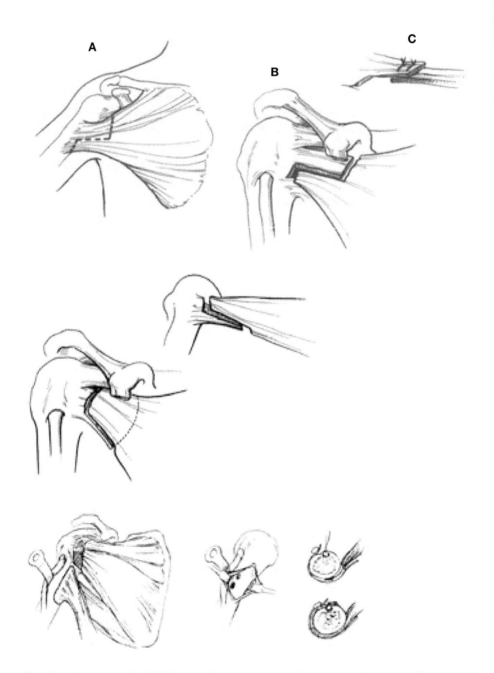

Fig. 13.1 For the modified L'Episcopo-Sever procedure, z-lengthening of the pectoralis major is performed (A), the subscapularis is lengthened on the 'flat' (B), and the latissimus dorsi and teres major are transferred to the posteriolateral humerus using one incision (C) or two incisions (not shown).

Source: Koman LA, editor. *Wake Forest University School of Medicine Orthopaedic Manual 2001*. Winston-Salem, NC: Orthopaedic Press. (© Wake Forest University Orthopaedic Press.)

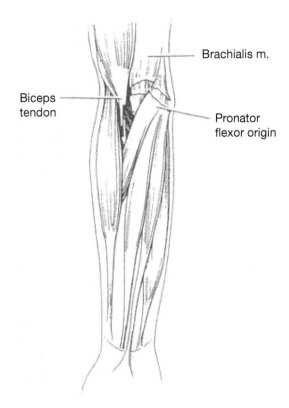

Biceps
tendon

Brachialis m.

Pronator
flexor origin

Fig. 13.2 Elbow flexion contractures
between 30 and 60 degrees.
Z-lengthening of the biceps tendon
and fractional lengthening of the
musculotendinous portion of the
brachialis with or without flexor
pronator release are appropriate.
Source: Koman LA, editor.
*Wake Forest University School of
Medicine Orthopaedic Manual 2001.*
Winston-Salem, NC: Orthopaedic
Press. (© Wake Forest University
Orthopaedic Press.)

complicating treatment. For elbow deformities between 30 and 60 degrees, soft tissue procedures (including lengthening of the biceps, brachialis and brachioradialis) are usually sufficient and will – when spasticity is present – reliably decrease the degree of deformity by approximately 50 per cent (Fig. 13.2). For deformities exceeding 60 degrees, release of the flexor pronator origin and elbow joint may also be required. Serial casting and/or external fixator-assisted correction may also be required in these cases for optimal results. Resection of a subluxed radial head may be beneficial in improving elbow flexion/extension and supination/pronation. Elbow fusion is reserved for patients who experience intractable pain. However, elbow fusion has never been required for the surgical management of our patients with cerebral palsy.

FOREARM

Forearm pronation deformities, commonly apparent, may be managed by: (1) release, lengthening, or rerouting of the pronator teres (PT); (2) release of the flexor-pronator origin; (3) resection of a subluxed or dislocated radial head; (4) osteotomy of the radius and/or ulna; and/or (5) alternative transfer routed to provide supination moment (e.g. flexor carpi ulnaris to extensor carpi radialis brevis). For a continuously active PT associated with passive supination, PT release, Z-lengthening, or fractional lengthening is appropriate. For

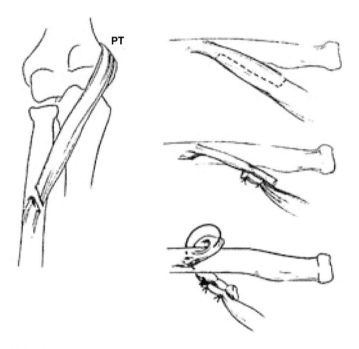

Fig. 13.3 The pronator teres may be detached from the radius and rerouted to provide a supination moment.

Source: Koman LA, editor. *Wake Forest University School of Medicine Orthopaedic Manual 2001.* Winston-Salem, NC: Orthopaedic Press. (© Wake Forest University Orthopaedic Press.)

patients with non-continuously firing or intermittent PT muscle activity, rerouting is the preferred surgical option at our institution (Fig. 13.3). Radial head resection is indicated when subluxation prevents supination and/or causes pain. Rerouting of the brachioradialis has been reported as another surgical technique to improve supination (Ozkan et al 2004). Radial and/or ulnar osteotomy is reserved for fixed, severe deformities; fusion is not generally performed.

WRIST

Significant wrist palmar flexion that interferes with function, produces pain, interferes with optimal caregiver activities, and/or elicits emotional distress is common. Management options for wrist palmar flexion include: (1) tendon transfer(s); (2) tendon lengthening or release; (3) proximal row carpectomy; and (4) arthrodesis. Wrist joint deformities may be fixed or dynamic with or without osseous deformities. Often, wrist deformity is interrelated with elbow and hand/finger deformities. Fixed wrist contractures associated with greater than 60 degrees of palmar flexion deformity may not respond to soft tissue release procedures. Tendon transfers may require concomitant bony procedures and/or gradual correction effected by serial casting or graduated external fixation, i.e. assisted distraction/angular deformity management using a multiplanar geared correction device.

Osseous options to correct significant wrist palmar flexion include proximal row carpectomy, radial shortening (shortening with or without angulation), wrist fusion (with or without carpal incisional resection), or a combination of the above. Wrist fusion procedures should be reserved for patients with good to excellent thumb–finger control with the wrist mobilized in or close to neutral, or for patients who require pain relief. Patients with functional extremities must be carefully evaluated before wrist fusion procedures are performed in order to prevent loss of the tenodesis effect on finger flexion and grasp and release (Omer and Capen 1976, Szabo and Gelberman 1985, Koman et al 1990).

Management of dynamic flexion deformities includes surgical procedures to transfer the flexor carpi ulnaris (FCU) to the extensor carpi radialis longus (ECRL), to the extensor carpi radialis brevis (ECRB) or to the extensor digitorum communis (EDC) (Fig. 13.4; Green 1942, Green and Banks 1962, Hoffer et al 1979, 1986). The choice of the most appropriate tendon transfer option is enhanced by pre-operative assessment of phasic, nonphasic and continuous muscle activity during wrist motion determined by careful clinical

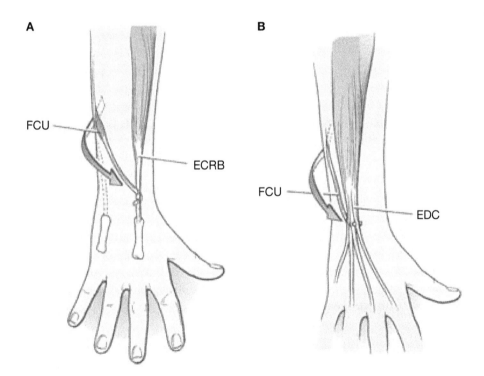

Fig. 13.4 Transfer of the flexor carpi ulnaris to the extensor carpi radialis brevis (A) or transfer of the flexor carpi ulnaris to the extensor digitorum communis (B) will improve wrist extension. The tendon may be transferred subcutaneously to provide a supination moment or through the interosseous membrane to provide more dorsiflexion without supination.

Source: Koman LA, editor. *Wake Forest University School of Medicine Orthopaedic Manual 2001*. Winston-Salem, NC: Orthopaedic Press. (© Wake Forest University Orthopaedic Press.)

Fig. 13.5 Transfer of the extensor carpi ulnaris (ECU) from its insertion on the fifth metacarpal to the fourth metacarpal will decrease ulnar deviation and assist flexion. The extensor retinaculum should be released to allow dorsal translation of the ECU tendon.

Source: Koman LA, editor. *Wake Forest University School of Medicine Orthopaedic Manual 2001*. Winston-Salem, NC: Orthopaedic Press. (© Wake Forest University Orthopaedic Press.)

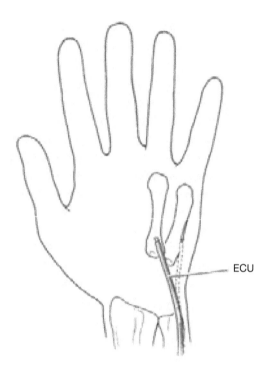

ECU

examination or electromyography evaluations (Hoffer et al 1979, 1986, Koman et al 1990). In patients with continuous FCU activation during wrist flexion and extension, transfer of the FCU to the ECRB/ECRL may produce a wrist extension deformity, and in this case, transfer to the EDC is preferable. The latter will eliminate FCU overpull, augment wrist and finger extension, permit finger flexion, and prevent wrist extension deformity (Hoffer et al 1979, Koman et al 1990). If the FCU contracts phasically, its transfer to the ECRB will improve voluntary wrist extension without creating any additional deformity. If significant ulnar deviation is an issue, transfer to the ECRL is appropriate. Concomitant Z-lengthening or fractional lengthening of the flexor carpi radialis (FCR) also may be necessary. For extremities with significant dynamic wrist flexion and ulnar deviation, transfer of the extensor carpi ulnaris (ECU) to the fourth metacarpal will often diminish ulnar deviation and facilitate wrist extension (Fig. 13.5).

THUMB AND FINGER DEFORMITIES

Finger flexion
Dynamic finger flexion secondary to spasticity of the flexor digitorum superficialis (FDS) and/or flexor digitorum profundus (FDP) can often be managed by augmenting EDC power by transfer of the FCU or the ring FDS to the EDC. One or two FDS motors may be utilized with the long and ring selected most frequently. Similarly, the extensor pollicis longus (EPL) may be reinforced using an FDS of the ring finger, long finger, or brachioradialis.

Fixed finger contractures require both extensor augmentation and lengthening of the shortened flexors. The normalization of the musculotendinous length of flexors may be achieved by one or more of the following interventions: serial muscle stretching after intramuscular botulinum A toxin (BoNT-A) injection(s); Z-lengthening of individual tendons; fractional lengthening of individual muscle-tendon units; transfer of the FDS proximally to the FDP distally (the superficialis to profundus (STP) transfer); and/or flexor-pronator slide procedures. For mild to moderate joint contractures, our management choice is fractional lengthening of the individual FDS muscles and injection of BoNT-A into both the lengthened FDS and the non-lengthened FDP. More severe deformities may require fractional or Z-lengthening of the FDP, fractional lengthening of the FDS, and intramuscular BoNT-A injections. Flexor-pronator slide procedures are reserved for severe deformities in patients with the potential for improved post-surgical function; superficialis to profundus transfers are used to manage severe deformities associated with pain and/or interference with hygiene concerns (Goldner 1955, Swanson 1966, Goldner 1974, Zancolli and Zancolli 1981, Szabo and Gelberman 1985, Koman et al 1990), but not when functional recovery is necessary (Goldner 1955, White 1972). An alternative procedure is a superficialis to profundus transfer using the proximal stump of the profundus to reinforce the superficialis.

Thumb flexion deformity
Dynamic thumb deformity is managed by augmenting thumb extensor power; this can be accomplished by a combination of plication, rerouting, and/or reinforcement using a brachioradialis or FDS tendon. Thumb deformities are rarely managed in isolation; procedures to address thumb deformities are associated with correcting fixed contractures of the flexor pollicis longus (FPL) muscle-tendon unit using Z- or fractional lengthening procedures. Ironically, the contracted and spastic FPL is often weak and reinforcement with either the brachioradialis or another tendon is an option to improve its overall strength (Koman et al 1990).

Thumb-in-palm deformity
Thumb-in-palm deformities develop as a result of multiple factors and may be related to soft tissue issues, joint instability, attenuation and weakness of the extensor tendons, dynamic and/or static deformities of the flexor pollicis longus, weakness of the abductor/opponens muscle(s), and dynamic or static deformity of the adductor pollicis brevis. Therefore, treatment for thumb-in-palm deformities must address all these factors. Metacarpal phalangeal joint (MCP) stability may be enhanced by volar plate capsulodesis for the management of pure hyperextension instability; however, combined hyperflexion and hyperextension, or global instability, is best corrected by MCP fusion. In addition, MCP fusion procedures reduce the number of motion segments, which, in turn, facilitates coordination of flexor extensor power (Goldner et al 1990, Koman et al 1990). Web space contractures are addressed by releasing contracted muscles (adductor pollicis brevis and first dorsal interosseous) and re-arranging of skin and soft tissue(s) (e.g. four-flap Z-plasty) (Figs 13.6, 13.7).

Thumb adduction deformities are managed by Z-plasty or myotomy of the adductor brevis. Abductor motor power can be managed using several techniques including: (1)

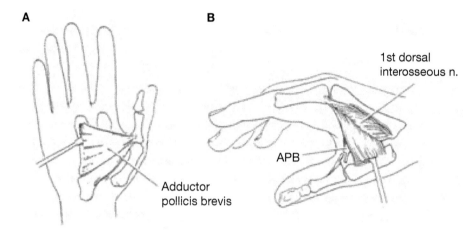

Fig. 13.6 The adductor pollicis brevis may be released from its origin on the third metacarpal through a volar incision (A); alternatively, the adductor tendon may be Z-lengthened or transferred proximally to the first metacarpal to increase the first web space; (B) the first dorsal interosseous may be released from the first metacarpal.

Source: Koman LA, editor. *Wake Forest University School of Medicine Orthopaedic Manual 2001*. Winston-Salem, NC: Orthopaedic Press. (© Wake Forest University Orthopaedic Press.)

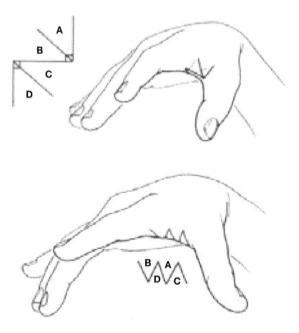

Fig. 13.7 Schematic representation of a four-flap Z-plasty.

Source: Koman LA, editor. *Wake Forest University School of Medicine Orthopaedic Manual 2001*. Winston-Salem, NC: Orthopaedic Press. (© Wake Forest University Orthopaedic Press.)

transfer of the brachioradialis (BR) to the abductor pollicis longus; (2) rerouting of the EPL to the radial side of Lister's tubercle with or without the BR or a flexor digitorum superficialis tendon; and/or (3) fusion of the MCP joint.

Thumb extensor tone is reduced by plication of the extensor pollicis longus (EPL), abductor pollicis longus (APL), and/or extensor pollicis brevis (EPB), while power is increased by tendon transfers using the brachioradialis or the flexor digitorum superficialis of the ring finger (Figs 13.8, 13.9). Management of FPL contractures is discussed under thumb flexion deformity above.

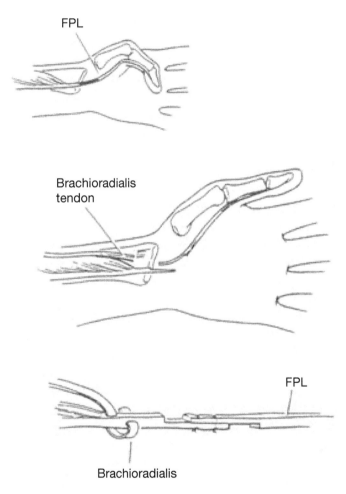

Fig. 13.8 A fixed contracture of the flexor pollicis longus may be managed by Z-lengthening as demonstrated, or more proximally by fractional lengthening (not demonstrated). Reinforcement may be achieved as demonstrated by transfer of the brachioradialis proximal to the Z-lengthening.

Source: Koman LA, editor. *Wake Forest University School of Medicine Orthopaedic Manual 2001*. Winston-Salem, NC: Orthopaedic Press. (© Wake Forest University Orthopaedic Press.)

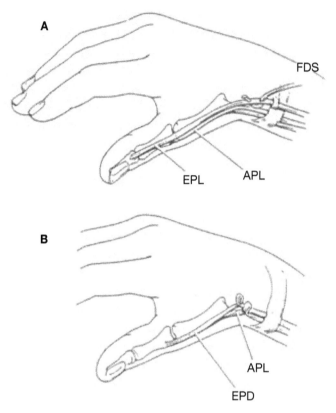

Fig. 13.9 The extensor pollicis longus may be rerouted radial to Lister's tubercle, plicated and reinforced, if necessary, with the flexor digitorum superficialis.

Source: Koman LA, editor. *Wake Forest University School of Medicine Orthopaedic Manual 2001*. Winston-Salem, NC: Orthopaedic Press. (© Wake Forest University Orthopaedic Press.)

Digital deformities

Swan neck deformities of the digit are managed by extensor tendon tenotomy (Carlson 2005), volar plate capsulodesis, FDS tenodesis, or PIP fusion. Contractures of the intrinsic muscles may adversely influence grasp and release. Effective treatment is difficult; however, intrinsic releases may be beneficial.

POST-OPERATIVE CARE

Post-operative care is crucial to maximize the child's post-operative outcomes. Pre-operative planning includes input from therapists regarding appropriate post-operative therapy modalities and splinting that will maximize surgical outcomes. In addition, intra-operative intramuscular neuromuscular blockade with botulinum A toxin is used to decrease post-operative pain, protect tendon repairs associated with lengthening and/or transfer procedures, permit earlier active motion, and prevent over-lengthening after fractional procedures. The initial three to four weeks of post-operative care are focused on protecting tendon transfers and maintaining or improving range of motion, combined with appropriate splinting at night and strengthening exercises.

HAND THERAPY

Post-operative hand therapy provided by occupational or physical therapists is crucial to the rehabilitation process and is necessary to ensure optimal outcomes in most patients. In the first three to four weeks after surgery, rigid splinting, pins and/or casts provide protection of the operative site. During this period, the therapist evaluates the patient in order to maintain proper joint position and range of motion of the proximal and distal joints. After the initial healing phase has occurred, active and passive range of motion protocols are implemented, and static splinting is utilized as indicated. At 6–10 weeks after surgery, strengthening is a crucial part of the rehabilitation programme, with the inclusion of a home programme as an important component of the rehabilitation process. Specific guidelines for post-operative therapy are outlined in Chapter 15. Evidence of the effectiveness of surgical intervention has largely been limited to case studies (see Chapter 26 for a review). Future multi-centre trials using functional classification systems pre- and post-surgery would assist in establishing evidence-based practice guidelines.

Summary

Although only a small percentage of children and adults with cerebral palsy are candidates for upper extremity surgery, judicious use of the surgical procedures discussed in this chapter can result in positive outcomes and improve patient health-related quality of life. However, proper patient selection is crucial to ensure reasonable post-operative results, and post-operative care must be coordinated with appropriately trained hand therapists for optimal results.

REFERENCES

Autti-Ramo I, Larsen A, Peltonen J, Taimo A, von Wendt L (2000) Botulinum toxin injection as an adjunct when planning hand surgery in children with spastic hemiplegia. *Neuropediatrics* 31: 4–8.
Boyce WF, Gowland C, Hardy S, Rosenbaum PL, Lane M, Plews N, Goldsmith C, Russell DJ, Wright V, Potter S, Harding D (1995) The gross motor performance measure: validity and responsiveness of a measure of quality of movement. *Phys Ther* 75: 603–613.
Carlson MG (2005) Cerebral palsy. In: Green DP, Hotchkiss RN, Pederson WC, Wolfe SW, editors. *Green's Operative Hand Surgery, 5th edn.* Philadelphia: Churchill Livingstone, pp. 1197–1234.
Carroll RE, Craig FS (1951) The surgical treatment of cerebral palsy. *Surg Clin North Am* 30: 385–396.
Goldner JL (1955) Reconstructive surgery of the hand in cerebral palsy and spastic paralysis resulting from injury to the spinal cord. *J Bone Joint Surg* 37: 1141–1153.
Goldner JL (1974) Upper extremity tendon transfers in cerebral palsy. *Orthop Clin North Am* 5: 389–414.
Goldner JL, Koman LA, Gelberman R, Levin S, Goldner RD (1990) Arthrodesis of the metacarpophalangeal joint of the thumb in children and adults. Adjunctive treatment of thumb-in-palm deformity in cerebral palsy. *Clin Orthop Relat Res* 253: 75–89.
Green WT (1942) Tendon transplantation of the flexor carpi ulnaris for pronation – flexor deformity of the wrist. *Surg Gynecol Obstet* 75: 337–342.
Green WT, Banks HH (1962) Flexor carpi ulnaris transplant and its use in cerebral palsy. *J Bone Joint Surg* 44A: 1343–1352.

Hoffer MM, Perry J, Melkonian GF (1979) Dynamic electromyography and decision-making for surgery in the upper extremity of patients with cerebral palsy. *J Hand Surg* 4A: 424–431.

Hoffer MM, Lehman M, Mitani M (1986) Long-term follow-up on tendon transfers to the extensors of the wrist and fingers in patients with cerebral palsy. *J Hand Surg* 1A: 836–840.

House JH, Gwathmey FW, Fidler MO (1981) A dynamic approach to the thumb-in-palm deformity in cerebral palsy. *J Bone Joint Surg* 63A: 216–225.

Johnson LM, Randall MJ, Reddihough DS, Oke LE, Byrt TA, Bach TM (1994) Development of a clinical assessment of quality of movement for unilateral upper-limb function. *Dev Med Child Neurol* 36: 965–973.

Koman LA, Gelberman RH, Toby EB, Poehling GG (1990) Cerebral palsy. Management of the upper extremity. *Clin Orthop* 253: 62–74.

Koman LA, Smith BP, Goodman A (2002) *Botulinum Toxin Type A in the Management of Cerebral Palsy.* Winston-Salem, NC: Wake Forest University Press.

Landi A, Cavazza S, Caserta G, Leti Acciaro A, Sartinni S, Gagliano MC, Manca M (2004) The upper limb in cerebral palsy: surgical management of shoulder and elbow deformities. *Hand Clin* 20: 345–347.

Manske PR, Langewisch KR, Strecker WB, Albrecht MM (2001) Anterior elbow release of spastic elbow flexion deformity in children with cerebral palsy. *J Pediatr Orthop* 21: 772–777.

Mowery CA, Gelberman RH, Rhoades CE (1985) Upper extremity tendon transfers in cerebral palsy: electromyographic and functional analysis. *J Pediatr Orthop* 5: 69–72.

Omer GE, Capen DA (1976) Proximal row carpectomy with muscle transfers for spastic paralysis. *J Hand Surg* 1A: 197–204.

Ozkan T, Tuncer S, Aydin A, Hosbay Z, Gulgonen A (2004) Brachioradialis re-routing for the restoration of active supination and correction of forearm pronation deformity in cerebral palsy. *J Hand Surg* 29B: 265–270.

Randall M, Carlin JB, Chondros P, Reddihough D (2001) Reliability of the Melbourne assessment of unilateral upper limb function. *Dev Med Child Neurol* 43: 761–767.

Swanson AB (1966) Treatment of the swan-neck deformity in the cerebral palsied hand. *Clin Orthop Relat Res* 48: 167–171.

Szabo RM, Gelberman RH (1985) Operative treatment of cerebral palsy. *Hand Clin* 1: 525–543.

Van Heest AE, House JH, Cariello C (1999) Upper extremity surgical treatment of cerebral palsy. *J Hand Surg* 24A: 323–330.

White WF (1972) Flexor muscle slide in the spastic hand: the Max Page operation. *J Bone Joint Surg* 54B: 453–459.

World Health Organization (2001) *International Classification of Functioning, Disability and Health.* Geneva: World Health Organization. http://www.who.int/icf

Zancolli EA, Zancolli ER Jr (1981) Surgical management of the hemiplegic spastic hand in cerebral palsy. *Surg Clin North Am* 61: 395–406.

14
ORTHOPAEDIC INTERVENTION IN THE MANAGEMENT OF CEREBRAL PALSY: BOTULINUM TOXINS

L. Andrew Koman, Zhongyu Li and Beth Paterson Smith

Chemodenervation and neuromuscular blockade in upper extremity cerebral palsy

Alcohol (45 per cent), phenol (5–7 per cent), and botulinum toxins are injectable agents that produce selective weakening of individual muscles or muscle groups. When injected into muscles, these parenteral agents primarily balance muscle forces across joints by selective and reversible flaccid muscle paralysis by neuromuscular blockade or chemodenervation; they have no direct anti-spasticity action(s). Alcohol and phenol denature protein and interrupt peripheral nerve transmission by denaturing axons and neuromuscular junctions, a form of chemodenervation. Botulinum toxin (BoNT) blocks acetylcholine vesicle-membrane fusion at the neuromuscular junction, thus preventing release of acetylcholine at the neuromuscular junction blocking neuronal signalling for muscle contraction (Koman et al 2002).

Therapeutic application of botulinum A toxin to manage spasticity in patients with cerebral palsy was envisioned by Koman in 1985, with the first patient injected in 1987. The first manuscript describing the initial clinical experience with intramuscular botulinum toxin injections for spasticity management was published in 1993 (Koman et al 1993). The first injections were administered in the upper extremity of a young adult with cerebral palsy. Since our preliminary experience, we have participated in numerous clinical trials to evaluate the safety and efficacy of BoNT injections. In addition, injections are currently used for managing patients and to facilitate post-operative care. The purpose of this chapter is to provide an overview of the role of botulinum toxin in the management of spasticity associated with upper extremity cerebral palsy based on our experience with this drug.

Pharmacology and pharmacokinetics of botulinum A toxin

Clostridium botulinum produces seven neurotoxin serotypes (A, B, C, D, E, F, G) (Schantz and Johnson 1992, Aoki 2001). By cleaving SNARE proteins (synaptobrevin, synaptosomal-associated protein 25, and syntaxin), normal fusion of the acetylcholine (ACh) containing vesicles with the nerve cell membrane is blocked, producing an incompetent neuromuscular junction (NMJ) (Fig. 14.1) (DePavia et al 1999, Arnon et al 2001, Koman et al 2002). The result of intramuscular toxin injection is paralysis of the motor unit and flaccid muscle paralysis (Arnon et al 2001). Toxins A, C and E cleave SNAP 25; B, D, F and G cleave synaptobrevin; and C cleaves both syntaxin and SNAP 25 (Fig. 14.2). A rat

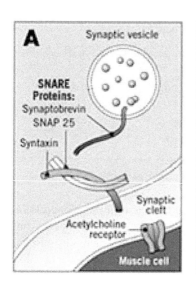
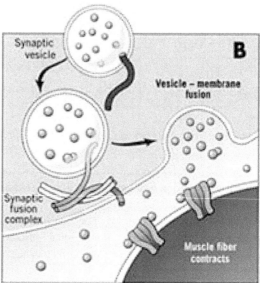

Fig. 14.1 Schematic depiction of normal vesicle–membrane fusion allowing release of acetylcholine (ACh) from the vesicle and stimulation of muscular contraction.

Source: Adapted from Arnon 2001. (Reproduced with permission from Koman LA, editor. *Wake Forest University School of Medicine Orthopaedic Manual 2001*. Winston-Salem, NC: Orthopaedic Press.)

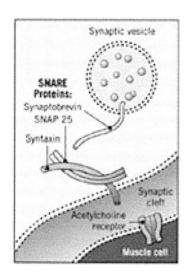
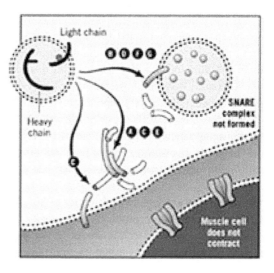

Fig. 14.2 Schematic representation of mechanism of action of botulinum toxins. Cleavage of SNARE proteins prevents vesicle–membrane fusion. The A toxin cleaves SNAP 25 producing flaccid paralysis of the motor unit.

Source: Adapted from Arnon 2001. (Reproduced with permission from Koman LA, editor. *Wake Forest University School of Medicine Orthopaedic Manual 2001*. Winston-Salem, NC: Orthopaedic Press.)

sciatic model was used to evaluate the effect of extrafascicular, infrafascicular and extra-neural injection of BoNT (Lu et al 1998). Histological and morphometric evaluations of the injected nerves demonstrated no damage to the nerves.

Toxin type A is the primary serotype that has been discussed in the peer-reviewed literature in relationship to spasticity management in paediatric cerebral palsy patients. Therefore, our discussion will be limited to the A toxin, produced commercially as a drug and marketed as BOTOX (Allergan Pharmaceuticals) and Dysport (Ipsen Limited). Currently, the only report in the literature describing the use of BoNT-B (Myobloc) in cerebral palsy describes B toxin combined with phenol injections for spasticity management (Gooch and Patton 2004).

Botulinum A toxin, a 150 kDa disulphide-linked dimer, consists of a 100 kDa 'heavy' chain and a 50 kDa 'light' chain (Fig. 14.3). The 'heavy' chain is similar among the toxin serotypes and is responsible for the irreversible binding and internalization of the toxin into the nerve terminus (Aoki 2001, 2003). The 50 kDa chain cleaves SNAP 25, a protein required for the release of ACh at the neuromuscular junction (Aoki 2005).

Neurotoxin serotype A is available commercially in 100 unit vials (BOTOX) and 500 unit vials (Dysport). Toxin units are defined using biologic assays in which 1 unit of toxin is injected intraperitoneally in a mouse resulting in the death of 50 per cent of the treated animals. *Units of BOTOX and Dysport are not equal or interchangeable.* The units are not equal because the methods for preparing BOTOX and Dysport are different, and the potency of their units is determined in different mouse strains using different testing protocols. Although the equivalency between BOTOX and Dysport has not been scientifically defined,

BOTOX© Structure

- Seven stereotypes: A, B, C1, D, E, F, G

- 150 kDa disulphide-linked dimer

  100 kDa membrane-binding
  heavy chain

  50 kDa zinc-dependent
  protease light chain

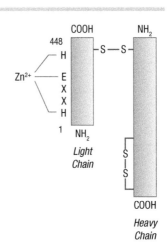

Fig. 14.3 Structure of botulinum A toxin displayed in two dimensions.

Source: Reproduced with permission from Koman LA, editor. *Wake Forest University School of Medicine Orthopaedic Manual 2001*. Winston-Salem, NC: Orthopaedic Press.

1 unit of BOTOX is approximately equivalent to 3 to 5 units of Dysport (Carr et al 1998). *Currently, no botulinum A toxin drug preparation is labelled for upper extremity use in the management of spasticity in cerebral palsy patients.* At the time of this manuscript, Botox was applying for upper extremity approval in Australia/New Zealand.

After parenteral injection, botulinum A toxin diffuses 2–3 cm within the muscle or until it binds irreversibly to specific membrane acceptors/receptors on cholinergic neurons (Black and Dolly 1986). When the toxin enters the cells, it cleaves SNARE proteins (Aoki 2001, 2003). Specifically, once internalized into the nerve terminal, the light chain of A toxin cleaves SNAP 25, inhibiting acetylcholine release at the neuromuscular junction with resultant flaccid paralysis (Fig. 14.2). The time course of muscle recovery after BoNT-A injection is known in the mouse but not in primates. The maximum effect of botulinum A toxin on muscle is evident at 36 to 72 hours (Ma et al 2004). At 30 days after toxin injection, muscle strength is 65 per cent of normal and at 180 days it has returned to 95 per cent of normal (Ma et al 2005) (Fig. 14.4).

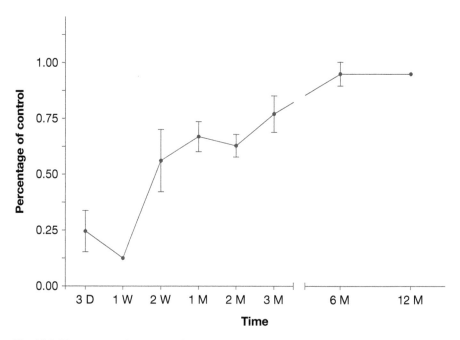

Fig. 14.4 Time course of recovery of muscle after injection of 4 units/kg body weight into the rat gastrocnemius.

Source: Reproduced with permission from Koman LA, editor. *Wake Forest University School of Medicine Orthopaedic Manual 2001.* Winston-Salem, NC: Orthopaedic Press.

Toxin injection

Botulinum A toxin preparations are reconstituted with physiological saline prior to intra-muscular injection. The volume of saline used to reconstitute the toxin is determined by the injecting physician and is based upon several factors including patient weight, number of muscles to be injected, size of the target muscle, and distribution of neuromuscular junctions in the target muscle. Toxicity associated with injected toxin occurs as a result of the spread of unbound toxin by direct diffusion outside the target muscle and/or through lymphatic channels to distant structures. However, following intramuscular injection of the toxin at the doses usually used in paediatric cerebral palsy patients, there is limited diffusion and/or systemic transportation of the toxin to areas outside the target injection area (Aoki 2003). This limited diffusion occurs because the toxin molecules bind with high affinity to specific acceptors/receptors on cholinergic neurons, thus limiting their spread outside the injection area (Black and Dolly 1986). *The human LD50 for BOTOX is estimated to be 39 to 50 units/kg body weight* (Aoki et al 1997).

Originally, the toxin dose per muscle used in our clinic was based upon patient body weight (Koman et al 1993). However, we now believe that dose calculations based on body weight are safe but imprecise, and, in fact, lead to toxin underdosage in younger and/or smaller patients while potentially utilizing more toxin than necessary in larger and/or older patients. We postulate that toxin dosages should be based upon the number of neuromuscular junctions present in the target muscle and that the volume of the injected toxin is more appropriately based on muscle size and the location of the neuromuscular junctions within the target muscle.

TOXIN RECONSTITUTION TECHNIQUES FOR BOTOX

1 *Constant concentration* is obtained by injecting 1, 2, 3 or more cc of physiological saline into the 100 unit vial of BOTOX. Frequently employed toxin concentrations are 100 units/cc, 50 units/cc, and 25 units/cc; however, any concentration may be appropriate depending on the desired post-injection level of muscle weakness.

2 *Constant volume* is achieved by determining the number of units to be injected and then diluting the units in a fixed volume of physiological saline. For example, 20 units or 80 units might be diluted in 4 cc. This technique was used in the European labelling study for the use of toxin to manage equinus foot deformity and is the basis for the initial clinical use of toxin injections for spasticity management in cerebral palsy patients (Koman et al 2000).

3 *Customized reconstitution* is based on the determination of the optimal number of units to achieve the desired result in a given muscle (e.g. 50 units in the pronator teres). In this case, the injected volume is based on the size of the muscle, the number of injection sites within the muscle, and the area over which the neuromuscular junctions are distributed (Koman et al 2002).

Localization of Injection

After the number of units and volume of toxin to be injected are determined for each patient, the toxin is injected into the target muscle as close to the neuromuscular junctions as possible. Although toxin will diffuse through fascial planes, optimal results occur when the toxin is injected within 1 to 2 cm of the neuromuscular junctions within the target muscle. The target muscle may be localized using: (1) palpation with or without stretch using anatomical landmarks; (2) active or passive electromyography (EMG); (3) ultrasound guidance; (4) direct vision (usually in the operating room as part of a surgical procedure); or (5) a combination of the aforementioned techniques. For large superficial muscle(s), palpation and anatomical landmarks are efficacious (Koman et al 1993, Fehlings et al 2000, Koman et al 2000, Fehlings et al 2001, Graham et al 2003). Muscle targeting using active EMG, ultrasound, or both, increases the accuracy of needle placement and is used to locate deep and/or small muscles (Koman et al 2002, Willenborg et al 2002, Chin et al 2005). At our institution, to administer upper extremity injections in awake, un-anaesthetized patients, the pectoralis major, latissimus dorsi, biceps, brachialis, brachioradialis, flexor carpi ulnaris, flexor carpi radialis, and adductor/first dorsal interosseous are injected using palpation under stretch and anatomical landmarks to identify the target muscles. However, deeper and smaller muscles (e.g. flexor pollicis longus, flexor digitorium superficialis) are targeted using ultrasound guidance. Under general anaesthesia, lack of muscle tone complicates targeting muscles using palpation. In this case, ultrasound or active EMG may be necessary to properly target the injections (author's experience). Direct visualization of the target muscle is possible intraoperatively and facilitates longitudinal injection of the muscle belly or multiple axial injections (Fig. 14.5). *It is important for the injecting physician to use the technique(s) with which they are most comfortable and which they consider to be the most effective. There is no rigid standard for the localization and targeting of toxin injections.*

Needle/Syringe Size/Injection Speed

A variety of needles and syringes are used for toxin injections; the final choice is based on physician preference. 22–27 gauge needles and 1 cc to 20 cc syringes are used commonly.

a) b)

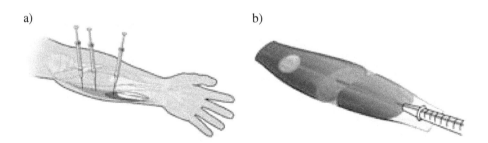

Fig. 14.5 (a) In the longitudinal technique a long 25 or 27 gauge spinal needle is inserted into the muscle belly and toxin is injected during withdrawal. (b) Close-up.

Source: Reproduced with permission from Koman LA, editor. *Wake Forest University School of Medicine Orthopaedic Manual 2001*. Winston-Salem, NC: Orthopaedic Press.

The use of smaller needles produces less muscle damage and provides less tactile feedback to the injecting physician. However, small needles are more difficult to control as the toxin is injected. Larger needles cause more soft tissue damage, and their use may result in post-operative pain. However, the use of larger needles also increases tactile feedback, and, because they are stiffer, larger needles maintain a more stable position in the muscle during the actual injection of the toxin. Although the rapidity of toxin injection affects the velocity of toxin delivery, the effect of speed-of-delivery on efficacy is unknown. Smaller syringes provide less resistance during injection than larger syringes. In general, at our institution, a 26 to 27G needle and a 10 cc control syringe are utilized. However, multiple 1 cc syringes and 27G needles may also be used.

ANAESTHESIA/ANALGESIA
There is no topic that is more hotly debated than the use of analgesia during toxin injections. Commonly used analgesia techniques include topical anaesthetics, conscious sedation, and general anaesthesia. However, many physicians prefer to administer injections without analgesia. When injecting my own abductor hallucis (LAK), the 25 gauge needle was barely perceptible as it penetrated the skin and entered the muscle; the injection was perceived as producing a 'cold' but not uncomfortable sensation. Based on my experience, the injection process was significantly less painful than a measles shot and was equivalent to a TB test in discomfort level. In over 20,000 upper and lower extremity injections administered in our clinics using palpation and muscle stretch guided with anatomical landmarks, over 99 per cent were well tolerated by the patient and were clinically effective.

Injection sessions that involve the injection of larger volumes and multiple needle insertions in order to treat all target muscles increase patient discomfort. Even so, the injections may be performed in an outpatient setting without sedation. In our practice, topical anaesthetics to numb the skin are used if requested by patients. Conscious sedation is reserved for hysterical patients or those with anxious parents. We have found that parental angst and injector anxiety are significant and often determine the type of analgesia utilized. Unquestionably, sedation is appropriate in selected patients, especially in patients who require multiple injections and/or patients whose target muscles require precise localization of needle placement (e.g. the need to use active EMG for muscle identification). Upper extremity injections of botulinum A toxin can be administered without conscious sedation using a combination of palpation, anatomical landmarks, and ultrasound to identify target muscles. The procedure is associated with manageable pain and anxiety levels in the majority of children. In fact, older children often request toxin injections to be administered without cold spray to numb the skin overlying the target muscle (personal experience).

Goal setting and target muscle selection
BoNT-A is a localized treatment for focal spasticity. Toxin injections are designed to: (1) decrease limb deforming forces; (2) improve specific function(s); (3) decrease pain; (4) enhance the ease of caregiving; and (5) improve self-esteem (Table 14.1).

Appropriate goal selection requires input from the patient, family, teachers, social workers, and health-care providers. The goals should be identified and agreed upon prior

TABLE 14.1
Goals

Decrease deformity

Improve specific functions
    shoulder rotation
    elbow flexion/extension
    wrist flexion/extension
    supination/pronation
    thumb abduction/adduction
    finger flexion/extension
    grasp/release

Decrease pain

Facilitate care

Improve self-esteem
    decrease posturing

to the initiation of the injection sessions. The World Health Organization's global goals include: altering CNS performance, increasing societal participation, and improving health-related quality of life (Boyd and Hays 2001). There are limitations associated with the temporary partial paralysis effected by toxin injections when they are used to balance muscle forces to alter global outcomes; these limitations must be recognized within this context. For example, it has been demonstrated that improving supination positively impacts single limb performance, is perceived generally by the patient as beneficial, and often increases self-esteem. However, these results may not only demonstrate changes at the body structure and function level of the World Health Organization criteria, but with the use of appropriate outcome instruments, changes in activity and participation levels may also be demonstrated.

The selection of the appropriate muscles to be injected is based upon each child's individual deformity after a thorough examination of the upper extremity to be treated (Table 14.2). Successful treatment of muscle spasticity effected by intramuscular toxin injections is determined by the actual impact of the degree of spasticity reduction produced in the specific target muscles. Clearly, reduction of focal muscle spasticity may or may not address more global spasticity issues. For example, decreased thumb adduction may not improve activities of daily living. Although reduction of muscle spasticity by BoNT-A addresses muscle imbalance and deformity, the impact of neuromuscular blockade on disability may vary significantly from patient to patient. Identical technical success (e.g. decreasing the deforming force of the flexor carpi ulnaris) may not improve function in one child yet it may enhance performance and health-related quality of life in another child. Therefore, it is important to establish both global and specific goals for each child and then use appropriate outcome instruments to assess the success or failure of the treatment for that child. The possibility that BoNT-A injections may stimulate cortical reorganization is intriguing, exciting, and demands additional study (Boyd et al 2004).

TABLE 14.2
Common patterns of deformity

Deformity	Muscle (deforming force)
Shoulder internal rotation	Pectoralis major
	Subscapularis
	Latissimus dorsi
Shoulder external rotation	Infraspinatus
	Teres minor
Elbow flexion	Biceps brachii
	Brachialis
	Brachioradialis
Forearm pronation	Pronator teres
Wrist flexion	Flexor carpi ulnaris
	Flexor carpi radialis
Wrist ulnar deviation and flexion	Extensor carpi ulnaris
Finger flexion	Flexor digitorium profundus
	Flexor digitorium superficialis
Thumb flexion	Flexor pollicis longus
Thumb-in-palm	Adductor pollicis brevis
	First dorsal interosseous

Selection of children for injections

Careful patient selection is important. Botulinum toxin produces flaccid paralysis and only indirectly affects spasticity. Careful assessment of the extent and magnitude of both spasticity and associated dystonia is crucial. We find the Tardieu scale (Tardieu et al 1954) more useful than the Ashworth scale (Ashworth 1964, Bohannon and Smith 1987). However, a qualitative and quantitative assessment of the type of hypertonicity is necessary for optimal evaluation. Although, there are dystonia scales, mild, moderate or severe assessments of chorea or athetosis are sufficient for BoNT injection planning.

Evaluation should include the effects of hypertonicity on symptoms, signs, active and passive range of motion, function, strength and performance of activities of daily living, and/or burden of external care. The magnitude of pain, if present, is assessed. Active and passive range of motion (ROM) is recorded, and functional capability determined using standardized measures. Video is helpful. Fixed joint deformities are noted; BoNT alone cannot correct fixed joint contracture. The modified Tardieu assessment measures the range of motion at the ankle and knee (Boyd and Graham 1999). The R1 measurement is made by moving the joint quickly through its range of motion in order to determine where in the range of motion the joint stops or catches. A goniometric measure of the angle as the first catch occurs is recorded in degrees of extension as R1. R2 is the goniometric range of motion measurement of the knee or ankle when the limb is moved slowly through its range of motion. R2 is recorded in degrees as the extent of passive motion. In normal individuals R1 equals R2. In a hypertonic patient, the interval between R1 and R2 is the potential gain.

Assuming adequate passive joint motion, in a good result R1 approaches R2. In order to improve function, reduction in tone must facilitate ROM; therefore, a significant fixed contracture or small R1–R2 interval is a relative contraindication. Similarly, excessive weakness is a relative contraindication. However, pain associated with hypertonicity is a relative indication for injection.

Current protocols for the frequency and precautions of repeated injections

Based on the time course of recovery, injections should be necessary at 2–3-month intervals (Ma et al 2004). However, the clinical need for injections ranges from 3 to 12 months and appears to be multifactorial. Multilevel injections, movement disorders contributing to a large percentage of hypertonicity, stretching, younger patients without muscle or joint contracture, and strengthening appear to increase the injection interval. To date, it is unclear if regular injections at fixed intervals provide better long-term results than reinjection based on loss of efficacy. In general, we reinject only after the beneficial effects of the last injection have ended. In addition, children only receive repeat injections if the preinjection spasticity reduction goals for the previous injection were reached. Antibody formation is of concern and, for this reason; the lowest efficacious dose, in units, should be used at the longest interval that maintains positive outcome(s). We evaluate the patient at 3–6-month intervals and inject as needed. Indications are dynamic upper extremity imbalance that interferes with physical functioning, that hampers the performance of activities of daily living, that produces discomfort, or that compromises caregiver activity. Exclusion criteria include: previous lack of efficacy; a small R1–R2 interval in the absence of pain; uncontrolled systemic disease; myasthenia gravis; concurrent use of aminoglycoside antibiotics or anticholinergic agents; fixed contractures or joint instability.

Clinical acumen predicts the potential for improvement of specific deformity pain, function, range of motion, appearance, self-worth, health-related quality of life, societal participation, and impact on society.

Injection of specific muscles

Toxin injections in the upper extremity are used to improve active and passive range of motion, to facilitate care, to improve function, to facilitate activities of daily living, and to maximize self-esteem. The muscles most frequently injected are the biceps, pronator teres, flexor carpi radialis, flexor carpi ulnaris, and adductor pollicis. However, any upper extremity muscle or muscle group may be injected. The muscles injected depend upon the individual patient's deformity; therefore, each patient must be analysed based on their individual post-injection goals. Upper extremity neuromuscular blockade requires precise needle localization to achieve maximized outcomes; muscle localization within the target muscle may be aided by ultrasound or active EMG techniques.

SHOULDER

Internal rotation and adduction deformity of the shoulder may be managed by injection of one or more of the following muscles: pectoralis major, subscapularis, and/or latissimus dorsi. Localization of the correct injection site in the pectoralis and latissimus dorsi can be

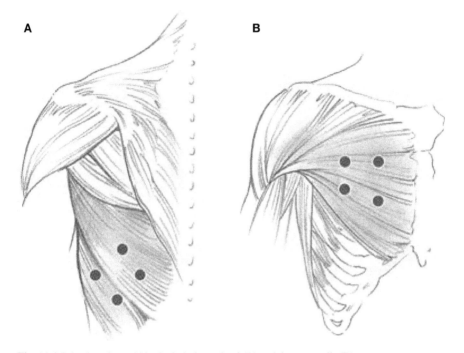

Fig. 14.6 Injection sites within the latissimus dorsi (A) and the pectoralis (B).

Source: Reproduced with permission from Koman LA, editor. *Wake Forest University School of Medicine Orthopaedic Manual 2001.* Winston-Salem, NC: Orthopaedic Press.

achieved reliably using palpation of the muscle under stretch (Fig. 14.6). However, subscapularis injections are best performed using active EMG or ultrasound guidance. Because the pectoralis major has segmental innervation, multiple injections are required to achieve an optimal clinical result. Occasionally, the teres major may require injection.

ELBOW

Elbow flexion deformity is generally secondary to overactivity of the biceps brachialis, and/or brachioradialis (Fig. 14.7). In addition, the pronator-flexor muscles may contribute to elbow deformity. Because the target muscle is determined by the patient's disability, the involved muscles vary from patient to patient. Injection of the biceps, often the most spastic muscle, weakens supination, leading some physicians to inject the brachialis. Localization of injection sites may be achieved reliably using muscle palpation in patients with well-defined biceps and brachialis muscles. However, active EMG and ultrasound techniques may be useful for patients with poorly defined muscles that are difficult to locate using palpation and anatomical landmarks.

Fig. 14.7 The injection sites within the biceps brachii are located in the area of neuromuscular junction distribution.

Source: Reproduced with permission from Koman LA, editor. *Wake Forest University School of Medicine Orthopaedic Manual 2001.* Winston-Salem, NC: Orthopaedic Press.

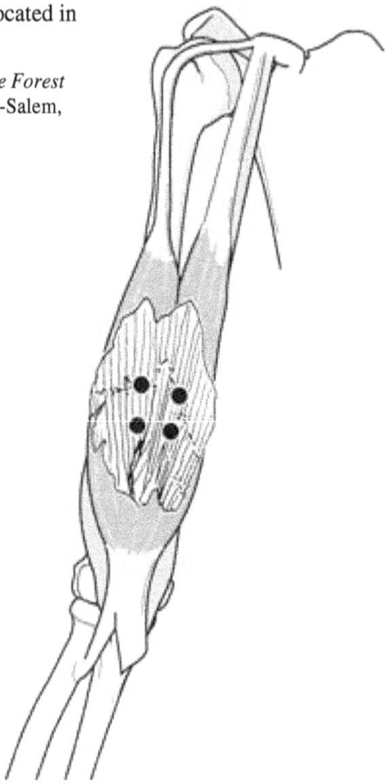

FOREARM/WRIST

Abnormal forearm pronation is secondary to pronator teres overactivity. Wrist flexion primarily results from spasticity of the flexor carpi ulnaris and flexor carpi radialis (Fig. 14.8). In addition, spasticity of the finger flexors (flexor digitorum superficialis and flexor digitorum profundus) may provide a secondary deforming force (Fig. 14.9). On occasion, overactivity of the palmaris longus is a factor causing wrist flexion. These forearm muscles are easily palpated, have consistent anatomical characteristics, and are amenable to injection without EMG or ultrasound guidance.

HAND

Frequent hand deformities observed in paediatric cerebral palsy patients include the following: thumb and finger flexion secondary to overactivity of the flexor pollicis longus, flexor digitorum superficialis, or flexor digitorum profundus (Fig. 14.9); and thumb-in-palm deformity secondary to overactivity of the adductor pollicis brevis or first dorsal interosseous muscles (Fig. 14.10). Because these muscles are located deep within the hand, they are difficult to palpate. Therefore, active EMG or ultrasound guidance is necessary to localize muscles for injections targeting these muscles. The exception is the adductor pollicis muscle because its consistent anatomy facilitates needle localization based on anatomical landmarks.

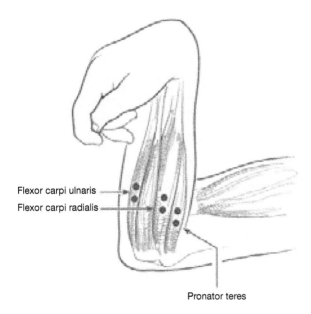

Fig. 14.8 Injection sites within the pronator teres, flexor carpi ulnaris, and flexor carpi radialis.

Source: Reproduced with permission from Koman LA, editor. *Wake Forest University School of Medicine Orthopaedic Manual 2001*. Winston-Salem, NC: Orthopaedic Press.

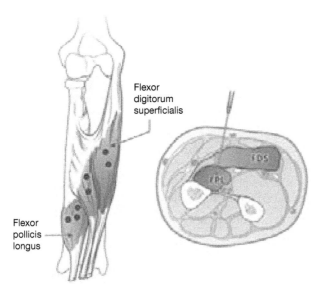

Fig. 14.9 Injection sites within the deep muscles of the forearm including the flexor digitorum superficialis, flexor digitorum profundus, and the flexor pollicis longus.

Source: Reproduced with permission from Koman LA, editor. *Wake Forest University School of Medicine Orthopaedic Manual 2001*. Winston-Salem, NC: Orthopaedic Press.

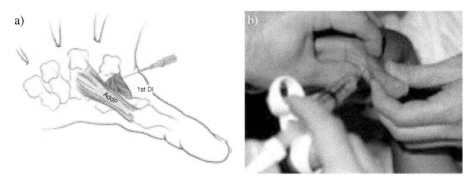

Fig. 14.10 Schematic representation (a) and photograph (b) of injection of the adductor and first dorsal interosseous.

Source: Reproduced with permission from Koman LA, editor. *Wake Forest University School of Medicine Orthopaedic Manual 2001*. Winston-Salem, NC: Orthopaedic Press.

Complications and concerns

Botulinum A toxins (BOTOX and Dysport) have safe pharmacological profiles. Following toxin injections, clinical efficacy is maintained for one to two years in approximately 50 per cent of patients; however, the patients require repeat serial injections. Complications associated with toxin injections include pain on injection, post-injection muscle soreness, and possible antibody formation to the toxin itself. The pain associated with toxin injections is less than that of an immunization (unpublished study). If post-injection muscle soreness occurs, it is easily managed with anti-inflammatory agents. Transient excessive muscle weakness may also occur. Although preferably avoided, this transient excessive weakness provides an opportunity for aggressive joint mobilization and stretching during the period of muscle weakness. The most common issue associated with the toxin injection procedure is patient and parent anxiety; this issue is best handled by a confident injector.

Indications and results

BoNT-A injections are indicated to reduce muscle spasticity that: (1) produces pain; (2) causes deformity; (3) interferes with function; (4) prevents optimal caregiving; and/or (5) negatively impacts self-esteem. In addition, toxin injections are indicated to decrease muscle tone after surgery or injury and to prevent or delay the onset of joint deformity or contracture (Wall et al 1993, Corry et al 1997, Van Heest 1997, Fehlings et al 2000, 2001, Koman et al 2004). Expected intermediate efficacy – similar to the lower extremity – is approximately 50 per cent.

Critical reviews of the literature relating to the use of intramuscular injections of botulinum toxin in cerebral palsy neither support nor refute its use (Wasiak et al 2004). Unresolved issues described in the literature support the need for future research examining functional outcomes of toxin-induced muscle weakness and the long-term effect of repeat injections (Hoare and Imms 2004). Four randomized trials demonstrate the short-term efficacy of toxin injections with documented reduction in muscle tone (Corry et al 1997), improved upper limb function one month after injection, and improved functional skills one and six months after injection (Fehlings et al 2000). Improved range of motion and function in moderately-involved children and enhanced ease of caregiving in severely involved patients have also been documented (Koman et al 2004). In a third randomized controlled trial comparing BoNT-A and therapy with therapy alone, function at one, three and six months after treatment was significantly improved with BoNT-A and therapy (Lowe et al 2006). Additional studies report positive findings but lack sufficient statistical power to support definitive conclusions (Wall et al 1993, Friedman et al 2000). A recent interventional case study of 16 children documented sustained improvement in functional outcomes after BoNT-A injections but noted increasing muscle tone after initial tone reduction (Wallen et al 2004). Our experience with a randomized, placebo-controlled trial supports the use of BoNT-A injections in the upper extremity in paediatric cerebral palsy patients in order to facilitate shoulder, elbow and wrist active or passive motion, reduce discomfort, and enhance care (Koman et al 2004).

Hand therapy

Rehabilitation strategies including home programmes combined with periodic 'hands-on' therapy by occupational or physical therapists are crucial for optimal post-BoNT-A treatment outcomes (in our opinion). Although irrefutable evidence-based support for the combined use of therapy and BoNT-A injections is limited (Hoare and Imms 2004, Lannin et al 2005), the anecdotal and peer-reviewed support for the therapy-augmented effects of BoNT-A is compelling (Koman et al 2002, Yang et al 2003, Carda and Molteni 2005, Speth et al 2005, Basciani and Intiso 2006, Lowe et al 2006, Wallen et al 2007). Therapy must be patient-oriented and may include static splinting, active and passive range of motion, strengthening, casting, taping, and/or electrical stimulation. In a study that compared BoNT-A injections and therapy versus placebo injections and therapy, Wallen et al demonstrated that BoNT-A and therapy 'resulted in accelerated attainment of functional goals . . .' (Wallen et al 2007). In this study, therapy was provided for one hour each week in both groups using patient-based therapy protocols ('aimed to mirror usual practice') rather than standardized protocols (Wallen et al 2007). In a randomized, controlled trial without placebo but with standard therapy and injection protocols, Fehlings et al demonstrated that BoNT-A and therapy was superior to therapy alone (Fehlings et al 2000). For additional review of studies in children with cerebral palsy receiving BoNT-A, see Chapters 13 and 23.

REFERENCES

Aoki KR (2001) Pharmacology and immunology of botulinum toxin serotypes. *J Neurol* 248(Suppl 1): 3–10.
Aoki KR (2003) Pharmacology and immunology of botulinum toxin type A. *Clin Dermatol* 21: 476–480.
Aoki KR (2005) Review of a proposed mechanism for the antinociceptive action of botulinum toxin type A. *NeuroToxicology* 26: 785–793.
Aoki KR, Ismail M, Tang-Liu D, Brar B, Wheeler LA (1997) Botulinum toxin type A: from toxin to therapeutic agent. *Eur J Neurol* 4: S1–S3.
Arnon SS, Schechter R, Inglesby TV, Henderson DA, Bartlett JG, Ascher MS, Eitzen E, Fine AD, Hauer J, Layton M, Lillibridge S, Osterholm MT, O'Toole T, Parker G, Perl TM, Russell PK, Swerdlow DL,

Tonat K (2001) Botulinum toxin as a biological weapon: medical and public health management. *JAMA* 285: 1059–1070.

Ashworth B (1964) Preliminary trial of carisoprodol in multiple sclerosis. *Practitioner* 192: 540–542.

Basciani M, Intiso D (2006) Botulinum toxin type-A and plaster cast treatment in children with upper brachial plexus palsy. *Pediatr Rehabil* 9: 165–170.

Black JD, Dolly JO (1986) Interaction of 125I-labeled botulinum neurotoxins with nerve terminals. I. Ultrastructural autoradiographic localization and quantitation of distinct membrane acceptors for types A and B on motor nerves. *J Cell Biol* 103: 521–534.

Bohannon RW, Smith MB (1987) Interrater reliability of a modified Ashworth scale of muscle spasticity. *Phys Ther* 67: 206–207.

Boyd RN, Graham HK (1999) Objective measurement of clinical findings in the use of botulinum toxin type A for the management of children with cerebral palsy. *Eur J Neurol* 6: S23–S35.

Boyd RN, Hays RM (2001) Outcome measurement of effectiveness of botulinum toxin type A in children with cerebral palsy: an ICIDH-2 approach. *Eur J Neurol* 8(Suppl 5): 167–177.

Boyd R, Bach T, Morris M, Imms C, Johnson L, Graham HK, Mit AS, Abbott D, Jackson GD (2004) A quantitative functional MRI study in children with congenital hemiplegia: a randomized trial of botulinum toxin A and upper limb training. *Dev Med Child Neurol* 46: 11.

Carda S, Molteni F (2005) Taping versus electrical stimulation after botulinum toxin type A injection for wrist and finger spasticity. A case-control study. *Clin Rehabil* 19: 621–626.

Carr LJ, Cosgrove AP, Gringras P, Neville BGR (1998) Position paper on the use of botulinum toxin in cerebral palsy. *Arch Dis Child* 79: 271–273.

Chin TY, Nattrass GR, Selber P, Graham HK (2005) Accuracy of intramuscular injection of botulinum toxin A in juvenile cerebral palsy: a comparison between manual needle placement and placement guided by electrical stimulation. *J Pediatr Orthop* 25: 286–291.

Corry IS, Cosgrove AP, Walsh EG, McClean D, Graham HK (1997) Botulinum toxin A in the hemiplegic upper limb: a double-blind trial. *Dev Med Child Neurol* 39: 185–193.

DePavia A, Neunier FA, Molgo J, Aoki KR, Dolly JO (1999) Functional repair of motor endplates after botulinum neurotoxin type A poisoning: biphasic switch of synaptic activity between nerve sprouts and their parent terminals. *Proc Natl Acad Sci USA* 96: 3200–3205.

Fehlings D, Rang M, Glazier J, Steele C (2000) An evaluation of botulinum-A toxin injections to improve upper extremity function in children with hemiplegic cerebral palsy. *J Pediatr* 137: 331–337.

Fehlings D, Rang M, Glazier J, Steele C (2001) Botulinum toxin type A injections in the spastic upper extremity of children with hemiplegia: child characteristics that predict a positive outcome. *Eur J Neurol* 8: 145–149.

Friedman A, Diamond M, Johnston MV, Daffner C (2000) Effects of botulinum toxin A on upper limb spasticity in children with cerebral palsy. *Am J Phys Med Rehabil* 79: 53–59.

Gooch JL, Patton CP (2004) Combining botulinum toxin and phenol to manage spasticity in children. *Arch Phys Med Rehabil* 85: 1121–1124.

Graham HK, Boyd RN, Fehlings D (2003) Does intramuscular botulinum toxin A injection improve upper-limb function in children with hemiplegic cerebral palsy? *Med J Aust* 178: 95–96.

Hoare BJ, Imms C (2004) Upper-limb injections of botulinum toxin-A in children with cerebral palsy: a critical review of the literature and clinical implications for occupational therapists. *Am J Occup Ther* 58: 389–397.

Koman LA, Mooney JF III, Smith B, Goodman A, Mulvaney T (1993) Management of cerebral palsy with botulinum-A toxin: preliminary investigation. *J Pediatr Orthop* 13: 489–495.

Koman LA, Mooney JF III, Smith BP, Walker F, Leon JM (2000) Botulinum toxin type A neuromuscular blockade in the treatment of lower extremity spasticity in cerebral palsy: a randomized, double-blind, placebo-controlled trial. BOTOX Study Group. *J Pediatr Orthop* 20: 108–115.

Koman LA, Smith BP, Goodman A (2002) *Botulinum Toxin Type A in the Management of Cerebral Palsy.* Wake Forest Cerebral Palsy Center. Winston-Salem, NC: Wake Forest University Press

Koman LA, Smith BP, Evans P, Williams R, Richardson R, Rushing J (2004) Placebo-controlled, double-blind, randomized clinical trial evaluating the effect of botulinum toxin A on upper extremity spasticity associated with cerebral palsy. *Dev Med Child Neurol* 46: 10.

Lannin N, Scheinberg A, Clark IC (2005) AACPDM Systemic review of the effectiveness of therapy for children with cerebral palsy following botulinum toxin-A injection. http//www.aacpdm.org.resources/botoxst.pdf

Lowe K, Novak I, Cusick A (2006) Low-dose/high-concentration localized botulinum toxin A improves upper limb movement and function in children with hemiplegic cerebral palsy. *Dev Med Child Neurol* 48: 170–175.

Lu L, Atchabahian A, Mackinnon SE, Hunter DA (1998) Nerve injection injury with botulinum toxin. *Plast Reconstr Surg* 101: 1875–1880.

Ma J, Elsaidi GA, Smith TL, Walker FO, Tan KH, Martin E, Koman LA, Smith BP (2004) Time course of recovery of juvenile skeletal muscle after botulinum toxin A injection: an animal model study. *Am J Phys Med Rehabil* 83: 774–780.

Ma J, Smith BP, Smith TL, Walker FO, Rosencrance EV, Koman, LA (2005) Juvenile and adult rat neuro-muscular junctions: density, distribution, and morphology. *Muscle Nerve* 26: 804–809.

Schantz EJ, Johnson EA (1992) Properties and use of botulinum toxin and other microbial neurotoxins in medicine. *Microbiol Rev* 56: 80–99.

Speth LA, Leffers P, Janssen-Potten YJ, Vles JS (2005) Botulinum toxin A and upper limb functional skills in hemiparetic cerebral palsy: a randomized trial in children receiving intensive therapy. *Dev Med Child Neurol* 47: 468–473.

Van Heest AE (1997) Applications of botulinum toxin in orthopedics and upper extremity surgery. *Tech Hand Upper Extremity Surg* 1: 27–34.

Wall SA, Chait LA, Temlett JA, Perkins B, Hillen G, Becker P (1993) Botulinum A chemodenervation: a new modality in cerebral palsied hands. *J Plast Surg* 46B: 703–706.

Wallen MA, O'Flaherty SJ, Waugh MC (2004) Functional outcomes of intramuscular botulinum toxin type A in the upper limbs of children with cerebral palsy: a phase II trial. *Arch Phys Med Rehabil* 85: 192–200.

Wallen MA, O'Flaherty SJ, Waugh MC (2007) Functional outcomes of intramuscular botulinum toxin type A in occupational therapy in the upper limbs of children with cerebral palsy: a randomized controlled trial. *Arch Phys Med Rehabil* 88: 1–10.

Wasiak J, Hoare B, Wallen M (2004) Botulinum toxin A as an adjunct to treatment in the management of the upper limb in children with spastic cerebral palsy. *Cochrane Database Syst Rev* 18: CD003469.

Willenborg MJ, Shilt JS, Smith BP, Estrada RL, Castle JA, Koman LA (2002) Technique for iliopsoas ultrasound-guided active electromyography-directed botulinum A toxin injection in cerebral palsy. *J Pediatr Orthop* 22: 165–168.

Yang TF, Fu CP, Kao NT, Chan RC, Chen SJ (2003) Effect of botulinum toxin type A on cerebral palsy with upper limb spasticity. *Am J Phys Med Rehabil* 82: 284–289.

15
THERAPEUTIC INTERVENTIONS AT THE BODY STRUCTURE AND FUNCTION LEVEL TO SUPPORT CHILDREN'S UPPER EXTREMITY FUNCTION

Patricia A. Burtner and Janet L. Poole

Introduction

For decades, clinicians have focused intervention efforts on the ameliorization of impairments in children with cerebral palsy (CP). More recently, there has been a shift away from impairment-based intervention to function-based intervention with an emphasis on increasing the participation level of the child in natural environments. This shift is reflected in the International Classification of Functioning, Disability and Health (ICF; World Health Organization 2001). Function-oriented intervention is not a new concept; however, the ICF provides a more systematic approach with greater emphasis on function and participation. While the emphasis on the child's functional skills is long overdue and compelling, intervention at multiple ICF levels and combination therapies may be most beneficial for some children. The two previous chapters outlined surgical approaches and the use of botulinum toxin in children with upper extremity deformity. This chapter will give an overview of the relationship between upper extremity deformity and function, and the rationale of using conservative treatments in conjunction with surgery or proactively to prevent/reduce deformity, as well as current evidence supporting their effects on upper extremity function. Suggestions for future directions for research and practice will be presented.

Relationship between upper extremity impairments and function

Most children with CP because of their neurological disability are at risk for musculoskeletal deformity. Prevention of deformity may not be a priority for some children who show functional skills that approximate those of their peers. However, when significant deformity has occurred, children often require orthopaedic surgery and/or non-surgical treatments to optimize benefits from function-based interventions.

Since cerebral palsy is a multifaceted disorder, it has been difficult to study how motor impairments impact the functional activities of children with CP. Major upper extremity studies have demonstrated relationships between impairments and hand function skills. Frieden and Lieber (2006) showed increases in key pinch and pronation following tendon transfer surgery in individuals with spinal cord injuries and hypothesize similar functional improvement in other populations post tendon transfer procedures at appropriate length and tension. Rameckers and associates (2007) reported changes in spasticity post botulinum toxin injections which resulted in more accurate arm movements during aiming tasks. Other researchers (Vaz et al 2006) documented moderate correlations between manual function as measured by tasks on the Jebsen-Taylor Hand Function test and muscle strength and stiffness. No upper extremity studies have related impairments to measures at the ICF Activity and Participation level.

Ostensjo and colleagues (2004) investigated the relationship between lower extremity motor impairments (spasticity, decreased passive range of motion, poor selective motor control) and the functional abilities of 95 children with CP. Their results suggested that selective motor control was the best predictor of a child's performance in gross motor functional skills and activities of daily living. While these results provide some information about the relationship between impairment and activity level functions, results may not easily be generalized to upper extremity impairment and functional abilities. This is because hand function in children is more complex than lower extremity function and is more closely associated with cognition, visual perception, sensation, arousal level and the individual's interests (motivation). Thus, further investigations are needed to determine what combination of therapies, as well as what intensity and duration of intervention, is required for children with different levels of upper extremity disability for best outcomes.

TYPES OF DEFORMITY
When we think of deformity we often visualize a child with contractures that severely limit joint range of motion. However, children with CP may exhibit 'dynamic' or 'static' deformities, with a blurring between the two conditions. Dynamic deformities are often observed during volitional movements of the upper extremity, but when examined the child has full passive range of motion. Dynamic deformities are often corrected by applying graded force against the body structures using interventions such as stretching, casting or splints. Static or 'fixed' deformity, in contrast, refers to a mechanical shortening of the muscle, tendon and often other soft tissue surrounding the joint, thus preventing full range of motion. These static contractures may require more aggressive intervention procedures including serial casting and orthopaedic surgery.

Within the diagnostic category of CP, an estimated 78–84 per cent of children have the spastic subtype (Bax and Brown 2004). The presence of spasticity in the upper extremity (UE) of these children often results in stereotypical movement patterns of adduction and internal rotation of the shoulder, elbow flexion with pronation of the forearm, ulnar deviation and flexion of the wrist and fingers (Carlson 1999, VanHeest et al 1999) and (adducted/opposed) thumb-in-palm deformities (Waters and VanHeest 1998). A continuum of deformity has been outlined by McNeill (2004). Mild deformity is primarily dynamic deformity posturing during active movement with no or minimal contracture. If the child uses upper extremity postures persistently, contractures can develop. Moderate deformity is often a combination of dynamic and fixed contractures which affect active and passive joint range of motion, with adjacent joints often biomechanically coupling with the contracted joint. Severe deformity involves fixed contractures of the muscle-tendon unit as well as related soft tissue. Changes in the joint and bone shape and position occur and discomfort and pain may be present.

CLASSIFICATION SYSTEMS OF UPPER EXTREMITY FUNCTION AND DEFORMITY

Although the deformity classification system outlined above is often used, it does not provide information about the child's functional hand use. Recently, functional classification systems of children's hand skills have become integrated into practice. To understand the effect of intervention at multiple ICF levels, a combination of classification systems may be utilized. At ICF Activity and Participation levels, the Manual Ability Classification System (MACS), described in the Introduction, is particularly useful (Eliasson et al 2006). This classification system is specifically designed to classify the child's ability to use two hands together during daily activities. In contrast, the Modified House Scale (House et al 1981, Koman 2000) and the Zancolli classification system (Zancolli and Zancolli 1987) are designed to document changes in hand deformity following hand surgery and may be more useful to document specific unilateral hand changes at the ICF Body Structure and Function levels. The latter classification scales are used post-surgery (Koman 2000) and for documenting hand grasp and release patterns post botulinum toxin injections (Speth et al 2005) and post electrical stimulation (Maenpaa et al 2004). However, all classification systems are appropriate for documenting change in children as well as for matching children to establish groupings of children at similar functional levels.

RATE-LIMITING FACTORS AFFECTING UPPER EXTREMITY FUNCTION

Clinicians are increasingly being challenged to provide a rationale and evidence of outcome studies when providing services. Underlying rationales for specific interventions targeting changes at the body structure/function level (and ultimately function) are based on evidence of the presence of rate-limiting factors affecting upper extremity function. Rate-limiting factors are considered to be different components affecting upper extremity development. Four critical rate-limiting factors are presented to justify interventions targeting impairments experienced by children with CP.

Growth factors affecting range of motion and deformity

Growth differences in the upper limb are often seen in children with CP. Since the spastic muscle grows more slowly than normal muscle in relation to bony growth (Ziv et al 1984), deformity may result. The slow growth in spastic muscles is thought to be related to the lack of full excursion of the muscle and joint during daily movement activities, as well as poor relaxation of the muscle during stretching and decreased force production during movement (Graham and Selber 2003). Berger and colleagues report mechanical changes in shortened spastic muscles over time (Berger et al 1982). Based on this research, interventions to counteract the effects of deformity by attending to muscle length in relation to bony growth (stretching) can be justified until the child reaches skeletal maturity (Boyd and Graham 1997). This research also supports the need for intervention that requires the child to produce increased force output followed by relaxation (strength training). Increasing the intensity of therapy during growth spurts should also be considered, based on the child's growth differences.

Muscle imbalance of agonist and antagonist muscles
Poor selective control of muscle activity in children with CP has been documented by numerous researchers (Damiano et al 1995, Gage 2004). Since typical smooth movement requires alternate phasing of agonist and antagonist muscle activation, excessive coactivation of agonist and antagonist muscles which limits free movement is often observed when spasticity is present. In children with CP, deficits in the muscle activation and sequencing (delayed onset and offset of muscles) have been reported, as well as the presence of high levels of agonist/antagonistic muscle coactivation (Nashner et al 1983, Brogren et al 1996, 1998, Burtner et al 1998). Although it is beyond the scope of this chapter to describe possible causes for the poor selective motor control of muscles and increased coactivation, failure of reciprocal inhibition and activation of agonist and antagonist muscles during voluntary movement has been well documented in children with CP (Berger et al 1982, Hallet and Alvarez 1983). These findings support the use of biofeedback, functional electrical stimulation and muscle re-education training to promote timing of muscles and increase selective motor control.

Muscle weakness
Weakness in antagonist muscles has long been recognized; however, with the introduction of selective dorsal rhizotomy surgery and the unmasking of the effects of spasticity, there has been a new appreciation for the underlying weakness in the child's spastic muscles (Giuliani 1991). Muscle weakness is now viewed as a significant problem for children with spasticity (Damiano and Abel 1998, Stackhouse et al 2005). Justification for strength training (McCubbin and Shasby 1985, Damiano et al 1995) and the use of neuromuscular electrical stimulation (Kerr et al 2004) for children with spasticity is based on the presence of this rate-limiting factor.

Decreased sensibility
As discussed in Chapter 9 decreased sensation is often more disabling than motor impairment for upper limb functional outcome in children with CP (Cooper et al 1995, Eliasson et al 1995, Gordon and Duff 1999). When analysing the components of interventions, sensory input is inherent in the treatment, whether prolonged stretch, pressure with casting/splinting or electrical stimulation etc. is used. However, constant sustained sensory input may result in habituation rather than sensory stimulation. Thus, specific sensory intervention may be warranted (Bumin and Kayihan 2001).

Pre- and post-operative rehabilitation of the upper extremity
Since the child with CP often exhibits a pattern of deformity by 3 years of age (Goldner 1988), early and ongoing monitoring is required to determine the impact of impairment on function. When reconstructive surgery is recommended, the orthopaedic surgeon, occupational therapist, parents and child collaborate throughout the pre- and post-operative stages. The goals of surgical reconstruction are to rebalance agonist/antagonist muscles to increase functional use, to correct deformity (Carlson 1999, VanHeest et al 1999) and to improve hygiene and appearance. Generally the surgical procedures include muscle release,

muscle transfer, tendon lengthening, arthrodesis or soft tissue release (see Chapter 13 for a review).

The occupational or hand therapist provides consultation to the orthopaedic surgeon during the pre-operative stages through functional performance tests, sensory testing, range of motion (ROM) testing, motion analysis studies and/or dynamic electromyography studies. Pre-operative therapy is provided only when maximum ROM of the child's UE is indicated to maximize functional outcome. Botulinum toxin A (BoNT-A) injections, in conjunction with serial casting or splinting, are often used in preparation for surgery (Koman et al 1993, Carlson 1999, Chin and Graham 2003). In some cases BoNT-A is injected in specific muscles to determine if a release will enhance function (Autti-Ramo et al 2001, Boyd et al 2001).

Gallagher and Lewin (2006) recently outlined guidelines for post-operative rehabilitative care for children with CP. The three phases of intervention outlined include specifics to consider according to the procedure the child received. During Postoperative Phase I (weeks 0–4) the authors stress the importance of immobilization to maintain rebalanced muscles at resting lengths while attending to oedema control and active/passive ROM of uninvolved joints. Postoperative Phase II (weeks 4–8) includes protective splinting and intensive therapy (clinic and home exercise programmes) to assist the child in regaining motor control over muscles of the rebalanced limb. Neuromuscular electrical stimulation may be introduced to activate lengthened or transferred muscles during this phase, and splints specific to the surgical procedure are worn by the child at all times except during therapy. Task-oriented massed practice unilaterally and bilaterally as well as extremity use during activities of daily living begins in Postoperative Phase III (week 8 to 6 months). During this phase, progressive muscle strengthening programmes are initiated and the child wears splints at night-time only. Discharge criteria are also outlined.

To date, evidence-based published studies of the effect of orthopaedic surgery and post-operative therapy have been limited to case studies or group designs with no concurrent control groups (Smeulders et al 2005). An overview of current evidence is presented in Chapter 26.

Conservative treatments for upper extremity management
Traditional views of motor development and body structure/function intervention for children with CP were based on neurophysiological studies in animals, with inferences made to developing humans. Based on the work of Sir Charles Sherrington (1947), John Hughlings Jackson and others (Magnus 1926, Schaltenbrand 1928), movement was hypothesized to be reflex-based and the CNS was thought to be organized hierarchically. This reflex-hierarchical theory of movement underpinned assumptions that influenced therapeutic intervention for children with CP during most of the twentieth century, primarily the neurodevelopmental treatment approach (NDT). More contemporary theories of motor control have changed our thinking. We now consider the interaction of the person, task and environment in a systems approach based on theoretical principles set forth by Bernstein (1967). Using contemporary motor control/motor learning theories, conservative therapeutic interventions impacting the body structure/function levels of the individual are used to

support functional activities of the child with cerebral palsy (For a complete review of these theories, see Shumway-Cook and Woollacott 2006.)

NEURODEVELOPMENTAL TREATMENT
In the early 1940s, a physical therapist and a neuropsychiatrist, Berta and Karel Bobath, began to develop the neurodevelopmental treatment (NDT) approach for children with cerebral palsy based on clinical observations and the current neuroscience theories at the time, the reflex-hierarchical theory (Bobath and Bobath 1985). Assumptions incorporated into the treatment approach that influenced upper extremity intervention were: (1) handling techniques were used to control sensory input, inhibit primitive reflex patterns and abnormal muscle tone/abnormal movement patterns, and facilitate normal muscle tone, equilibrium responses and voluntary movement patterns; (2) cephalo-caudal development was emphasized with head control development preceding trunk and extremity control; and (3) proximal to distal development with an emphasis on developing shoulder and hip control prior to arm/hand and leg/foot control. The assumption that proximal control precedes distal control discouraged clinicians from providing early eye–hand coordination training to infants with cerebral palsy, and often therapists waited until children were older before concentrating efforts on improving hand function. In later years, the Bobaths recognized that their rigid adherence to developmental sequence had not resulted in carry-over to daily activities. Many handling techniques were incorporated into daily routines of dressing, eating and play (Finnie 1997); however, the focus was more on tone reduction and normal movement pattern than on independence in self-care. This technique might still be useful for children with severe CP who continue to require intensive assistance with their daily care.

The effectiveness of NDT for children with CP was systematically reviewed in an American Academy of Cerebral Palsy and Developmental Medicine (AACPDM) evidence report (Butler and Darrah 2001). Best evidence was examined in literature published between 1956 and 2001, resulting in 21 studies (out of 61 citations) that met the criteria. The authors concluded that, with the exception of immediate improvement in dynamic range of motion, there was no consistent evidence of NDT effectiveness in changing abnormal motor responses, preventing contractures, or facilitating more normal motor development or functional motor outcomes. Studies with greater intensity of NDT intervention did not show greater benefit and there was no clear evidence of increases in social-emotional, language or cognitive development.

CONTEMPORARY APPROACHES TO BODY STRUCTURE/FUNCTION INTERVENTION
Using a similar approach, we identified therapeutic interventions commonly used to address the body structure and function systems of children with CP and conducted systematic reviews of the literature. Reviews were limited to studies of children and adolescents with the diagnosis of CP, and published studies from 1983 to the present with full-text articles available in English. Electronic databases included: Medline, Cochrane Library and CINAHL. Additional references were obtained by reviewing the reference lists in articles identified in the search. Guidelines developed by the American Academy of Cerebral Palsy and Developmental Medicine (AACPDM) provided the format for classifying the levels of

evidence assigned to each study (Butler et al 2005). Both authors reviewed the studies and agreed on the classifications. Although initially the reviews were to be limited to studies of levels I–III and to include studies where intervention at the impairment level (ICF Body Structure/Function level) demonstrated functional changes (ICF Activity and Participation level), the authors soon found few studies meeting these criteria. Thus, studies at all levels of evidence were included.

STRETCHING/CASTING

Stretching is a technique designed to lengthen pathologically shortened soft tissue in order to increase range of motion (Kisner and Colby 1996). Applying an external force, such as a cast, to lengthen the shortened muscles, is referred to as passive stretch (Kisner and Colby 1996). When a joint is held in a position of stretch, it is thought that the number of sarcomeres in series increase, subsequently resulting in more permanent increases in muscle or tendon length (Gossman et al 1982, Threlkeld 1992). Serial casting has been used in children with cerebral palsy to provide a passive stretch to position a muscle in a lengthened state in order to obtain increases in motion at a joint (Brouwer et al 2000).

The evidence on the effectiveness of stretching via casting to improve upper extremity function in children with cerebral palsy is limited (see Table 15.1). The casts in the studies varied from long casts extending from the mid-humerus to distal to the MCP joints, to short casts extending from below the elbow to distal to the MCP joints. Studies also varied in the length of time the casts were worn per day, ranging from 4 hours to 24 hours. In addition, the intervention time ranged from 48 hours to 12 months. As seen in Table 15.1, the majority of the studies are case reports with one to three subjects. Only two randomized control studies were found, but in these studies the casting was accompanied by intensive therapy so it is difficult to determine whether improvements were primarily due to the casts (Law et al 1991, 1997).

Studies have examined the effects of casts on range of motion, hand function and quality of upper limb movements. Range of motion has been found to increase at both the wrist and elbow. Muscle tone decreased in one study (Copley et al 1996). However, the two studies by Law and colleagues showed conflicting results regarding improvements in quality of movement after casting, which may have been due to the ages of the children in the studies. Law suggested that quality of movement appears to be more sensitive to change in children over 4 years of age (Law et al 1997). In regard to hand function, Law et al showed that while there were no differences between an intensive NDT programme plus casting and regular occupational therapy, hand function did improve over time. There does not appear to be consensus on how many hours a day a cast should be worn, or on the duration of treatment. One study on the lower limb showed that the soleus muscle required stretching for at least six hours daily to prevent contracture progression in children with cerebral palsy (Tardieu et al 1988).

Guidelines for intervention
Casting alone has limited evidence for improving hand function in children with cerebral palsy. Thus, casting should be used in conjunction with occupational or physical therapy,

236

TABLE 15.1

Evidence-based studies examining effects of stretching/serial casting on children's upper extremity function

Reference	N	Level of evidence	Intervention protocol	Measurements	Results
Copley et al 1996	11 children 5 hemiplegic 6 quadriplegic 5.3–17.8 yrs	IV pre-post test	Casting worn 4 hrs/day and at night for 4–6 weeks followed by 6 months post-casting programme Weekly OT, daily weight bearing of affected limb, passive joint ROM, active movement of affected limb with cast removed	Range of motion Muscle tone Individual/family functional goals	Increased ROM and decreased tone immediately after casting (6 achieved full or nearly full ROM, 4 improved in ROM ranging from 42–130°) 4 children who had active motion at the beginning increased active ROM from 20 to 80° After 6 months, most children maintained ROM gains 8 children fully achieved functional goals, 2 partially achieved goals and 1 none
Cruickshank and O'Neill 1990	1 spastic quadriplegia 11 yrs	V case report	Circular bivalve cast worn 4 hrs/day at school and 2–3 hrs/day at home on both upper limbs for 5 months Cast extended from mid-humerus to just proximal to wrist joint but was modified with hand splint at 5–8 months Hand splint eliminated at 8 months	Elbow range of motion	After 5 months, an increase of 20° of extension noted in right elbow and 16° in left 5–8 months, loss of extension was 13° to 17° After hand splint eliminated, 13° of extension was gained in both elbows
Law et al 1991	73 children 44 spastic quadriplegia 28 spastic hemiplegia 18 months–8 yrs	II RCT	6 month intervention 4 treatment groups: (1) Intense NDT (45 mins 2×/wk + 30 mins daily home programme) and casting (short arm bivalve cast worn 4 hrs/day); cast below elbow to palm of hand (2) Intense NDT (45 mins 2×/wk + 30 mins daily home programme) (3) Regular NDT (1/wk or 1/month + 15 mins home program 3×/wk) and casting (short arm bivalve cast worn 4 hrs/day) (4) Regular NDT (45 mins 2×/wk + 30 mins daily home program) and no casting	Peabody Fine Motor Scales Quality of Upper Extremity Skills Test (QUEST) Wrist range of motion	No significance differences between treatment groups for the Peabody After 6 months of cast use, quality of movement (p = .03) and wrist extension (p < .02) increased significantly in the groups wearing the casts After 3 months, the changes were no longer significant

237

TABLE 15.1 (continued)

Evidence-based studies examining effects of stretching/
serial casting on children's upper extremity function

Reference	N	Level of evidence	Intervention protocol	Measurements	Results
Law et al 1997	50 children Spastic 18 months–4 yrs (mean = 33 months)	II Randomized crossover design	4 months Intensive NDT plus casting (45 mins 2×/wk) + 30 mins daily home program + short arm bivalved cast worn 4 hrs, 2×/day Regular occupational therapy (45 mins 1×/wk)	Peabody Fine Motor Scales Quality of Upper Extremity Skills Test (QUEST) COPM Parent perception of hand function	No significant difference between treatment groups for the Peabody, QUEST, COPM, or parent perception Significant improvements on the Peabody (p = .0001), QUEST (p = .007), and the COPM (p = .0001) over time
Smith and Harris 1985	1 Spastic quadriplegia 5 yrs, 6 months	V Case study	Circular bivalve cast worn 3 hrs/day on both upper limbs for 12 months Cast extended from mid-humerus to just proximal to wrist joint	Range of motion of elbow	Contracture reduced in left elbow, remained the same in right
Tona and Schneck 1993	1 Spastic AB 8 yrs, 6 months	IV Case study	Circular cast worn for 48 hrs Cast extended from distal 2/3 of humerus to distal to the MCP joints	Quality and quantity of movement Modified Ashworth Scale (MAS) Resistance during constant velocity passive movement (Biodex System)	Increased quality of movement, increased use Trend toward decreased spasticity on MAS Decrease in resistance to passive movement (p < .05)
Yasukawa et al 2003	3 Spastic all 7 yrs	IV Case study	Botulinum toxin injection to biceps and brachioradialis in both upper limbs and serial bivalve cast mid-humerus to distal MCP joints Casts worn 4 hrs/day for 8 months	Modified Ashworth Scale (MAS) Passive range of motion Caregiver questionnaire	Range of motion for extension increased but the increase was temporary Decreased spasticity on MAS but decrease temporary

as studies combining the two interventions have been shown to be effective in improving motion and hand function. In addition, casts should be worn 4–6 hours/day.

Serial casting to increase range of motion is used primarily at the elbow joint to lengthen hypoextensible elbow flexors, increasing range of motion and decreasing contracture caused by spasticity. Typically the affected joint is cast in submaximal range (5–10 degrees below maximum passive range). Cast change schedules range from every day for recent contractures to every 10 days for chronic contractures. Serial casting requires careful monitoring of blood circulation, oedema, skin condition and sensation. Final casts are usually bivalved and applied daily to maintain range of motion (Lohman 2001).

ORTHOSES
The use of orthoses is one approach often recommended to prevent shortening in spastic muscles over time (Koman et al 1990) and to assist in motor control functions such as grip, pinch and release of objects (Flegle and Leibowitz 1988). Because of the short lever arms and complex arches of the hand, the decreased sensation inherent in orthotic use, and the limitation of function when the wrist is immobilized, wrist/hand orthoses are prescribed selectively for children with moderate to severe deformity. Thus, research studies are limited by small sample sizes (see Table 15.2). The types of splint designs commonly used are: dynamic orthoses (providing positioning with some mobility) and static orthoses (providing complete mobilization at the joint splinted), as shown in Fig. 15.1 (Feldman 1990). In the past decade, there has been an increase in commercially available orthoses (resting hand orthoses and the Pedi Comfy splints which provide flexibility in changing the orthotic angles as the child increases ROM). For children with minimal involvement, small opponens hand orthoses are often used, which are colourful, made of soft material, and removable and washable (see Fig. 15.2).

Since dynamic orthoses have moving parts that allow the individual a range of voluntary controlled movement, it has been proposed that their use may prevent contractures and allow opposing antagonist muscle force to counter the force of the spastic muscle (Kaplan 1962). Three studies with control comparison data support the use of dynamic orthoses in children with CP to improve grip and dexterity (Exner and Bonder 1983, Flegle and Leibowitz 1988, Burtner et al 2008). Static orthoses are designed to be rigid for controlled support (immobilization) of the involved joint in order to maintain muscle length and improve hand function (Coppard and Lohman 2001). Although several case reports document subjective changes in children with CP using static orthoses (Exner and Bonder 1983, Currie and Mendiola 1987, Carmick 1997), only one study documented specific hand function changes (Goodman and Bazyk 1991).

Other orthotic interventions
Therapists also use neoprene, a thick stretchy material, and more recently Lycra for garments that provide postural support. Two studies (Blair et al 1985, Nicholson et al 2001) report some positive results in children with CP, but generally this intervention remains questionable due to the impact on the child and family (Nicholson et al 2001, Knox 2003). Another recent study (Yasukawa et al 2006) reported significant effects of shoulder and upper limb

TABLE 15.2

Evidence-based studies examining effects of wrist/hand orthoses on children's upper extremity function

Reference	N	Level of evidence	Intervention protocol	Measurements	Results
Burtner et al 2008	10 children with hemiplegic CP 5 age-matched controls without CP 4–13 yrs	Level III Cohort with control group Randomized splint order	Surface electrode electromyography (EMG) recorded 8 UE muscles during force and dexterity tasks 3 orthotic (dynamic, static, no) conditions in randomly assigned order	Grip strength Pinch strength (lateral) Modified 9 Hole Peg Test Average integrated EMG (IEMG) expressed as % of maximum voluntary contraction (MVC) for each muscle	Children with CP scored significantly ↓ than controls in grip, pinch, peg in all orthotic conditions Children with CP in dynamic orthoses had ↑ grip strength ($p < 0.008$) and ↓ peg time scores ($p = .02$) Children with CP had ↑ pinch ($p = .04$) with no orthoses than with static splint All children had ↓ wrist IEMG with static orthoses Children with CP had ↑ shoulder EMG activation in no and static splint conditions
Currie and Mendiola 1987	5 children with spastic hemiplegia 20–26 months	Level V Case Descriptive	Cortical thumb orthosis of Polyform and velcro to position thumb MP joint from adducted 'thumb-in-palm' position	Descriptive observations of prehension patterns with and without orthosis	With thumb orthosis, child changed from ulnar raking pattern to 3-jaw chuck grasp with cube and lateral pinch with pellet With orthosis, bimanual activities changed from unilateral or fisted hand assist to cylinder grasp with both hands on glass and bimanual exploration
Exner and Bonder 1983	12 children with hemiplegic CP	Level IV Prospective before/ after design with no control group	Three splint designs studied (orthokinetic cuff, short opponens thumb splint and MacKinnon splint) Children wore each splint 8 hrs/day for 6 wks with 2 wks of no splint use between each trial splint	Descriptive observations of spontaneous bilateral hand use Descriptive observations of spontaneous grasp patterns	Grasp improved in all children wearing the MacKinnon splint Changes most dramatic in child with poorest hand function prior to wearing splint Small opponens splint less frequently associated with changes in grasp or bilateral hand use

240

Study	Subjects	Design	Method	Measures	Results
Flegle and Leibowitz 1988	3 children with hemiplegic CP	Level V Prospective AB single subject design Descriptive	Grasp skills measured during 15 sessions with MacKinnon splint use initiated at different times for each child	Descriptive data of grasp patterns	Grasp improved with all subjects wearing MacKinnon splint Child with poorest grasp had most change
Goodman and Bazyk 1991	4-year-old child with moderate spastic quadriparesis	Level V Prospective AB single subject design	Baseline measures taken without splint 2×/wk for 4 wks Intervention was child wearing short opponens splint 3 hrs am and pm for 4 wks with measures taken 2×/wk	Active ROM of CMP joint Grip strength Pinch strength (lateral, palmar, 2 pt) Blocks & Box Test (dexterity) Block stacking Erhardt Developmental Prehension Assessment	Significant improvements in: Palmar and radial abduction; thumb opposition Grip strength Blocks & Box scores of dexterity Cube stacking Lateral pinch
Reid and Sochaniwskyj 1992	10 children with quadriplegic or athetoid CP	Level IV Prospective before/ after design with no control group	Reaching and visual motor skills measured with hand positioning splint on and off over 3 sessions	Electromyography (EMG) of UE muscles Measure of visual motor skills	NS on all measures Some evidence of more normal muscle activation during reaching with splint Trend in improved visual motor performance

CP = cerebral palsy; UE = upper extremity; NS = not significant

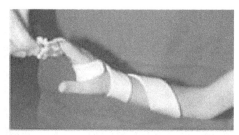

Dynamic splint

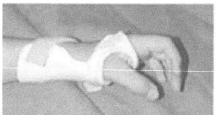

Static splint

Fig. 15.1 Dynamic spiral splint and static splint.

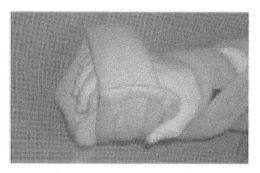

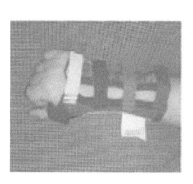

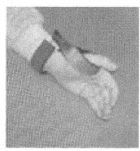

Fig. 15.2 Commercially available splints: Pedi-Comfy wrist hand splint. Neoprene wrist hand orthoses and small opponens Joe Cool™ splint.

kinesio-taping on Melbourne Assessment scores in 15 children with acute brain injury. No studies investigating the effects of kinesio-taping on functional skills of children with CP were found.

Guidelines for intervention

Before fabrication, the therapist first plans the orthosis according to the therapeutic purpose (Charest 2003). If the orthosis is to provide positioning to prevent contractures, to provide correct alignment with strong joint stability, or to provide a resting position for the hand, a low-temperature thermoplastic splinting material should be used. Use of a hand pattern is recommended to decrease the fabrication time on the actual arm of the child. After creating the pattern, try it on the child's hand prior to tracing and cutting the thermoplastic material. Once the orthosis is fabricated and the child has worn the splint for the first time, remove the splint, wait 20 minutes and check for pressure areas (redness that has not gone away). Low-temperature thermoplastic materials may not be strong enough to counteract mechanical forces in some cases of strong spasticity or rigidity in the wrist and hand. In such cases, referral to an orthotist is recommended. For thumb-in-palm deformity caused by minimal spasticity, the orthosis may be used to position the thumb out of adduction into a more functional abducted/extended position for good finger–thumb opposition. Soft neoprene orthoses or commercially available Joe Cool™ splints may provide enough support.

Orthoses may be used to augment existing function by substituting for weak muscles. The therapist can design an orthosis to hold an eating utensil or pencil or to support the index finger for access to a communication device or a computer. Other common uses of orthoses are for hygiene and for protection. Skin breakdown, accompanied by low grade infection, is not uncommon when the hand is held tightly in a flexed position secondary to spasticity. By splinting a child's fisted hand into a more extended position, the airflow is increased to the palm of the hand to minimize skin breakdown from constant contact with the finger and thumb to palm. Bivalve splints may be used for protection post-surgery when the hand is not to be touched or moved excessively.

Since children often do not like the idea of wearing an orthosis, the therapist should take time to introduce the splint as a positive experience. Whenever possible, the therapist and parents should explain to the child why the orthosis is needed, in terms he or she will understand. Some preparatory time should be included to allow the child to participate in choosing colours for the splint and straps, or to splint a stuffed animal, or to decorate their own splint with stickers – activities which may greatly increase the child's compliance. If the child has strong sensitivity in his hands, a hand desensitization programme prior to splinting may be required for the child to accept the splint. To maximize orthotic compliance, a user-friendly wearing schedule that matches the child's routine should be designed. For example, the child could apply the splint at breakfast and remove it at lunchtime, rather than having a schedule of 2–3 hours on and 2–3 hours off.

STRENGTHENING

Children with cerebral palsy have been shown to have deficits in strength, and movement disorders in children with cerebral palsy have been shown to be due in part to skeletal muscle weakness (Stackhouse et al 2005). A recent review by Dodd et al (2002) examined whether strength training increased strength and motor activity in persons with cerebral palsy without adverse effects. They reviewed studies of both the upper and lower limb and concluded that, although there is evidence to support strength programmes in children and young adults with cerebral palsy, the methodological limitations and insufficient information in the articles prevented them from drawing firm conclusions about the effectiveness of strengthening exercises. For the purpose of this chapter, we have included only the studies involving strengthening of the upper limbs, and single case studies. Table 15.3 shows that the sample sizes in the majority of studies were small, ranging from 1 to 23 subjects. Only one study, by O'Connell et al (1992), examined the effect of strengthening on gains in activities. Wiley and Damiano (1998) have published recommendations for strength training for the lower limb, but there are not enough studies for the upper limb to develop guidelines.

Guidelines for intervention
The following guidelines on strengthening individual muscles using free weights are based on Damiano and Abel (1998) but should be used with caution as they have not been tested in clinical studies on the upper extremities. The recommended protocol uses 65 per cent of the maximum voluntary contraction and involves performing four sets of five repetitions each, with a one-minute rest between sets. The training frequency recommended is three times per week for six weeks.

In addition, children can be encouraged to participate in recreational activities to promote strengthening, such as climbing, paddling a canoe or rowing a boat, gymnastics, swimming, pushing and pulling toys, and propelling hand-propelled bikes or self-propelled riders.

BOTULINUM TOXIN A COMBINED WITH THERAPY
The use of botulinum toxin A (BoNT-A) in children with CP was first introduced by Koman in 1993 to reduce spasticity and improve lower extremity function (Koman et al 1993). Controlled studies and observations have further refined the intervention. Wasiak and colleagues (2004) in a Cochrane Review found insufficient evidence to support the use of BoNT-A as an adjunct to treatment of the upper limb in children with spastic CP. Table 15.4 presents the two studies meeting inclusion criteria of the Cochrane Review and three additional randomized control studies since the review. An in-depth review of current practice is presented in Chapter 14 and more recent studies presented in Table 15.4 outline therapy protocols. Based on recent studies (Speth et al 2005, Lowe et al 2006, Wallen et al 2007), protocols using BoNT-A combined with therapy appear to be more efficacious in promoting functional hand use in children than BoNT-A injections alone. However, additional studies are required to determine the frequency, intensity and duration of therapy for children classified at the different levels of functional ability. Evidence-based studies using a combination of botulinum toxin A and therapy to improve upper extremity function are also presented in Chapter 26.

TABLE 15.3

Evidence-based studies examining effects of strengthening exercises on children's upper extremity function

Reference	N	Level of evidence	Intervention protocol	Measurements	Results
Darrah et al 1999	23 children 13 hemiplegia, 5 diplegia 2 quadriplegia 2 ataxia 1 dystonia 11–20 yrs (mean = 14.2)	IV	Targeted muscles: shoulder flexors, knee extensors, hip extensors and abductors Flexibility and aerobics Free and fixed weights, aerobics (3 sets 12 reps, 3x/wk for 10 wks)	Maximum isometric contraction Flexibility Perceived physical appearance Other measures of cardiovascular fitness, i.e. heart rate and energy expenditure	Shoulder flexion strength increased ($p < .01$) Flexibility increased significantly ($p < .05$) Positive perception of physical appearance increased significantly ($p < .00$)
Horvat 1987	1 patient with spastic, hemiplegia 21 yrs	V Single case	Targeted muscles: upper and lower limb Free weights and training machines (10 reps, 3×/wk for 8 wks)	Strength Range of motion (ROM) Endurance	Shoulder flexion, extension, internal rotation, external rotation strength increased Shoulder ROM increased Shoulder endurance increased
McCubbin, and Shasby 1985	30 children 24 spastic 4 mixed 2 athetoid 10–20 yrs	II RCT	Targeted muscle: triceps 3 treatment groups: 1 control 2 isokinetic resistance (3 sets of 5 reps, 3×/wk for 6 wks) 3 repetitive practice no resistance (3 sets of 5 reps, 3×/week for 6 wks)	Rate of torque development, movement times	Isokinetics group showed a significant decrease in movement time ($p < .05$) as compared to the other 2 groups Isokinetic group showed a significant increase in torque production ($p < .05$) as compared to the other 2 groups
Mulligan et al 2004	1 child with spastic diplegia 13 yrs, male	V Single case	6 wk circuit type functional exercise training programme Aerobic activities and, for strengthening, body weight used as resistance (3 sets of 10 reps) Training 1×/wk with PH and 3×/wk with home program	Strength of upper and lower limb muscles using hand-held dynamometer 6-min walk test Gross motor function measure Energy expenditure VO2 max	Upper limb strength increased in elbow and shoulder muscles with more improvements in the left or non-dominant upper limb

245

TABLE 15.3 (continued)

Evidence-based studies examining effects of strengthening exercises on children's upper extremity function

Reference	N	Level of evidence	Intervention protocol	Measurements	Results
O'Connell et al 1992	6 children 3 with CP: 2 spastic 1 ataxic CP: 7–14 yrs (mean = 11.8) 3 with myelomeningocele	IV	Free weights (3 sets of 6 reps maximum (RM), 3×/wk for 9 wks)	Change in weight over 6 RM Fastest of 3 times for 50 metre wheelchair propulsion dash Distance travelled in wheelchair in 12 mins	Children with CP and myelomeningocele analysed together Significant improvements in upper extremity muscles ($p < .05$) Significant improvement in the 12-min test ($p < .05$)

TABLE 15.4

Evidence-based studies examining effects of botulinum toxin A on children's upper extremity function

Reference	N	Level of evidence	Intervention protocol	Measurements	Results
Wasiak et al 2004	2 studies met criteria (Corry et al 1997, Fehlings et al 2000)	Level I Review of RCTs			Insufficient evidence to support or refute use of BoNT-A in UE
Corry et al 1997	14 children/ adolescents with hemiplegic, triplegic or quadriplegic CP 4–19 yrs (mean = 9 yrs)	Level II Double blind RCT Control (n < 100)	BoNT-A injections (Botox = 4–7 U/kg; Dysport = 8–9 U/kg body weight) in identified muscles with measures at 0, 2 and 12 wks Control group saline solution, later BoNT-A No ongoing therapy reported	Modified Ashworth Scale (MAS) Thumb, MCP and UE ROM Caregiver ratings of UE changes Grasp/release Pinch (coin transfer) Wrist stiffness – resonant frequency	MAS ↓ elbow at 2 wks (p = .01); wrist at 2 and 12 wks (p < .01) ROM ↑ elbow (p = .03) and thumb (p = .04) at 2wks Caregiver ratings – trend ↑ Grasp/release = 2 wks, NS; 12 wks (p = .01) Pinch = NS Wrist stiffness = ↓ 2wks (p = .02); 12 wks (p = .05)
Fehlings et al 2000	30 children with hemiplegia 2.5–10 yrs	Level II Single blind RCT (n < 100)	BoNT-A injections (Botox = 2–6 U/kg body weight) in identified muscles with measures at 0, 1, 3 and 5 months Also received occupational therapy Control group OT only	Quality of Upper Extremity Skills Test (QUEST) Modified Ashworth Scale (MAS) Pediatric Evaluation of Disability Inventory (PEDI) Passive ROM elbow, wrist and thumb	QUEST scores significantly ↑ in BoNT-A group than in control group (p = .039) MAS = NS Passive ROM = NS PEDI Self Care scores significantly ↑ in BoNT-A group than in control group (p = .04)
Lowe et al 2006	42 children with hemiplegic CP (GMFCS level I) 2–8 yrs (mean = 4 yrs)	Level II Evaluator blinded RCT (n < 100)	Low dose/high concentration localized BoNT-A (Botox) did not exceed 8 U/kg body weight for injections based on estimated muscle size Both groups of children received occupational therapy	Quality of Upper Extremity Skills Test (QUEST) Modified Ashworth Scale (MAS) Pediatric Evaluation of Disability Inventory (PEDI)	Average treatment effects at 1, 3 and 6 months favoured BoNT-A group: QUEST (p < .001) MAS (p < .001) PEDI (p = .03) COPM Performance (p = .002); Satisfaction (p = .007) GAS (p < .001)

TABLE 15.4 (continued)

Evidence-based studies examining effects of botulinum toxin A on children's upper extremity function

Reference	N	Level of evidence	Intervention protocol	Measurements	Results
				Canadian Occupation Performance Measure (COPM) Goal Attainment Scale (GAS) for selected goals in dressing, leisure, eating and school functional skills	
Speth et al 2005	20 children with hemiplegia; excluded Zancolli III 4–16 yrs	Level II RCT non-blinded subjects matched by Zancolli level	BoNT-A (Botox) injections: 1–6 muscles; dose = 5.8 U/kg of body weight, with measures taken at 0, 2 and 6 wks and 3, 6 and 9 months All children received occupational therapy and physical therapy 3×/wk for 6 months	Modified Ashworth Scale (MAS) Melbourne Assessment Pediatric Evaluation of Disability Inventory (PEDI) 9 Hole Peg Test	Clinically relevant changes in active wrist extension and wrist flexor tone on the MAS No significant changes in BoNT-A group vs control group on functional measures (Melbourne, PEDI and 9 Hole Peg scores)
Wallen et al 2004	16 children: 8 quadriplegia 7 hemiplegia 1 triplegia 2–12 yrs (mean = 6.4 yrs)	Level IV Prospective cohort study with no control group	BoNT-A (Botox) injections: 1–4 muscles; article says children received 1–4 but there was a possibility of 5 muscles (mean total dose/child = 7.16 U/kg of body weight) with measures taken at 0 and 2 wks, and 3 and 6 months Maintained existing levels of occupational and physical therapy	Canadian Occupation Performance Measure (COPM) Goal Attainment Scale (GAS) for selected goals in dressing, leisure, eating and school functional skills Melbourne Assessment Child Health Questionnaire (CHQ) Parent questionnaire Modified Ashworth Scale (MAS) Tardieu scale for UE UE ROM	Significant changes in COPM Performance Ratings (3 months, $p < .004$; 6 months, $p < .002$) and Satisfaction Ratings (3 months, $p < .01$; 6 months, $p < .003$) Significant changes in GAS (T score < 50) in 3 participants at 3 months and 8 participants at 6 months NS = Melbourne scores, CHQ MAS and Tardieu significant difference at 2 wks and gradual return to baseline except Tardieu at elbow UE active ROM and passive ROM no change

Guidelines for intervention
As stated previously, specific occupational therapy guidelines post botulinum toxin A injections based on different MACS levels of function are needed. It is common practice to apply bivalve casts post-intervention to provide support to weakened muscles. The duration of casting is individualized for the child; however, the average length of time is approximately two weeks post-injection. Strengthening exercises for weak antagonist muscles to the muscle injected are implemented during the casting period, as well as beginning a strengthening regime for the agonists that have received injections. With increased motor control on the part of the child, the active interplay of the injected muscles and the opposing muscles is emphasized. In addition to strengthening exercises, therapy also includes massed practice of fine motor coordination training, and age-appropriate activities of daily living and play, with emphasis on elbow and wrist extension, forearm supination and grasp/ release patterns.

NEUROMUSCULAR ELECTRICAL STIMULATION
The use of electrical stimulation has been reported with increased frequency over the past decade. Underlying rationales for use of electrical stimulation are: to reverse multiple rate-limiting factors by increasing strength (Dubowitz et al 1988, Hazelwood et al 1994), to increase range of motion (Hazelwood et al 1994), to increase sensation and to improve motor skills (Steinbok et al 1997, Wright and Granat 2000). A systematic review by Kerr et al (2004) identified evidence primarily for lower extremity muscle electrical stimulation. Generally, threshold electrical stimulation (TES) studies (low subcontraction electrical stimulation as the child sleeps, over a period of several months) have produced disappointing results (Sommerfelt et al 2001, Dali et al 2002). However, one study (Steinbok et al 1997) strongly supported the use of TES in children post dorsal rhizotomy surgery for increasing their muscle strength. More positive results are reported with neuromuscular electrical stimulation (NMES), which is electrical stimulation strong enough to elicit contraction and is used in conjunction with active exercise to assist weak muscles in contraction. NMES is also referred to as functional electrical stimulation (FES) when used in conjunction with a task. FES is regulated to stimulate a muscle in phase with the task requirements.

Evidence-based studies to improve upper extremity function are presented in Table 15.5. Studies by Kamper and colleagues (2006) as well as by Wright and Granat show the most promising results of NMES in this population. Continued research in this area of intervention is needed in order to weigh the benefits of NMES against the inconvenience of intensive therapy. More definitive studies based on functional level of the child may assist in determining the best candidates for NMES.

Guidelines for intervention
Upper and lower arm protocols for NMES have been developed over years of experience (Logan 2006). Children must be aged 2 years or more and must be cooperative and able to provide accurate feedback about stimulation intensity and comfort. The severity of the child's involvement is considered when choosing candidates for NMES intervention. Original guidelines recommend children at levels I, II and III on the Gross Motor Function

TABLE 15.5
Evidence-based studies examining effects of electrical stimulation on children's upper extremity

Reference	N	Level of evidence	Intervention protocol	Measurements	Results
Atwater et al 1991	10 children with spastic CP: only 2 in UE group 5.5–16 yrs	Level IV Case series	8-wk intervention (45–60 min sessions 3×/wk) of electromyography-triggered electrical muscle stimulation (EMG-EMS) 2 children received UE stimulation with traditional therapeutic exercise No ongoing OT and PT	Active ROM of wrist extension Peabody Fine Motor Developmental Scales (PDMS) Videotape of UE quality of movement on 6 UE tasks by blind reviewer with inter-rater reliability established	Movement times in 5 of 6 UE tasks ↓ significantly in both children receiving UE stimulation ROM approximated neutral wrist joint angle on 4 of 6 UE tasks Global ratings of videotapes of UE were positive for ↑ movement quality PDMS scores stayed the same or were lower
Carmick 1993	Two children with hemiplegic CP 1.6 and 6.7 yrs	Level V Case reports	Case 1: after 11 months of therapy, NMES 15 min triceps during crawling; NMES 15 min wrist/finger flexors during grasp/release Case 2: 2×/wk for 5 wks, NMES to triceps, wrist and thumb extensors/abductors and finger flexors	Descriptive observation of changes in hand function	Case 1: crawling on extended arm during session 1 of NMES with carry-over at home and over 5 wks. With NMES to wrist and fingers, immediate bilateral hand use and ↑ grasp/release Case 2: 2 wks of NMES ↑ sensation and ↓ non-use. 7 sessions of NMES ↑ use of hand as assist and spontaneous reach and grasp
Carmick 1997	6-year-old child with spastic hemiparetic CP	Level V Case report	38 sessions of NMES to wrist extensors, finger flexor/extensors followed by 24 sessions with a combination of NMES and dorsal wrist splint Weekly therapy sessions with NMES amplitude by child tolerance with rise time of 0.5/1 s and pulse width at 300 ms	Descriptive observations of: Spontaneous hand use Active ROM Bilateral hand use	Splint use discontinued after 9 months, and child could: actively extend wrist and maintain position to hold object; press toy object with index finger and pick up small objects; perform shoe lacing independently without splint

Study	Subjects	Design	Intervention	Outcome measures	Results
Kamper et al 2006	8 children with spastic hemiparesis 5–15 yrs	Level IV Prospective pre/post design with no control	3 months of NMES to wrist extensors and flexors; performed in home, 15 mins 5 days/wk first 6 wks. Second 6 wks, session length extended to 30 mins and targeted only wrist extensors with therapy added (grasping objects, lifting weights). Measurement: 2 sessions pre-, 1 at 6 wks, and 2 post-intervention	Peak active ROM of wrist extension against gravity. Spasticity measures of velocity-dependent stiffness recorded using a servomotor. Voluntary wrist extensor on servomotor. Isometric wrist extensor and flexor torque	Active ROM significantly ↑ ($p = .002$). No significant changes in spasticity or passive resistance as a group, some individual differences. Seven children significantly ↑ in wrist extensor strength; wrist flexor strength changes NS
Scheker et al 1999	19 subjects with spastic CP 4–21 yrs	Level V Prospective pre/post cohort design	Treatment length ranged from 3 to 43 months. 30-min sessions of NMES to antagonist forearm extensor and triceps muscles combined with dynamic orthotic traction device in home setting	Zancolli classification scale of hand function. Patient compliance ratings	All subjects ↑ 1–3 levels on the Zancolli classification scale. Description of marked upper extremity improvement in subjects. Children with high compliance showed faster improvement within the first 4–6 weeks
Wright and Granat 2000	8 children with hemiplegic CP mean age = 10 yrs	Level IV Prospective pre/post cohort design	Baseline of 3 wks, 6 wks of intervention, 6-week follow-up. Cyclic FES applied 30 mins daily during the treatment phase	Jebsen Hand Function Test. Active wrist extension. Wrist extension moment	Significant ↓ in time scores on 3 Jebsen subtests during intervention ($p = .03$) and 6 wks post ($p = .04$). Significant ↓ in active wrist extension during intervention ($p = .03$) and 6 wks post ($p = .04$). Wrist extension moment = NS

CP = cerebral palsy; UE = upper extremity; OT = occupational therapy; PT = physical therapy; ROM = range of motion; NMES = neuromuscular electrical stimulation; s = seconds; ms = milliseconds; NS = not significant; FES = functional electrical stimulation

Classification System (GMCFS; Palisano et al 1997). These functional levels are considered to be similar to levels I, II and III on the MACS (Eliasson et al 2006). Children at functional level IV on the MACS and GMCFS may not be optimal for NMES intervention since the stimulation of very high tone muscles may damage the tissues.

Figs 15.3 and 15.4 show placement of the electrodes on the upper and lower arms (Logan 2006). The NMES training programne for the elbow or wrist is approximately 2500 repetitions during a 3–4-month period, with useful carry-over to a higher level of fine motor function. Stimulus parameters are generally considered to be 35–45 Hz with a pulse width of 280 and contraction time of 5 seconds, ramp-up at 0.5 seconds. The aim of the home programme for the high tone individual is to decrease tone in spastic elbow or wrist flexors and to teach the child to turn the opposing muscles 'on' and 'off'. Since specific protocols outlining upper extremity positioning and increases in stimulation repetition have been developed, consultation with an experienced therapist is recommended.

BIOFEEDBACK/AUGMENTED FEEDBACK

Electromyographic (EMG) biofeedback and augmented feedback involve supplementing feedback that is intrinsic in an activity. The feedback may be provided through tactile, auditory and/or visual pathways (Talbot and Junkala 1981, van Dijk et al 2005). EMG biofeedback involves the application of external electrodes to muscles in order to activate motor unit electrical potential, while augmented feedback provides visual or auditory feedback about the state of the neuromuscular system being monitored (James 1992).

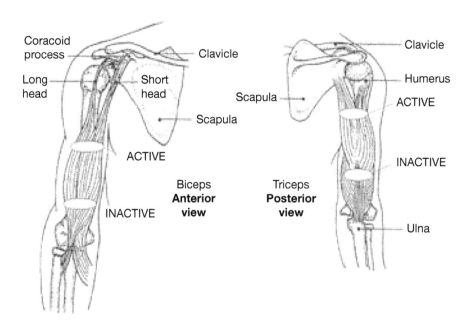

Fig. 15.3 Electrode placement for neuromuscular electrical stimulation of upper arm.

Source: Adapted from K Pape, tascnetwork.net.

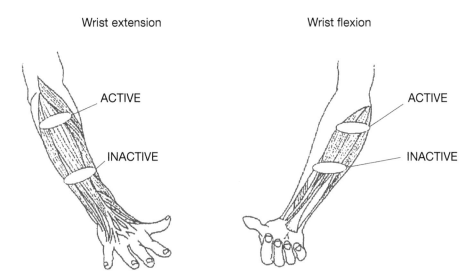

Fig. 15.4 Electrode placement for neuromuscular electrical stimulation of forearm.

Source: Adapted from K Pape, tascnetwork.net.

Table 15.6 shows the results from the few studies that have examined the effectiveness of biofeedback on upper extremity function in children with cerebral palsy. James (1992) conducted the only review of biofeedback studies and found studies that used biofeedback for head and limb control, sitting posture control, ankle joint control, gait training, eye–hand coordination, and drooling. He reported that while the results from the studies were promising, more control studies with a greater number of subjects were needed, as well as studies of the effectiveness of carry-over to real-life situations (James 1992).

Guidelines for intervention
Candidates for biofeedback or augmented feedback should have intact cognition in order to be able to understand cause/effect relationships, and a good attention span. Biofeedback paradigms for children with cerebral palsy have included visual feedback for movement accuracy or effort on a computer screen, and electromyography-based biofeedback which causes toys to move once the child reaches a targeted muscle contraction threshold. However, at the moment, the limited evidence regarding biofeedback makes it impossible to establish specific guidelines for intervention. Positive results have been reported, but since this intervention had limited carry-over and is time-consuming (James 1992), clinicians are cautioned to document outcomes and generalization to real-life situations.

Future directions for research and practice
In summary, therapeutic interventions to improve upper extremity function in children with CP at the ICF Body Structure/Function level consist of stretching/casting, orthoses, botulinuum toxin A combined with therapy, functional electric stimulation and biofeedback.

TABLE 15.6

Evidence-based studies examining effects of biofeedback on children's upper extremity function

Reference	N	Level of evidence	Intervention protocol	Measurements	Results
Reid and Koheil 1987	1 child with spastic hemiplegic CP 2 yrs 6 months, male	V Case study	$A_1/B/C/A_2$ 2 consecutive sessions of 1 hr of biofeedback training to make toy train move forward, 15 mins 2×/day, 5 days/wk for 2 months	*Clinical observations:* Left arm position in walking/play Active wrist extension Spontaneous use of left hand Holding a bead	Elbow carried at 45 degree angle with hand below waist level; fingers loosely flexed in walking/play Able to slowly actively extend wrist Used left arm spontaneously in play Able to stabilize 1 in. bead in left hand while right hand inserted thread
Talbot and Junkala 1981	59 individuals with spastic CP 7–21 yrs (mean = 14 yrs 3 months)	II RCT	40 training sessions 3 treatment groups: tracing with auditory augmented feedback; tracing alone; control – no tracing, no feedback	Southern California Motor Accuracy Test (SCMAT) accuracy and speed	Group with tracing with auditory training scored significantly higher than the other two groups (p < .05) There was a trend toward significance for speed (p < .059) in favour of the tracing and feedback group After 3 months group differences were no longer significant

CP = cerebral palsy; RCT = randomized controlled trial

254

The evidence for these interventions is primarily single case studies with limited randomized control studies. These evidence-based studies show mixed results in regard to improvements, and only a few examine the effect of impairment-based intervention on functional outcomes at the Activity and Participation level of the ICF. Future studies are needed to examine the relationship between body structure/function intervention for children with CP and the activity/participation outcomes they experience. The following guidelines should be considered for future studies:

1 Studying changes in children with CP by functional groupings using systems such as the Manual Ability Classification System (MACS, see Introduction), the Modified House Scale and/or the Zancolli classification system
2 Using reliable, valid measures designed to measure functional changes in children with CP (see Chapter 12 for review).
3 Creating systematic intervention protocols to test the intensity, duration, and age of children at different functional levels to determine intervention outcomes.
4 Establishing multi-centre studies (perhaps internationally) to increase sample sizes and generalization of results.

REFERENCES

Atwater SW, Tatarka ME, Kathrein JE, Shapiro S (1991) Electromyography-triggered electrical muscle stimulation for children with cerebral palsy: a pilot study. *Ped Phys Ther* 8: 190–199.
Autti-Ramo I, Larsen A, Taimo A, vonWendt L (2001) Management of the upper limb with botulinum toxin type A in children with spastic type cerebral palsy and acquired brain injury: clinical implications. *Eur J Neurol* 8(Suppl 5): 136–144.
Bax M, Brown JK (2004) The spectrum of disorders known as cerebral palsy. In: Scutton J, Damiano D, Mayston M, editors. *Management of Motor Disorders in Children with Cerebral Palsy.* Clinics in Developmental Medicine 161. London: Mac Keith Press, pp 9–21.
Berger W, Quintern J, Deitz V (1982) Pathophysiology of gait in children with cerebral palsy. *Electroenceph Clin Neurophys* 53: 538–548.
Bernstein N (1967) *Coordination and Regulation of Movements.* New York: Pergamon.
Blair E, Ballantyne J, Horsman S, Chauvel P (1985) A study of a dynamic proximal stability splint in the management of children with cerebral palsy. *Dev Med Child Neurol* 37: 544–554.
Bobath K, Bobath B (1984) The neuro-developmental treatment. In: Scrutton D, editor. *Management of the Motor Disorders of Children with Cerebral Palsy.* Philadelphia, PA: J.B. Lippincott, pp 6–17.
Bobath K, Bobath B (1985) *Abnormal Postural Reflex Activity Caused by Brain Lesions.* Rockville, MD: Aspen.
Boyd R, Graham HK (1997) Botulinum toxin A in the management of children with cerebral palsy: indications and outcomes. *Eur J Neurol* 4(Suppl 2): 515–522.
Boyd RN, Morris ME, Graham HK (2001). Management of upper limb dysfunction in children with cerebral palsy: a systematic review. *Eur J Neurol* 8(Suppl 5): 150–166.
Brogren E, Hadders-Algra M, Forssberg H (1996) Postural control in children with spastic diplegia: muscle activity during perturbations in sitting. *Dev Med Child Neurol* 38: 379–388.
Brogren E, Hadders-Algra M, Forssberg H (1998) Postural control in sitting children with cerebral palsy. *Neurosci Biobehav Rev* 22: 591–596.
Brouwer B, Davidson LK, Olney SJ (2000) Serial casting in idiopathic toe-walkers and children with spastic cerebral palsy. *J Pediatr Orthop* 20: 221–225.
Bumin G, Kayihan H (2001) Effectiveness of two different sensory-integration programmes for children with spastic diplegic cerebral palsy. *Disabil Rehabil* 23: 394–399.
Burtner PA, Qualls C, Woollacott MH (1998) Muscle activation characteristics for stance balance in children with spastic cerebral palsy. *Gait Posture* 41: 748–757.

Burtner PA, Poole JL, Torres T, Medora SM, Keene J, Qualls C (2008) Effect of splints on grip, pinch, manual dexterity and muscle activation in children with spastic hemiplegia. *J Hand Ther* 21: 36–42.

Butler C, Darrah J (2001) Effects of neurodevelopmental treatment (NDT) for cerebral palsy: an AACPDM evidence report. *Dev Med Child Neurol* 45: 1–13.

Butler C, Chambers H, Goldstein M, Harris S, Leach J, Campbell S et al (2005) Evaluating research in developmental disabilities: a conceptual framework for reviewing treatment outcomes. http://www.aacpdm.org/index?service=page/treatmentOutcomesReport (accessed May 2005).

Carlson MG (1999) Cerebral palsy. In: Hotchkiss R, editor. *Green's Operative Hand Surgery*. New York Elsevier.

Carmick J (1993) Clinical use of neuromuscular electrical stimulation for children with cerebral palsy. *Phys Ther* 73: 523–527.

Carmick J (1997) Use of neuromuscular electrical stimulation and a dorsal wrist splint to improve the hand function of a child with spastic hemiparesis. *Phys Ther* 77: 661–671.

Charest E (2003) The pediatric patient. In: Jacobs M, Austin N, editors. *Splinting the Hand and Upper Extremity: Principles and Process*. Philadelphia: Lippincott, Williams & Wilkins.

Chin TY, Graham HK (2003) Botulinum toxin A in the management of upper limb spasticity in cerebral palsy. *Hand Clin* 19: 591–600.

Cooper J, Majnemer A, Rosenblatt B, Birnbaum R (1995) The determination of sensory deficits in children with hemiplegic cerebral palsy. *J Child Neurol* 10: 300–309.

Copley J, Watson-Will A, Dent K (1996) Upper limb casting for clients with cerebral palsy: a clinical report. *Aust Occup Ther J* 43: 39–50.

Coppard BM, Lohman H (2001) *Introduction to Splinting: A Clinical Reasoning and Problem Solving Approach*. St Louis, MO: Mosby.

Corry IS, Cosgrove AP, Walsh EG, McClean D, Graham HK (1997) Botulinum toxin A in the hemiplegic upper extremity: a double blind trial. *Dev Med Child Neurol* 39: 185–193.

Cruickshank DA, O'Neill DL (1990) Upper extremity inhibitive casting in a boy with spastic quadriplegia. *Am J Occup Ther* 44: 552–555.

Currie DM, Mendiola A (1987) Cortical thumb orthosis for children with spastic hemiplegic cerebral palsy. *Arch Phys Med Rehabil* 68: 214–216.

Dali C, Hansen FJ, Pedersen SA, Skov L, Hilden J et al (2002) Threshold electrical stimulation (TES) in ambulant children with CP: a randomized double-blind controlled clinical trial. *Dev Med Child Neurol* 44: 364–369.

Damiano DL Abel MF (1998) Functional outcomes of strength training in spastic cerebral palsy. *Arch Phys Med Rehabil* 79: 119–125.

Damiano DL, Kelly LE, Vaughn CI (1995) Effects of quadriceps femoris muscle strengthening on crouch gait in children with spastic diplegia. *Phys Ther* 75: 658–667.

Darrah J, Wessel J, Nearingburg P, O'Connor M (1999) Evaluation of a community fitness program for adolescents with cerebral palsy. *Pediatr Phys Ther* 11: 18–23.

Dodd K, Taylor N, Damiano DL (2002) Systematic review of strengthening for individuals with cerebral palsy. *Arch Phys Med Rehabil* 83: 1157–1164.

Dubowitz L, Finnie N, Hyde SA, Scott OM, Vrbova G (1988) Improvement of muscle performance by chronic electrical stimulation in children with cerebral palsy. *Lancet* 1: 587–588.

Eliasson AC, Gordon AM, Forssberg H (1995) Tactile control of isometric fingertip forces during grasping in children with cerebral palsy. *Dev Med Child Neurol* 37: 72–84.

Eliasson A-C, Gordon AM, Forssberg H (2005) Tactile control of isometric fingertip forces during grasping in children with cerebral palsy. *Dev Med Child Neurol* 37: 72–84.

Eliasson AC, Krumlinde-Sundholm L, Rosblad, B, Beckung E, Arner M, Ohrvall AM, Rosenbaum P (2006) The Manual Ability Classification System (MACS) for children with cerebral palsy: scale development and evidence of validity and reliability. *Dev Med Child Neurol* 48: 549–554.

Exner CE, Bonder BR (1983) Comparative effects of three hand splints on bilateral hand use, grasp, and arm-hand posture in hemiplegic children: a pilot study. *Occup Ther J Res* 3: 75–92.

Fehlings D, Rang M, Galzier J, Steele C (2000) An evaluation of botulinum-A toxin injections to improve upper extremity function in children with hemiplegic cerebral palsy. *J Pediatr* 137: 331–337.

Feldman P (1990) Upper extremity splinting and casting. In: Glenn MB, Whyte J, editors. *The Practical Management of Spasticity in Children and Adults*. Malvern, PA: Lea & Febiger, pp 59–166.

Finnie N (1997) *Handling the Young Cerebral Palsied Child at Home, 3rd edn*. Oxford: Butterworth Heinemann.

Flegle JH, Leibowitz JM (1988) Improvement in grasp skill in children with hemiplegia with the MacKinnon splint. *Res Dev Disabil* 9: 145–151.

Frieden J, Lieber RL (2006) Spastic muscle cells are shorter and stiffer than normal cells. *Muscle Nerve* 27: 157–164.

Friedman A, Diamond M, Johnston MV, Daffner C (2000) Effects of botulinum toxin A on upper limb spasticity in children with cerebral palsy. *Am J Phys Med Rehabil* 79: 53–59.

Gage JR (2004) *The Treatment of Gait Problems in Cerebral Palsy*. Clinics in Developmental Medicine 164–5. London: Mac Keith Press.

Gallagher KG, Lewin JP (2006) Upper extremity surgical intervention in patients with cerebral palsy: musculotendinous procedures. In: Cioppa-Mosca J, Cahil JB, Cavanaugh JT, Corradi-Scalise D, Rudnick H, Wollf AL, editors. *Postsurgical Rehabilitation Guidelines for the Orthopedic Clinician*. St Louis, MO: Mosby Elsevier.

Giuliani CA (1991) Dorsal rhizotomy for children with cerebral palsy: support for concepts in motor control. *Phys Ther* 71: 248–259.

Goldner JL (1988) Surgical reconstruction of the upper extremity in cerebral palsy. *Hand Clin* 4: 223–265.

Goodman G, Bazyk S (1991) The effects of a short thumb opponens splint on hand function in cerebral palsy: a single-subject study. *Am J Occup Ther* 45: 726–731.

Gordon AM, Duff SV (1999) Fingertip forces during object manipulation in children with hemiplegic cerebral palsy. 1. Anticipatory scaling. *Dev Med Child Neurol* 41: 166–175.

Gossman M, Sharmann S, Rose S (1982) Review of length-associated changes in muscle: experimental evidence and clinical implication. *Phys Ther* 62: 1799–1808.

Graham HK, Selber P (2003) Musculoskeletal aspects of cerebral palsy. *J Bone Joint Surg* 85B: 157–166.

Graham HK, Aoki KR, Autti-Ramo I, Boyd R, Delagado M et al (2000) Recommendations for the use of botulinum toxin A in the management of cerebral palsy. *Gait Posture* 11: 67–79.

Hallet M, Alvarez N (1983) Attempted rapid elbow flexion movements in patients with athetosis. *Neurosurg Psychiatry* 46: 745–750.

Hazelwood ME, Brown JK, Rowe PJ, Slater P (1994) The use of therapeutic electrical stimulation in the treatment of hemiplegic cerebral palsy. *Dev Med Child Neurol* 36: 661–673.

Horvat M (1987) Effects of a progressive resistance training program on an individual with spastic cerebral palsy. *Am Corrective Ther J* 41: 7–11.

House JH, Gwathmey FW, Fidler MO (1981) A dynamic approach to thumb-in-palm deformity in cerebral palsy. *J Bone Joint Surg Am* 63: 216–225.

Hurvitz EA, Conti GE, Brown SH (2003) Changes in movement characteristics of the spastic upper extremity after botulinum toxin injection. *Arch Phys Med Rehabil* 84: 444–454.

James R (1992) Biofeedback treatment for cerebral palsy in children and adolescents: a review. *Pediatr Exerc Sci* 4: 198–212.

Kamper DG, Yasukawa AM, Barrett KM, Gaebler-Spira DJ (2006) Effects of neuromuscular electric stimulation treatment of cerebral palsy on potential impairment mechanisms: a pilot study. *Pediatr Phys Ther* 18: 31–38.

Kaplan N (1962) Effect of splinting on reflex inhibition and sensorimotor stimulation in treatment of spasticity. *Arch Phys Med Rehabil* 43: 563–569.

Kerr C, McDowell B, McDonough S (2004) Electrical stimulation in cerebral palsy: a review of effects on strength and motor function. *Dev Med Child Neurol* 46: 205–213.

Kinghorn J, Roberts G (1996) The effect of an inhibitive weight-bearing splint on tone and function: a single case study. *Am J Occup Ther* 50: 805–815.

Kisner C, Colby LA (1996) Stretching. In: Kisner C, Colby LA, editors. *Therapeutic Exercise: Foundations and Techniques, 3rd edn*. Philadelphia, PA: F.A. Davis Co.

Knox V (2003) The use of lycra garments in children with cerebral palsy: a report of a descriptive clinical trial. *Brit J Occup Ther* 66: 71–77.

Koman LA (2000) Cerebral palsy: House Classification modified. In: Orthopaedic care: medical and surgical management of musculoskeletal disorders: a comprehensive, peer-reviewed internet textbook. *J South Orthop Ass*. http://www.orthotextbook.net

Koman LA, Gelberman RH, Toby EB, Poehling GG (1990) Cerebral palsy. Management of the upper extremity. *Clin Orthop* 253: 62–74.

Koman LA, Moooney JF, Smith BP, Goodman A, Mulvaney T (1993) Management of cerebral palsy with botulinum toxin A: a preliminary investigation. *J Pediatr Orthop* 253: 62–74.

Law M, Cadman D, Rosenbaum P, Walter S, Russell D, DeMatteo C (1991) Neurodevelopmental therapy and upper-extremity casting for children with cerebral palsy. *Dev Med Child Neurol* 33: 379–387.

257

Law M, Russell D, Pollock N, Rosenbaum P, Walter S, King G (1997) A comparison of intensive neurodevelopmental therapy plus casting and a regular occupational therapy program for children with cerebral palsy. *Dev Med Child Neurol* 39: 664–670.

Logan L (2006). Personal communication: Upper extremity protocols for neuromuscular electrical stimulation (NMES). Syracruse, NY: SUNY Upstate Medical University.

Lohman M (2001). Antispasticity splinting. In: Coppard BM, Lohman HC. *Introduction to Splinting: A Clinical-Reasoning and Problem Solving Approach.* St Louis, MO: Mosby.

Lowe K, Novak I, Cusik A (2006) Low dose/high dose-concentration localized botulinum toxin improves upper limb movement and function in children with hemiplegic cerebral palsy. *Dev Med Child Neurol* 48: 170–175.

McCubbin JA, Shasby GB (1985) Effects of isokinetic exercise on adolescents with cerebral palsy. *Adapt Phys Ed Q* 2: 56–64.

McNeill S (2004) The management of deformity. In: Scutton J, Damiano D, Mayston M, editors. *Management of Motor Disorders in Children with Cerebral Palsy.* Clinics in Developmental Medicine 161. London: Mac Keith Press, pp 130–146.

Maenpaa H, Jaakkola R, Sandstrom M, Airi T, vonWendt L (2004) Electrostimulation at sensory level improves function of the upper extremity in children with cerebral palsy: a pilot study. *Dev Med Child Neurol* 46: 84–90.

Magnus R (1926) Some results of studies in the physiology of posture. *Lancet* 2: 531–585.

Mulligan H, Abbott S, Clayton S, McKegg P, Rae P (2004) The outcome of a functional exercise programme in an adolescent with cerebral palsy: a single case study. *NZ J Physiol* 32: 30–38.

Nashner LM, Shumway-Cook A, Marin O (1983) Stance postural control in select groups of children with cerebral palsy: deficits in sensory organization and muscular organization. *Exp Brain Res* 49: 393–409.

Nicholson JH, Morton RE, Attfield S, Rennie D (2001) Assessment of upper limb function and movement in children with cerebral palsy wearing lycra garments. *Dev Med Child Neurol* 43: 384–391.

O'Connell DG, Barnhard R, Parks L (1992) Muscular endurance and wheelchair propulsion in children with cerebral palsy or myelomeningocele. *Arch Phys Med Rehabil* 73: 709–711.

Ostensjo S, Carlberg EB, Vollestad NK (2004) Motor impairments in young children with cerebral palsy: relationship to gross motor function and everyday activities. *Dev Med Child Neurol* 46: 580–589.

Ozer K, Chesher SP, Scheker LR (2006) Neuromuscular electrical stimulation and bracing for the management of upper-extremity spasticity in children with cerebral palsy. *Dev Med Child Neurol* 48: 559–563.

Palisano R, Rosenbaum P, Walter S, Russell D, Wood E, Galuppi B (1997) Development and reliability of a system to classify gross motor function in children with cerebral palsy. *Dev Med Child Neurol* 39: 214–223.

Rameckers EA, Speth LA, Duysens J, Vles JS, Snits-Engelsman BC (2007) Kinematic aiming task: measuring functional changes in hand and arm movements after botulinum toxin-A injections in children with spastic hemiplegia. *Am J Phys Med Rehabil* 86: 538–547.

Reid D, Koheil R (1987) EMG biofeedback training to promote hand function in a cerebral palsied child with hemiplegia. *Occup Ther Health Care* 4: 97–107.

Reid DT, Sochaniwskyj A (1992) Influences of a hand positioning device on upper-extremity control of children with cerebral palsy. *Int J Rehabil Res* 15: 15–29.

Schaltenbrand G (1928) The development of human motility and motor disturbances. *Arch Neurol Psychiatry* 20: 720–730.

Scheker LR, Chesher SP, Ramirez S (1999) Neuromuscular electrical stimulation and dynamic bracing as the treatment for upper-extremity spasticity in children with cerebral palsy. *J Hand Surg* 24B: 226–232.

Sherrington CS (1947) *The Integrative Action of the Nervous System.* New Haven, CT: Yale University Press.

Shumway-Cook A, Woollacott MH (2006) *Motor Control: Translating Research into Clinical Practice, 3rd edn.* Baltimore, MD: Lippincott, Wilkins & Williams.

Smeulders M, Coester A, Kreulen M (2005) Surgical treatment for the thumb in palm deformity in patients with cerebral palsy. *Cochrane Database Syst Rev* 19: CD004093.

Smith L, Harris S (1985) Upper extremity inhibitive casting for a child with cerebral palsy. *Phys Occup Ther Pediatr* 5: 71–75.

Sommerfelt K, Markestad T, Berg K, Saetesdal I (2001) Therapeutic electrical stimulation in cerebral palsy: a randomized controlled crossover trial. *Dev Med Child Neurol* 43: 609–613.

Speth LAWM, Leffers P, Janssen-Potten YJM, Vles JSH (2005) Botulinum toxin A and upper limb functional skills in hemiparetic cerebral palsy: a randomized trial in children receiving intensive therapy. *Dev Med Child Neurol* 47: 468–473.

258

Stackhouse SK, Binder-Macleod SA, Lee SC (2005) Voluntary muscle activation, contractile properties and fatigability in children with and without cerebral palsy. *Muscle Nerve* 31: 594–601.

Steinbok P, Reiner A, Kestle JRW (1997) Therapeutic electric stimulation following selective dorsal rhizotomy in children with spastic diplegic cerebral palsy: a randomized clinical trial. *Dev Med Child Neurol* 39: 515–520.

Talbot ML, Junkala J (1981) The effects of auditorally augmented feedback on the eye–hand coordination of students with cerebral palsy. *Am J Occup Ther* 35: 525–528.

Tardieu C, Lespargot A, Tabary C, Bret MD (1988) For how long must the soleus muscle be stretched each day to prevent contracture? *Dev Med Child Neurol* 30: 3–10.

Threlkeld AJ (1992) The effects of manual therapy on connective tissue. *Phys Ther* 72: 893.

Tona J, Schneck C (1993) The efficacy of upper extremity inhibitive casting: a single-subject pilot study. *Am J Occup Ther* 47: 901–910.

van Dijk H, Jannink MJA, Hermens HJ (2005) Effect of augmented feedback on motor function of the affected upper extremity in rehabilitation patients: a systematic review of randomized controlled trials. *J Rehabil Med* 37: 202–211.

VanHeest AE, House JH, Cariello C (1999) Upper extremity treatment of cerebral palsy. *J Hand Surg* 24A: 323–330.

Vaz DV, Cotta Mancini M, Fonseca ST, Vieira DS, de Melo Pertence AE (2006) Muscle stiffness and strength and their relation to hand function in children with cerebral palsy. *Dev Med Child Neurol* 48: 728–733.

Wallen MA, O'Flaherty SJ, Waugh MA (2004) Functional outcomes of intramuscular botulinum toxin type A in the upper limbs of children with cerebral palsy: a phase II trial. *Arch Phys Med Rehabil* 85: 192–200.

Wallen MA, O'Flaherty SJ, Waugh MA (2007) Functional outcomes of intramuscular botulinum toxin type A in the upper limbs of children with cerebral palsy: a randomized control trial. *Arch Phys Med Rehabil* 88: 1–10.

Wasiak J, Hoare B, Wallen M (2004) Botulinum toxin A as an adjunct to treatment in the management of the upper limb in children with spastic cerebral palsy. *Cochrane Database Syst Rev* 18: CD003469.

Waters PM, VanHeest A (1998) Spastic hemiplegia of the upper extremity in children. *Hand Clin* 14: 119–133.

Wiley ME, Damiano DL (1998) Lower extremity strength profiles in spastic cerebral palsy. *Dev Med Child Neurol* 40: 100–107.

World Health Organization (2001) *International Classification of Functioning, Disability and Health*. Geneva: World Health Organization.

Wright PA, Granat MH (2000) Therapeutic effects of functional electrical stimulation of the upper limb of eight children with cerebral palsy. *Dev Med Child Neurol* 42: 724–727.

Yasukawa A, Malas BS, Gaebler-Spira DJ (2003) Efficacy for maintenance of elbow range of motion of two types of orthotic devices: a case series. *J Prosth Orthot* 15: 72–77.

Yasukawa A, Patel P, Sisung C (2006) Pilot study: Investigating the effects of kinesiotaping in an acute pediatric rehabilitation setting. *Am J Occup Ther* 60: 104–110.

Zancolli EA, Zancolli E (1987) Surgical rehabilitation of the spastic upper limb in cerebral palsy. In: Lamb DW, editor. *The Paralyzed Hand*. Edinburgh: Churchill Livingstone, pp 153–160.

Ziv I, Blackburn N, Rang M, Koreska J (1984) Muscle growth in normal and spastic mice. *Dev Med Child Neurol* 26: 94–99.

16

MOTOR LEARNING IN CHILDREN WITH CEREBRAL PALSY: IMPLICATIONS FOR REHABILITATION

Shailesh S. Kantak, Katherine J. Sullivan and Patricia Burtner

Learning movement skills is an important part of normal development in children. Throughout their childhood and adolescence, children continue to learn motor tasks of increasing complexity associated with their expected social roles. In contrast, children with cerebral palsy (CP) are limited in their activity performance and participation due to multiple sensorimotor and cognitive impairments (Beckung and Hagberg 2002, Schenker et al 2005a, 2005b). A major purpose of physical rehabilitation in children with cerebral palsy is to provide a therapeutic intervention that includes motor skill learning to increase independence and participation in daily routines. Advances in rehabilitation research have led to a better understanding of the processes associated with neurorecovery and motor learning. Understanding and incorporating this evidence into practice can lead to more effective rehabilitation strategies. Having an insight into the processes associated with motor skill performance and learning will enable the therapist to conduct more effective practice by helping their clients to better learn a wide variety of movement skills. The purpose of this chapter is to review the findings emerging from the motor learning literature in order to understand the implications that they may have in physical rehabilitation of children with cerebral palsy.

Motor skill acquisition is the *process* by which an individual learns a motor skill. A child has achieved a motor skill when the movement task can be performed efficiently, accurately, consistently and with considerable flexibility. Starkes and Allard (1993) propose that skill acquisition involves both cognitive and motor processes. For example, throwing a basketball accurately requires certain decision-making processes such as anticipation, planning, and regulation of force. The mental work involved in decision making requires cognitive effort (Sherwood and Lee 2003). Given that motor skill acquisition requires both motor processes and cognitive effort, effective skill learning results from the interaction of motor and cognitive systems with the task and environmental demands.

Children with cerebral palsy have multiple motor system impairments, such as weakness, decreased movement selectivity and spasticity. Additional challenges include the sensory and cognitive-perceptual deficits commonly present in these children. It is likely that the combined motor, sensory, and cognitive-perceptual impairments associated with cerebral palsy have a profound influence on the processes involved in motor learning in these children. Current literature provides some insights into the processes involved during motor learning in young healthy adults; however there is little research investigating these processes in children, especially those with cerebral palsy. Further, we do not have a satisfactory understanding of how multiple sensorimotor and cognitive impairments affect the process of skill acquisition.

Motor learning: definition and learning–performance distinction

Motor learning has been defined as a set of processes associated with practice or experience leading to *relatively permanent changes* in the capability for movement (Schmidt and Lee 2004). In a clinical or a real-world setting, learning cannot be directly measured because it is a set of internal neural events, such as the enhanced efficacy of existing synapses within a neural network that develops with repetition. Therefore, motor learning is inferred by observing motor performance. In the clinic, improvements in the ability to perform motor skills, which are retained between treatment sessions, would indicate that the client has learned.

The learning–performance distinction is an important concept which discriminates between the observed motor behaviour (i.e. motor performance) and the resilience of this behaviour which develops over practice and is sustained over time (i.e. motor learning). Performance is influenced by a number of temporary factors, such as motivation or mood, and hence does not reflect the 'relatively permanent change' in the capability to produce the desired movement. Therefore, motor learning is inferred when the learner accurately and consistently performs a motor skill in different settings and across various points in time. In other words, learning refers to the processes involved in the 'carry-over' of the skill that has been learned. This learning–performance distinction is of utmost significance because conditions of practice and feedback that improve performance can interfere with cognitive processes that promote motor learning (Schmidt and Bjork 1992). It is important that the therapist sets up the practice environments in a manner that would maximally facilitate long-term functional changes (learning) rather than immediate performance (Winstein 1991).

The process of motor learning

Motor learning is an active, problem-solving process, during which the learner uses motor and cognitive resources to acquire a skill. For example, a child learning to hit a baseball needs to actively learn the strategies for anticipating the exact time to hit the ball as well as for deciding the exact amount of force that needs to be used as the ball passes over the plate. Therefore, the child has to make decisions based on the task and environmental constraints to produce the most efficient and effective motor output.

This decision making requires active information processing on the part of the learner. The ability of the learner to use task-related cognitive processes is an important determinant of how well the skill is learned (Sherwood and Lee 2003). Information-processing demands change as the learner acquires motor skills. In the next section, we will discuss the stages of information processing that evolve over the course of motor skill learning as well as how different impairments in motor and cognitive systems influence those stages.

Information processing involves cognitive processes, whereby information from the environment and task is analysed for its relevance and related to past memories of movements and respective outcomes. In other words, it is an elaboration of sensorimotor information that evolves from attention to perception, and ultimately to meaning or goal relevance. In addition, motor learning includes specific processes associated with the selection of a motor response and appropriate force and timing parameters to execute the response. According to Schmidt and Lee (2004), information processing involves three stages: (1) stimulus identification, (2) response selection, and (3) response programming.

The *stimulus identification* stage involves detection, recognition and interpretation of a stimulus from the environment. Detection of a relevant stimulus requires selective attention, while recognition and interpretation involve memory processes and ability to evaluate the significance of the stimulus for task performance. Evidence exists to indicate that the ability to selectively attend to relevant stimuli and inhibit irrelevant stimuli improves with age (Tipper et al 1989). Identification of relevant task-related stimuli in children with cerebral palsy is further challenged by significant attention deficits (Katz et al 1998), visuoperceptual disorders (Marozas and May 1985, Menken et al 1987, Stiers et al 2002) and movement-related memory deficits (Lesny et al 1990, White and Christ 2005).

Therapists can assist these children by providing necessary cues to recognize an appropriate environment to attend to relevant stimuli, as well as important sources of task-related information. Specific therapy for treatment of perceptual disorders may promote the child's ability to explore the environment for task-related information. With deficits in memory, learning may be slower in children with cerebral palsy and may require extended bouts of practice for retention.

In the *response selection* phase, the learner makes decisions about selection of movement strategy based on the stimulus identification and recognition. For example, in order to pick up a pencil, use of a lateral pinch grip is more appropriate than other kinds of grasp. In the *response programming* phase, the learner organizes the motor system to produce the motor response. In this phase, the learner selects appropriate parameters to execute the movements.

If the learner is new to the task, the process of response selection and programming will involve more cognitive and decision-making processes, and this may delay execution. For example, in order to lift a novel object, we utilize information about object properties such as size and shape to select and programme our responses. On the other hand, if we have prior experience with the task, we rely on our past experience or memory representations (internal model) to produce a response in a feed-forward manner (Gordon et al 1993). These anticipatory (or feed-forward) mechanisms use prior knowledge or experience to produce or modify automatic and voluntary movements (Winstein et al 2000).

Evidence from studies investigating grip forces during prehension suggests that children with cerebral palsy are unable to use information about object properties effectively to scale the rate of grip and load forces during prehension of novel objects (Eliasson et al 1992). Compared to typically developing healthy controls, children with hemiplegic CP demonstrate deficient anticipatory control for complex grasping tasks and use on-line control for complex movement performance (Mutsaarts et al 2005). However, they are able to use appropriate anticipatory forces to grasp objects that are familiar to them in their daily use (Duff and Gordon 2003). Several studies have demonstrated that with extended practice children with CP have the capability to form internal representational models of movements (Gordon and Duff 1999, Duff and Gordon 2003).

The process of response selection and programming in children with cerebral palsy is further challenged by the limited number of movement repertoires available to them (Mutsaarts et al 2004, Mackey et al 2005). Therefore, they may not be able to choose the most appropriate and economical movement pattern for a response. The therapist may help such children to enhance their resources – i.e. the movement-related range of motion and strength available to them – by applying interventions targeted to treat these impairments (Damiano and Abel 1998, Blundell et al 2003, Lyon et al 2005, Morton et al 2005). These enhanced movement-related resources may then be incorporated into practice of functional skills (Blundell et al 2003).

STAGES OF MOTOR LEARNING
Information-processing demands change during the process of motor learning. Fitts and Posner (1967) propose that the process of motor learning occurs in stages, described as the cognitive phase, the associative phase and the autonomous phase.

During the *cognitive phase*, the learner is new to the task and tries out different strategies to attain success. During this phase, the learner makes frequent errors and displays variable performance. This stage requires considerable cognitive processing in order to determine appropriate strategies to achieve success. Successful strategies are retained while inappropriate ones are discarded, thus leading to higher performance gains during this phase. In this stage of learning, feedback serves as an important source of information for selection and modification of strategies.

The second phase of the motor learning process is the *associative phase*. By this time, the learner has selected the optimal strategy to solve the motor problem and attempts to refine the skill. Error is gradually reduced and performance becomes more consistent. It is proposed that, during this stage, the learner begins to rely less on augmented feedback and tries to attend more to his own intrinsic feedback mechanisms. With further extended practice, the learner shifts to the *autonomous phase*, in which the motor skill is performed more automatically with minimal error. The cognitive effort required during this stage is less than that required in the earlier stages.

In summary, understanding that motor learning occurs in stages that require different levels of cognition is important when planning a therapeutic session for a child with cerebral palsy. It is also important to acknowledge that the phase of learning and corresponding performance proficiency will vary in relation to different factors such as skill level of the learner, task complexity and environmental demands.

Factors affecting performance and learning
Many factors – such as task, skill level of the learner, practice and instruction – influence the process of motor learning. Of these, practice and feedback are the most significant and

well-studied. Motor learning research demonstrates that schedules of practice and feedback which may be effective in improving performance during practice may not be optimal for promoting learning (Winstein 1991, Schmidt and Bjork 1992). Clinically, we observe motor performance when the patient practises the task during a therapy session. Learning is inferred by observing the patient's performance in the following therapy session, with no feedback or cueing provided. Performance at this moment would reveal the task-related learning that occurred as a result of the previous therapy session and any practice at home. Another measure of learning is the ability of the patient to generalize what was learned to other tasks or environments.

Consistently, motor learning studies of healthy young adults demonstrate that motor learning is enhanced when conditions of practice and feedback that require greater cognitive effort are used. Cognitive effort refers to the mental processes that are involved in decision making during learning (Sherwood and Lee 2003). While increased cognitive effort is associated with increased evidence of motor learning, it is not clear if this finding can be generalized to children – whether typically developing or with cerebral palsy – as there are known differences in information processing in children.

Designing a therapeutic practice session to enhance motor skill learning involves making decisions about task selection, practice and feedback schedules. Further, as therapists, we also want to know how instruction and physical guidance during therapy influence learning. Providing absolute answers to these questions is a very difficult task. This section of the chapter will review the literature that investigates the effects of different practice and feedback variables on motor learning in healthy young adults, typically developing children and children with cerebral palsy. Theoretical constructs of information processing that underlie these effects and subsequent therapeutic implications will be discussed. Understanding these principles will assist the therapist in making informed decisions during the structuring of practice sessions.

PRACTICE STRUCTURE AFFECTS LEARNING
The single most important variable that significantly influences motor learning is *practice*. Practice is different from rote repetition, where a movement is repeated without aiming for a functional goal. During therapy, practice is comprised of purposeful repetition with the aim of improving the child's skill in functional task performance. This is achieved by making practice a problem-solving process in which the child is presented with a task-related problem that forces them to plan and execute a purposeful goal-directed movement. Thus, a therapeutic practice session aimed at enhancing motor learning makes the child an active participant in therapy rather than just a passive recipient (Marley et al 2000).

Practice-related factors such as the scheduling of activities during practice or the variability of practice are examples of practice conditions that can promote greater problem solving, and hence enhance motor learning in children. The following sections describe how these factors can be manipulated during therapy to increase skill acquisition and learning.

Part- vs whole-task practice

When training in a new skill, the therapist is often presented with the question of whether the skill should be practised as a whole or whether it should be broken down into component parts and each component practised separately. Often, it is assumed that practising parts of the skill will ultimately improve the child's capacity to perform the whole skill. For example, isolated elbow extension or the opening and closing of the hand are practised as parts of the whole functional skill of reaching and grasping.

The effectiveness of part- vs whole-task practice depends on the type of task being practiced, and therefore on the underlying motor control mechanisms of the criterion task. Learning of a serial task that can be broken down into components can be enhanced by practising the components of the task in a specific order. It is suggested that part-task practice can be effective when learning tasks that can be naturally broken down into units that reflect the inherent goals of the task (Winstein 1991). For example, donning and doffing a shirt may be broken down into parts, which include buttoning and unbuttoning the shirt, and putting the shirt on and taking it off. On the other hand, a task such as reach-to-grasp requires coordination and timing which allow for smooth and accurate motor control between the reach and grasp components of this discrete task. Tasks such as these, which require learning the relationship between critical phases of a movement, do not benefit from part-task practice (Marley et al 2000). For instance, having a child practise scooping food at the same time as learning to eat with a spoon may be more effective in developing independence in eating than learning the tasks separately.

Constant vs variable practice

Variable practice involves practising a task under a variety of conditions, such as throwing bean bags at a target set at different distances. This is in contrast to constant practice where the task is practised under the same conditions (e.g. putting blocks on a shelf at one height). There is evidence to suggest that variable practice leads to more effective learning than practice under constant conditions, in healthy young adults (Shea and Kohl 1990, 1991) and in typically developing children (Kerr and Booth 1978, Shapiro and Schmidt 1982). Unfortunately, this has not been tested in children with cerebral palsy. It is thought that practice with different parameter conditions (i.e. different sizes, shapes, weights, heights) leads to a better capacity on the part of the learner to form an abstract 'rule' about the relationship between the movement outcome and the parameters used for the movement. Learning a 'movement rule', such as how to throw a ball overhand, under various 'movement parameter specifications', such as different distances, increases the likelihood of generating an accurate movement in a novel movement situation.

In children with cerebral palsy, it has been suggested by some authors that an adapted variable practice schedule may be beneficial to learning (Valvano 2004). It is proposed that practice under constant conditions may be beneficial in the earlier stages of learning when information-processing resources are directed towards attaining the basic coordination of movement. Once the movement coordination is attained, varying the parameter conditions may be beneficial in promoting the child's capacity to produce the movements under different conditions. This, however, has not been empirically tested.

Random vs blocked practice

During therapy, a child practises a number of tasks, such as throwing, pushing/pulling, pouring, sorting to practise grasp/release, etc. Therapists often face the decision of the optimal order in which these tasks should be practised so as to maximize learning. Practice of multiple tasks (e.g. A, B, C) can be scheduled in blocks such that practice of task A is followed by practice of task B, followed by practice of task C (e.g. AAA . . . BBB . . . CCC). Alternatively, the order of these three tasks can be random across the practice session (e.g. ACBCABCBA . . .). It has been demonstrated in young able-bodied adults that random practice is effective in promoting motor learning, evident in retention and transfer tests, even though it degrades performance during acquisition (Shea and Morgan 1979).

The greater effectiveness of random practice compared to blocked-order practice is attributed to the contextual interference (CI) effect, which refers to the cognitive interference due to trial-to-trial instability. Thus, blocked practice causes less CI while random practice results in high interference. In random practice, the switching between tasks induces a 'forgetting' of the action plan of the first task as the interspersed task is planned and executed. In other words, each interspersed task induces interference that requires reconstruction of the subsequent task's action plan (Lee and Magill 1983). This reconstruction is not necessary in blocked practice conditions where the action plan stays in working memory. The higher cognitive effort required during random order practice facilitates motor learning.

Research investigating the CI effect in children has yielded mixed results. Some studies (Pollock and Lee 1997, Granda Vera and Montilla 2003) have demonstrated the superiority of random practice in promoting learning in children, while others (French et al 1990, Jarus and Goverover 1999) have shown no difference between the effects of blocked and random practice. Still others have demonstrated that blocked practice leads to better learning in children (Pinto-Zipp and Gentile 1995, Farrow 1997, Jarus and Gutman 2001). These studies collectively suggest that the effect of the order of practice on motor learning in children depends upon multiple factors, such as the complexity of the task, level of skill, and age of the children (Jarus and Gutman 2001, Wulf and Shea 2002). In general, it has been observed that blocked-order practice leads to more effective learning than random practice in younger and less skilled children, especially when the tasks are complex. When the tasks are more complex, with high memory, attentional and motor demands, random-order practice may 'overload' the system, thereby limiting the ability to learn the skills. In such situations, blocked practice may be better at promoting motor learning (Albaret and Thon 1998, Wulf and Shea 2002).

Few studies have evaluated the effects of random and blocked practice schedules in children with cerebral palsy. Duff and Gordon (2003) investigated the effects of random and blocked schedules on the ability of children with cerebral palsy to develop an internal model for grasping. Children practised grasping and lifting three object shapes (with identical volumes), each having a different weight, either in a blocked or in a random order of practice. Children with cerebral palsy were able to develop and retain an internal memory representation of the novel objects for anticipatory control irrespective of the type of practice schedule employed. However, these results cannot be generalized to all forms of learning as this particular task was employed to investigate learning of internal representation and involved the same movement (grasping) but different object-weight and force associations.

It is not clear how brain injury in children affects various higher level cognitive processes such as memory for reconstruction, ability to contrast tasks, etc. More research is needed to make inferences about these cognitive processes by investigating the type of practice schedule that would be most beneficial for learning in children with cerebral palsy.

FEEDBACK-RELATED VARIABLES INFLUENCE LEARNING

Feedback has a strong influence on motor performance and learning. While practising a task, a child receives intrinsic feedback from visual, proprioceptive and auditory systems about their performance. This information is often supplemented by augmented feedback in the form of knowledge of results (KR) and/or knowledge of performance (KP) as the therapist provides verbal, visual or tactile information and encouragement and reward during training. KR consists of terminal feedback about the outcome of the movement in terms of the environmental goal, while KP consists of information about the quality of the movement performed.

Research has demonstrated developmental differences in the use of feedback during motor skill acquisition (Barclay and Newell 1980, Gallagher and Thomas 1980). For instance, Gallagher and Thomas (1980) demonstrated that younger children process feedback information more slowly than adults. They also suggested that too much information contained in extremely precise KR may interfere with skill acquisition.

Augmented feedback helps motor skill acquisition by giving the learner information about the movement such that errors in the movement can be corrected while the successful aspects may be retained. However, if the feedback is given frequently or continuously, it interferes with problem-solving cognitive processes that should occur during practice and 'guide' the learner to the optimal response. Studies examining the effects of different feedback frequencies in healthy young adults (Winstein and Schmidt 1990), older adults (Behrman et al 1992) and adults with stroke (Winstein et al 1999) demonstrate that less frequent feedback during practice promotes motor learning. It is proposed that reduced frequency of augmented feedback allows the learner to attend to the processing of intrinsic feedback, leading to better error detection strategies, which may help promote learning.

There is a scarcity of evidence related to effects of different schedules of feedback presentation in both typically developing children and children with cerebral palsy. A recent study (Kantak et al 2006) evaluated the effect of reduced relative frequency of feedback on motor learning of a discrete arm movement task in typically developing children compared to healthy young adults. In this study, children (average age 9 years) were assigned to one of two groups. One group received feedback about task error and accuracy after every arm movement (100 per cent feedback frequency). The other group received feedback after every trial for the first 50 trials of practice, but the feedback was then reduced until they received feedback only 25 per cent of the time for the last 50 trials, out of 200 total trials of practice. The researchers reported that motor learning benefits were more evident in children who received frequent feedback, particularly during a retention test on the next day when no feedback was presented. Children who received less frequent feedback did not demonstrate evidence of learning during the no-feedback retention test. However, evidence of motor learning was present in the reduced feedback group. When additional practice was provided, performance was just as accurate as the 100 per cent feedback group. This finding demonstrates that there is a critical point when feedback reduction interferes with motor learning in children, which is not demonstrated in adults. It appears that typically developing children need longer periods of practice with more frequent feedback compared to adults before feedback can be reduced during practice.

Few studies have investigated how children with cerebral palsy use feedback for motor learning. In a study by Thorpe and Valvano (2002) 13 children with diplegic or quadriplegic cerebral palsy practised riding a therapeutic vehicle in a backward direction. The participants received no augmented feedback, KP or cognitive strategies in the course of the practice session. It was observed that children with cerebral palsy benefited from practice. Some (eight) of the children were able to use cognitive strategies and KP for learning.

It is not known what kind of feedback schedules enhance motor learning in children with cerebral palsy. However, some predictions can be made about the effects of reducing relative frequency of feedback by reviewing the mechanisms that underlie the beneficial effect of reduced feedback frequency. Bruechert et al (2003) proposed that reducing the feedback frequency challenges the error detection capacity in healthy young adults. Harbourne (2001) demonstrated that the ability to detect errors was affected in children with cerebral palsy, compared to healthy age-matched controls, leading to more errors in a linear positioning task. If error detection is one of the reasons that account for the beneficial effects of reduced feedback frequency on learning, it may be hypothesized that with deficient error detection capability, children with cerebral palsy may benefit from more frequent feedback. This needs to be tested empirically.

One manner of scheduling feedback which has been shown to be effective is the use of bandwidth feedback. In this method, the therapist provides feedback only when the performance is outside an accepted tolerance level. For instance, in a child with spastic quadriplegia, feedback about accuracy during a writing task may only be provided when errors go beyond a defined space width. This could be done by setting a writing task with wide-ruled paper. When the number of errors (i.e. writing outside the lines) is reduced to a predetermined threshold, then narrower-ruled paper can be introduced. The concept of bandwidth feedback can be used in temporal tasks (completing a task within a given time limit) as well as in spatial tasks as in this example. This manner of reducing the frequency of feedback has been shown to be very effective in healthy adults because it is tailored to individual skill level. However, its effectiveness has not been tested in the paediatric population.

Another common form of feedback used in a therapeutic setting is continuous or concurrent feedback. Biofeedback, computer-assisted feedback and continuous guidance by a therapist are some examples of concurrent feedback observed in a clinical environment. In studies in adults, concurrent feedback has been shown to be detrimental to motor learning, although it benefits performance during acquisition (Winstein et al 1996). There is little research investigating the effects of concurrent feedback on motor learning in children with and without neuromuscular disorders. However, clinical trials have demonstrated the effectiveness of biofeedback as an adjunct to rehabilitation in cerebral palsy in improving impairments such as tone (O'Dwyer et al 1994) and range of motion (Toner et al 1998) as well as gait parameters (Colborne et al 1994, Dursun et al 2004). Thus, it is not clear how typically developing children and children with brain damage use feedback for motor skill acquisition. There is a need for systematic motor learning studies which examine the cognitive processes underlying the use of feedback in children with cerebral palsy.

ROLE OF INSTRUCTIONS

An important component of the practice schedule which affects performance and learning is instruction. Since we conceptualize practice as a problem-solving event, instructions need to be directed to the goals of the task to be practised. Too much information in the instructions may benefit performance but hinder learning.

Instructions have an effect on motor performance and learning by directing the learner's attention to the important aspects of the task and/or movement. Directing the focus of attention during delivery of instructions has been shown to influence learning in adults. It has been demonstrated that instructions that direct the learner's attention to the movement outcome in the environment are more beneficial for learning than instructions that direct the learner's attention to their own movements (Wulf and Prinz 2001). Van der Weel et al (1991) demonstrated that children with cerebral palsy responded with greater range of movement during concrete instructions than during abstract instructions, as compared to non-disabled children, who showed no difference in their response to the two types of instructions.

INFLUENCE OF PHYSICAL ASSISTANCE

Physical assistance is the most common form of guidance used by therapists when treating patients with neurological disorders. Even though guidance techniques have long been regarded as an effective means to teach movement skills (Howle 2002) research in motor learning suggests otherwise. It has been consistently demonstrated that physical assistance or handling techniques aimed at leading the learner to the optimal movement have strong performance-enhancing effects during practice; however, these effects are temporary. That is, when the guidance is withdrawn, the learner demonstrates poor performance, indicating that the learner becomes 'dependent' on the guidance (Schmidt 1991). This suggests that physically guiding a child to perform a task may not be the most effective method of promoting motor learning.

Does this mean that any physical assistance during therapy is detrimental to learning? The answer is 'no'. Wulf and Shea (2002) propose that physical assistance during practice may be conducive to learning of a complex skill as long as it allows the learner to explore the 'perceptual-motor workspace'. In other words, the therapist may provide assistance to allow the child to explore multiple solutions to the task, rather than guiding the child to the optimal movement. For example, a therapist may provide assistance to optimize the biomechanical alignment of the child during sitting, as the child actively performs a reaching task. This may allow the child to explore more degrees of freedom by performing the task actively, thus promoting better learning.

Do motor learning principles apply to learning of fine motor skills?

During therapy, a child practises tasks that incorporate gross motor as well as fine motor skills. It has been proposed that fine motor skills such as in-hand manipulation are highly dependent on cognition (Exner 1995). Therefore, training fine motor functions needs to involve an active problem-solving approach. It has been suggested that training of fine motor skills must involve training of cognitive strategies used to perform the task successfully (Eliasson 2005). For example, to train a child to put a book in a book-bag, each step in the task must be explicitly memorized and executed. Despite the limited literature investigating fine motor skill acquisition, we present evidence and a rationale to support the idea that the principles of motor learning emerging from investigations using experimental tasks can be applied to the learning of fine motor skills.

In addition to using cognitive strategies, there is evidence to demonstrate that physical practice of fine motor tasks leads to improvements in children with cerebral palsy (Eliasson et al 2003). In a study by Eliasson and colleagues (2003) nine adolescents with hemiplegic cerebral palsy practised an in-hand manipulation task for 15–20 minutes daily for two weeks. Learning was measured at the baseline, at retention (at the end of two weeks) and at a follow-up after five months. The researchers observed a significant improvement in the performance of the practised in-hand manipulation task after two weeks of practice and even at the five-month follow-up. This study provides evidence to support the idea that physical practice benefits acquisition of fine motor skills.

In order to further enhance the process of skill acquisition, the practice session and feedback can be scheduled such that we optimally challenge the problem-solving capability. This optimal challenge and the subsequent cognitive effort have been demonstrated to allow the learner to better retain fine motor skills. For example, in a study by Ste-Marie et al (2004), elementary school children showed better retention of handwriting skills when they practised tasks in a random order. This suggests that the manner in which the tasks are scheduled during practice affects the retention of fine motor skills.

Feedback forms an important part of learning – more so in fine motor skill acquisition because of high accuracy constraints. However, if the feedback takes the form of guidance instead of information, the process of learning is adversely affected. This was well illustrated by Naka (1998), who compared the effects of repeated writing with feedback, repeated writing without any feedback, and tracing on memory for pseudo-characters and foreign letters in three groups of children. Results demonstrated that children who practised repeated writing with feedback had better recall than those who practised tracing or repeated writing without feedback. Of the three groups, the children who traced the letters had the worst recall. This suggests that practice of a fine motor skill can be made more effective by scheduling feedback in a manner that provides optimal information to the learner *without* guiding him/her to the optimal outcome.

In conclusion, we propose that the effectiveness of a therapeutic practice session to train fine motor skills can be enhanced by invoking optimal cognitive effort through appropriate manipulation of variables related to practice and feedback. More research is needed to gain a better insight into the process of fine motor skill acquisition and how cognitive effort affects it.

Conceptual algorithm to enhance motor learning in children with cerebral palsy

The therapeutic practice session is complex. The effectiveness of a therapeutic practice session depends on the dynamic interaction of multiple variables that can influence both motor performance and motor learning. Therefore, the principles that emerge from behavioural research in motor learning can be used as guidelines for clinical practice since there is limited research that translates basic science findings into clinical practice. Fig. 16.1

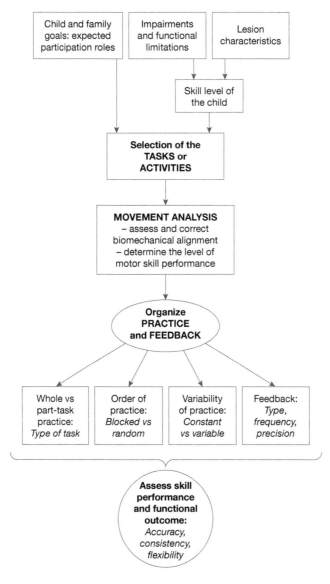

Fig. 16.1 Algorithm for designing a therapeutic intervention for enhancing motor learning.

proposes an algorithm to incorporate motor learning principles into the design of therapeutic interventions that aim to enhance motor skill learning. The algorithm outlines four major levels of decision making to enhance motor skill acquisition in rehabilitation: task selection, movement analysis, organizing practice and feedback, and assessing appropriate outcomes.

Task Selection: Significance of Patient's Goals and Skill Level

The therapist is responsible for developing task-related goals that will increase participation and improve the child's quality of life (Valvano 2004). These goals should be set in accordance with the recent conceptual models for management of cerebral palsy which emphasize family-centred care and participation in family, school and community activities (Bartlett and Palisano 2000).

Another important factor that influences task selection is the level of skill of the child. Given that the severity of CP varies widely, the skill level of the child will depend on lesion characteristics and impairments in sensorimotor and cognitive systems. A specific functional task would represent different challenge levels for children with differing abilities and skill levels (Wulf and Shea 2002, Guadagnoli and Lee 2004). Evidence emerging from the literature suggests that in order to ensure effective motor learning, practice conditions should be modified in relation to the difficulty of the task and the skill level of the performer (Guadagnoli and Lee 2004). Thus, it is important to match the difficulty level of the task to the skill level of the child in order to provide an optimal challenge to the child.

Movement Analysis

Movement analysis is an important tool which allows for an assessment of how system impairments (primary and secondary) and environmental factors affect functional task performance. It also reveals different planning, execution and compensatory strategies that the child employs to achieve the task. Movement analysis also allows determination of the skill level of the learner and relative task complexity.

Movement analysis helps in planning specific strategies directed at treating system impairments and enhancing movement-related resources. In addition, it allows for making appropriate decisions about scaling the task and environmental demands during practice so as to provide an optimal challenge to the child.

Organizing Practice and Feedback

To maximize learning benefits, a therapeutic practice session must pose an optimal cognitive-motor challenge to the child. Practice and feedback conditions, as well as relative task complexity, interact to provide this challenge. Given that practice and feedback are the two most significant variables that influence motor skill acquisition, they should be organized in a manner that will invoke optimal information processing and cognitive effort. An understanding of how different schedules/variability of practice and feedback affect skill acquisition in children with CP will help the therapist make informed decisions about the organization of practice and feedback.

272

Skill is an ability to perform a task with accuracy, consistency and flexibility. The functional outcome measures used to assess the efficacy and effectiveness of a therapeutic practice session must evaluate the acquisition of the skill. In other words, they should assess the accuracy, consistency and flexibility of the task performance.

Summary and future directions
In the current era of evidence-based practice, it is unfortunate that there is very limited literature on motor learning in typically developing children and children with neurological disorders. The challenge for researchers in the field is to conduct experiments to understand the information-processing and motor control processes that implement behavioural improvements following practice in the paediatric population. From a therapeutic perspective, research must focus on the dynamic interaction of multiple impairments, task complexity, and practice and feedback variables, and how these factors affect learning. Further, all these principles need to be integrated with principles of neural plasticity while designing clinical trials to provide the highest level of evidence to the clinical practitioner. The challenge for the clinician is to incorporate an evidence-based approach into designing interventions for their paediatric patients. The art of therapy emerges from the ability of the therapist to integrate the scientific principles of motor learning and neural plasticity by designing a goal-oriented task practice that is optimally complex and challenging for the patient's level of skill. Such evidence-based interventions will enhance our patients' ability to maximize their independence and participation in daily routines.

REFERENCES

Albaret JM, Thon B (1998) Differential effects of task complexity on contextual interference in a drawing task. *Acta Psychol* 100: 9–24.

Barclay CR, Newell KM (1980) Children's processing of information in motor skill acquisition. *J Exp Child Psychol* 30: 98–108.

Bartlett DJ, Palisano R J (2000) A multivariate model of determinants of motor change for children with cerebral palsy. *Phys Ther* 80: 598–614.

Beckung E, Hagberg G (2002) Neuroimpairments, activity limitations, and participation restrictions in children with cerebral palsy. *Dev Med Child Neurol* 44: 309–316.

Behrman AL, Vander Linden DW, Cauraugh JH (1992) Relative frequency knowledge of results: older adults learning a force-time modulation task. *J Hum Mov Stud* 23: 233–250.

Blundell SW, Shepherd RB, Dean CM, Adams RD, Cahill BM (2003) Functional strength training in cerebral palsy: a pilot study of a group circuit training class for children aged 4–8 years. *Clin Rehabil* 17: 48–57.

Bruechert L, Lai Q, Shea CH (2003) Reduced knowledge of results frequency enhances error detection. *Res Q Exerc Sport* 74: 467–472.

Colborne GR, Wright FV, Naumann S (1994) Feedback of triceps surae EMG in gait of children with cerebral palsy: a controlled study. *Arch Phys Med Rehabil* 75: 40–45.

Damiano DL, Abel MF (1998) Functional outcomes of strength training in spastic cerebral palsy. *Arch Phys Med Rehabil* 79: 119–125.

Duff SV, Gordon AM (2003) Learning of grasp control in children with hemiplegic cerebral palsy. *Dev Med Child Neurol* 45: 746–757.

Dursun E, Dursun N, Alican D (2004) Effects of biofeedback treatment on gait in children with cerebral palsy. *Disabil Rehabil* 26: 116–120.

Eliasson AC (2005) Improving the use of hands in daily activities: aspects of the treatment of children with cerebral palsy. *Phys Occup Ther Pediatr* 25: 37–60.

Eliasson AC, Gordon AM, Forssberg H (1992) Impaired anticipatory control of isometric forces during grasping by children with cerebral palsy. *Dev Med Child Neurol* 34: 216–225.

Eliasson AC, Bonnier B, Krumlinde-Sundholm L (2003) Clinical experience of constraint induced movement therapy in adolescents with hemiplegic cerebral palsy – a day camp model. *Dev Med Child Neurol* 45: 357–359.

Exner C (1995) *Cognition and Motor Skill.* St Louis: Mosby.

Farrow DMW (1997) The effects of contextual interference on children learning forehand tennis groundstrokes. *J Hum Mov Stud* 33: 47–67.

Fitts PM, Posner MI (1967) *Human Performance.* Belmont, CA: Brooks-Cole.

French KE, Rink JE, Werner PF (1990) Effects of contextual interference on retention of three volleyball skills. *Percept Mot Skills* 71: 179–186.

Gallagher JD, Thomas JR (1980) Effects of varying post-KR intervals upon children's motor performance. *J Mot Behav* 12: 41–56.

Gordon AM, Duff SV (1999) Fingertip forces during object manipulation in children with hemiplegic cerebral palsy. I: anticipatory scaling. *Dev Med Child Neurol* 41: 166–175.

Gordon AM, Westling G, Cole KJ, Johansson RS (1993) Memory representations underlying motor commands used during manipulation of common and novel objects. *J Neurophysiol* 69: 1789–1796.

Granda Vera J, Montilla MM (2003) Practice schedule and acquisition, retention, and transfer of a throwing task in 6-yr-old children. *Percept Mot Skills* 96: 1015–1024.

Guadagnoli MA, Lee TD (2004) Challenge point: a framework for conceptualizing the effects of various practice conditions in motor learning. *J Mot Behav* 36: 212–224.

Harbourne RT (2001) Accuracy of movement speed and error detection skills in adolescents with cerebral palsy. *Percept Mot Skills* 93: 419–431.

Howle J (2002) *Neurodevelopmental Treatment Approach: Theoretical Foundations and Principles of Clinical Practice.* Laguna Beach, CA: Neuro-Developmental Treatment Association.

Jarus T, Goverover Y (1999) Effects of contextual interference and age on acquisition, retention, and transfer of motor skill. *Percept Mot Skills* 88: 437–447.

Jarus T, Gutman T (2001) Effects of cognitive processes and task complexity on acquisition, retention, and transfer of motor skills. *Can J Occup Ther* 68: 280–289.

Kantak SS, Sullivan K, Burtner PA (2006) Effects of reduced frequency feedback on motor performance and learning in children. *Pediatr Phys Ther* 18: 76.

Katz N, Cermak S, Shamir Y (1998) Unilateral neglect in children with hemiplegic cerebral palsy. *Percept Mot Skills* 86: 539–550.

Kerr R, Booth B (1978) Specific and varied practice of motor skill. *Percept Mot Skills* 46: 395–401.

Lee TD, Magill RA (1983) The locus of contextual interference in motor skill acquisition. *J Exp Psychol: Learn Mem Cogn* 9: 730–746.

Lesny I, Nachtmann M, Stehlik A, Tomankova A, Zajidkova J (1990) Disorders of memory of motor sequences in cerebral palsied children. *Brain Dev* 12: 339–341.

Lyon R, Liu X, Schwab J, Harris G (2005) Kinematic and kinetic evaluation of the ankle joint before and after tendo achilles lengthening in patients with spastic diplegia. *J Pediatr Orthop* 25: 479–483.

Mackey AH, Walt SE, Lobb GA, Stott NS (2005) Reliability of upper and lower limb three-dimensional kinematics in children with hemiplegia. *Gait Posture* 22: 1–9.

Marley TL, Ezekiel HJ, Lehto NK, Wishart LR, Lee TD (2000) Application of motor learning principles: the physiotherapy client as a problem-solver. II. Scheduling practice. *Physiother Can* 52: 315–320.

Marozas DS, May DC (1985) Effects of figure-ground reversal on the visual-perceptual and visuo-motor performances of cerebral palsied and normal children. *Percept Mot Skills* 60: 591–598.

Menken C, Cermak SA, Fisher A (1987) Evaluating the visual-perceptual skills of children with cerebral palsy. *Am J Occup Ther* 41: 646–651.

Morton JF, Brownlee M, McFadyen AK (2005) The effects of progressive resistance training for children with cerebral palsy. *Clin Rehabil* 19: 283–289.

Mutsaarts M, Steenbergen B, Meulenbroek R (2004) A detailed analysis of the planning and execution of prehension movements by three adolescents with spastic hemiparesis due to cerebral palsy. *Exp Brain Res* 156: 293–304.

Mutsaarts M, Steenbergen B, Bekkering H (2005) Anticipatory planning of movement sequences in hemiparetic cerebral palsy. *Motor Control* 9: 439–458.

Naka M (1998) Repeated writing facilitates children's memory for pseudocharacters and foreign letters. *Mem Cognit* 26: 804–809.

O'Dwyer N, Neilson P, Nash J (1994) Reduction of spasticity in cerebral palsy using feedback of the tonic stretch reflex: a controlled study. *Dev Med Child Neurol* 36: 770–786.

Pinto-Zipp G, Gentile AM (1995) Practice schedules in motor learning: children vs. adults. *Soc Neurosci Abstracts* 21: 1620 (AQ1627).

Pollock BJ, Lee TD (1997) Dissociated contextual interference effects in children and adults. *Percept Mot Skills* 84: 851–858.

Ste-Marie DM, Clark SE, Findlay LC, Latimer AE (2004) High levels of contextual interference enhance handwriting skill acquisition. *J Mot Behav* 36: 115–126.

Schenker R, Coster WJ, Parush S (2005a) Neuroimpairments, activity performance, and participation in children with cerebral palsy mainstreamed in elementary schools. *Dev Med Child Neurol* 47: 808–814.

Schenker R, Coster W, Parush S (2005b) Participation and activity performance of students with cerebral palsy within the school environment. *Disabil Rehabil* 27: 539–552.

Schmidt RA (1991) Frequent augmented feedback can degrade learning: evidence and interpretations. In: Reequin R, Stelmach GE, editors. *Tutorials in Neuroscience.* Dordrecht: Kluwer.

Schmidt RA, Bjork RA (1992) New conceptualization of practice: common principles in three paradigms suggest new concepts for training. *Psychol Sci* 3: 207–217.

Schmidt RA, Lee TD (2004) *Motor Control and Learning: A Behavioral Emphasis, 4th edn.* Champaign, IL: Human Kinetics.

Shapiro DC, Schmidt RA (1982) The schema theory: recent evidence and developmental implications. In: Kelso JAS, Clark JE, editors. *The Development of Movement Control and Co-ordination.* New York: Wiley, pp. 113–150.

Shea CH, Kohl RM (1990) Specificity and variability of practice. *Res Q Exerc Sport* 61: 169–177.

Shea CH, Kohl RM (1991) Composition of practice: influence on the retention of motor skills. *Res Q Exerc Sport* 62: 187–195.

Shea JB, Morgan RL (1979) Contextual interference effects on the acquisition, retention, and transfer of a motor skill. *J Exp Psychol: Learn Mem Cogn* 5: 179–187.

Sherwood DE, Lee TD (2003) Schema theory: critical review and implications for the role of cognition in a new theory of motor learning. *Res Q Exerc Sport* 74: 376–382.

Starkes J, Allard F (1993) *Cognitive Issues in Motor Expertise.* Amsterdam: North Holland.

Stiers P, Vanderkelen R, Vanneste G, Coene S, De Rammelaere M, Vandenbussche E (2002) Visual-perceptual impairment in a random sample of children with cerebral palsy. *Dev Med Child Neurol* 44: 370–382.

Thorpe DE, Valvano JA (2002) The effects of knowledge or performance and cognitive strategies on motor skill learning in children with cerebral palsy. *Pediatr Phys Ther* 14: 2–15.

Tipper SP, Bourque TA, Anderson SH, Brehaut JC (1989) Mechanisms of attention: a developmental study. *J Exp Child Psychol* 48: 353–378.

Toner LV, Cook K, Elder GC (1998) Improved ankle function in children with cerebral palsy after computer-assisted motor learning. *Dev Med Child Neurol* 40: 829–835.

Valvano J (2004) Activity-focused motor interventions for children with neurological conditions. *Phys Occup Ther Pediatr* 24: 79–107.

van der Weel FR, van der Meer AL, Lee DN (1991) Effect of task on movement control in cerebral palsy: implications for assessment and therapy. *Dev Med Child Neurol* 33: 419–426.

White DA, Christ SE (2005) Executive control of learning and memory in children with bilateral spastic cerebral palsy. *J Int Neuropsychol Soc* 11: 920–924.

Winstein C (1991) Designing practice for motor learning: clinical implications. In: Lister MJ, editor. *Contemporary Management of Motor Control Problems: Proceedings of the II-STEP Conference.* Alexandria, VA: Foundation for Physical Therapy, pp. 65–76.

Winstein C, Schmidt RA (1990) Reduced frequency of knowledge of results enhances motor skill learning. *J Exp Psychol: Learn Mem Cogn* 16: 677–691.

Winstein CJ, Pohl PS, Cardinale C, Green A, Scholtz L, Waters CS (1996) Learning a partial-weight-bearing skill: effectiveness of two forms of feedback. *Phys Ther* 76: 985–993.

Winstein CJ, Merians AS, Sullivan KJ (1999) Motor learning after unilateral brain damage. *Neuropsychologia* 37: 975–987.

Winstein CJ, Horak FB, Fisher BE (2000) Influence of central set on anticipatory and triggered grip-force adjustments. *Exp Brain Res* 130: 298–308.

Wulf G, Prinz W (2001) Directing attention to movement effects enhances learning: a review. *Psychon Bull Rev* 8: 648–660.

Wulf G, Shea CH (2002) Principles derived from the study of simple skills do not generalize to complex skill learning. *Psychon Bull Rev* 9: 185–211.

17
A COGNITIVE PERSPECTIVE ON INTERVENTION

Cognitive orientation to daily occupational performance (CO-OP) in the child with upper extremity spasticity

A.D. Mandich, H.J. Polatajko and Ann Zilberbrant

Introduction

Children with cerebral palsy (CP) have motor-based difficulties that affect the performance of the activities of everyday living, incuding actiivites at home, in school and at play. Therapists are frequently consulted to assist these children with these motor-based activities. Various therapeutic approaches have been used in treatment, including neurodevelopmental treatment (NDT), conductive education, electrical stimulation, strength training, hippother-apy and saddle riding, targeted training, swimming, and pelvic positioning (Siebes et al 2002). However, a comprehensive review reported inconclusive results on the efficacy of these interventions (Steultjens et al 2004). One issue, as explained by Siebes et al (2002), is that the focus of treatment has been mainly on the children's impairments rather than limitations in skill performance. In their conclusions, Steultjens et al (2004) highlighted the need for intervention to focus on functional and social goals as outcome measures. Indeed, researchers have emphasized the importance of focusing interventions on enabling independent functioning in everyday life (Rosenbaum 2003).

Some researchers have emphasized the need to involve children and parents in the treatment, an approach that has been shown to be more effective (Barrera et al 1986, Shonkoff and Hauser-Cram 1987, Short et al 1989). Valvano (2004) has also suggested activity-focused treatment involving functional tasks for children with neurological impairments. Early evidence suggests such approaches may be effective in increasing motor function (e.g. Knox and Evans 2002). One such approach – cognitive orientation to daily occupational performance (CO-OP) – is unique among performance-based approaches because of its emphasis on the role of cognition in skill acquisition, its involvement of children and their parents and its focus on evidence. CO-OP has been shown to be effective in improving the performance of children with motor-based performance problems, specifically developmental coordination disorder (Polatajko et al 2001a). Early studies of the use of CO-OP with children with cerebral palsy and traumatic brain injury show the promise of this approach for these populations (Samonte et al 2004, Solish et al 2005).

This chapter will introduce CO-OP for use during intervention with children with motor problems. This approach involves a shift in the therapist's general approach to intervention, from components-based to performance-based assessment and from remediation to guided discovery. Intervention using cognitive orientation centres on identifying effective cognitive strategies that will increase motor competence. A case study will be used to illustrate the results of the application of CO-OP to assist a child with CP.

Cognitive orientation to daily occupational performance (CO-OP)
'CO-OP is a client-centred, performance-based, problem solving approach that enables skill acquisition through a process of strategy use and guided discovery' (Polatajko and Mandich 2004: 24). Embedded in a learning paradigm, CO-OP breaks from traditional, deficit-based views on motor performance and adopts a contemporary, learning-based perspective on motor skill acquisition.

CO-OP embraces the shift of the World Health Organization (WHO) from a disability model to a new framework for health and disability, the International Classification of Functioning, Disability and Health (ICF) (WHO 2001). Developed within a research context, CO-OP draws on the knowledge of a number of disciplines, including behavioural and cognitive psychology, health, human movement science and occupational therapy, to achieve its objectives (Polatajko and Mandich 2004).

OBJECTIVES OF CO-OP
Cognition forms the foundation of CO-OP and enables the achievement of the four objectives of CO-OP:

- Skill acquisition
- Cognitive strategy use
- Generalization
- Transfer of learning

The primary objective of CO-OP is **skill acquisition**. Congruent with the ICF model, CO-OP focuses at the level of activity and participation and enables the child to learn to perform three specific ecologically valid skills, over ten intervention sessions. The specific motor-based skills learned by the child are those identified by the child, in collaboration with their parents, and may include activities such as riding a bike, handwriting, tying shoe-laces or cutting.

Cognitive strategies are used to solve motor-based performance problems and acquire motor-based skills. The second objective of CO-OP is to teach the child how to use strategies to achieve their motor-based goals. Children are actively taught a problem-solving strategy and are enabled to discover additional strategies that will support their motor-based skill acquisition.

The third objective of CO-OP is to facilitate generalization of the motor-based skill to other settings including home and school. Once the child has acquired the desired motor-based skill, the focus of therapy shifts to facilitating generalization of the learning beyond the therapy situation.

The final objective of CO-OP is the transfer of the learning to other similar skills. Since only three skills are addressed in the course of a CO-OP intervention, it is important that the children learn to adapt their skills and strategies to the demands of new situations that they encounter in everyday life. The aim of intervention is for the child to leave therapy with the ability to **generalize and transfer** the problem-solving strategies and skills that have been learned in therapy into everyday life.

THE KEY FEATURES OF CO-OP

Critical to the effectiveness of CO-OP is that the child and therapists are fully engaged in the approach as it has been specified in the intervention protocol. The CO-OP protocol, described in detail by Polatajko and Mandich (2004), is comprised of seven key components, referred to as key features.

The key features of CO-OP are:

1 Client-chosen goals
2 Dynamic performance analysis
3 Cognitive strategy use
4 Guided discovery
5 Enabling principles
6 Parent/significant other involvement
7 Intervention structure

Each of the key features addresses one or more of the four objectives of CO-OP. The first key feature is the identification of child-chosen goals; that is, the goals are set in collaboration with child and family and focus on activities the child wants to, needs to, or is expected to perform. The child is actively engaged in the goal-setting process to ensure motivation and ecological validity. Once the child has chosen the goals, the therapist observes the quality of the child's motor-based performance, and begins a dynamic process of analysis.

The second key feature of CO-OP is dynamic performance analysis (DPA) (Polatajko et al 2000). Developed specifically for use in CO-OP, DPA is a dynamic, interactive process that is applicable to any performance situation. DPA is based on the understanding that performance is the product of the interaction of person, environment and activity, and thus highly individualistic. DPA is carried out while observing performance; points and sources of performance problems or performance breakdown are noted. This requires careful attention to various aspects of the fit between client abilities, skills and actions and the task and environmental demands and supports. The focus of CO-OP is on performance, and correcting performance problems or breakdown, not underlying components. The DPA process supports this by focusing the analysis on the observed performance of the child, the observed demands of the skill, and the environmental variables that affect the performance. Underlying components are only considered as background information to help identify potential solutions. Once the therapist has identified the initial performance breakdown points, he or she uses cognitive strategies to bridge the gap between ability and skill proficiency.

Cognitive strategies – the third key feature – are used to support skill acquisition, generalization and transfer. Cognitive strategies are cognitive operations over and above those that are inherent to the task itself (Pressley et al 1987). The CO-OP approach uses strategies to facilitate this process. The strategies help the child engage in problem solving a performance issue and monitoring the outcome – in other words the strategies promote metacognition, thinking about one's thinking (Flavell 1979). In CO-OP two types of strategies are used to facilitate the use of metacognition in solving performance problems and promoting competence, generalization and transfer: global and domain-specific.

The child is specifically taught the CO-OP global strategy and is guided to discover domain-specific strategies. The global strategy used in CO-OP is the GOAL–PLAN–DO–CHECK strategy developed by Camp, Blom, Herbert and Van Doorwick (1976) and used by Meichenbaum (1977, 1991). In CO-OP, the child is taught to use the mnemonic GOAL–PLAN–DO–CHECK, to support the solving of performance problems. In the very first session after goal setting, the child is introduced to the GOAL–PLAN–DO–CHECK strategy and is directly taught to use it. While this can be done in a number of ways, in CO-OP the child is generally taught the strategy through the use of a puppet. The global strategy remains at the centre of each intervention session. Initially, the therapist takes the lead in using the GOAL–PLAN–DO–CHECK strategy. As the child becomes familiar with the strategy, the child gradually begins to initiate strategy use.

The second type of strategy used in CO-OP is called domain-specific. Domain-specific strategies (DSS) are strategies that are specific to a particular task or part of a task. Domain-specific strategies are embedded in the global strategy; they are task-, child-, and situation-specific; and they are often used only for a short time. The child is taught the global strategy, whereas domain-specific strategies emerge in the context of skill acquisition. In CO-OP, the DPA process is used to identify the need for a DSS and the therapist's knowledge about task performance is used to identify potential DSSs that will solve the particular motor performance problem.

The next key feature of CO-OP is guided discovery. Guided discovery is the process whereby the therapist guides the child to discover answers to problems. In CO-OP, the process of guided discovery is closely entwined with the process of strategy use. It is used in conjunction with the DPA process primarily to identify when the child becomes 'stuck' and to elucidate the plan, and within the GOAL–PLAN–DO–CHECK problem-solving process. Guiding the child to discover the PLAN and the DSSs increases the likelihood that he will attribute the success of the PLAN to himself, positively impacting his self-efficacy.

In conjunction with guided discovery the therapist uses four enabling principles to facilitate motor skill acquisition. The enabling principles, the fifth key feature, are an integral part of the approach, and are used throughout the intervention. CO-OP has its foundation in the client-centred philosophy of occupational therapy, which focuses on enabling people to perform the occupations they want to, need to, or are expected to perform. Four enabling principles have been identified for use in CO-OP to support skill acquisition, strategy use, generalization and transfer. The principles are in addition to guided discovery, which, in essence, is also an enabling principle. The enabling principles are captured in four imperatives:

- Make it fun
- Promote learning
- Work towards independence
- Promote generalization and transfer

The next key feature is the involvement of parents or significant others. The primary role of parents or significant others is to support the child in the acquisition of new skills and to facilitate the generalization and transfer of these to the home and other settings. Throughout the intervention, the therapist shares information with the parents or significant others, so that they can celebrate successes with the child and support the child's use of newly learned skills and strategies in environments beyond the intervention sessions. The therapist also assigns homework so that the child can practise his new skills and strategies in their natural settings, between sessions. Parents and significant others are encouraged to support the child in the homework.

The final feature of CO-OP is the format of the intervention sessions. The CO-OP programme involves a preparation phase, ten intervention sessions and a re-evaluation phase. In the preparation phase of the CO-OP process, the child, in collaboration with their parent(s), identifies three goals to address during intervention, and then the therapist base-lines the child's performance on these chosen goals. Subsequently, in the first intervention session, the therapist teaches the child the GOAL–PLAN–DO–CHECK strategy and then it is applied to the child's three goals. The GOAL–PLAN–DO–CHECK strategy is, in the following nine intervention sessions, used throughout to identify the DSSs. Once the ten intervention sessions are complete the therapist re-evaluates the child's performance.

The following case study illustrates the use of CO-OP.

CASE EXAMPLE
Noah is a 6-year-old boy diagnosed with spastic diplegia, a form of cerebral palsy (CP) affecting his lower extremities. He currently attends kindergarten and is experiencing difficulties performing various activities at school and at home. Noah is very sociable and does not like to be left out in class. His challenges include: getting dressed to go out for recess (playtime), printing, colouring, and other table-top activities required in kindergarten. After much consideration, the CO-OP approach was chosen to assist Noah in performing some of these motor tasks.

Preparation phase
- Establishing communication with parent(s)
- Explain the CO-OP approach to parents/teachers/educators, etc. and their involvement in the therapy

First visit with Noah at school
Assessment of Noah's fine and gross motor skills was completed. Discussions with his parents, teachers and educators enabled the therapist to have a better understanding of the everyday challenges for Noah. During these discussions, the Manual Ability Classification

System (MACS) was used to describe Noah's level of performance. MACS is a classification system used for children with cerebral palsy between the ages of 4 and 18 years. This system allows a therapist to allocate a level that represents the child's usual ability to handle various objects in the home environment, in the school environment and in the community. The best level that represents Noah's usual ability to perform activities is level 3. Motivation and need for encouragement were large factors in determining this level. When given plenty of time, much encouragement and, at times, a pre-arranged environment (e.g. pencils/crayons and paper set up in front of him and some assistance to get started with the activity), Noah is able to complete most activities with few difficulties. The Pediatric Activity Card Sort (PACS) (Mandich et al 2004) was administered during the assessment. The PACS is a client-centred, occupation-focused assessment tool, consisting of photographs of children participating in usual childhood activities. The Canadian Occupational Performance Measure (COPM) (Law et al 1998) was also completed.

Using the COPM, Noah identified some goals, which included printing and dressing to go outside at recess. On the *Importance* scale, Noah rated these goals as 10 (indicating they were very important to him). However, on the *Performance* and *Satisfaction* scales, the score in both cases was 1 (not being able to do it at all, and not at all satisfied with his performance). Although Noah was having difficulties in these areas, he was not completely incapable of performing these tasks. From his general demeanour and answers to some questions, it was clear that Noah's confidence and self-esteem were very low and fragile. When asked to perform an activity, he automatically said that he could not do it and he needed assistance. Upon further investigation, his mother revealed that having an older sibling and being the only child with a disability in the family, Noah was used to having things done for him.

When demonstrating his printing, Noah was able to form only one letter, N, but was really motivated to know how to print the rest of his first name and last name. The Performance Quality Rating Scale (PQRS) (Polatjko and Mandich 2004) was used to measure his performance, with its scale from 1 (not able to perform the task) to 10 (able to perform the task), where Noah's score for printing was set at 2. When dressing himself in his winter clothes for recess, Noah was able to perform parts of the task independently but needed assistance for other tasks. However, it took 15 minutes for him to accomplish this task, while recess only lasts 20 minutes. His PQRS score on this task was set at 3.

Dynamic performance analysis (DPA) was conducted on each task to allow the therapist to understand the breakdown points of each task.

Intervention phase

SESSION 1
The first step was to teach Noah the global strategy, GOAL–PLAN–DO–CHECK. After this task was completed, the therapist and Noah began to work on specific goals and develop various strategies.

While promoting the global strategy of GOAL–PLAN–DO–CHECK, domain-specific strategies were also implemented. Encouraging parents, teachers and educators to use the global and domain-specific strategies, at home and in school, was very important.

For printing, the first strategy was seating and posture. Proper seating and support for a child with CP is crucial, but at this school the only equipment available was the tables and chairs already present in the classroom. After the proper height of the desk and chair were determined, Noah's feet did not touch the ground. A foot support was provided to accommodate for this. However, Noah also needed to do his part to keep his posture. Noah came up with a strategy of sitting like 'Mr Incredible' from the Disney film *The Incredibles* (dir. Brad Bird, 2004), that is, sitting straight and tall.

A similar strategy, focusing on posture, was identified to address a breakdown point in dressing. Being quite 'floppy' and lacking balance, Noah needed some supports for him to dress. All children were required to sit on the bench to get dressed and Noah's 'cubby' was right in the middle. When he tried to get dressed, he would fall over on to other children sitting next to him. When Noah was asked where would be the best place for him to get dressed, he said away from all the other kids because he was embarrassed about falling on them. However, he could not identify which place would be best. Several scenarios were tried during the session – on his chair in the classroom, at the end of the bench, on another bench, and on the floor leaning against the wall. After trying all these different places, the therapist and Noah reached a collaborative decision: the floor with the wall at his back was the ideal place.

Other strategies developed to help Noah's printing were:

- Explicit instruction for the letters in the name
- Where to start when printing letters
- Various letter stroke mnemonics (e.g. around, around, around we go, just like a race track . . . for the letter O)
- Different media to make practising the letters fun, e.g. using paints, water, markers, crayons, chalk, etc.

Other strategies developed for Noah's 'Getting dressed for recess' goal were:

- Remind mom to send all items of winter clothing to school (a home checklist was produced to be hung by the front door)
- Make sure mom bought proper size clothing
- Order of dressing:

    Snow pants
    Boots
    Neck warmer
    Jacket
    Hat
    Mittens

TABLE 17.1

Goal	COPM						PQRS	
	Importance		Performance		Satisfaction			
	Pre-test	Post-test	Pre-test	Post-test	Pre-test	Post-test	Pre-test	Post-test
Printing	10	9	1	8	1	7	2	7
Dressing	10	10	1	9	1	9	3	9

Re-evaluation phase

The COPM and PQRS were re-administered at school. Interviews with parents, teachers and educators were also completed. Both the COPM and PQRS scores showed significant improvement for the specified goals (see Table 17.1). Noah was very happy that he was able to print his name like the other children and that he had time to play outside at recess with his friends. Noah's parents, teachers and educators were pleased with his progress and the improvement in his performance.

Summary and conclusion

CO-OP was developed over the course of ten years as an alternative to the traditional approaches for the treatment of children with motor-based performance problems, specifically children with developmental coordination disorder (Polatajko et al 2001a, 2001b, Polatajko and Mandich 2004). Early studies elucidated the essential features of CO-OP and provided evidence to support its further development and evaluation. A number of additional formal and informal studies were carried out to determine the effectiveness of CO-OP (for a more detailed discussion, see Polatajko et al 2001a, 2001b). The findings of these studies clearly indicated that a new approach had been found for the treatment of motor-based performance problems in children: an approach that (1) meets the demands of parents, in that it is effective in helping children to succeed; (2) meets the demands of therapists, in that it is client-centred and performance-based; and (3) meets the demands of administrators, in that it is cost-effective, efficient and evidence-based. Currently a pilot randomized clinical trial is being conducted with children with CP (Dawson et al 2007).

In general, the findings from the application of a cognitive approach to motor performance problems suggest that skilled performance arises from a dynamical interaction of a variety of factors, and that cognition can be a mediating factor in facilitating the learning of new motor skills. Further research is needed, but these findings suggest that cognition ought to be given a more prominent role in the design of interventions that are based on a dynamical systems perspective.

REFERENCES

Barrera M, Rosenbaum P, Cunningam C (1986) Early home intervention with low-birthweight infants and their parents. *Child Dev* 57: 20–33.
Camp B, Blom G, Herbert F, Van Doorwick W (1976) Think Aloud: a program for developing self-control in young aggressive boys. Unpublished manuscript, University of Colorado School of Medicine, Denver, Colorado, USA.

Dawson D, Polatajko H, Cameron D (2007) A contextualized, meta-cognitive rehabilitation approach for enhancing participation in adults and children with acquired brain injury. Course presented at the 2007 Joint Education Conference of the American Congress of Rehabilitation Medicine and American Society of Neurorehabilitation, Washington DC, 5 October.

Fitts PM, Posner MI (1967) *Human Performance*. Belmont, CA: Brooks/Cole.

Flavell JJ (1979) Metacognition and cognitive monitoring: a new area of cognitive-developmental inquiry. *Am Psychol* 34: 906–911.

Kaplan BJ, Polatajko HJ, Wilson BN, Faris P (1993) Re-examination of sensory integration therapy: a combination of two efficacy studies. *J Learn Disabil* 26: 342–347.

Kavale K, Mattson PD (1983) 'One jumped off the balance beam': meta-analysis of perceptual-motor training. *J Learn Disabil* 16: 165–173.

Knox V, Evans AL (2002) Evaluation of the functional effects of a course of Bobath therapy in children with cerebral palsy: a preliminary study. *Dev Med Child Neurol* 44: 447–460.

Law M, Polatajko H, Schaffer R, Miller J, Macnab J (1991) The impact of heterogeneity in a clinical trial: motor outcomes after sensory integration therapy. *Occup Ther J Res* 11: 177–189.

Law M, Baptiste S, Carswell A, McColl MA, Polatajko H, Pollock N (1998) *Canadian Occupational Performance Measure, 3rd edn*. Toronto: CAOT Publications ACE.

Mandich A (1997) Cognitive strategies and motor performance in children with developmental coordination disorder. Unpublished master's thesis, University of Western Ontario, London, Ontario, Canada.

Mandich A, Polatajko H (2003) Developmental coordination disorder: mechanisms, measurement and management. *Hum Mov Sci* 22: 406–411.

Mandich A, Polatajko HJ, Macnab JJ, Miller LT (2001a) Treatment of children with developmental coordination disorder: what is the evidence? *Phys Occup Ther Pediatr* 20: 51–68.

Mandich A, Polatajko HJ, Missiuna C, Miller L (2001b) Cognitive strategies and motor performance in children with developmental coordination disorder. *Phys Occup Ther Pediatr* 20: 125–144.

Mandich A, Polatajko H, Rodger S (2003) Rites of passage: understanding participation of children with developmental coordination disorder. *Hum Mov Sci* 22: 583–595.

Mandich A, Polatajko HJ, Miller L, Baum C (2004) *The Paediatric Activity Card Sort*. Toronto: CAOT Publications ACE.

Marchiori GE, Wall AE, Bedingfield EW (1987) Kinematic analysis of skill acquisition in physically awkward boys. *Adap Phys Activity Q* 4: 305–315.

Martini R (1994) Verbal self-guidance as an approach to the treatment of children with developmental coordination disorder: a systematic replication study. Unpublished master's thesis, University of Western Ontario, London, Ontario, Canada.

Martini R, Polatajko HJ (1998) Verbal self-guidance as a treatment approach for children with developmental coordination disorder: a systematic replication study. *Occup Ther J Res* 18: 157–181.

Meichenbaum D (1977) *Cognitive-Behavior Modification: An Integrative Approach*. New York: Plenum Press.

Meichenbaum D (1991) Cognitive-behavior modification. Workshop presented at the Child and Parent Research Institute symposium, London, Ontario, Canada.

Miller LT, Polatajko HJ, Missiuna C, Mandich AD, Macnab JJ (2001) A pilot trial of a cognitive treatment for children with developmental coordination disorder. *Hum Mov Sci* 20: 183–210.

Mulder T (1991) A process-oriented model of human motor behaviour: toward a theory-based rehabilitation approach. *Phys Ther* 71: 157–164.

Polatajko HJ (1999) Developmental coordination disorder (DCD): alias the clumsy child syndrome. In: Whitmore K, Hart H, Willems G, editors. *A Neurodevelopmental Approach to Specific Learning Disorders*. London: Mac Keith Press, pp 119–133.

Polatajko HJ, Mandich A (2004) *Enabling Occupation in Children: The Cognitive Orientation to Daily Occupational Performance (CO-OP) Approach*. Ottawa, Ontario: CAOT Publications ACE.

Polatajko HJ, Law M, Miller J, Schaffer R, Macnab J (1991) The effect of a sensory integration program on academic achievement, motor performance and self-esteem in children identified as learning disabled: results of a clinical trial. *Occup Ther J Res* 11: 155–176.

Polatajko HJ, Kaplan BJ, Wilson BN (1992) Sensory integration treatment for children with learning disabilities: its status 20 years later. *Occup Ther J Res* 12: 323–341.

Polatajko HJ, Macnab J, Anstett B, Malloy-Miller T, Murphy K, Noh S (1995) A clinical trial of the process-oriented treatment approach for children with developmental co-ordination disorder. *Dev Med Child Neurol* 37: 310–319.

Polatajko HJ, Mandich AD, Martini R (2000) Dynamic performance analysis: a framework for understanding occupational performance. *Am J Occup Ther* 54: 65–72.

Polatajko HJ, Mandich AD, Miller L, Macnab J (2001a) Cognitive Orientation to daily Occupational Performance: Part II – The evidence. *Phys Occup Ther Paediatr* 20: 83–106.

Polatajko HJ, Mandich AD, Missiuna C, Miller L, Macnab J, Malloy-Miller T, et al (2001b) Cognitive Orientation to daily Occupational Performance (CO-OP): Part III – The protocol in brief. *Phys Occup Ther Pediatr* 20: 107–124.

Pressley M, Borkowski JG, Schneider W (1987) Cognitive strategies: good strategy users coordinate metacognition and knowledge. In: Vasta R, editor. *Annals of Child Development*. London: JAI Press, pp 89–129.

Rosenbaum P (2003) Cerebral palsy: what parents and doctors want to know. *BMJ* 326: 670–674.

Samonte S, Solish L, Delaney L, Polatajko H (2004) Cognitive Orientation to daily Occupational Performance: beyond developmental coordination disorder. Student paper presented at the Canadian Association of Occupational Therapists Conference, Charlottetown, PEI, 25 June.

Schmidt RA, Wrisberg CA (2000) *Motor Learning and Performance: A Problem-Based Learning Approach, 2nd edn*. Champaign, IL: Human Kinetics Publishers.

Segal R, Mandich A, Polatajko H, Cook JV (2002) Stigma and its management: a framework for understanding social isolation of children with developmental coordination disorder. *Am J Occup Ther* 56: 422–428.

Shonkoff J, Hauser-Cram P (1987) Early intervention for disabled infants and their families: a quantitative analysis. *Pediatrics* 80: 650–658.

Short D, Schkade J, Herring J (1989) Parent involvement in physical therapy: a controversial issue. *J Pediatr Orthop* 9: 444–446.

Shumway-Cook A, Woollacott MH (1995) *Motor Control: Theory and Practical Application*. Baltimore, MD: Williams & Wilkins.

Siebes RC, Wijnrok L, Vermeer A (2002) Qualitative analysis of therapeutic motor intervention programmes for children with cerebral palsy: an update. *Dev Med Child Neurol* 44: 593–603.

Sigmundsson H, Pedersen AV, Whiting HT, Ingvaldsen RP (1998) We can cure your child's clumsiness! A review of intervention methods. *Scan J Rehabil Med* 30: 101–106.

Solish L, Samonte S, Polatajko H (2005) Cognitive Orientation to daily Occupational Performance (CO-OP): a six month follow-up. Poster presentation at the Canadian Association of Occupational Therapists Conference, Vancouver, BC, 26 May.

Steultjens EMJ, Dekker J, van de Nes JCM, Lambregts BLM, van den Ende CHM (2004) Occupational therapy for children with cerebral palsy: a systematic review. *Clin Rehabil* 18: 1–14.

Thelen E (1995) Motor development: a new synthesis. *Am Psychol* 50: 79–95.

Valvano J (2004) Activity-focused motor interventions for children with neurological conditions. *Mov Sci* 79–107.

Wilcox A (1994) Children with mild motor problems: exploring a client-centred, cognitive approach in OT intervention. Unpublished master's thesis, University of Western Ontario, London, Ontario, Canada.

Wilcox A, Polatajko H (1993) Verbal self-guidance as a treatment technique for children with developmental coordination disorder. *Can J Occup Ther*, Conference Supplement, p 20.

Wilcox A, Polatajko HJ (1994) The impact of verbal self-guidance on children with developmental coordination disorder. 11th International Congress of the World Federation of Occupational Therapists Congress Summaries, 3, 1518–1519.

World Health Organization (2001) *ICF: International Classification of Functioning, Disability and Health*. Geneva: WHO.

18
GOAL-ORIENTED TRAINING OF DAILY ACTIVITIES – A MODEL FOR INTERVENTION

Ann-Christin Eliasson and Birgit Rösblad

Goal-oriented training is a therapeutic approach that promotes increased independence in daily life by addressing those goals that children and their families have identified as being important to them (Matos et al 2007). The rationale for the therapy is predominantly influenced by the ecological Person–Environment–Occupation model focusing on the interdependence of variables (Law et al 1996, CAOT 2002). The goal-oriented model for intervention outlined in this chapter is based on principles of motor learning.

A review of the recent literature on this topic lends strong support for the use of activity-based approaches, as opposed to component-driven ones, to achieve important functional goals in a child's daily life (Law et al 1996, Fisher 1998). Five steps of goal-oriented training will be discussed: (1) the selection of meaningful goals; (2) analysis of the child's task performance; (3) the intervention/practice regime required to achieve the goal; (4) evaluation of the child's attainment of the goal after the intervention; and (5) the transfer of learning to other activities (see Fig. 18.1).

Selection of goals

FAMILY-CENTRED SERVICE

The provision of services to children does not occur in isolation, but through interaction with the families. It is important to note that there has been a move during recent decades from a professional-centred model of service delivery to a family-centred model in which the parents are always considered to be the experts on their own child. The family works together with service providers to make informed decisions about the services and support to be given to the child and family. In a family-centred service, the strength and needs of all the family members are considered (Law et al 1998, McGibbon et al 2003). A widely adopted conceptual framework for family-centred services has been developed by the CanChild group (at the Center for Childhood Disability Research, McMaster University, Hamilton, Ontario, Canada). The concept is based on the belief that parents know their children best and want the best for them; that families are different and unique; and that optimal functioning for the child occurs in a supportive family and community context (Rosenbaum et al 1998). The overall goal is to enhance the quality of life of all family members, and to involve them in decision-making, collaboration and partnership.

Family-centred intervention has become an approach to service delivery the value of which no one today would dispute. However, to provide these services, professionals need to have a broad acceptance of the family's choice. This change of service model also means that professionals need to develop new areas of expertise, to enable them to discuss and explain the advantages and disadvantages of different types of intervention with families. As family resource professionals, practitioners need to be informed about the best evidence for decision-making about care options available for individual children.

CHILD-CENTRED GOALS

In the family/child-centred model, therapists actively facilitate participation of the family in intervention planning to support the goals chosen by, with or for the child, and to ensure that these are important and meaningful for the child. This means that the therapist needs to develop an understanding of each family's preferred activities and the environment in which these activities take place. Recent authors have pointed out the importance of supporting the child's own ability to set the goals and recognizing that the child's goals may differ from those that the parents think are most important (Missiuna et al 2006). Some children, however, cannot express their wishes because they are too young or have cognitive delay that limits their decision-making abilities. Under such circumstances, family members or significant others may identify therapeutic goals. Most children or families express more than one desired outcome and, in such cases, the practitioner helps them to rank the goals to determine which activity is the most important. Other families may find it difficult to come up with a goal or, in some cases, it may take them some time to decide what the most important goal is for intervention. Thus, the goal-setting process requires time for discussion, to avoid stress on family members and to ensure that the whole intervention is built upon the desired goal. Once the goal has been selected, the therapist then discusses the characteristics of the goal. In this discussion, the acronym 'SMART' – highlighting the important characteristics of a goal – may be helpful. The goal needs to be Specific, Measurable, Attainable, Realistic and Time-limited.

The types of goals may differ – they can be activity-based or movement-based – but the desired outcomes must be clearly expressed and accepted by all team members. O'Neill and Harris (1982) were amongst the first to point out the importance of being able to define measurable goals for treatment. Although they promoted the use of functional goals, their examples reflected neuromaturational orientation and focused on presumed movement components of functional skills (such as maintaining a prone-on-elbow position with the head in midline, or righting the head when tipped laterally while sitting on a therapy ball). While therapists need to address impairments during treatment, there is increasing agreement that the goals of therapy should be functional and related to the ability to perform meaningful activities in daily life (Bower 2004).

Each step in the goal-oriented training process is illustrated in the case study of Sara.

Case Study: Selection of Goals

Sara is 9 years old and has diplegia. Her functional level of MACS is III and of GMFCS IV. She mainly uses a powered wheelchair for mobility. She was referred to occupational therapy since she has difficulty with several daily activities related to manual ability. After some short discussion, it became obvious that Sara would like to learn how to use scissors to cut more efficiently. This skill was important to Sara because her friends at school did a great deal of cutting both at school and in their leisure activities. Sara's parents were also in favour of the activity since it meant that if she could cut properly she would have some regular leisure activities she could do at home. The goal of intervention was therefore expressed as 'To be able to cut paper with a pair of scissors'. Sara and her family were clear about their goal for the treatment, therefore no special goal-setting tools were used.

ASSESSMENT FOR GOAL SETTING

There are several tools available that might facilitate the goal-setting process. For example, the Canadian Occupational Performance Measure (COPM) is widely used. This is a semi-structured interview where participants rate the most important issues in the areas of self-care, work and leisure. Each identified activity is than rated a second time according to the client's satisfaction and perceived performance of the activity, thus giving the therapist insight into the participant's perceived competence (Law et al 1994, 1998). Since young children usually find it difficult to answer such questions, parents are often asked to speak for their child by identifying and rating the most important functional skills to be addressed as intervention goals. More recently, professionals have discouraged parent reporting for the child and have recognized the importance of self-chosen goals that are intrinsically motivating to the child. To maximize the child's successful outcomes, it is important to give the child their own voice in goal selection.

New assessments are now available which attempt to determine the child's own opinion of his or her activity performance. The Perceived Efficacy and Goal Setting (PEGS) assessment is a card sorting system designed for use with children aged 5–11 years (Missiuna et al 2006). When using PEGS, the child is asked to sort picture cards showing play, school and self-care activities in daily life. Cards which describe activities that the child is able to do are sorted into one pile, and cards which show activities they feel are difficult to perform are sorted into another pile. The pile of cards describing difficult activities can then be used for discussing goals for intervention.

The Pediatric Evaluation of Disability Inventory (PEDI) is an additional assessment that can be used for goal setting (see Chapter 21) in the areas of self-care, mobility and social skills. Since all items are presented in sequential developmental steps, it is easy to discuss what the next step will be if the child is to learn to perform the activity.

The Goal Attainment Scale (GAS) is an individualized assessment suitable for evaluation of goal-directed training (see case study). GAS has been widely used to evaluate

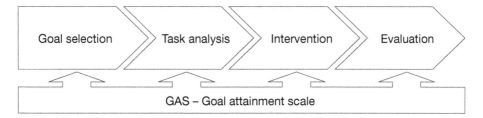

Fig. 18.1 The goal-directed training process.

Source: Reproduced with permission from Matos et al, Goal directed training: linking theories of treatment to clinical practice for improved functional activities in daily life. *Clinical Rehabilitation* 21: 1–9, Copyright (© Sage Publications, 2007), by permission of Sage Publications Ltd.

health services, educational programmes, and social services (Kiresuk and Sherman 1968, King et al 1999, Cusick et al 2006). GAS uses a five-step scale as follows: baseline (–2), less than expected outcome (–1), expected outcome (0), greater than expected outcome (+1), and much greater than expected outcome (+2). Since GAS is criterion-referenced, rather than norm-referenced, it is potentially responsive to small changes that are perceived by children and families to be important for daily activities. The flexibility of the GAS approach is particularly useful for children with low cognitive and motor functioning, since standardized measures are rarely sensitive to the small, but meaningful, changes targeted for these individuals. Other potential advantages of GAS include improved clarity of the objectives of therapy for the therapist, and for the child and their family, as well as improved conceptualization and delivery of the intervention. If the child is videotaped when trying to perform the goal activities – prior to as well as after intervention – this strengthens the reliability of the outcome.

Analysis of task performance
The rationale for the analysis of task performance is also influenced by the ecological Person–Environment–Occupation (PEO) model, emphasizing the interdependence of variables (Law et al 1996). This means that, if a person is skilled, the task can generally be performed in any environment, but also that the environment affects the performance, especially if the person has a reduced functional capacity. It is, for example, more difficult to carry a tray in a restaurant than in an empty room. So, when asking a child with hemiplegia if she can carry a tray, the answer will probably be 'It depends'. In addition, the type of occupation can also influence the performance. When asking a child if she can eat independently, the answer might be 'It depends if you mean pancake or steak.' Thus, when analysing the child's task performance, it is important to investigate how the environment and the chosen activity contribute to or limit the child's ability. For many therapeutic approaches, the first step of any analysis involves the identification of performance problems, whereupon a leap is typically made straight into assessing underlying body functions and impairments. However, this neglects the task performance analysis that is necessary for goal-oriented training.

When the goal for intervention has been decided upon, an analysis must be made of the task, the environment and the person's capacity. The influence of the environment and structure of the task need to be analysed first before investigating the person components. Adaptations of environment and activity are typically easier to carry out than changing a child's capacity. By adapting the environment or activity first, the intervention also supports the child's self-esteem and problem-solving skills. The message to the child is that any problems that arise are external rather than being the result of the child's impairment. Adaptation of an environment and of tasks can facilitate the performance and learning procedure. Such adaptation may include the use of technical aids or simplification of the activity in question, depending on the child's wishes and ability to perform the activity. Adaptations and simplifications are usually made in the early learning phase, and can be altered with improved performance of the activity.

Simplification of an activity and, if possible, breaking down the activity into different steps are crucial. An activity includes several tasks, performed in a certain order. Any task is built up from a sequence of movements. The sequences need to be executed in a certain order, forming a successful strategy for the task. Each sequence also needs to have a certain quality of skilled performance. The order in which the sequences are conducted and the quality of the individual's movements will influence the result (Gentile 1987). The complexity of the movement patterns required, the temporal and spatial demands and force control are parameters that determine the quality of the performance, as has been extensively investigated in experimental research (Eliasson 2006).

Kimmerle and coworkers (2003) have introduced the 'Functional Repertoire of the Hand Model', which is useful for analysis of the person's ability to perform the task. The model consists of four key components that can be used to delineate theoretically different aspects of hand function. The first component of the model, *Personal constraints*, refers to physical and psychological impairment; its analysis gives information on which are the key elements for activity limitations. The second key component, *Hand roles*, identifies what each hand has to do within the activity, which is essential since daily activities typically involve the collaborative use of two hands, and the requirements of each of the hands are different (Krumlinde-Sundholm et al 2007). Children with cerebral palsy often exhibit decreased collaborative use of their hands, which is not solely related to hemiplegia because it is also evident in children with diplegia. The third key component concerns *Object-related hand actions*, and is divided into the categories reaching, grasping and manipulating. These fundamental actions comprise the hand skills, applied and carried out in many different combinations in a variety of contexts. The last key component is called *Task parameters*. This includes the handling of objects representing different challenges, due to their variation in size, shape or surface, as well as different demands on spatial, temporal and force performance. The *Object-related hand actions* category identifies what the hand can actually do with the object, while the *Task parameters* clarify how skilfully the objects are manipulated. Analysing the child's 'Functional Repertoire of the Hand' when performing certain tasks, rather than making an assessment of the child's general limitations, gives the therapist a tool for planning treatment and for defining the different steps in the GAS.

Case Study: Analysis of Task Performance

When Sara tried to cut along a straight line, it resulted in erratic cutting, and cutting out figures was very difficult. She cut a lot of small pieces instead of adjusting the paper for continuous cutting. Sara sat in her wheelchair with her arms held up in the air, the scissors and the paper close to her eyes. She commonly lost postural control, falling over to her right, but continued to do the cutting. As Sara imposes high demands on the result, she corrected herself endlessly, but she was still not satisfied.

When analysing Sara's performance, the Person–Environment–Task model was used. Some adaptation had already been made to the **environment** since Sara was using an adapted pair of scissors with a 'spring handle'. From the **task** perspective, she was able to cut, but doing so resulted in uneven and jagged cutting and it was time-consuming. From a **personal** perspective, it was obvious that she understood the concept of cutting, but the 'hand roles' aspect was unclear; it was difficult for her to feed the paper with one hand and cut with the other hand. She held the scissors with a good grasp, but the paper was held with a static pronated grasp, informing us that 'Object-related hand actions' were used, but in an inflexible manner. The tooth-edged cutting indicated that 'Task parameters' such as force coordination and direction of the cutting movement were inefficient. Moreover, Sara was continually falling over to the right, and she did not seem to be aware of this.

When using the same model for planning treatment, it was obvious that the **environmental** aspects needed further consideration. Her tendency to fall over might be reduced by providing other chairs and tables. Arranging how and where the training should be performed is also an environmental issue. The **task** itself needed to be graded, and Sara needed to be started off with very simple cutting tasks in which she would feel more satisfied. It might be beneficial to try thicker paper than before, and paper of a smaller size. On a **personal** level, Sara understood the cutting procedure, but by discussing strategies that she could adopt, she would become more efficient in figure cutting. The training needed to be arranged in such a way that Sara would retain her high level of motivation to practise. If Sara is motivated, she will repeat the task, and it is only by repetition that 'Task parameters' and 'Object-related hand actions' will be improved and her cutting behaviour become more flexible. 'Object-related hand actions' and 'Task parameters' are implicit behaviour and are refined by practice. To improve the figure cutting her cutting strategies needed to be highlighted and discussed. In addition, her unawareness of the falling over needed to be discussed. Usually posture is an unconscious form of behaviour, but the first step to changing one's behaviour is to make it conscious.

Sara and the therapist decided to start to work on cutting simple shapes, to increase the speed with which she could cut, with the short-term goal being to cut a heart. After some discussion, Sara agreed to include improving balance as a goal, to enable her to become more aware of her behaviour.

GAS for cutting
-2   Handling a pair of scissors with a spring handle and cutting a straight line 2 cm long
-1   Handling a pair of scissors with a spring handle and cutting along a line 10 cm long, whether straight or bent
0   Cutting out two drops
+1   Cutting out a heart, with some help in the middle when changing the direction of cutting
+2   Cutting out a heart without assistance

GAS for postural control
-2   Falling over to the right
-1   Being able to correct her posture if falling, and ceasing to cut until she is upright again
0   Quickly correcting her posture if tending to fall over, without stopping cutting
+1   Being able to cut a heart and keep a good posture
+2   Being able to keep a good posture when performing any task

Intervention
Motor skill acquisition is facilitated by helping children to develop the cognitive processes associated with functional movements (Smith and Wrisberg 2000). The child's conscious involvement is vital to the learning process, and they need to be involved at the highest level they are capable of, which is dependent on their age and stage of development. The main idea is to consider the children as problem solvers who use their personal characteristics or resources to the greatest possible extent to interact meaningfully and adaptively with the environment (Horak 1990, Missiuna et al 2001, Eliasson 2005). Recent research has revealed that more permanent changes in motor performance are promoted through practice and repetition, problem solving and feedback, as is extensively described in Chapter 16. The child's conscious involvement is paramount in the learning process. Thus, the role of the therapist is not to treat the child in a passive sense, but to design learning situations that will facilitate this problem solving and promote the exploration of alternative strategies, to regard children as competent individuals, and to focus on each child's strengths in an individualized and flexible way. This child-centred approach can be applied with children of different ages and with disabilities of different degrees of severity, highlighting the importance of meeting the child with the right level of expectations.

The three-stage model of motor learning, initially described by Fitts and Posner, is a good guide for planning treatment (Fitts and Posner 1967). The three stages are as follows: (1) *verbal-cognitive stage*; (2) *motor stage*; and (3) *autonomous stage* (see Chapter 16). The *early verbal-cognitive stage* relies on external physical and/or verbal assistance to enable the child to understand the explicit demands imposed by the task. In this explicit learning phase, the child needs to practise various strategies to find the optimal solution to a motor problem and develop skilled performance. The children need to be active problem solvers who use their personal characteristics or resources to the greatest possible extent to interact meaningfully and adaptively with the environment. In this stage of learning the therapist has an active role: to discuss, demonstrate and/or guide the child through the activity, which is adjusted to the child's age, cognitive level and other needs. The therapist is an important collaborator and coach, using cues to help the child to remember what to do, and giving feedback, i.e. informing them of the result and the performance. The main idea is to help the child to find the most efficient strategy to adopt to accomplish the task.

In the *intermediate motor stage*, the child begins to perform the activity in a more consistent manner, and the focus shifts to improving the quality of the movement through practice. The implicit learning that occurs through successive attempts allows the child to anticipate how to complete the task. In this phase the role of the therapist is to arrange the environment, giving the child the opportunity to practise the task, supporting and encouraging him or her. Children with cerebral palsy may remain in this phase for an extended period of time since they may have limited learning ability and this underlying impairment may hinder them from moving on to the next phase. In the *final autonomous stage*, movement patterns are refined and diversified. Children demonstrate consistency by performing the relevant task spontaneously and efficiently, and they are able to draw on their previous problem-solving experiences to perform variations of the task in novel situations. At this stage, the therapist has to be there, but primarily as a coach. The coaching procedure needs to be tailored to each child, perceiving efficacy and behavioural competence in the situation. Being able to coach children at the right level is very important.

Case Study: Intervention

Session I and planning for the first homework: Sara understood the cutting procedure, but the quality of her cutting was poor, which indicated that Sara was in the second phase of learning, the motor stage. Therefore practising cutting was the focus of training; Sara agreed to practise every day over a period of five weeks. She wanted to be responsible for the training herself, although her parents were involved in the process. She received a diary in which she could makes notes about the amount of time spent on training, and she looked upon the training as a kind of homework. The first step in the training procedure was to reach level +1on the GAS. The plan was that Sara should meet the therapist once a week to receive new homework, based on her updated performance. A strategy for improved posture was awareness of and attention to her behaviour. Sara made a sign which said 'lean the elbow towards the table' to put in front of her when practising, making the posture an explicit behaviour. She was told to cut strips of paper 2–10 cm long for ten minutes every day, an easy task, with the aim being to improve the quality of her cutting performance. She was given special coloured paper to work with, making it fun and increasing her motivation.

Session II: Sara had done her homework every day but one and she also brought back all the papers she had cut. She could easily gain feedback on her cutting accuracy from the papers themselves, but she also told us that she was now cutting much faster. This time she tried a forearm support, an assistive device adjusted to provide support in a sideways direction since the therapist was not sure the elbow on the table was the best strategy. *Homework II*: The next cutting task was somewhat more difficult, Sara was asked to cut a half moon, including the curved lines. In doing this shape, Sara needed to increase the flexibility of her cutting skills. She was also asked to try to use the forearm support at home. Again, the task was to practise for ten minutes every day.

Session III: As before, Sara had done her homework; she had used the assistive device, but typically she stabilized her arms by keeping them close to her body, a strategy she had discovered herself. Now Sara was able to adjust the position of the paper more efficiently and was satisfied with the result. She also made fewer corrections to her cutting. *Homework III* (for two weeks): to cut two drops every day in order to increase the demands of the task and, hopefully, to continue to improve the speed. She was encouraged to find out the best strategy for keeping her posture.

Evaluation of goals

Evaluation is the critical element of any intervention, but in goal-oriented training it is simplified since evaluation is directed at the self-selected functional goals (Mathiowetz and Haugen 1994, King et al 1999). Since goals are highly individualized, we recommend that the Goal Attainment Scale (GAS) (Kiresuk and Sherman 1968) or another individualized criterion-referenced measure, such as the COPM, is used. Standardized assessments of function are often designed to measure general capacity of, for example, fine motor skills, which may result in no change in the child's score, even though a certain goal has been achieved.

The GAS procedure involves defining a unique goal, specifying a range of possible outcomes on a scale (see p. 288) and using this for planning the intervention. The same GAS scale is used to evaluate the child's change in performance after the specified period of intervention. This type of evaluation is easily understood by children, which is, of course, important.

Case Study: Evaluation of Goals

Sara came to the last session with 24 drops and wanted to try to cut out a real heart. She was able to do so with the help of verbal instructions and she achieved a score of +1 on the GAS. She had a good strategy, cutting first one side then the other, leaving the trickiest part in the middle to the end. At that point she received some verbal instructions on how to turn the paper. Her speed increased, she made fewer corrections and she was also able to talk at the same time as cutting. The grip she used to hold the paper had changed from a pronated to a supinated grasping pattern. Sara had recognized that, by performing this grasp, it was easier to adjust the paper forward herself during cutting. She kept herself in an upright position almost all the time, and when falling, she quickly corrected herself, making it less fatiguing; this resulted in a score of 0 on the GAS. She liked the idea of stabilizing herself by holding her arms against her body and was proud of the results.

Transfer of learning

A previous assumption regarding treatment was that obtaining an improved quality of movement will automatically lead to increased mastery of skills. Current theorists question this assumption of automatic transfer of learning (see Gentile 1987). It is even difficult to find evidence of the transfer of learning from a specific task in a specific environment to a more global ability. The only obvious result of practice is that children learn what they are practising (Eliasson 2005). For transfer or generalization of motor skills to occur, a child probably needs to progress to the autonomous stage of learning where flexible task performance is observed in new situations (Smith and Wrisberg 2000).

Another possible approach to transfer of learning or generalization of skills might be to use cues or strategies as general guidelines to facilitate problem solving and encourage the child to establish internal procedures of motor sequences and tasks. By developing a strategy in one motor task the child may draw upon the strategy in new situations and adapt the learned strategy to master new skills. If the result of the training is close to the child's expectations about their own capability, reinforcing feedback emphasizes the child's own achievements, and a gradual experience of mastery over important aspects of everyday life helps the child to predict and manage everyday life situations despite barriers. Thus, the child's self-efficacy in performing activities associated with everyday life increases over the course of treatment.

Case Study: Transfer of Learning

At a two-year follow-up, Sara was still satisfied with her cutting ability, but there had not been an obvious transfer of her cutting skills to other activities. She also continued to have difficulty with her postural control, typical falling over in other activities.

Conclusion

The objective of goal-oriented training is to help children to learn specific activities that are important in daily life. This approach is individualized to the child and suitable for children with a range of physical and cognitive abilities. Intervention is directed towards functional tasks in natural settings, rather than focusing on sensory stimuli or movement patterns, since we cannot take it for granted that there will be transfer from movements learned and practised to other activities. Essential elements include collaborative goal setting, task analysis, and engagement of the child as an active problem solver while undertaking repetitive practice with structured feedback. The GAS is an effective tool for conceptualizing goal-oriented training and for evaluating the outcome of an intervention. A greater emphasis is placed on activities and environmental adaptations than on body impairments, to ensure that the child achieves the goal. This approach is congruent with the principles of a top-down approach, whereby intervention strategies and outcomes are guided by an analysis of activity performance problems rather than of component body impairments.

REFERENCES

Bower E (2004) Goal setting and the measurement of change. In: Scrutton D, Daminiano D, Maystone M, editors. *Management of the Motor Disorders of Children with Cerebral Palsy*. London: Mac Keith Press, pp 32–51.

CAOT (2002) *Enabling Occupation: An Occupational Therapy Perspective, rev edn*. Ottawa: Canadian Association of Occupational Therapists.

Cusick A, McIntyre S, Novak I, Lannin N, Lowe KA (2006) Comparison of goal attainment scaling and the Canadian Occupational Performance Measure for pediatric rehabilitation research. *Pediatr Rehabil* 9: 149–157.

Eliasson AC (2005) Improving the use of hands in daily activities: aspects of treatment of children with cerebral palsy. *Phys Occup Ther Pediatr* 25: 37–60.

Eliasson AC (2006) Sensorimotor integration of normal and impaired development of precision movement of the hand. In: Henderson A, Pehoski C, editors. *Hand Function in the Child: Foundations for Remediation, 2nd edn*. St Louis: Mosby.

Eliasson AC, Bonnier B, Krumlinde-Sundholm L (2003) Experience of forced use of upper extremity in adolescents with hemiplegic cerebral palsy: a day camp model. *Dev Med Child Neurol* 45: 357–359.

Fisher AG (1998) Uniting practice and theory in an occupational framework: Eleanor Clarke Slagel Lecture. *Am J Occup Ther* 52: 509–521.

Fitts PM, Posner MI (1967) *Human Performance*. Belmont: Brooks/Cole Publishing Co.

Gentile AM (1987) Skill acquisition: action, movement and neuromotor processes. In: Carr JH, Shepherd RB, editors. *Movement Science: Foundations for Physical Therapy in Rehabilitation*. Gaithersburg, PA: Aspen Publications, pp 111–188.

Gentile AM (1998) Implicit and explicit processes during acquisition of functional skills. *Scan J Occup Ther* 5: 7–16.

Gordon J (1987) Skill acquisition: assumptions underlying physical therapy intervention: theoretical and historical perspectives. In: Carr JH, Shepherd RB, editors. *Movement Science: Foundations for Physical Therapy in Rehabilitation*. Gaithersburg, PA: Aspen Publications, pp 1–24.

Horak FB (1990) Assumptions underlying motor control for neurologic rehabilitation. In: Lister MJ, editor. *II STEP: Contemporary Management of Motor Control Problems*. Norman, OK: Foundation for Physical Therapy, Oklahoma University, pp 11–28.

Kielhofner G, editor (2002) *A Model of Human Occupation: Theory and Application, 3rd edn*. Baltimore, MD: Lippincott Williams & Wilkins.

Kimmerle M, Mainwaring L, Borenstein M (2003) The functional repertoire of the hand and its application to assessment. *Am J Occup Ther* 57: 489–498.

King GA, McDougall J, Palisano RJ, Gritzan J, Tucker MA (1999) Goal attainment scaling: its use in evaluating pediatric therapy programs. *Phys Occ Ther Pediatr* 19: 31–52.

Kiresuk TJ, Sherman RE (1968) Goal Attainment Scaling: a general method for evaluating comprehensive community mental health programs. *Community Ment Health J* 4: 443–453.

Krumlinde-Sundholm L, Holmefur M, Kottorp A, Eliasson AC (2007) Current evidence of validity, reliability and responsiveness to change concerning the Assisting Hand Assessment. *Dev Med Child Neurol* 49: 259–264.

Law M, Polatajko H, Pollock N, McColl MA, Carswell A, Baptiste S (1994) Pilot testing of the Canadian Occupational Performance Measure: clinical and measurement issues. *Can J Occup Ther* 61: 191–197.

Law M, Cooper BA, Strong S, Stewart D, Rigby P, Letts L (1996) The Person–Environment–Occupation Model: a transactive approach to occupational performance. *Can J Occup Ther* 63: 9–23.

Law M, Darrah J, Pollock N, King G, Rosenbaum P, Russell D, Palisano R, Harris S, Armstrong R, Watt J (1998) Family-centred functional therapy for children with cerebral palsy: an emerging practice model. *Phys Occup Ther Pediatr* 18: 83–102.

McGibbon Lammi B, Law M (2003) The effects of Family-Centred Functional Therapy on the occupational performance of children with cerebral palsy. *Can J Occup Ther* 70: 285–297.

Mathiowetz V, Haugen JB (1994) Motor behavior research: implications for therapeutic approaches to central nervous system dysfunction. *Am J Occup Ther* 48: 733–745.

Matos M, Miller K, Eliasson AC, Imms C (2007) Goal directed training: linking theories of treatment to clinical practice for improved functional activities in daily life. *Clin Rehabil* 21: 1–9.

Missiuna C, Mandich AD, Polatajko H, Malloy-Miller T (2001) Cognitive orientation to daily occupational performance (CO-OP): Part 1 – theoretical foundation. *Phys Occup Ther Pediatr* 20: 69–81.

Missiuna C, Pollock N, Law M, Walter S, Cavey N (2006) Examination of the Perceived Efficacy and Goal Setting System (PEGS) with children with disabilities, their parents, and teachers. *Am J Occup Ther* 60: 204–214.

O'Neill, Harris SR (1982) Developing goals and objectives for handicapped children. *Physical Ther* 62: 295–298.

Rosenbaum P, King S, Law M, King G, Evans J (1998) Family-centered service: a conceptual framework and research review. *Phys Occup Ther Pediatr* 18: 1–20.

Smith RA, Wrisberg CA, editors (2000) *Motor Learning and Performance. A Problem-based Learning Approach, 2nd edn*. Baltimore, MD: Human Kinetics.

19
VOLITION: CHILD-ORIENTED INTERVENTION FOR THE UPPER EXTREMITY

Susan M. Cahill and Gary Kielhofner

The child's ability to use hand skills to successfully handle objects symbolizes an evolutionary ability distinctive of the behaviour unique to higher life forms (Pehoski 2006). We rely on our hands as primary tools to participate in activities that are the essence of daily life (Eliasson 2006). Our ability to use our hands in this manner is closely tied to our volition to engage in activities that give our life meaning.

The multifaceted relationship between a child's inherent characteristics and abilities and a multitude of environmental factors come together to influence development (Humphry 2002). When a child has cerebral palsy, the child's inherent abilities may require intervention to support development, and adapted environments may be required that provide occupational opportunities. The development of volition must be supported and, if necessary, volition must be cultivated.

The origins of volition

Infants are focused on getting their basic physiological needs met and an inherited neurological drive to act (Kielhofner 2007). This drive becomes more and more pronounced as children grow up. It manifests as a curiosity about people, objects, and events that take place around them, along with a nearly insatiable drive to produce effects. Early on, this drive is manifest in such simple behaviours as attending, looking around, kicking, and moving the arms. These movements quickly take on an intentional quality so that the child is soon lifting their head to look at things, reaching for an intended object and so on. Shortly after, children begin to participate in occupations that have a component of shared value with others, such as purposeful play.

Each new form of occupational engagement enables the child to develop capacity and learn new skills as well as to internalize new habits and acquire roles. Whether they are learning social reciprocity or handling objects successfully, a child's volition for occupation is developing.

The nature of volition

Volition is realized though occupation. By engaging in occupations, each child builds up their own volition. Moreover, since the process of occupation is ongoing, the child is constantly re-developing their volition. Therefore, volition is an evolving collection of thoughts and feelings that a child has about their occupational engagement. Moreover, these thoughts and feelings drive future choices for action.

The thoughts and feelings that comprise volition in childhood are concerned with personal competence and control, enjoyment and pleasure in doing, and value assigned to doing. Thus it is argued that volition is made up of personal causation, values, and interests. Personal causation refers to one's sense of competence and effectiveness. Values refer to what one finds important and meaningful to do. Interests refer to what one finds enjoyable or satisfying to do. Some occupations the child chooses to engage in will be driven by pleasure, some by a desire to achieve more control or mastery, and some by what others in the social context value.

Personal causation in childhood

Personal causation is made up of two components (Kielhofner 2007). The first of these is the sense of capacity; this refers to what the child believes they can and cannot do, or what capacities they have. The second component, sense of efficacy, is the child's perception of their relative success in achieving desired ends and in doing what others expect of them.

Positive thoughts and feelings related to personal causation support the development of a sense of personal control and independence. Positive personal causation shapes the child's sense of confidence and motivates them to seek new experiences and take on new challenges. On the other hand, when personal causation is compromised (i.e. when a child is convinced they do not have abilities, or when they feel that they are not effective in certain situations), the child will tend to avoid engaging in action. Self-assessment or knowledge of personal capacity plays a major role in their decision to act (Kielhofner 2007).

If the child with cerebral palsy, functioning at MACS Level III, were unable to open a box of cookies efficiently, he might negatively judge his capacity to get a cookie independently. If this were to happen, the child would recognize that he does not have the capacity to successfully and easily handle the box without adaptations. However, if this child has a strong sense of efficacy, he is likely to look for another way to accomplish his desired end. He may, for instance, opt to find his mother and ask for help, or attempt to use an assistive device. However, a child with compromised personal causation, with or without cerebral palsy, may tend to see this as one more 'failure' and give up, feeling distressed and unable. On the other hand, if the child is able to open the box and get the cookie, he will experience success. He will not only realize he has a new ability, but also feel a sense of accomplishment and therefore a strong sense of self-efficacy. Additionally the child will develop the view that he could again experience this outcome.

The interrelationship between the child and the environment, as well as the child's true abilities and sense of personal causation, will determine the child's level of proficiency with tasks. It may also establish the child's level of participation in occupations. How a child responds to perceived success or failure will depend on how the child's personal causation has developed. If he generally experiences himself to have capacity and feel efficacious, he will be more likely to accept failure as a specific instance in which he does not have enough capacity to be effective. Such a child can go on and seek out other opportunities where success can be experienced. Children with a strong sense of personal causation are more able to pick themselves up and go on after failure. Conversely, a child who has a history of failure and poor sense of capacity and efficacy will have a tendency to generalize the failure to an overall view of self, contributing to a downward cycle. Children with poor personal causation are less resilient to frustrations, may give up easily and may even develop a widespread sense of hopelessness and avoidance of action.

Values in childhood

Kielhofner (2007) explains that values are based on convictions, or 'views of life that define what matters'. The values of children are influenced by extrinsic factors and develop over time. For example, cultural and societal influences affect a child's disposition and guide their beliefs about values (Kielhofner 2007). Values in childhood are also driven by the desire to please adults (Kielhofner 2007). Caregivers, and more specifically parents, shape children's understanding of right and wrong. As social beings, children are hungry for acceptance and approval from persons in authority. Children begin to shape their behaviour to match the values of the adults in their world; they often adopt these values to be their own.

Regardless of race or ethnicity, for most children, being able to exert will and complete actions with intention is valued. The child who opened the box of cookies and reached in independently was excited by the notion that he could exert his will and get the cookie on his own. Many of our values related to work, leisure and self-care are dependent on our skill in handling objects and using tools successfully. For example, a child with cerebral palsy, at MACS Level IV, who is able to easily manage only a few objects or requires many adaptations, may feel obligated to relinquish ownership of an activity tied to his values. In this instance, the child may value autonomy and wish to brush his own teeth. However, if he needs physical assistance or adapted equipment to complete the task, he may feel like he is giving up his independence.

Interests in childhood

Children are born with an innate desire to explore, discover and learn about the world they live in. They seek to have new experiences and try out their skills. Children gain pleasure from engaging in activities that they are successful at. Often, the time spent being occupied with such activities causes them to be cultivated into interests. Interests provide individuals with satisfaction and pleasure throughout life (Kielhofner 2007). Put simply, we like to do what we are good at and what we think is fun. Children use interests as an avenue to experiment with their abilities and increase their capacities within the context of occupations that they prefer.

When the occupational performance of children with disabilities is examined, we may discover that they lack the necessary opportunities to experience adequate investment and satisfaction (Kielhofner 2007). Their prospects for experiencing enjoyment may be limited. Furthermore, the fear of being rejected due to diminished capacities may cause them to ignore the opportunities that they are presented with (Kielhofner 2007). For example, a 9-year-old child with cerebral palsy at GMFCS Level I who enjoys playing sports may pass up the opportunity to try out for the local tennis team. Despite his ability to perform the basic gross motor tasks necessary to play tennis, he might prefer to stand at the sidelines rather then allow his peers to see him struggle with coordination and timing while engaged in a match.

The impact of volition in upper extremity intervention

Decreased volition to participate in occupations may further result in delayed skill development, as well as a lack of independence (Andersen et al 2005). If a child is not motivated or engaged, he may choose to be a passive participant in intervention. Children with cerebral palsy who demonstrate a low sense of efficacy may assume a passive role in daily occupations. The inability to effectively execute movements related to hand function, and the presence of high or low tone, as well as sensory impairments, may present obstacles to efficient occupational performance for children with cerebral palsy (Skold et al 2004). If failure and ineffectiveness dominate their experiences, motivation to engage in occupations is likely to decrease.

Children who are passive and possess deficient skills related to independence may develop learned helplessness. Due to a low sense of personal causation, they may begin to suspect that their actions do not impact their environment in the ways in which they would hope (Deitz et al 2002). The relationship between actual abilities, personal causation and challenges may cause unnecessary reliance on other individuals, such as caregivers.

Besides learned helplessness, a child with cerebral palsy who presents with functional limitations related to hand use may not have enough confidence to initiate exploration of their environment. Consequently, children with functional limitations may experience fewer opportunities to fine-tune their motor, communication and process skills. In fact, a trend in the literature suggests that children with physical impairments are less persistent in play. Their play is shorter, less complex, and developmentally inappropriate; they are, as a result, less engaged (Smidt and Cress 2004). Ultimately, children with physical impairments, such as those that are a result of cerebral palsy, may have very limited interests. For example, they may choose to engage only in activities that are passive, such as watching television.

In order to address functional limitations, a clinician must understand a child's volition so that intervention is meaningful. Rather then merely working on increasing range of motion or building strength in the affected hand, the therapist should structure treatment so that it is driven not only by the child's needs, but also by the child's values and interests. The clinician must also take into consideration the child's sense of personal causation, and structure activities related to the development of hand function, as well as the environment, in a manner supportive of success.

Children with special needs may have developed inadequate investment and satisfaction in occupational performance due to fewer opportunities, related to their disabilities (Kielhofner 2007). Decreased personal capacity and decreased sense of efficacy may have caused them to experience dislike of or dissatisfaction with certain occupations. A child with cerebral palsy at MACS Level I may wish to play with a certain toy, such as Legos, but because of decreased fine motor control may not be able to do so to the degree that they wish. Larger Legos or other building blocks may not offer the same sense of gratification, and as a result they may choose not to engage in play at all.

Supporting the development of volition in upper extremity intervention

The use of assessment tools based on the Model of Human Occupation (MOHO) can provide insights that give the clinician a better understanding of a child's volition, in addition to supporting the development of meaningful and child-centred goals and treatment sessions. By exploring the child's values and interests, as well as their sense of personal causation, the therapist may succeed in eliciting increased participation from the child. Integrating the child's desires and needs into treatment may increase the child's volition and lead to functional gains (Basu et al 2004) towards upper extremity intervention goals. Table 19.1 explains the purposes and administration of three MOHO-based assessments.

Christina: a case study

Christina is aged 6 years 2 months and has a medical diagnosis of spastic cerebral palsy and mild intellectual impairment. Christina is functioning at MACS Level IV and GMFCS Level IV. She recently moved to a new school district. She uses an augmentative communication device to participate in calendar as well as other classroom activities. A paraprofessional assists Christina with wheelchair mobility, table-top activities, and school-related self-care tasks, such as feeding and toileting.

USING ASSESSMENT TOOLS TO EXAMINE VOLITION

The occupational therapist decided to complete the SCOPE, the PVQ and the COSA with Christina to learn more about her motivation and skill level, as well as the impact that the environment has on her patterns of performance. In order to complete the assessments, the clinician reviewed Christina's records and scheduled a time to work with her on a one-to-one basis and two opportunities to observe her in the natural context, once in her classroom and again in the cafeteria during lunch.

USING VOLITION TO SUPPORT FUNCTIONAL UPPER EXTREMITY GAINS

Christina expressed that she often has difficulty using her hands to work with things and making her body do what she needs to do, as shown in the COSA assessment. She has difficulty with using feeding utensils and with using her name stamp. Based on the assessment findings, it was recommended that Christina arrive early at the cafeteria to practise her self-feeding skills before the other students arrived, so that she would be more available to interact with them. In addition, it was recommended that she communicate, with a hand signal, when she would like help with feeding or would like to take a break from self-feeding and be fed. This would give Christina the opportunity to continue to develop self-feeding skills while supporting her desire to engage in social interactions with peers in the lunchroom. The therapist also suggested that Christina bring her communication device to the cafeteria so that she could communicate with other students over lunch. It was recommended that Christina be included in the process of choosing a more appropriate name stamp by exploring several different options and indicating her preference.

The therapist learned that Christina's desire to explore, enjoy, and demonstrate preferences facilitated her participation in occupation (see results on the PVQ and SCOPE). However, Christina's response to challenges restricted her participation because she did not

TABLE 19.1

Assessment tools based on the Model of Human Occupation (MOHO)

Assessment	Purpose	Age range	Administration	Reporting
Pediatric Volitional Questionnaire (PVQ)	Assesses the volitional characteristics of young children and those who have limitations in cognitive, verbal or physical abilities (Basu et al 2002)	Primarily used with children between 2 and 6 years of age and with older children who experience developmental delay	Completed during a minimum of two observations (15 minutes in length or longer) in the child's natural contexts	The information from the PVQ can be reported on the standardized summary form which shows the ratings the child achieved for each item. It can alternatively be reported as part of regular case notes which characterize the child's volitional strengths and weaknesses as well as factors in the environment that support or attenuate volition
Child's Occupational Self-Assessment (COSA)	A client-centred tool which provides information regarding a child's personal sense of occupational competence (Keller et al 2002)	Primarily used with children between 8 and 13 years of age or those who demonstrate insight and wish to collaborate	Two versions available: a checklist format and a card sort system. The child rates each statement based on significance and own sense of efficacy with the occupation	The COSA form can be included as a component of the assessment or it can be summarized in a narrative note. What is critical in documenting the COSA process is: to acknowledge the child's perceptions of his/her own strengths/weaknesses and what is important to the child; to identify major gaps between what is important to the child and how the child sees his/her performance; and to incorporate the child's priorities into the treatment goals planning process
Short Child Occupational Profile (SCOPE)	Provides an overview of a child's functioning and determines how the environment supports or limits occupational participation (Bowyer et al 2004)	Administered across treatment settings. Appropriate for all ages and levels of ability	Data are gathered primarily through observation, caregiver interview, and review of records	The SCOPE can be used as a screening tool or as an interdisciplinary evaluation. Information gained from the SCOPE can be used to collect baseline data about a child's functional abilities, as an outcome measure, and to develop trans- and interdisciplinary goals and treatment interventions

303

PVQ Assessment – Summary Form (Form B)

Name:	Christina Sulin
Date of Birth:	1-11-00
Sex:	☐ Male ☒ Female
Examiner:	J. Buckley, OTR/L

Ratings:

Session I Date: 3-20-06 Setting: Classroom

Shows curiosity	Initiates actions	Task directed	Shows preferences	Tries new things	Stays engaged	Expresses mastery pleasure	Tries to solve problems	Tries to produce effects	Practices skill	Seeks challenges	Modifies environment	Pursues activity to completion	Uses imagination
S	S	S	S	S	S	S	S	S	S	S	S	S	S
I	I	I	I	I	I	I	I	I	I	I	I	I	I
H	H	H	H	H	H	H	H	H	H	H	H	H	H
P	P	P	P	P	P	P	P	P	P	P	P	P	P

Session II Date: 3-22-06 Setting: Cafeteria

Shows curiosity	Initiates actions	Task directed	Shows preferences	Tries new things	Stays engaged	Expresses mastery pleasure	Tries to solve problems	Tries to produce effects	Practices skill	Seeks challenges	Modifies environment	Pursues activity to completion	Uses imagination
S	S	S	S	S	S	S	S	S	S	S	S	S	S
I	I	I	I	I	I	I	I	I	I	I	I	I	I
H	H	H	H	H	H	H	H	H	H	H	H	H	H
P	P	P	P	P	P	P	P	P	P	P	P	P	P

Key: P = Passive   H = Hesitant   I = Involved
S = Spontaneous

Summary:

During the second observation, Christina was initially task-directed. However, as lunch progressed, Christina lost the desire to remain involved in self-feeding due to her desire to interact with the other students, the effort involved and the time constraints placed on her. The lunchroom environment may not be supporting her to problem solve or try to produce effects. In addition, students must finish their lunch in a designated amount of time, which may make it more challenging since she eats more slowly. The additional challenge of having to perform this ADL task more quickly over-challenges her sense of capacity. Christina is an active participant in classroom activities. Possible reasons for this may be that she is familiar with peers in her class and comfortable with the structure of the class routine, as well as the time allotted for each task. In addition, Christina may feel that there is a good match between her abilities and the task demands.

Fig. 19.1 Christina's Pediatric Volitional Questionnaire.

Myself	I have a big problem doing this	I have a little problem doing this	I do this OK	I am really good at doing this	Not really important to me	Important to me	Really important to me	Most important of all to me
Watch a movie				X			X	
Make my body do what I want it to do	X						X	
Use my hands to work with things	X						X	

Fig. 19.2 Christina's COSA (Child's Occupational Self-Assessment) record form. Christina's therapist completed the card sort version of the COSA with her. (The COSA contains 25 items or statements – the items represented here are those that are relevant to Christina's case.)

Short Child Occupational Profile (SCOPE)
Summary Sheet

Client: Christina Sulin	Assessor: J. Buckley, OTR/L
Age: __6__ Years __2__ Months Date of Birth:__1_/_1__00_	Date of Evaluation: __3_/__22__/__06__
Sex: Male ___ Female _X_	___ Intial _X_ Re-evaluation
Date of referral/admission: __2_/__21/_06_	Treatment Setting: ... School...
Dx./Reason for referral: CP	COUNTERINDICATIONS (Allergies, etc.): none

Background Information

Primary caregiver/s: Mr. and Mrs. Smith

Where does the client live? Ranch style home in the northwest suburbs of Chicago

Who else lives in the household? Christina's older sister

School/day care information: Christina attentds a full day special education kindergarten program.

Comments: Christina uses an augmentative communication device and has a manual wheelchair. The team is exploring power options. Currently she does not self-propel her wheel chair.

F	Facilitates	Facilitates participation in occupation
A	Allows	Allows participation in occupation
I	Inhibits	Inhibits participation in occupation
R	Restricts	Restricts participation in occupation

Analysis of Strengths and Limitations:

Christina uses adapted scissors & built up crayons with maximum assistance to complete an art project.

She can bring a wash cloth up to her face, but requires assistance to complete the task.

Christina is able to hold a tambourine, but requires adult assistance to shake it. She attempts to push down

elastic pants for toileting, but requires assistance to get them past her hips. Christina recognizes familiar

people, enjoys novel activities, and makes choices at snack time and through the day.

Summary of Ratings

	Volition				Habituation				Communication and interaction skills				Process skills				Motor skills				Environment				
	Exploration	Enjoyment	Preferences	Response to challenge	Daily activities	Response to transitions	Routines	Roles	Non-verbal communication	Vocal/verbal expression	Conversation	Relationships	Understands & uses objects	Orientation to environment	Makes decisions	Problem solving	Posture & mobility	Coordination	Strength	Energy/endurance	Physical space	Physical resources	Social groups	Occupational demands	Family routine
F	**F**	**F**	F	F	F	**F**	F	F	F	**F**	F	F	F	F	F	F	F	F	F	F	F	F	F	F	F
A	A	A	**A**	A	A	A	**A**	**A**	**A**	A	A	**A**	A	A	**A**	A	A	A	A	A	A	**A**	A	A	**A**
I	I	I	I	I	**I**	I	I	I	I	I	I	I	**I**	**I**	I	I	**I**	I	**I**	I	I	I	**I**	I	I
R	R	R	R	**R**	R	R	R	R	R	R	R	**R**	R	R	R	**R**	R	R	R	R	R	R	R	R	R

Fig. 19.3 Christina's Short Occupational Profile.

feel effective and gave up. The therapist advised the team to provide Christina with increased opportunities to be successful by downgrading upper extremity task requirements. Their careful matching of Christina's current abilities with appropriate task demands would support Christina in the development of a stronger sense of efficacy and provide her with successful experiences. Once Christina had developed confidence, the team could then increase task demands and introduce her to experiences that previously she may have perceived as too challenging.

REFERENCES

Andersen S, Kielhofner G, Lai J (2005) An examination of the measurement properties of the Pediatric Volitional Questionnaire. *Phys Occup Ther Pediatr* 25: 39–57.

Basu S, Kafkes A, Geist R, Kielhofner G (2002) *A User's Guide to the Pediatric Volitional Questionnaire (PVQ) (Version 2.0)*. Chicago: Model of Human Occupation Clearinghouse, University of Illinois at Chicago.

Basu S, Jacobson L, Keller J (2004) Child-centered tools: using the Model of Human Occupation framework. *School System Special Interest Section Quarterly* 11: 1–3.

Bowyer P, Ros M, Schwartz O, Kielhofner G (2004) *A User's Guide to the Short Child Occupational Profile (SCOPE) (Version 2.0)*. Chicago: Model of Human Occupation Clearinghouse, University of Illinois at Chicago.

Deitz J, Swinth Y, White O (2002) Powered mobility and preschoolers with complex developmental delays. *Am J Occup Ther* 56: 86–96.

Eliasson A (2006) Normal and impaired development of force control in precision grip. In: Henderson A, Pehoksi C, editors, *Hand Function in the Child: Foundations for Remediation*. St Louis: Elsevier, pp 45–61.

Humphry R (2002) Young children's occupations: explicating the dynamics of developmental processes. *Am J Occup Ther* 56: 171–179.

Keller J, Kafkes A, Basu S, Federico J, Kielhofner G (2002) *The Child Occupational Self Assessment (COSA) (Version 2.0)*. Chicago: Model of Human Occupation Clearinghouse, University of Illinois at Chicago.

Kielhofner G (2007) *A Model of Human Occupation: Theory and Application, 4th edn*. Baltimore, MD: Lippincott Williams & Wilkins.

Pehoski C (2006) Cortical control of hand–object interaction. In: Henderson A, Pehoksi C, editors. *Hand Function in the Child: Foundations for Remediation*. St Louis: Elsevier, pp 3–20.

Skold A, Josephsson S, Eliasson A (2004) Performing bimanual activities: the experience of young persons with hemiplegic cerebral palsy. *Am J Occup Ther* 58: 416–425.

Smidt ML, Cress CJ (2004) Mastery behaviors during social and object play in toddlers with physical impairments. *Educ Train Dev Disabil* 39: 141–152.

20
CONSTRAINT-INDUCED MOVEMENT THERAPY FOR CHILDREN WITH HEMIPLEGIA

Ann-Christin Eliasson and Andrew M. Gordon

Constraint-induced movement therapy (CI therapy) has recently regained attention as a potential intervention for children with hemiplegic cerebral palsy (CP). The main principle of the treatment is twofold: restraint of the uninvolved hand and intensive practice with the involved hand during a specified time period. The number of studies of this intervention with children is increasing. Although the results so far are mainly positive, more information is needed before the intervention can be considered to be evidenced-based. This chapter will give an overview of the knowledge in the area, and discuss what is known about the effect of the treatment, the various modifications that have been made to make the intervention child-friendly, and how CI therapy fits in relation to other types of interventions.

Principles of constraint-induced movement therapy

The principle of CI therapy was developed through neurophysiological research by Dr Edward Taub during the 1950s (see Taub 1980). Somatic sensation was unilaterally abolished in monkeys using dorsal rhizotomy. This caused the monkeys to stop using the affected arm unless the intact limb was restrained, in combination with practising tasks using the deafferented limb for one to two weeks. Since these monkeys regained functional use of the deafferented limb, the initial lack of use of the involved limb was interpreted to occur as a result of behavioural suppression. Taub defined this as 'learned non-use' and proposed that restraint of the intact limb and use of special training techniques would overcome the learned non-use and even lead to increased function in the involved limb (Taub 1980). Further studies with deafferented monkeys were conducted to delineate the learned non-use and forced use paradigms (Taub et al 1980, 1994).

Constraint-induced movement therapy in adults

The monkey experiments formed the basis for experimentation in adult humans who had sustained a stroke. The first clinical attempt to examine the effect of restricting the use of the intact upper extremity in humans was performed more than 25 years ago in a 50-year-old woman with hemiplegia, by Ostendorf and Wolf (1981). The woman reported that it was easier to use her affected extremity after the period of restraint. This was followed up by a larger study of forced use (Wolf et al 1989). Subsequent studies involving adults who had sustained a stroke utilized restraint in addition to various training techniques to examine changes in involved upper extremity function (e.g. Taub et al 1993, Taub and Wolf 1997).

Gradually the intervention was refined and eventually termed 'constraint-induced movement therapy' (Taub et al 1999). Subsequent studies of CI therapy examined the efficacy of this intervention for improving involved upper extremity use with various types of restraints, interventions and outcome measures, and in people with chronic, acute and sub-acute stroke (for a review see Wolf et al 2002). Today, for adults, restraint for 90 per cent of waking hours is typically used, together with a structured training programme.

Neuroimaging and transcranial magnetic stimulation studies of the brain prior to and after CI therapy have demonstrated cortical reorganization around the infarct site after the intervention. These differences led to hypotheses regarding central nervous system (CNS) plasticity and the role of CI therapy in cortical reorganization (Liepert et al 1998, 2000, Levy et al 2001, Schaechter et al 2002, Park et al 2004). Overall, the results of these adult studies suggest that, following stroke, CI therapy may improve upper extremity function (see Wolf et al 2002 for a review, Wolf et al 2006).

Constraint-induced therapy/forced use in children

OVERVIEW OF STUDIES

There have been a considerable number of case studies of CI therapy in children, but recently there have also been several larger studies as well (Table 20.1; for an extensive review of the literature see Charles and Gordon 2005, Hoare et al 2007). One study (Willis et al 2002) involved forced use, i.e. restraint of the involved upper extremity without training. All of the other studies engaged children in training during the restraint period. Various outcome measures were used, although all of these studies reported positive results of the intervention. Thus, CI therapy seems to be a promising intervention method to improve involved hand and arm function in children with hemiplegia.

However, only four studies used a randomized design (Willis et al 2002, Taub et al 2004, Sung et al 2005, Charles et al 2006), and none of these studies can readily be designated level I (AACPDM, Evidence Report, based on Sackett 1989) since they were small randomized clinical trials. Of the remaining studies, one was a prospective study with a control group (Eliasson et al 2005), three were studies with an ABAA design (Eliasson et al 2003, Naylor and Bower 2005, Gordon et al 2006), and one was a study with an ABA design (Karman et al 2003). Hence, these studies were all level II and III or lower. Thus, despite its promise, the evidence to date is tentative at best. The variability in the type of restraint, the restraint duration, the length of the intervention, the intensity of practice, and evaluation measures further weakens the evidence and makes it difficult to draw conclusions about efficacy and dosage (Gordon et al 2005).

A number of issues regarding use of CI therapy in pediatric populations have been raised by these studies.

INCLUSION CRITERIA

All of the participants in these studies had hemiplegia, although the causes included cerebral palsy, acquired head injury and stroke. Thus, across these studies, the distribution of impairment was discussed but the etiology was not suggested as an indicator of the appropriateness

309

TABLE 20.1
Summary of pediatric constraint-induced therapy and forced use studies

Year	Authors	Participants	N	Ages	Intervention	Design	Outcome measures
2002	Willis et al	Hemiplegia (stroke, CM, trauma, unknown aetiology)	25 Tx = 12 Cont = 13	1–8 yrs	1 mo cast	RTC Pre- and 1 mo post-intervention & 6-mo follow-up	PDMS and parent interview
2003 letter 2006 full article	Eliasson et al Bonnier et al	Hemiplegia (CP)	9	13–18 yrs	10/12 d, 7 h/d, mitt-like splint, group intervention	ABAA Pre- and post-intervention 5-mo follow–up tests	B-Os, J-T Test, AMPS, grip strength, in-hand manipulation, Novel Motor Task Performance
2003	Karman et al	Hemiplegia (TBI, AV malformation, stroke)	7	7–17 yrs	10/14 d, Posey mitt during waking hrs + 6 hrs shaping	ABA Pre- and post-intervention	AAUT, MAL
2004	Taub et al	Hemiplegia (CP)	18 Tx = 9 Cont = 9	7–96 mo	3 wk, bi-valved full-arm cast during waking hrs, including 15 d shaping, 6 h/d	RTC Pre- and post-intervention, 3 wk & 3 mo post-intervention 6-mo follow-up (Tx group only)	EBS, PMAL, TAUT
2005	Eliasson et al	Hemiplegia (CP)	41 Tx = 21 Cont = 20	18 mo–4 yrs	Restraint glove 2 h/d over 2-mo period	Prospective + control Pre- and post-intervention 6-mo follow-up	AHA
2005	Naylor & Bower	Hemiplegia (CP)	9	21–61 mo	1-hr sessions 2×/wk Duration = 4 wk gentle physical restraint + verbal instruction	ABAA Pre- & post-intervention 4-wk follow-up	QUEST
2005	Sung et al	Hemiplegia (CP)	31 Tx = 18 Cont = 13	>8 yrs	6 wk, short arm cast, training 2× 30min/wk	RTC Pre- & post-intervention	Box and blocks WFIM EDPA
2006	Charles et al	Hemiplegia (CP)	22 Tx = 11 Cont = 11	4–8 yrs	10 of 12 consecutive days, sling 6 h/d	RTC Pre- & post-intervention. 1-mo & 6-mo follow-up	J-T Test B-Os CFUS

| 2006 | Gordon et al | Hemiplegia (CP) | 19 Younger = 11 Older = 8 | 4–8 yrs 9–14 yrs | 10 of 12 consecutive days, sling 6 h/d | RTC Pre- & post-intervention. 1- & 6-mo follow-up | J-T Test B-Os CFUS |

Source: Adapted from Gordon and Charles 2005.

Abbreviations: CP = cerebral palsy, CM = cerebral malformation, TBI = traumatic brain injury, AV malformation = arterio-venous malformation, UE = upper extremity, Tx = treatment, J-T Test = Jebsen-Taylor Test of Hand Function, PDMS = Peabody Developmental Motor Scales, AMPS = Assessment of Motor Processing Skills, B-Os = Bruininks-Oseretsky Test of Motor Proficiency, AAUT = Actual Amount of Use Test, MAL = Motor Activity Log, PMAL = Pediatric Motor Activity Log, TAUT = Toddler Arm Use Test, EBS = Emerging Behavior Scale, AHA = Assisting Hand Assessment, QUEST = Quality of Upper Extremity Skills Test, CFUS = Caregiver Functional Use Survey, EDPA = Erhardt Developmental Prehension Assessment

of the intervention. In addition, sensory integrity and/or amount of motor function were described and almost all the children across the studies were fairly mildly to moderately impaired. Only one study included children with varying severity of hand function impairment (Eliasson et al 2005). To date, the extent to which specific impairments and the severity level are predictive of efficacy is not known, although there is some evidence that CI therapy is less effective in older individuals with more severe hand function impairment (Charles et al 2006). Children below the age of 4 years with severely impaired hand function showed improvements. Specifically, they learned to use the hand more efficiently during bimanual tasks (Eliasson et al 2005).

AGE APPROPRIATENESS AND CNS PLASTICITY
The potentially greater CNS plasticity in young children could mean that CI therapy is more efficacious in younger children than in older children. Thus, promoting early use could conceivably enhance the development of spared circuitry, optimizing developmental motor skill potential. Yet, restricting movement or motor activity during such a critical period could have the opposite effect on the non-involved extremity, leading to impoverished corticospinal termination and motor behaviour (e.g. Martin et al 2004). Although the extent to which such critical periods exist in humans is not known, caution should still be exercised in restraining children by casting them for a longer period at too young an age. Therefore the adapted two-hours-a-day model introduced by Eliasson et al (2005) may be less invasive in this regard.

The ages of the children who participated in the studies ranged from 7 months to 17 years. The optimal age for CI therapy and forced use is not possible to determine since the methodologies differed across all studies. However, a general 'earlier is better' rule can be questioned. Eliasson and coauthors demonstrated that older children (around 4 years old) improved more than younger ones (around 18 months old). However, Gordon et al (2006) found no difference in improvement between 4–8-year-old children and 9–13-year-old children, suggesting that there might well be other factors influencing the optimal age (e.g. severity, attention span; see Charles at al 2006). But the stage of development does influence the type of tasks that may be employed that sustain interest. Adolescents often demonstrate high motivation to improve their motor function (Bonnier et al 2006), and their improvements may be due to greater effort. Younger children learn to incorporate the arm into the body frame and use the arm for reaching and initiating movements more naturally, potentially explaining the positive results in the studies in young children (Eliasson et al 2005). This may be related to the learned non-use phenomenon, while pure hand dysfunction such as poor dexterity and precision may be improved in older children or adolescents (Eliasson et al 2003, Charles et al 2006, Gordon et al 2006). There might be different advantages to the therapy depending on age, which suggests that the treatment might be provided more than once during childhood.

TYPE OF RESTRAINT

The restraints in these studies are worn for extended periods (from 2 to 24 hours/day). Therefore it is important that the restraint is comfortable and adapted to the child's needs. Several types of restraint have been used in adult studies, including a sling (sometimes combined with a resting hand splint), a half-glove and a mitt. Intensive practice without a restraint is also used. It has been suggested that a restraint that allows some use of the non-involved extremity results in less intensive practice because the non-involved arm can still be used to complete tasks (Taub and Wolf 1997); however, it is unclear if this affects the efficacy. There are, however, relevant safety considerations when using slings, in case of loss of balance or falls.

The following types of restraints have been used for children: casts (Willis et al 2002, Sung et al 2005), gloves (Eliasson et al 2003, 2005), slings (Charles et al 2001, 2006, Gordon et al 2006), mitts (Karman et al 2003), and gentle intermittent physical restraint (Naylor and Bower 2005). In two studies (Eliasson et al 2003, 2005) the children were allowed to use the restraint hand as an assist (without grasping, which was prevented by the glove). This resulted in an increase in the number of activities that could be included in the training, and reduced verbal prompting. It is likely that the type of restraint is less important for efficacy than for comfort and safety. To wear a cast for 24 hours a day is not child-friendly and the advantages are not obvious. Furthermore, the dropout rate seems to be higher, although this is not clearly reported (Willis et al 2002, Taub et al 2004).

PROGRAMME INTENSITY

Programme intensity is commonly related to the time spent wearing the restraint. For children above the age of 4 years, the training period was mainly concentrated into two weeks (10 days) and the restraints were mainly worn during the practice hours, and never less than six hours per day (see Table 20.1). In this respect, the length of time of active programming and the duration of the intervention generally followed the protocol in adult CI therapy studies. For younger children, a modified version with fewer hours per day over a longer time period was used (Eliasson et al 2005, Naylor and Bower 2005). The advantage of less intensive training is that it is easier to find appropriate activities for two hours a day compared to six hours a day, especially for young children and children with severely impaired hand function. It also gives the child the opportunity to immediately integrate the 'new' ability into everyday activity. However, reduced continuity over longer time periods may reduce the efficacy of the training in older children (Charles et al 2006). Variations in duration have been made to make the intervention more child-friendly. Three studies (Willis

312

et al 2002, Taub et al 2004, Sung et al 2005) required the children to wear a cast for 24 hours per day for 3–6 weeks. Even if they received therapy six hours a day, the frustration associated with their limited ability to complete tasks may harm more than facilitate the child's motivation to learn to use the hand. Furthermore, it is difficult to maintain the high intensity of the training. In a recent study, children were found to spend less than 60 per cent time-on-task using the six hours/day model (Charles et al 2006).

Although compliance is assured, the frustration for children, in all age groups, and their families, could be excessive, particularly for children with more severe impairment and those whose attention span on a task is typically short. If the child does not want to cooperate and complete the desired tasks, it is essential to terminate the programme. Since efficacy is reported to be independent of age, it may be possible to convince caregivers that it is better to stop the programme and wait until the child is better prepared and motivated. Although difficult to prove, intensity is probably the critical factor for improvement, but the precise dose response is unknown.

The importance of practice

CI therapy and forced use both involve restraint of the non-involved extremity and practice using the involved extremity. Although restraint is common to both techniques, the types of practice provided during the restraint period differ. By definition, placing a restraint on the non-involved upper extremity results in practice of the involved hand and arm for any movement performed. The difference between forced use and CI therapy lies in the extent to which the practice is structured and organized (Charles and Gordon 2005). Most studies have used CI therapy with some sort of modification in order to make it child-friendly. Of the largest studies, only Willis and coauthors clearly used forced use by just casting the children. CI therapy involves a structured practice period which includes shaping and repetitive task practice, or activity-based practice (see Winstein et al 2003, Eliasson et al 2005, Bonnier et al 2006).

FORCED USE

Forced use involves casting without structured or activity-based practice. There is no help in selection of appropriate activities adapted to the child's abilities. Since the results of the various studies were positive regardless of the type of practice provided during the restraint period, we cannot see any advantages of forced use over more active treatment – the risks of frustration are not worth saving the cost of the treatment. When forced use is combined with casting, unexpected harm may be done since the treatment may coincide with activity-dependent critical periods for hand function (see Gordon et al 2005). Accordingly, the dropout rates of participants receiving CI therapy (Eliasson et al 2005, Charles et al 2006, Gordon et al 2006) are likely to be much lower than in studies using forced use.

STRUCTURED PRACTICE

Shaping and repetitive task practice are used in interventions involving structured practice. Shaping is a behavioural technique, similar to adaptive or part practice described in the motor learning literature (Winstein 1991, Schmidt and Lee 1999), in which a motor objective is approached in small steps through successive approximation; the task may then be made more difficult or the speed of performance increased progressively. Specific activities are selected by considering the joint movements with the greatest deficits. The activities are also chosen on the assumption that they have the greatest potential for improvement. The choice of specific activities is viewed as less important than the movements that result. For example, board games can be used to encourage wrist supination and extension, precision grasp, and grasp stability.

Structured practice involves clear instructions for the child to follow regarding how the activity should be performed. Although the movements are important, the child's preferences for activities are taken into account, as long as the activities have similar potential for improving identified movements. Feedback about performance is provided frequently, and only positive reinforcement is given. The intensity of the practice is dependent on the individual's ability. The environment can be manipulated to vary the task requirements, elicit specific movements, or increase the difficulty, and it is always monitored so that frequent successes can be achieved.

Repetitive task practice involves games or functional tasks that are performed continuously over a specific period, and overall feedback is provided at the end of the task (Winstein et al 2003). Most games include repetitive components that could be used for this type of practice. Thus, movements are embedded in the context of tasks.

Both shaping and repetitive practice provided through play activities are thus child-friendly, although this type of practice may be too difficult for young children. Structured practice that includes shaping is described in several studies (DeLuca et al 2003, Karman et al 2003, Taub et al 2004, Charles et al 2006, Gordon et al 2006).

Structured practice through group training has been developed primarily at Teachers College, Columbia University. The environment is easy to modify to meet the children's needs, to control the tasks, to minimize distractions, and to allow children to interact with each other, thus increasing social support. The intervention is conducted with groups of two to four children, with each child being assigned to at least one trained interventionist. This team approach allows interventionists and supervisors to meet and discuss each child, review progress, solve problems, and plan for the next day (Gordon et al 2005).

ACTIVITY-BASED PRACTICE
Activity-based practice focuses mainly on the activity performance, but is also based on the motor learning literature (Trombly 1989, Schmidt and Wrisberg 2000, Missiuna et al 2001). The activities are practised only as whole movements and they are intended to be meaningful and motivating, providing the child with the possibility of using their hand in a variety of situations. As in structured practice, the most important thing for the child is to have fun. The activities are also similar to those in structured practice, but do not, as earlier described, focus on specific types of movements, such as wrist supination and extension during a board game. Instead attention is focused on task completion and any kind of movement strategy is allowed. Problem solving is encouraged in order for the child to discover the most efficient strategies. The main idea is that children should improve basic components of hand function and work on cognitive strategies rather than practising specific types of movements. The

goal is to teach the child how their impaired movement can still be utilized functionally. For example, during board games, the focus is on successfully grasping the card, positioned so that they can read it, and then progressing to the next step, such as moving a board piece within a reasonable amount of time. It is the ability to play the game that is important, despite irregular movements.

The activities must be of appropriate difficulty level and the motor component difficulty is progressively increased to be on the edge of the child's ability, as in structured practice. Activities include repetition as long as it is meaningful for the child. Motivation for using the hemiplegic hand may be the most important agent in attaining intense practice. Most activities are typically unimanual, but the child can occasionally use the dominant hand as a supporting limb if a glove is used as the restraint (Eliasson et al 2005).

Activity-based practice has been provided for young children using individualized home training (Eliasson et al 2005). For young children it is important that the training takes place in the child's customary environment (at home and/or in their preschool setting), since the intervention duration needs to be adapted to the child's routine (i.e. eating, napping) and their short attention span. Having a rich natural environment in which a wide variety of different activities would be encountered is important to facilitate the learning process. Unlike in structured practice, the parents and/or preschool teachers are responsible for providing the intervention daily, with supervision from an experienced therapist once a week. Supervision includes discussion of the child's progress and grading the activities for the following week, and encouragement and support to continue the programme. Extensive training of parents and teachers is required (Eliasson et al 2005).

A recreational day-camp has also been used for activity-based practice (Bonnier et al 2006). The camp programme primarily consists of performing common daily and recreational activities. It takes place in a motivating setting, an open recreational area, very different from traditional treatment settings. As part of the daily programme the adolescents, engage in various recreational activities, including frisbeegolf, basketball, boules, canoeing, water games, and various fine motor board games and dice and card games. The participants are also engaged in the preparation of meals, eating, and washing the dishes. All activities are specifically selected to include the use of gross motor function of the upper extremity as well as hand manipulation tasks. The day camp programme is designed to take advantage of the group setting, keeping motivation high. Adolescents can actively help each other with problem solving. One member of staff for every three participants is sufficient for adolescents, while one staff member for every two participants is needed for younger children (8–12 years).

By highlighting these three models of intervention, we want to show that there are various possibilities for treating a child with the assistance of a restraint. The intervention has been provided in various environments. There have been individualized programmes and group programmes. The decision on which programme to use will depend on the health service options in various countries. However, motor learning principles seem to be an appropriate theoretical framework to use in defining a CI therapy intervention (Schmidt and Lee 1999, Gordon et al 2005), although they are utilized in a slightly different manner, and the optimal ingredients for successful practice are as yet unknown.

315

Assessment to be used

In the studies to date, the outcome measures vary from study to study. This diversity of measures is in part due to the age range of the children (toddler to late adolescence) and the lack of availability of appropriate outcome tools. Most existing tests of paediatric hand function were not designed for children with unilateral impairments, and the psychometric properties of the instruments in this population are limited (see Chapter 12).

Using the International Classification of Functioning (ICF: WHO 2001) as the framework, the outcome has to be assessed at the level the intervention took place (i.e. in this case the activity domain). We propose that assessment should take place from at least three perspectives. First, changes in quality of unimanual hand function should be measured, since that is what is trained, i.e. the best capacity of hand function. This requires standardized measurements that are valid, reliable and sensitive to changes in children with hemiplegia. Second, changes in bimanual hand performance (i.e. the quality of task performance when both hands are required) should be examined. This is important since we do not expect children to use the hemiplegic hand as the dominant hand after treatment. This needs to account for the different roles of the dominant and non-dominant hands (Fagard and Jacquet 1989; see Chapter 11). Of course, this raises the issue of whether bimanual practice might be more effective (see Chapter 11). The assessments should measure both capacity (i.e. what the child can do) and performance (i.e. what the child actually does). Finally, perceived changes by parents/caregivers and children need to be evaluated. Clarification of intervention goals, consistent with the needs of the intended population, is important in the selection of appropriate evaluation tools (Palisano et al 2000).

To date, evaluation of outcome has mainly been related to the capacity of the impaired limb. The Jebsen-Taylor Test of Hand Function is the most frequently used test. It is a timed-task test measuring dexterity in unilateral tasks. Subtests of the Bruininks-Oseretsky Test of Motor Proficiency have also been used, although modified so that the unimanual items are executed with the hemiplegic hand instead of the stipulated preferred hand. For younger children, QUEST has also been used. QUEST has its limitations since the aim is to measure the effect of neurodevelopmental treatment (NDT) in which protective reaction and weight-bearing have a more dominant role compared to manipulatory skills. This means there are few items in QUEST directly related to hand skills. The only test so far that evaluates the affected hand in bimanual activities is the Assisting Hand Assessment (AHA; see Chapter 12). AHA was developed to measure the usefulness of the affected hand during bimanual performance and is a promising new tool.

Core concept of CI therapy and its relation to other interventions of upper limb function

The goal of CI therapy, as well as all other treatments for children with hemiplegia, should be to learn how to use the two hands as efficiently as possible when needed in bimanual activities, since people with unilateral hand involvement will always use the non-involved hand whenever possible. The non-involved hand will always have better precision, speed and accuracy.

Based on the literature, CI therapy appears to be a promising method for improving hand function in children with hemiplegic CP, although there are various ways to administer it. During childhood and adolescence, different forms of CI therapy may be useful depending on the child's ability and circumstances (economic, social, etc.). However, even if there are modifications, it is important to point out that the key elements – intensive practice during a specified time period and restraint of the non-involved hand – are required when providing CI therapy. Therefore the training should not be performed in the short time available in the course of usual and customary care (typically one hour or less). The most important factor is likely to be the intensity.

Skilled therapists and other involved providers are another important ingredient of the programme. The therapist needs to understand the concept of CI therapy before starting treatment and have theoretical and practical knowledge of motor-learning principles of skill acquisition, as well as pedagogic skills – i.e. the therapist needs to know how to teach children to learn, and how to supervise parents and preschool teachers if involved. An important consideration is that it is not the restraint that induces change; rather, it is the environment that is used to solicit intensive practice.

We would like to point out that CI therapy should be used in addition to other treatments of the upper extremity throughout the child's long-term paediatric programme since it can only be used for a short period. It may be repeated during childhood (Charles and Gordon 2007) since children show additional improvement with a second period of training. They might also benefit in different ways at different ages.

The extent to which children improve is multifactorial and not easy to determine. The child's motivation, attention span and severity of impairment may all impact on the results. In general, treatment of hand function in children with hemiplegia is poorly investigated. Although there are more studies on CI therapy than on other treatment approaches, there is still much that is not known and further research is required.

It is important to recognize the individual child's needs. The overall goal for treatment must be guided by the person's own life situation. Improvements following CI therapy are usually sustained at follow-up, helping the child and family to feel confident about the child's own competence. After the intensive treatment the child and family can then focus on other important aspects of the child's life situation such as their social and academic skills.

REFERENCES

Bonnier B, Eliasson AC, Krumlinde-Sundholm L (2006) Effects of constraint-induced movement therapy in adolescents with hemiplegic cerebral palsy: a day camp model. *Scan J Occup Ther* 13: 13–22.

Charles J, Gordon AM (2005) A critical review of constraint-induced movement therapy and forced use in children with hemiplegia. *Neural Plast* 12: 245–261.

Charles J, Gordon AM (2007) Repeated doses of constraint-induced movement therapy results in further improvement. *Dev Med Child Neurol* 49: 770–773.

Charles J, Lavinder G, Gordon AM (2001) The effects of constraint-induced therapy on hand function in children with hemiplegic cerebral palsy. *Pediatr Phys Ther* 13: 68–76.

Charles J, Wolf SL, Schneider J, Gordon AM (2006) Efficacy of a child-friendly form of constraint-induced movement therapy in hemiplegic cerebral palsy: a randomized control trial. *Dev Med Child Neurol* 48: 635–642.

DeLuca SC, Echols K, Ramey SL, Taub E (2003) Pediatric constraint-induced movement therapy for a young child with cerebral palsy: two episodes of care. *Phys Ther* 83: 1003–1013.

Duque J, Thonnard JL, Vandermeeren Y, Sebire G, Cosnard G, Olivier, E (2003) Correlation between impaired dexterity and corticospinal tract dysgenesis in congenital hemiplegia. *Brain* 126: 732–747.

Eliasson AC, Bonnier B, Krumlinde-Sundholm L (2003) Clinical experience of constraint-induced movement therapy in adolescents with hemiplegic cerebral palsy – a day camp model. *Dev Med Child Neurol* 45: 357–359.

Eliasson AC, Krumlinde-Sundholm L, Shaw K, Wang C (2005) Effects of constraint-induced movement therapy in young children with hemiplegic cerebral palsy: an adapted model. *Dev Med Child Neurol* 47: 266–275.

Fagard J, Jacquet A (1989) Onset of bimanual coordination and symmetry versus asymmetry of movement. *Infant Behav Dev* 12: 229–235.

Gordon AM, Charles J, Wolf SL (2005) Methods of constraint-induced movement therapy for children with hemiplegic cerebral palsy: development of a child-friendly intervention for improving upper extremity function. *Arch Phys Med Rehabil* 86: 837–844.

Gordon AM, Charles J, Wolf SL (2006) Efficacy of constraint-induced movement therapy on involved upper-extremity use in children with hemiplegic cerebral palsy is not age-dependent. *Pediatrics* 117: 363–373.

Hoare BJ, Wasiak J, Imms C, Carey L (2007) Constraint-induced movement therapy in the treatment of the upper limb in children with hemiplegic cerebral palsy (Review). *The Cochrane Library*. Issue 2.

Karman N, Maryles J, Baker RW, Simpser E, Berger-Gross P (2003) Constraint-induced movement therapy for hemiplegic children with acquired brain injuries. *J Head Trauma Rehabil* 18: 259–267.

Levy CE, Nichols DS, Schmalbrock PM, Keller P, Chakeres DW (2001) Functional MRI evidence of cortical reorganization in upper-limb stroke hemiplegia treated with constraint-induced movement therapy. *Am J Phys Med Rehabil* 80: 4–12.

Liepert J, Miltner WH, Bauder H, Sommer M, Dettmers C, Taub E, Weiller C (1998) Motor cortex plasticity during constraint-induced movement therapy in stroke patients. *Neurosci Lett* 250: 5–8.

Liepert J, Bauder H, Wolfgang HR, Miltner WH, Taub E, Weiller C (2000) Treatment-induced cortical re-organization after stroke in humans. *Stroke* 31: 1210–1216.

Martin JH, Choy M, Pullman S, Meng Z (2004) Cortico-spinal system development depends on motor experience. *J Neurosci* 24: 2122–2132.

Missiuna C, Mandich AD, Polatajko H, Malloy-Miller T (2001) Cognitive orientation to daily occupational performance (CO-OP): Part 1 – theoretical foundation. *Phys Occup Ther Pediatr* 20: 69–81.

Naylor CE, Bower E (2005). Modified constraint-induced movement therapy for young children with hemiplegic cerebral palsy. *Dev Med Child Neurol* 47: 365–369.

Ostendorf CG, Wolf SL (1981) Effect of forced use of the upper extremity of a hemiplegic patient on changes in function. *Phys Ther* 61: 1022–1027.

Palisano RJ, Campbell SK, Harris SR (2000) Decision making in pediatric physical therapy. In: Campbell SK, Vander Linden DW, Palisano RJ, editors. *Physical Therapy for Children, 2nd edn*. Philadelphia, PA: W.B. Saunders Co, pp 198–224.

Park SW, Butler AJ, Cavalheiro V, Alberts JL, Wolf SL (2004) Changes in serial optical topography and TMS during task performance after constraint-induced movement therapy in stroke: a case study. *Neurorehabil Neural Repair* 18: 95–105.

Sackett DL (1989) Rules of evidence and clinical recommendations on the use of antithrombotic agents. *Chest* 95(Suppl 2): 2–4.

Schaechter JD, Kraft E, Hilliard TS, Dijkhuizen RM, Benner T, Finklestein SP, et al (2002) Motor recovery and cortical reorganization after constraint-induced movement therapy in stroke patients: a preliminary study. *Neurorehabil Neural Repair* 16: 326–338.

Schmidt RA, Lee TD (1999) *Motor Control and Learning: A Behavioral Emphasis*. Champaign, IL: Human Kinetics Publishers.

Schmidt RA, Wrisberg CA (2000) *Motor Learning and Performance. A Problem-based Learning Approach, 2nd edn*. Champaign, IL: Human Kinetics Publishers.

Sung, IY, Ryu JS, Pyun SB, Yoo SD, Song WH, Park MJ (2005) Efficacy of forced-use therapy in hemiplegic cerebral palsy. *Arch Phys Med Rehabil* 86: 2195–2198.

Taub E (1980) Somatosensory deafferentation research with monkeys: implications for rehabilitation medicine. In: Ince LP, editor. *Behavioral Psychology in Re-habilitation Medicine: Clinical Applications*. Baltimore, MD: Williams & Wilkins, pp 371–401.

Taub E, Wolf SL (1997) Constraint induction techniques to facilitate upper extremity use in stroke patients. *Top Stroke Rehabil* 3: 38–61.

318

Taub E, Harger M, Grier HC, Hodos W (1980) Some anatomical observations following chronic dorsal rhizotomy in monkeys. *Neurosci* 5: 389–401.

Taub E, Miller NE, Novack TA, Cook EW, Fleming WC, Nepomuceno CS, et al (1993) Technique to improve chronic motor deficit after stroke. *Arch Phys Med Rehabil* 74: 347–354.

Taub E, Crago JE, Burgio LD, Groomes TE, Cook EW 3rd, et al (1994) An operant approach to rehabilitation medicine: overcoming learned nonuse by shaping. *J Exp Anal Behav* 61: 281–293.

Taub E, Uswatte G, Pidikiti R (1999) Constraint-induced movement therapy: a new family of techniques with broad application to physical rehabilitation – a clinical review. *J Rehabil Res Dev* 36: 237–251.

Taub E, Ramey SL, DeLuca S, Echols K (2004) Efficacy of constraint-induced movement therapy for children with cerebral palsy with asymmetric motor impairment. *Pediatrics* 113: 305–312.

Trombly C (1989) Carr and Shepherd approach: motor relearning programme for stroke patients. In: Trombly C, editor. *Occupational Therapy for Physical Dysfunction*. Baltimore, MD: Williams & Wilkins, pp 155–160.

WHO (2001) *International Classification of Functioning, Disability and Health*. Geneva: World Health Organization.

Willis JK, Morello A, Davie A, Rice JC, Bennett JT (2002) Forced use treatment of childhood hemiparesis. *Pediatrics* 110: 94–96.

Winstein CJ (1991) Designing practice for motor learning: clinical implications. In: Lister MJ, editor. *Contemporary Management of Motor Control Problems: Proceedings of the II Step Conference*. Alexandria, VA: Foundation for Physical Therapy.

Winstein CJ, Miller JP, Blanton S, Taub E, Uswatte G, Morris D, et al (2003) Methods for a multisite randomized trial to investigate the effect of constraint-induced movement therapy in improving upper extremity function among adults recovering from a cerebro-vascular stroke. *Neurorehabil Neural Repair* 17: 137–152.

Wolf SL, Lecraw DE, Barton LA, Jann BB (1989) Forced use of hemiplegic upper extremities to reverse the effect of learned nonuse among chronic stroke and head-injured patients. *Exp Neurol* 104: 125–132.

Wolf SL, Blanton S, Baer H, Breshears J, Butler AJ (2002) Repetitive task practice: a critical review of constraint-induced movement therapy in stroke. *Neurology* 8: 325–338.

Wolf SL, Winstein CJ, Miller JP, Taub E, Uswatte G, Morris D, Giuliani C, Light KE, Nichols-Larsen D (2006) Effect of constraint-induced movement therapy on upper extremity function 3 to 9 months after stroke. The EXCITE randomized clinical trial. *JAMA* 17: 2095–2104.

21
SELF-CARE AND HAND FUNCTION

Anne Henderson and Ann-Christin Eliasson

Introduction

Participation in all societies includes expectations for independence in basic self-care. Self-care activities are among the first achievements of childhood and their accomplishment engenders both a sense of competence and social approval. The mastery of self-care increases a child's control of both home and school environments, freeing the child from dependence on the convenience of caregivers (Amato and Ochiltree 1986). Only when disease or disability interrupts the timely achievement of self-care abilities, do we become aware of how important they are in our daily life – e.g. deficient self-care skills are a problem for schooling, as the child entering school is expected to be self-sufficient in eating, dressing, washing, and toilet activities. As skilled manipulatory actions highly influence self-care activities, independence in basic self-care is difficult to achieve without fine motor skill (Dellatolas et al 2005), and a typical child practises a skill over months and years before the skill is mastered. Maturation plays a major role in a child's achievement and, if not interrupted by intellectual or physical disability, the achievement of self-care skills follows an orderly progression of cognitive and motor development (Gesell et al 1940).

Children are highly variable in the chronological ages at which they acquire self-care skills, and a three- to four-year span may separate the earliest and latest age at which a particular skill is mastered (Haley et al 1992, Carruth and Skinner 2002). Cultural, societal, class and family variables have all been shown to influence timing (e.g. Bott et al 1928, Tsuji et al 1999, Gannotti and Handwerker 2002, Wong et al 2002, Henderson 2006), as have personal qualities of persistence and self-reliance (Wagoner and Armstrong 1928, Key et al 1936, Hauser-Cram et al 2001).

Children with cerebral palsy have, as a group, a pronounced deficit in self-care ability (Ostensjo et al 2004), although this ability has not been thoroughly investigated in its relationship to different levels of functional limitation. Gross motor function and learning disability have been identified as important factors influencing independence in self-care and the particular problems depend on both the topography and the severity of disability (Ostensjo et al 2004). Fine motor skill is also an important factor in self-care ability (Dellatolas et al 2005), but the lack of good assessments has hampered investigation into its relationship to independence and identification of the particular problems of children with cerebral palsy.

The recently developed Manual Ability Classification System (MACS) is now making it possible to review the differing abilities of a heterogeneous group of children with cerebral

palsy in relation to their ability to use their hands in daily activities (Eliasson et al 2006). Although MACS is not specifically an assessment of activities of daily living, it is designed to describe children's ability to use their hands in daily activities including self-care (for details of MACS, see Introduction). Relating MACS levels to ability in self-care, the most competent children (at MACS level I) are independent even in advanced self-care activities, like grooming, although they might need to spend more time than their peers learning certain skills. Children at MACS level II can also learn to manage almost all self-care activities, even fasteners and cutting food, but need a lot of practice to become skilful. Furthermore, they might avoid wearing clothes that are hard to manage, such as jeans with difficult buttons. Children at MACS levels I–II are typically independent in self-care but only if their gross motor function is also adequate, as they usually need to be at level I or II on the Gross Motor Function Classification System (GMFCS; Palisano et al 2000). There is a high correlation between GMFCS and MACS but different levels are also common (Eliasson et al 2006; see also Fig. I.3 in the Introduction).

Children at MACS level III typically need help with activities like cutting food but can eat independently if the environment is arranged to meet their needs and technical aids are introduced. Children at MACS level III also have trouble with fasteners, but their dressing independence is to a great extent dependent on their gross motor ability, which may vary from GMFCS level I to level IV. For children at MACS level IV, independence probably occurs only for simple tasks like pulling off a hat and eating with an adapted spoon. Children at level V do not achieve independence in any self-care activities. Children at lower levels in MACS and GMFCS are typically very dependent on caregivers. However, self-care can always be improved by training, although the goals depend on children's functional limitation (Ketelaar et al 2001, Wong et al 2004, Eliasson et al 2005).

This chapter reviews the typical development of self-care skills in relation to the upper extremity and the way functional limitation impacts on the self-care capabilities of children with cerebral palsy. We will discuss intervention based on task-oriented approaches and goal-directed training, and give examples of actual occupational therapy case studies which demonstrate the way goals can be organized in respect to a child's level of functional limitation (see also Chapter 17).

Measurement of self-care
Two assessments, the Wee Functional Independence Measure (WeeFIM; State University of New York at Buffalo 1994) and the Pediatric Evaluation of Disability Inventory (PEDI; Haley et al 1992), are widely used paediatric functional assessments of children. As they both include sections on self-care they are discussed here. These instruments were developed in the United States but have been validated or normed in other countries, e.g. Japan (Liu et al 1998), China (Wong et al 2002), Puerto Rico (Gannotti and Cruz 2001), Sweden (Nordmark et al 1999), Slovenia (Srsen et al 2005), Holland (Custers et al 2002), and Norway (Ostensjo et al 2003, Berg et al 2004). Both instruments have been demonstrated to reliably measure responsiveness to change following surgery (e.g. Loewen et al 1998) or rehabilitation (e.g. Dumas et al 2001, Knox and Evans 2002, Ekström-Ahl et al 2005).

The WeeFIM was standardized for children ranging in age from 6 months to 7 years. However, its companion, the Functional Independence Measure (FIM; Uniform Data System for Medical Rehabilitation 1987), can be used as children get older. The WeeFIM is concise and simple and can be administered by observation or interview. There are 18 items in three sections, on self-care, mobility and cognition. Seven of the 18 items are on self-care and the seven-point ordinal scale yields a single score for the level of independence in each of the domains of eating, grooming, bathing, dressing upper body, dressing lower body and toileting.

The PEDI is standardized on children aged from 6 months to 7 years 6 months. It includes three measurement dimensions: ability in functional skills, the amount of caregiver assistance, and the equipment and modifications needed for function. The functional skills assessment provides great detail in three content domains: self-care, mobility and social function. The self-care functional skill section includes the domains of eating, dressing, bathing, toileting and grooming, encompassing 15 areas that are further broken down into skill items. For example, dressing includes the four areas of pullover/front opening garment, pants, shoes/socks, and fasteners, each of which has five items. Normative standard scores for self-care are available at six-month intervals from the age of 6 months to 7 years 6 months. Raw scores can also be converted to Scale Scores ranging from 1 to 100. Scale Scores reflect increasing levels of self-care achievement, and as they estimate achievement regardless of age, they can be used as a summary score for older children. Total self-care scores can be used to measure the overall progress of children or scores can be obtained for separate domains and for individual items. This latter feature is useful in clinical decision making when a treatment programme is directed toward teaching a specific skill. Age expectations are also given for items, and the user can select the level of expectation desired, such as the age range at which 10 per cent, 25 per cent, 50 per cent, 75 per cent, or >90 per cent of children without disabilities achieve a skill.

In summary, the WeeFIM and the PEDI, the most commonly used norm-referenced assessments of self-care independence, have been found to be valid and reliable and to responsively measure change over time. The WeeFIM has the advantage of being easy and fast to administer. The PEDI, though more complex to administer and score, is more comprehensive, and provides a depth of information that can be useful in treatment planning as well as in programme evaluation.

Self-care acquisition in children

The development of adult self-care activity spans many years, from early infancy to adolescence, and adult-level proficiency requires the maturation of cognition, perception and motor skill. The following pages present developmental sequences in the self-care performance of typical children, together with an analysis of the capabilities that affect their achievement in self-care, and examples of use of the information in children with cerebral palsy. The tables present the approximate ages at which typical children become self-sufficient in discrete skills. Pre-skills, attempts at skills and partial skills are included as they show steps in learning. The items from the PEDI (Haley et al 1992) use the ages at which 75 per cent of the children studied achieved mastery. Other ages are those given by the sources identified.

EATING

The acquisition of eating behaviour begins at 6 months when the infant holds a bottle, and continues for 10 years, at which time self-feeding is completely independent.

Basic eating skills

Table 21.1 presents the eating and drinking skills that enable infants to feed themselves. These early skills require only the basic hand skills that are functional before 1 year of age: bilateral hold, gross grasp and pincer grasp. Infants drink from a closed cup and feed

TABLE 21.1
Basic self-feeding skills

Skill	Age
FINGER FOODS	
Reaches to mouth while sitting	6 mo[1]
Feeds self cracker, whole hand grasp	7 mo[1]
Feeds self finger foods, pincer grasp	10 mo[1]
Takes bite-size pieces from plate, delicate grasp,	
appropriate force, with demonstrated release	1 yr[1]
DRINKING	
Holds bottle and brings to mouth	6 mo[1]
Tips bottle to drink	10 mo[2]
Drinks from bottle/spout cup with lid	1 yr[3]
Holds cup alone, hands pressed on side	1 yr[2]
Grasps with thumb and fingertips and tilts	1 yr 3 mo[2]
Lifts cup to mouth, drinks well, may drop	1 yr 6 mo[1]
Lifts open cup securely with two hands	2 yrs[3]
SPOON USE	
Pre-skills while being fed	
Mouth open, head moves toward spoon	3–6 mo[4]
Removes food by lip compression	3–6 mo[2]
Spoon skills	
Grasps spoon in fist	10–11 mo[2]
Dips spoon in food, lifts to mouth	1 yr 3 mo[2]
Fisted grasp, pronated forearm, turns spoon	1 yr 3 mo[1]
Fills spoon, turns in mouth, spilling	1 yr 6 mo[1]
Spoon angled slightly toward mouth	1 yr 6 mo[2]
Tilts spoon handle up as removes from mouth	1 yr 6 mo[2]
Scoops food, lifts with spilling	2 yrs[3]
Point of spoon enters mouth without turning	2 yrs[2]
Fills by pushing point of spoon into food	2 yrs[4]
Uses spoon well with minimal spilling	2 yrs 6 mo[3]

Notes:

[1] Coley 1978
[2] Gesell and Ilg 1943
[3] Haley et al 1992
[4] Gesell and Ilg 1937

themselves, first a cracker in the whole hand, and then bite-size pieces of food picked up with a precise pincer grasp. At first, grasp force is unregulated and the cracker breaks, but by 1 year the child has learned to use appropriate force in both hand and pincer grasps (Coley 1978). The spoon is the first tool used by infants and has thus been the subject of several detailed developmental studies (Bott et al 1928, Gesell and Ilg 1937, Connolly and Dalgleish 1989). The basic components of spoon use – understanding of the spoon as a tool, head control, removing food with the lips, filling the spoon, and carrying it to the mouth with little spilling – are well established before 3 years of age. Over this time, the spoon is held in a fisted grasp with the arm pronated and children gradually learn to flex their wrists to avoid spilling.

Advanced eating skills
Table 21.2 shows the chronology of continued development in the use of eating tools (cups, spoons, forks, and knives). The adult finger grip of the spoon requires new patterns of grasp and movement and more motor control and dexterity (Haley et al 1992), and as spoon grasp changes from fisted to finger grasp the associated patterns of arm and shoulder movements change from pronation to supination and shoulder rotation. The adult finger grip does not

TABLE 21.2
Advanced eating skills

Skill	Age
DRINKING	
Holds cup with one hand, free hand poised to help	2 yrs[1]
Holds small glass with one hand	2 yrs[2]
Drinks with a straw	2 yrs[2]
Cup held by handle, drinks securely, one hand	3 yrs[1]
Obtains drink from tap	3 yrs 6 mo[1]
Pours self drink from large pitcher or carton	4 yrs 6 mo[3]
SPOON	
Adult grasp of spoon with fingers (girls supinate)	3 yrs[1]
Fills spoon by pushing point or rotating spoon	3 yrs[1]
Holds spoon with fingers for solid foods	4 yrs[2]
Eats liquids, spoon held with fingers, few spills	6 yrs[2]
FORK	
Spears and shovels food, little spilling	2 yrs 6 mo[3]
Fork held in fingers	4 yrs 6 mo[2]
KNIFE	
Uses knife to cut soft foods (sandwich)	5 yrs 6 mo[3]
Spreads with knife	7 yrs[2]
Cuts meat with knife	7–8 yrs[2]

Notes:

[1] Gesell and Ilg 1943.
[2] Coley 1978.
[3] Haley et al 1992.

develop until 3 years in girls and even later in boys (Gesell et al 1940). By 4 years a child can handle liquids in spoons or cups and uses two hands to serve himself/herself from the tap or pitcher. The 5-year-old develops greater strength and precision in finger grasp of tools and acquires new bilateral skills with a knife, spreading and cutting soft foods. A fisted grasp is used in early attempts to cut meat with a knife and fork, as it appears that the force needed for holding and cutting requires hand and finger power that is not developed until a child is 7 or 8. The 5-year-old is skilful but slow; self-feeding takes concentration, and it is not until later that the skill is sufficiently automatic to allow eating and talking at the same time (Hurlock 1964, Klein 1999). The child becomes deft and graceful at 8 or 9 years of age (Gesell and Ilg 1946), and at 10 years observes adult cultural standards of eating behaviour (Hurlock 1964).

Eating in children with cerebral palsy
Early eating skills demand relatively simple motor capabilities yet they are a challenge to the child with cerebral palsy. The typical collaborative use of two hands when holding the bottle or cup is difficult for many children with cerebral palsy and is not usual for children with hemiplegia. Low tonus, poor head control and chewing and swallowing problems complicate the eating skills of a large group of children with cerebral palsy. Nevertheless, even with limited upper extremity use, most children with cerebral palsy can learn to eat certain things themselves. Training of their hand to mouth movements can be facilitated by the caretaker's guidance of the child's hand as it grasps food or a spoon (Finnie 1997), as well as by the child's own trial and error. The children start to learn to finger feed by eating crackers, as do their peers.

The adult grip on utensils requires coordinated arm and shoulder movements that are difficult for many children with cerebral palsy. However children at MACS level I will have only minor problems in stressful situations. Children at MACS level II manage almost all eating skills with only minor alternative strategies or adaptations. Their success typically depends on the capacity in the most involved hand (hemiplegia and diplegia) since bilateral finger grips are crucial for cutting food with a knife and fork. Ataxic and uncoordinated movements also have a major impact on the ability to cut food. Cutting food is highly influenced by force regulation as well as by strategy. A typical treatment goal is to determine with the child their most efficient strategy for cutting food of different textures and then to practise that strategy with force control.

Children at MACS level III typically need adaptation and preparation: for example, use of an adapted fork, or help cutting and serving food. Children at MACS level IV are very dependent on environmental aids when eating. They have a poor repertoire of hand movements, making it difficult to shovel food onto the fork and then to supinate the forearm to get the fork into the mouth. It is also worth noting that children with cerebral palsy at several levels may eat so slowly that it negatively influences their independence in many situations.

Example of learning to cut food

The way treatment can be structured can be illustrated by telling the story of Anna. She is 8 years old and she often asked for help when eating because she had difficulty cutting food. She also felt that her eating skills were not as neat as those of her peers, e.g. she dropped food from her fork. Anna has diplegia, and, with a greater than typical skill difference between her hands, functions at MACS level II and GMFCS level III. By analysing her eating, the occupational therapist found that Anna had no clear strategy for cutting food: when she tried, she continually changed her grasp patterns. The strategy Anna tried most of the time was to use her right hand for the knife and the left for the fork. However, the fork was often too upright, making it difficult to stabilize the food when cutting, and the cut pieces of food were too large.

Anna, her parents, and an assistant at school agreed to work on her eating skills for five weeks, starting with her cutting strategy and using both lunch and dinner as a natural environment for training. At the beginning, Anna needed continual reminders: (1) to keep the knife in the right hand, (2) to hold the fork in a more horizontal position, and (3) not to cut big pieces. Anna and her assistant at school met the occupational therapist once a week and cooked a light meal. At the same time they discussed the progress of Anna's learning. During the third week Anna's behaviour became more consistent: she had chosen an efficient strategy for cutting and holding the utensils. A new aspect of training was added to make her eating style more elegant. She needed to learn to hold the fork in a more dynamic and flexible way, and to put food on the fork securely so as not to lose it on the way to her mouth. During the following week she again needed continual reminders of how to adjust the fork, but over time the assistant and the parents were able to minimize verbal instruction and cueing. After five weeks Anna became more confident and satisfied in her eating situations. Anna, the family and the assistant agreed that having a defined goal, and a time-limited period during which they got continuous support and supervision from the therapist, had had a remarkably successful impact on Anna's eating skills.

DRESSING

Dressing skill proceeds from undressing, to dressing, to managing fasteners. Taking off an item of clothing is far easier than putting it on because the latter requires both greater motor skill and new perceptual abilities. It is easy to pull off a sock, but two hands and a foot must work together to put a sock on and the heel of the sock must be rotated correctly to match the heel to the foot. Pulling up pants requires more hand strength and bilateral coordination than pushing them down and kicking them off. Most dressing fasteners require a high level of finger strength and dexterity.

Undressing

Table 21.3 lists approximate ages at which children achieve undressing skills. The 6-month-old infant uses grasp and simple motor sequences for the inappropriate removal of hats and socks. Undressing continues to be interesting and by 2½ years most children can and want to take off their clothes. Undressing requires minimal perceptual skills and hand use requires little more than gross grasp, pulling, and pushing with one or both hands. With assistance in unfastening, the toddler can take off most articles of clothing (Coley 1978), and by 3 years undressing is performed well and rapidly (Gesell and Ilg 1943).

TABLE 21.3
Undressing: clothes unfastened

Skill	Age
HAT	
Pulls off hat	6 mo[1]
Pulls off hat appropriately on request	1 yr 6 mo[2]
MITTENS	
Removes mittens	14 mo[3]
SOCKS	
Pulls off bootie, socks	6–9 mo[2]
Reaches to toes while sitting	1 yr 4 mo[3]
Removes socks on request	2 yrs[4]
SHOES	
Removes untied/unfastened shoes	2 yrs[4]
Unties shoes and removes	3 yrs[3]
PANTS/PULL-DOWN GARMENTS	
Pushes off pants if soiled	1 yr[2]
Helps push down pants	2 yrs[3]
Pushes down underpants/shorts	2 yrs[2]
Removes long pants, elastic top, clearing over bottom	2 yrs 6 mo[4]
SHIRT/COAT/SWEATER	
Removes second arm from coat	1 yr[5]
Removes unbuttoned coat	1 yr[5]
PULLOVER GARMENT	
Removes pullover garment, needs assistance	3 yrs[3]
Removes T-shirt, dress	3 yrs[4]
Removes pullover garment with little assistance	4 yrs[3]

Notes:

[1] Vulpe 1979
[2] Gesell and Ilg 1943
[3] Coley 1978
[4] Haley et al 1992
[5] Brigance 1978

Dressing

The infant begins to help by pushing with arms or legs while being dressed, and demonstrates understanding of the process by holding out arms or lifting legs (Gesell and Ilg 1943, Haley et al 1992). As shown in Table 21.4, children learn rapidly between 1½ and 3½ years (Key et al 1936, Gesell et al 1940), but as Key and her associates (1936) noted, the learning of dressing skills is continuous, increasingly difficult, and unstable in these preschool years.

TABLE 21.4
Self-dressing without fasteners

Skill	Age
HAT	
Puts on, may be backwards	2 yrs[1]
SOCKS	
Puts on with help on heel orientation	3 yrs[2]
Puts on heel correctly oriented	3–3 yrs 6 mo[3]
Pulls socks to full extension	4 yrs[4]
SHOES	
Gets shoe on halfway	1 yr 6 mo[1]
Puts on, may be on wrong feet	3 yrs 6 mo[3]
Puts on correct feet	5 yrs[3]
Puts on independently with Velcro fastenings	5 yrs[3]
COAT/OPEN-FRONT SHIRT	
Holds arm out	9 mo[2]
Finds large armholes	2 yrs[2]
Puts on coat with help	2 yrs 9 mo[2]
Adjusts collar to neck	3 yrs[4]
Puts on open-front shirt	4 yrs[3]
PULLOVER GARMENT/T-SHIRT/DRESS	
Reaches above head; bilaterally/unilaterally	2–5 yrs[2]
Puts head through hole	2 yrs[4]
Pulls down over trunk	3 yrs[4]
Puts arm through hole	3 yrs 6 mo[4]
Puts on pullover garment	3 yrs 6 mo[3]
Distinguishes front/back, inside out	4 yrs[2]
PANTS/PULL-UP GARMENT	
Helps pull pants up	2 yrs[1]
Puts on if oriented verbally	3 yrs 6 mo[3]
Orients correctly and puts on	4 yrs[2]
Can turn right side out	4 yrs[2]

Notes:

[1] Gesell et al 1940
[2] Coley 1978
[3] Haley et al 1992
[4] Key et al 1936

Putting on clothes makes great demands on both motor and perceptual skills. Bilateral motor skills and hand and finger power grasps are needed to pull on most clothes, and hands and fingers work in unison to pull socks up to full extension, pull on boots, and pull up trousers or skirts (Thornby and Krebs 1992). Hands work cooperatively to hold a shirt or coat with one hand while finding the armhole with the other. Manoeuvring an arm into a second dress hole is a difficult motor task (Finnie 1997).

Nevertheless, the age at which particular dressing skills are achieved is in good part a reflection of the challenging perceptual skills needed. The child learns the motor skills of dressing one to two years before he or she learns to distinguish the front and back of garments or the left and right shoes.

Dressing and undressing in children with cerebral palsy
Participation in dressing and undressing should begin with assisted movements in infancy. The child should be encouraged to help by extension and flexion of arms and legs at the appropriate time during the dressing procedure, and to gradually take over the actions. This capability is the first of many steps of skills that precede and are necessary for independent self-dressing. Caretakers should be alerted to the readiness of a child to participate and incorporate their capability into daily routines. Attention to these part skills (see Tables 21.3 and 21.4) is important in dressing training of the child with cerebral palsy. It might be that most children at MACS levels IV–V are able to learn some part skills, while children at MACS levels I–III can proceed further.

Hand function always influences the child's dressing and undressing performance, but the child's gross motor performance is sometimes the greatest problem: increased lower extremity tone and decreased postural control in a child with diplegic or quadriplegic cerebral palsy make it difficult for them to be independent in self-dressing (Finnie 1997, Eliasson et al 2000, Knox and Evans 2002). This is a typical problem for children at GMFCS levels IV–V, and sometimes at level III. Commonly, these children wear casts on their feet and increased tension in their legs and ankles makes it difficult for them to reach their feet. Furthermore, manipulatory skills are needed to put on or remove casts. Gross motor problems complicate the use of hands for removing pants, socks and shoes, and the risk of losing balance makes it hard to lift clothing over the head (Coley 1978). In this case the need for positioning should be discussed and determined before the actual training starts. In addition to the motor dysfunction influencing the training procedure, learning and perceptual problems make the dressing process difficult to learn, as clothes have to be arranged in a certain way and the procedure remembered.

There are other typical upper-limb problems of dressing for children with cerebral palsy. One is the inability to move the arms in different directions – that is, to have the difficult bilateral control needed to hold with one hand and pull or push with the other hand. For a child with spastic hemiplegia, gross motor problems rarely influence tasks but typically spasticity in one of their upper limbs results in a need to develop special strategies for success. Then, too, much dressing must be learned well enough to be done without visual control, and learning problems highly influence performance. For many reasons, therefore, young children with hemiplegic cerebral palsy typically need more time for practice, encouragement and support to learn dressing activities early. However, as adolescents these children are almost always independent.

Example of learning to put on a jacket

Emma is only 3 years old but her parents wanted her to be more engaged in dressing. She has hemiplegic cerebral palsy and it was difficult for her to put her hemiplegic arm into the sleeve of a jacket. Typically she started with her dominant arm and then asked for help with the hemiplegic arm. She needed to learn to start by putting the hemiplegic arm into the sleeve. To help her to remember this, her mother sewed a marker inside the jacket close to the sleeve and Emma also got a temporary tattoo on her hemiplegic hand. These aids showed Emma how to put on the jacket, helping her to overcome her learning and perceptual problems. By the first week she was able to perform the procedure and in the following weeks she became less dependent on the markers and tattoo. After a few weeks of training she was able to put on any jacket without markers.

FASTENERS: SNAPS, BUTTONS, ZIPPERS AND TIES

Fastening and unfastening clothing is challenging for children (see Table 21.5). Fasteners are tools, involving the manipulation of one object relative to another (Parker and Gibson 1977), and, in general, self-care with tools matures later than other types of self-care. Tools require understanding of purpose and procedural memory of the actions involved in their use. A spoon is a relatively simple tool and its use is accomplished in infancy. Most fasteners, however, are complex tools and require mature perceptual skill to see relationships of both the separated and the combined parts of the fasteners and to follow changes in the relationship of parts as fastening is accomplished. Advanced cognitive skill is also needed to analyse what went wrong when errors are made and to develop strategies that lead to success.

Dressing fasteners also require advanced levels of motor skill, including precision grip, in-hand manipulation, and the learning of complex motor sequences: for the most part these capabilities must be bilateral and strength is essential (Koch and Simenson 1992). For example, hooking and separating a zipper requires gross power grasp in one hand and a precision and power finger grip with the other, making it a difficult bilateral task (Thornby and Krebs 1992, Sköld et al 2004).

Buttons and bows require spatial perceptual skill as well as power and precision in finger grips and in-hand manipulation in both hands. Because hands must work cooperatively through different manipulative sequences, and loops and strings have complex spatial relationships, tying shoes is an especially challenging self-care task, and achievement is a milestone of special importance for a child's sense of mastery and independence from adult help. Finally, tying a necktie is one of the last skills learned, because it requires every

TABLE 21.5
Fasteners: snaps (Velcro), buckles, buttons, zippers, laces, and ties

Skill	Age
SNAPS	
Snaps most front and side snaps	4 yrs[1]
Snaps back snaps	6 yrs[2]
BUCKLES	
Unbuckles belt or shoe	3 yrs 9 mo[2]
Buckles belt or shoe	4 yrs[2]
Inserts belt in loops	4 yrs 6 mo[2]
BUTTONS	
Buttons one large front button	2 yrs 6 mo[2]
Unbuttons most front and side buttons	3 yrs[2]
Reaches behind head, hands together	6 yrs[2]
Buttons back buttons	6 yrs 3 mo[2]
ZIPPERS	
Zips and unzips, locked tab	2 yrs 6 mo[1]
Opens front separating zipper	3 yrs 6 mo[2]
Zips front separating zipper	4 yrs 6 mo[2]
Opens back zipper	4 yrs 9 mo[2]
Closes back zipper	5 yrs 6 mo[2]
Zips, unzips, hooks, unhooks separating zipper	6 yrs[1]
SHOE LACES/TIES	
Laces shoes	5 yrs[2]
Ties overhand knot	5 yrs 3 mo[2]
Ties bow on shoes	6 yrs 6 mo[1]
SASHES	
Unties back sash of apron or dress	5 yrs[2]
Reaches behind back, hands together	6 yrs[2]
Ties front sash of apron or dress	6 yrs[2]
Ties back sash of apron or dress	8 yrs[2]
NECKTIE	
Ties necktie	10 yrs[2]

Notes

[1] Haley et al 1992
[2] Coley 1978

skill – multiple complex motor sequence learning, complementary use of two hands, and perceptual and cognitive skill, all of which must be learned with mirror vision.

Children need visual guidance to master the use of fasteners, and must practise several years with vision before they can perform a skill such as buttoning without the aid of the eyes (Wagoner and Armstrong 1928). Considerable visually guided practice is needed for any fastener before it can be mastered in awkward positions or with only touch for guidance.

Fastening the side or back of garments is especially difficult both because it is done without vision and because it requires shoulder rotation.

Use of fasteners in children with cerebral palsy

Many children with cerebral palsy will never have the finger strength and prehension or the bilateral skill needed for managing fasteners (Fedrizzi et al 2005). Children with hemiplegia at MACS levels II–III have a hard time holding pants or jackets in place while zipping, and alternating hands in the grasp of fabric and finger grip on the button to first insert and then pull the button through the hole. They may need help to develop a personal technique. Fortunately there are many adaptations of clothing fasteners using Velcro, rings on zippers, elasticated waists, etc., and adaptive clothing can be introduced early and serve a lifetime need (Coley and Procter 1989, Case-Smith 2000). When tactile sensation is compromised, a child will be more than usually dependent on watching their hands and will be slow to learn a skill. Back, neck and side fastenings that require tactual guidance may not be feasible. However, most children at MACS levels I and II are able to learn fastener skills, although they may need both help in developing strategies and extensive practice. Usually managing fasteners is the last part of dressing procedure to be learned, taking the child from dependence to independence in self-care.

Example of learning to button jeans

Jens is 9 years old and has hemiplegic cerebral palsy, MACS level II and GMFCS level II. He is independent in self-care except for buttoning his trousers. He didn't wear jeans to school because he would have needed help in buttoning his trousers when going to the toilet – therefore, Jens was motivated to learn this task. The therapist decided to use video for task analysis and recorded his attempt to unbutton and button up. When looking at the video it became obvious that Jens had no idea of how to hold the trousers and get the button through the hole at the same time, even when his mother tried to guide him. The therapist and Jens looked at the video recordings, and then they looked at another video recording of a person who succeeded in the buttoning. By looking at the videos and discussing the procedure it become obvious to Jens where to place his fingers in relation to the button. Jens was than asked to put on his largest jeans, sit on a chair and lean backward in order to see what he was doing. Jens agreed to go home and work on buttoning his trousers five minutes each day. After a week of training Jens could sometimes button the jeans in a few seconds but sometimes it took longer. After the second week he was prepared to wear the jeans to school, and manage going to the toilet and changing clothes for sports.

Looking back at this successful training, it was important first to involve Jens in the analysis of the problem by helping him to see the difference between success and failure. The second step was to establish a time-limited home training programme, to involve his parents and to continuously discuss his progress.

HYGIENE, TOILETING AND GROOMING

Most of the hygiene skills listed in Table 21.6 are achieved between the ages of 4 and 7 years. As with dressing, most hygiene tasks are bilateral: hands are washed together, soap and washcloth are held in different hands, and the towel is passed from hand to hand while

TABLE 21.6
Hygiene and grooming

Skill	Age
WASHING HANDS/FACE	
Dries hands with help	1 yr 6 mo[2]
Rubs hands together to clean them	2 yrs[1]
Turns tap on/off	3 yrs[1]
Disposes of paper towel or replaces towel	4 yrs[2]
Washes and dries thoroughly	4 yrs[1]
Washes/dries face thoroughly	6 yrs[1]
Washes ears	9 yrs[1]
BATHING BODY	
Tries to wash body	2 yrs[1]
Bathes down front of body	3 yrs[2]
Soaps cloth and washes	4 yrs 6 mo[2]
Washes back	7 yrs[3]
TEETH BRUSHING	
Opens mouth for teeth to be brushed	2 yrs[1]
Brushes teeth, not thoroughly	2 yrs 6 mo[1]
Prepares brush, wets and applies paste	5 yrs[1]
Thoroughly brushes teeth	5 yrs[1]
NOSE CARE	
Attempts to blow nose	2 yrs[1]
Wipes on request	2 yrs 6 mo[1]
Blows and wipes alone	6 yrs 6 mo[1]
TOILETING	
Assists with clothing management	2 yrs 6 mo[1]
Manages clothes before and after toileting	3 yrs 6 mo[1]
Tries to wipe self after toileting	3 yrs 6 mo[1]
Manages toilet seat, toilet paper, flushes	3 yrs 6 mo[1]
Wipes self thoroughly	6 yrs[1]
HAIR	
Brushes or combs hair; combs with supervision	3 yrs[1]
Brushes without rumpling	3 yrs[3]
Manages tangles/parts hair	7 yrs[1]
Combs using mirror to check style	7 yrs[2]
Uses rollers, hairspray	12 yrs[2]

Notes:

[1] Haley et al 1992.
[2] Coley 1978.
[3] Hurlock 1964.

drying hands and body. Even teeth brushing is a bilateral activity, as the toothbrush must be stabilized while applying toothpaste on the brush (Thornby and Krebs 1992, Sköld et al 2004). Once a child can sit alone in and climb into the bath, they can bathe themselves partially, and by 4 years the child is independent except for washing their back.

Toileting independence requires the learning of many sub-skills that develop over the preschool years. By the time a child is 3½ years old they are sufficiently aware of their bowel and bladder needs to obtain timely assistance in using a potty, but it is not until 5 years that they can get on and off an adult-size toilet, and complete independence in toileting is not achieved until a child is 6 years of age. The hand skills required for toileting include the management of clothing that often has fasteners, tearing paper from the roll, and flushing. The most difficult upper extremity skill, and the last to be achieved, is reaching behind to wipe oneself thoroughly. It requires wrist flexion, internal rotation, and arm extension.

Hair care for girls can be a difficult grooming activity, depending a lot on style. The 4- to 7-year-old child learns the basics of combing and brushing hair, but braids and the use of curlers, pins and dryers are teenage accomplishments. These and other grooming skills require a high level of bilateral dexterity and many must be performed without vision or with mirror vision.

HYGIENE, TOILETING AND GROOMING IN CHILDREN WITH CEREBRAL PALSY

Children with cerebral palsy who are functioning at MACS and GMFCS levels I and II should be able to achieve independence in most hygiene tasks at the same age level as their peers. Children whose hand skills are more compromised might only be independent in simple hygiene tasks such as washing their hands. They are typically dependent on an adaptive environment and simple adjustments. An automatic toothbrush might, for example, increase participation in hygiene.

Independence in toileting skills requires secure sitting balance and a high level ability to transfer in addition to hand skills. Hand actions are made more difficult by the need to combine them with transfer skills, e.g. holding a dress up while climbing on the toilet. Thoroughly cleaning oneself after going to the toilet is a late achievement for all children and is particularly difficult for children at GMFCS levels III–IV because of the difficulty maintaining balance while reaching behind. It should be recognized that children with cerebral palsy might take longer to learn toileting skills. For more information see Coley and Procter (1989), Finnie (1997), and Shepard (2001).

Complete independence in grooming is typically rare for children with cerebral palsy, and only expected for children at MACS level I. Grooming requires complex bilateral manipulation of many tools, and sensory inadequacy may hamper automatic and vision-free function. Adolescents with hemiplegic cerebral palsy can master many grooming skills but some skills, such as cutting nails on the dominant hand, may be too difficult. Adolescents also want to learn skills such as shaving, using make-up, shampooing and setting hair, and manicure. They should be encouraged to develop alternative strategies for themselves in order to manage many of these small tasks (Sköld et al 2004).

Summary of motor skills needed for self-care

There are high demands on the capabilities of the hands for the attainment of discrete self-care skills. The basic capabilities include: (1) power, precision, and force control in whole hand grips; (2) power, precision, and force control in finger grips; (3) complex finger dexterity and in-hand manipulation; (4) bilateral hand use including both complementary and cooperative action; (5) arm and shoulder control including positioning the hands in reaching to the feet, above the head, or behind the back while maintaining trunk stability; (6) eye–hand coordination followed by the ability to use the hands without visual feedback. Skilled acquisition rests on the adequate hand sensation that is needed for finger dexterity, force control, automaticity, and vision-free performance. In addition, gross motor functions, cognitive abilities, motivation and attention influence behaviour (Guidetti and Söderback 2001, Ostensjo et al 2004, Eliasson et al 2005). These capabilities combine into multiple and increasingly complex self-care action sequences that typically reach an automatic level of skill execution in adolescence. Any or all of these capabilities may be compromised in children with cerebral palsy and the potential for mastery of discrete self-care abilities differs from child to child. The sequence in which skills are learned will differ from that of typical children and also differ among functional levels and types of disability in cerebral palsy. Nevertheless, the sequences of learning shown in the tables above can provide clues for planning intervention.

Current research in self-care

Therapists have analysed the steps and motor skills involved in many self-care activities and these have served to determine necessary adaptations of equipment and teaching methods. Sources of information on adaptive equipment, clothing and methods are available in textbooks (e.g. Coley 1978, Finnie 1997, Klein 1999, Case-Smith 2000, Shepard 2001, Crepeau et al 2003, Christiansen 2004). However, little research has been done on the effect of training of self-care or on the way in which self-care develops in the presence of the different functional limitations caused by cerebral palsy.

Only minor improvements in self-care have been related to botulinum toxin and selective posterior rhizotomy in combination with training (e.g. Loewen et al 1998, Lowe et al 2006). Two studies focusing on goal-directed training have reported changes in self-care as measured by the PEDI (Ketelaar et al 2001, Ekström-Ahl et al 2005). Although the focus of training was on mobility, there were goals related to self-care and, after 18 months, the median increase of PEDI functional skill was 5 per cent in one of the studies and 10 per cent in the other. These results must be considered from the perspective that a clinically meaningful difference has been shown to be about 11 per cent on the PEDI (Lakshmi et al 2003).

One small study demonstrated that occupational therapy directed to a child's needs in self-care showed improvement (Guidetti and Söderback 2001). The most positive results of training in all of the above studies occurred when the training was directed to particular goals: in these cases goal fulfilment was high. However, the impact of the changes found in these studies is difficult to interpret since we do not know what progress should be expected during a year of typical development for children with different types of cerebral palsy.

335

Guidelines for treatment

Early independence is always a goal and adaptations that foster participation in skills or part skills should be introduced in infancy in both typical children and those with cerebral palsy (Shepard 2001). In the typical child, self-care skills appear to emerge following the development of motor skills. Self-care is a natural exercise. However, in children with cerebral palsy you cannot take it for granted that they will learn tasks without specific training. Therapists have to develop treatment plans but must also take into account that motor skill development facilitates participation in self-care activities, but participation in self-care also fosters motor skill development (Finnie 1997).

Training in self-care can follow two approaches. First, families should use the usual times for eating, dressing, etc. in their daily schedules for practice, just as they do for the typical infant and child. Therapists and caretakers must be alert to signs that a child is ready to cooperate in a skill activity, and encourage the child to attempt tasks, and never interfere when the child spontaneously initiates an attempt (Finnie 1997). Whatever a child can do, they should be expected to do, and their participation should be incorporated into their daily routine. Such participation is important for the development of early habits of self-care and for engendering a sense of responsibility. A typical child practises parts of a skill over months and years before the skill is mastered. A child with cerebral palsy needs to do the same.

The second approach is to consider the specific self-care difficulties that children may have, depending on their functional limitations. There might be a need for an intervention period to help children overcome a specific self-care limitation. That is, there might be certain problems within certain tasks that need to be worked on – different types of problems at different ages. This is when self-care becomes a challenge for the therapist and family. Goal-oriented training is a good model for intervention – i.e. a specific individualized intervention programme should be created, carried out and evaluated in order to help the child to be as independent as possible in self-care (see Chapter 17). With the availability of the MACS, research will lead to a better understanding of the relationship of self-care to different levels of upper extremity functional limitation in children with cerebral palsy, and of the timing and sequence of self-care skills in the presence of different levels of MACS.

REFERENCES

Amato PR, Ochiltree G (1986) Children becoming independent: an investigation of children's performance of practical life-skills. *Aust J Psychol* 38: 3, 13, 59–68.

Berg M, Jahnsen R, Froslie KF, Hussain A (2004) Reliability of the Pediatric Evaluation of Disability Inventory (PEDI). *Phys Occup Ther Pediatr* 24: 61–77.

Bott EA, Blatz WE, Chant N, Bott H (1928) Observation and training of fundamental habits in young children. *Genet Psychol Monogr* 4: 1–161.

Brigance AH, editor (1978) *Diagnostic Inventory of Early Development.* North Billerica, MA: Curriculum Associates.

Carruth BR, Skinner JD (2002) Feeding behaviors and other motor development in healthy children (2–24 months). *J Am College Nutr* 21: 88–89.

Case-Smith J (2000) Self-care strategies for children with developmental disabilities. In: Christiansen C, editor. *Ways of Living: Self-Care Strategies for Special Needs.* Bethesda, MD: American Occupational Therapy Association, pp 81–121.

Christiansen C, editor (2004) *Ways of Living: Self-Care Strategies for Special Needs*. Bethesda, MD: American Occupational Therapy Association.

Coley IL, editor (1978) *Pediatric Assessment of Self-Care Activities*. St Louis: Mosby.

Coley I, Procter S (1989) Self-maintenance activities. In: Pratt PN, Allen AS, editors. *Occupational Therapy for Children, 2nd edn*. St Louis: Mosby.

Connolly K, Dalgleish M (1989) The emergence of a tool-using skill in infancy. *Dev Psychol* 25: 894–912.

Crepeau EB, Cohn ES, Schell BB, editors (2003) *Willard and Spackman's Occupational Therapy, 10th edn*. Philadelphia: Lippincott, Williams & Wilkins.

Custers JW, Wassenberg-Severijnen JE, Van der Net J, Vermeer A, Hart HT, Helders PJ (2002) Dutch adaptation and content validity of the 'Pediatric Evaluation of Disability Inventory (PEDI)'. *Disabil Rehabil* 24: 250–258.

Dellatolas G, Filho GN, Sousa L, Nunes LG, Braqga LW (2005) Manual skill, hand skill asymmetry, and neuropsychological test performance in schoolchildren with spastic cerebral palsy. *Laterality* 10: 161–182.

Dumas HM, Haley SM, Fragala MA, Steva BJ (2001) Self-care recovery of children with brain injury: descriptive analysis using the Pediatric Evaluation of Disability Inventory (PEDI) functional classification levels. *Phys Occup Ther Pediatr* 21: 7–27.

Ekström-Ahl LE, Johansson E, Granat T, Carlberg EB (2005) Functional therapy for children with cerebral palsy: an ecological approach. *Dev Med Child Neurol* 47: 613–619.

Eliasson AC, Ohrvall AM, Borell L (2000) Parents' perspectives of changes in movement affecting daily life following selective dorsal rhizotomy in children with cerebral palsy. *Phys Occup Ther Pediatr* 19: 91–109.

Eliasson AC, Krumlinde-Sundholm L, Shaw K, Wang C (2005) Effects of constraint-induced movement therapy in young children with hemiplegic cerebral palsy: an adapted model. *Dev Med Child Neurol* 47: 266–275.

Eliasson AC, Krumlinde-Sundholm L, Rosblad, B, Beckung E, Arner M, Ohrvall AM, Rosenbaum P (2006) The Manual Ability Classification System (MACS) for children with cerebral palsy: scale development and evidence of validity and reliability. *Dev Med Child Neurol* 48: 549–554.

Fedrizzi E, Pagliano E, Andreucci E, Oleari G (2005) Hand function in children with hemiplegic cerebral palsy. *Dev Med Child Neurol* 44: 85–91.

Finnie NR (1997) *Handling the Young Child with Cerebral Palsy at Home*. Edinburgh: Butterworth Heinemann.

Gannotti ME, Cruz C (2001) Content and construct validity of a Spanish translation of the Pediatric Evaluation of Disabilities Inventory for children living in Puerto Rico. *Phys Occup Ther Pediatr* 20: 7–24.

Gannotti ME, Handwerker WP (2002) Puerto Rican understandings of child disability: methods for the cultural validation of standardized measures of child health. *Soc Sci Med* 55: 2093–2105.

Gesell A, Ilg F, editors (1937) *Feeding Behavior of Infants*. Philadelphia: J.B. Lippincott.

Gesell A, Ilg F, editors (1943) *Infant and Child in the Culture of Today*. New York: Harper & Row.

Gesell A, Ilg F, editors (1946) *The Child From Five to Ten*. New York: Harper & Row.

Gesell A, Halverson HM, Thompson H, Ilg FL, Castner BM, Ames LB, Amatruda CS, editors (1940) *The First Five Years of Life: A Guide to the Study of the Preschool Child*. New York: Harper & Row.

Guidetti S, Söderback I (2001) Description of self-care training in occupational therapy: case studies of five Kenyan children with cerebral palsy. *Occup Ther Int* 8: 38–48.

Haley SM, Coster WL, Ludlow LH, Haltiwanger JT, Andrellos PJ (1992) *Pediatric Evaluation of Disability Inventory*. Boston: New England Medical Center Hospital Inc and PEDI Research Group.

Hauser-Cram P, Warfield ME, Shonkoff JP, Krauss MW (2001) Children with disabilities: a longitudinal study of child development and parent well-being. Overton WF, editor. *Monogr Soc Res Child Dev* (Serial No 266) 66(3): 1–126.

Henderson A (2006) Self care and hand skill. In: Henderson A, Pehoski C, editors. *Hand Function in the Child: Foundations for Remediation, 2nd edn*. St Louis: Mosby.

Hurlock EB, editor (1964) *Child Development, 4th edn*. New York: McGraw-Hill.

Ketelaar M, Vermeer A, Hart H, van Petegem-van Beek E, Helders PJ (2001) Effects of a functional therapy program on motor abilities of children with cerebral palsy. *Phys Ther* 81: 1534–1545.

Key CB, White MR, Honzik WP, Heiney AB, Erwin D (1936) The process of learning to dress among nursery-school children. *Genet Psychol Monogr* 18: 67–163.

Klein M, editor (1999) *Pre-dressing Skills*. San Antonio: Psychological Corporation.

Knox V, Evans AL (2002) Evaluation of the functional effects of a course of Bobath therapy in children with cerebral palsy: a preliminary study. *Dev Med Child Neurol* 44: 447–460.

Koch BM, Simenson RL (1992) Upper extremity strength and function in children with spinal muscular atrophy type II. *Arch Phys Med Rehabil* 73: 241–245.

Lakshmi VI, Haley SM, Watkins MP, Dumas HM (2003) Establishing minimally clinically important differences for scores on the Pediatric Evaluation of Disability Inventory for inpatient rehabilitation. *Phys Ther* 83: 888–897.

Liu M, Toikawa H, Seki M, Domen K, Chino N (1998) Functional Independence Measure for Children (WeeFIM): a preliminary study in nondisabled Japanese children. *Am J Phys Med Rehabil* 77: 36–44.

Loewen P, Steinbok P, Holsti L, Mackay M (1998) Upper extremity performance and self-care changes in children with spastic cerebral palsy following selective posterior rhizotomy. *Pediatr Neurosurg* 29: 191–198.

Lowe K, Novak I, Cusick A (2006) Low-dose/high-concentration localized botulinum toxin A improves upper limb movement and function in children with hemiplegic cerebral palsy. *Dev Med Child Neurol* 48: 170–175.

Nordmark E, Orban K, Hagglund G, Jarnlo GB (1999) The American Pediatric Evaluation of Disability Inventory (PEDI): applicability of PEDI in Sweden for children aged 2.0–6.9 years. *Scan J Rehabil Med* 31: 95–100.

Ostensjo S, Carlberg EB, Vollestad NK (2003) Everyday functioning in young children with cerebral palsy: functional skills, caregiver assistance, and modifications of the environment. *Dev Med Child Neurol* 45: 603–612.

Ostensjo S, Carlberg EB, Vollestad NK (2004) Motor impairments in young children with cerebral palsy: relationship to gross motor function and everyday activities. *Dev Med Child Neurol* 46: 580–589.

Palisano RJ, Hanna SE, Rosenbaum PL, Russell DJ, Walter SD, Wood EP, Raina PS, Galuppi BE (2000) Validation of a model of gross motor function for children with cerebral palsy. *Phys Ther* 80: 974–985.

Parker ST, Gibson KR (1977) Object manipulation, tool use and sensorimotor intelligence as feeding adaptations in cebus monkeys and great apes. *J Hum Evol* 6: 623–641.

Shepard J (2001) Self-care and adaptations for independent living. In: Case-Smith J, editor. *Occupational Therapy for Children*. St Louis: Mosby.

Sköld A, Josephsson S, Eliasson AC (2004) Performing bimanual activities: the experiences of young persons with hemiplegic cerebral palsy. *Am J Occup Ther* 58: 416–425.

Srsen KG, Vidmar G, Zupan A (2005) Applicability of the pediatric evaluation of disability inventory in Slovenia. *J Child Neurol* 20: 411–416.

State University of New York at Buffalo (1994) *Functional Independence Measure for Children (WeeFim)*. Buffalo, NY: State University of New York at Buffalo.

Thornby MA, Krebs DE (1992) Bimanual skill development in pediatric below-elbow amputation: a multicenter, cross-sectional study. *Arch Phys Med Rehabil* 73: 697–702.

Tsuji T, Liu M, Toikawa H, Hanayama K, Sonoda S, Chino N (1999) ADL structure for nondisabled Japanese children based on the Functional Independence Measure for children (WeeFIM). *Am J Phys Med Rehabil* 78: 208–212.

Uniform Data System for Medical Rehabilitation (1987) *Functional Independence Measure*. Buffalo, NY: State University of New York.

Vulpe SG (1979) *Vulpe Assessment Battery for the Atypical Child*. Toronto: National Institute on Mental Retardation.

Wagoner LC, Armstrong EM (1928) The motor control of children as involved in the dressing process. *J Genet Psychol* 35: 84–97.

Wong V, Wong S, Chan K, Wong W (2002) Functional Independence Measure (WeeFIM) for Chinese children: Hong Kong cohort. *Pediatrics* 109: 317–319.

Wong V, Chung B, Hui S, Fong A, Lau C, Law B, Lo K, Shum T, Wong R (2004) Cerebral palsy: correlation of risk factors and functional performance using the Functional Independence Measure for Children (WeeFIM). *J Child Neurol* 19: 887–893.

338

22
WRITTEN COMMUNICATION: CLINICAL DECISION-MAKING FOR HANDWRITING IN CHILDREN WITH CEREBRAL PALSY

Sonya Murchland, Alison Lane and Jenny Ziviani

> . . . the pen is mightier than the sword.
> (Bulwer-Lytton 1839)

To be able to pick up a pen, pencil or brush loaded with ink, graphite or pigment, and direct the actions of these tools purposefully onto a surface such as paper, remains one of the most universal methods of communicating thoughts, feelings, or knowledge. The formation of written communication that is meaningful and understandable is a key occupation of childhood which permits participation in areas of education, leisure and socialization. Handwriting enables forms of creative expression to be read, distributed and interpreted by others. In addition, handwriting remains a way of personalizing greetings, legalizing documents through a signature, and verifying authenticity, and is an essential learning task of education (Hammerschmidt and Sudsawad 2004). While computers and other forms of information and communication technology are rapidly emerging and developing to provide alternative and complementary methods of written communication and expression, they are not yet readily available to all and are not always able to be customized to individual needs. This chapter will provide a guide for occupational therapists, teachers and others working with children with cerebral palsy to help them understand the performance components of handwriting and determine the best methods of supporting the development of handwriting in this population of children.

Within the framework of the World Health Organization's International Classification of Functioning, Disability and Health (ICF), handwriting is an activity that relies on interrelationships at all levels. It requires the integration of an individual's body structure and function (motor, sensory, visual and cognitive) with activities applying learning, knowledge and communication to enable participation in the life areas of school and education, social relationships, community and civic life. It occurs within a physical environment (e.g. in a classroom, at a table, with pencil/pen and paper) and social context (expectations, demands). Individuals with cerebral palsy may have impairments of body structure and functioning, limitations in capacity to complete activities and restricted participation in life roles that impact on their production of meaningful communication in a written form. The environment in which they operate may provide additional barriers to hinder their potential to generate written material. To facilitate the acquisition and production of writing, occupational therapists are uniquely skilled to determine the impact of an individual's personal skills, environmental demands and occupational requirements, and provide strategies and interventions to enable fulfilment of occupational roles where writing is required (Schwellnus and Lockhart 2002).

Success in handwriting is indicated by a child having appropriate letter formations, neatness of execution and adequate speed of production for their age and school year level to enable them to complete tasks within time, quantity and quality parameters relative to classroom peers. To be able to write, the child must have sufficient cognitive functioning to understand the requirements of the task, and the ability to direct the hand to form consistent symbols to which linguistic meaning is attached. Developing competence in handwriting is a major focus of the early years of schooling, with a variety of teaching strategies employed to support children's learning of this skill. Teachers and therapists have access to resources related to the development, assessment and teaching of handwriting. Similarly there is information on intervention strategies used by occupational therapists to support children with handwriting difficulties (see Appendix).

Despite the wealth of information on handwriting in children who are developing typically, little has been written on the handwriting abilities of children with cerebral palsy, and even less on appropriate methods of intervention (Rigby and Schwellnus 1999). DuBois et al (2004) found that handwriting difficulties were reported in the majority of children with hemiplegia (parents' report: 75 per cent; teachers' report: 69 per cent). The difficulties identified by parents and teachers included maintaining neatness, writing from dictation, writing at a functional speed, writing for long periods, and maintaining appropriate posture. Murchland and Kernot (2005) found that within a sample of 46 children with hemiplegia attending mainstream school, 71 per cent were experiencing difficulties with handwriting relating to speed, neatness or a combination of both, based on formalized assessment results.

The focus of this chapter will be on how therapists can utilize a clinical problem-solving method to help children with cerebral palsy who have handwriting difficulties. Specifically, through the use of case studies, the objectives of this chapter are to:

1   Describe the performance components necessary for readiness and participation in written communication via handwriting and the potential impact of cerebral palsy.
2   Propose a decision-making framework to assist practitioners to evaluate written communication needs of children with cerebral palsy.
3   Describe through the use of case scenarios common written communication difficulties experienced by children with cerebral palsy and identify intervention goals for each.

Performance components required for handwriting
To draw, write or type involves using the hands to control a tool, to form a series of marks on a surface to convey a message. While drawing tends to use images, colour and shapes in an infinite variety of possibilities, writing relies on an individual being able to form and consistently reproduce a series of predetermined symbols, in recognizable order to meet

340

the rules of spelling, syntax and grammar of a given language. Writing tasks may involve copying, completing familiar words within context, or composing original text. Writing is also a means of communicating and is the end product of many complex, interrelated skills that involve cognitive, visual, motor and language skills (Schneck and Henderson 1990, Bonney 1992, Cornhill and Case-Smith 1996, Murchland and Kernot 2005). To be ready to write, a child needs to have adequate postural control, visual and visual-motor skills, hand skills, cognition, attention and organizational skills. How graphomotor skills relevant to drawing and writing develop in typically developing children is clearly described in Ziviani and Wallen (2006) and will not be duplicated here.

IMPACT OF CEREBRAL PALSY ON HANDWRITING

Approximately two-thirds of all children with cerebral palsy have spastic diplegia or hemiplegia (Cerebral Palsy Register 2005), and attend mainstream school settings. In this group of children their dominant hand often appears minimally affected and the expectation that they will learn to write and become fluent in this task is common. However, these children's performance is often compromised due to a number of factors. Children with cerebral palsy experience disordered muscle tone and stereotyped movement patterns, and may be compromised in their ability to process sensory information. Cognitive difficulties in the form of specific learning difficulties are experienced by many children with cerebral palsy, unrelated to their intellectual ability. Difficulties with cognitive processing abilities may:

- delay the child's readiness for learning to write;
- restrict memory of shapes, letters, or words;
- interfere with the planning and organizational skills needed for task initiation, sequencing and completion;
- affect the child's motivation to participate in writing activities.

Further, difficulties in sensory processing may influence:

- visual motor integration;
- visual organization needed for directing and refining control of the writing tool to produce neat, legible writing;
- modulation and maintenance of appropriate pressure on the writing tool;
- development of consistent 'motor memory maps' needed for letter formations.

Muscle tone and movement difficulties are likely to impact on the child's ability to:

- maintain an appropriate posture for writing;
- grasp and control a writing tool;
- stabilize the work with the assisting hand;
- consistently form recognizable letters;
- write at speed and for long periods.

341

Language disorders or dyslexia may coexist with cerebral palsy, compounding the challenges associated with the early learning process of writing. However, the motivation to participate at school in ways similar to their peers can encourage even children with the most significant physical disabilities to learn to write.

The child with cerebral palsy has to manage within a physical environment that may or may not facilitate their participation in writing tasks. The furniture may impede postural stability and motor control, tools may be difficult to grasp and direct, and paper challenging to stabilize on a smooth desk surface. The social environment determines the expectations of speed and quantity of writing, the familiarity of demands, the class teaching and learning systems utilized, and peer abilities. All of these environmental factors require consideration, along with the person's performance competencies, to optimize their written output.

Clinical decision making to support participation in written communication
The Tool for Optimising Written Productivity (TOW-P) has been developed by Schwellnus and Lockhart (2002) as a means of assisting occupational therapists to plan and select appropriate interventions. This tool further developed work initially undertaken by Rigby and Schwellnus (1999) which was targeted at occupational therapy interventions for children with cerebral palsy who were experiencing difficulties with handwriting. It is based on the Person–Environment–Occupation Model (Law et al 1996), and uses these same three terms to group possible interventions. It provides a model that is consistent with the ICF, emphasizing that assessment and intervention not only need to consider the individual's functioning, but also the physical environment and context of the activity. The TOW-P utilizes a matrix structure where the issues identified at assessment (horizontal rows) are matched with interventions (vertical columns). Fig. 22.1 gives an abbreviated example of the structure of this tool.

For each assessment issue, a primary and a number of secondary interventions have been identified, with shading indicating the frequency of choice for use by occupational therapists. These interventions have been identified over four phases of testing and development of this tool with occupational therapists in Ontario, Canada. Readers are referred to Rigby and Schwellnus (1999) and Schwellnus and Lockhart (2002) for more details of the TOW-P, which is not yet available, but provides a promising framework for interventions.

The following sections discuss in more detail how cerebral palsy can impact on children in the performance of handwriting, using the TOW-P as a framework for discussion.

POSTURAL CONTROL
The ability to maintain a stable trunk is a prerequisite for freeing the arm and hand to engage in tasks requiring skilled grasp, release and manipulation. Without adequate postural control, one or both hands are needed to stabilize the body. This hand support in turn further restricts the ability to stabilize tasks and engage in bilateral hand activities. Ensuring correct sitting posture is therefore one of the first steps in handwriting training (Benbow 2006) for all children.

The child with cerebral palsy frequently experiences disorders of both muscle tone and movement which have a primary impact on postural balance and alignment, and a secondary

342

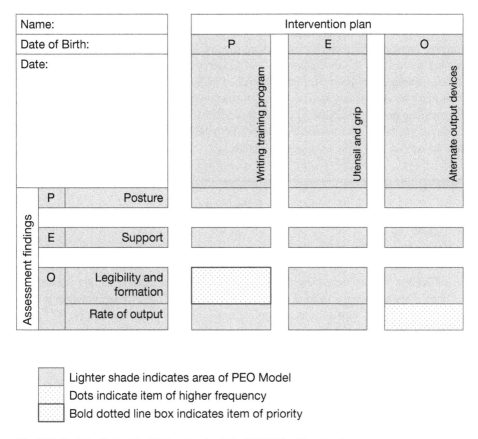

Lighter shade indicates area of PEO Model
Dots indicate item of higher frequency
Bold dotted line box indicates item of priority

Fig. 22.1 Tool for Optimizing Written Productivity (TOW-P): abbreviated example.

Source: Schwellnus and Lockhart 2002.

Note:
Within each category of assessment findings or intervention plan, generally only one of the options is given in this example. Within each assessment category (Person–Environment–Occupation), there are a number of possible subcategories (e.g. Person category includes posture, U/E physical components, in-hand manipulation, utensil grasp and force, motor coordination, visual-motor integration, visual-perception, organization, attention span, motivation; Environment/occupation category includes furniture, expectations, instructional methods, legibility and formation, spatial organization, rate of output, physical tolerance). For each of these subcategories, primary and secondary interventions have been identified and selected to reflect the most common practice items used by occupational therapists based on their research (e.g. intervention strategies for rate of output – writing training programme (primary intervention), expectations, task/process modifications, alternative output devices (secondary interventions)).

impact on the ability to isolate and control the trunk separately from the limbs. While this is most obvious in children with a significant degree of motor impairment who require assistive devices such as walking frames or wheelchairs for mobility (levels 3–5 on the Gross Motor Function Classification Scale (Palisano et al 1997)), impaired postural control is also apparent in children with less severe physical impairment. A study of handwriting abilities in children aged 8–13 years with hemiplegia attending mainstream school

(Murchland and Kernot 2005) found that there was a significant difference between children who had stable sitting postures and smooth arm movements across the page, and those who did not. Those children who were described as moving frequently in their chair had lower legibility scores on the Evaluation Tool of Children's Handwriting (ETCH; Amundson 1995), compared to those who were described as having stable or supported postures. Children who were observed to have smooth arm movements across the page (an indication of adequate postural stability to enable freedom of isolated arm and hand movement) achieved greater scores for word legibility on both the ECTH and an extended handwriting task than those with jerky or stop–start patterns.

Scenario 1: Postural control

Case 1: Jai

Jai is a 4-year-old boy with spastic diplegia, upper limb involvement, and asymmetry in his trunk and upper limb involvement. He was born preterm and has visual difficulties. Jai is independently mobile in a manual wheelchair and is able to walk short distances with a walking frame (GMFCS level IV). Jai's hand function is at MACS level III, with assistance required to modify and prepare activities. He has started kindergarten and participates in most activities, and is expected to engage in those involving pencil and paper. Jai is able to sit independently, albeit briefly, but then as he fatigues, due to associated reactions he falls further and further to his left side, consciously needing to recorrect his posture (see Fig. 22.2). Jai has low muscle tone in his trunk, and increased muscle tone in his limbs (legs more than arms, left more than right side).

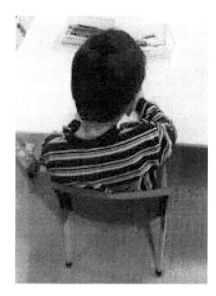

Fig. 22.2 Asymmetrical trunk and head position, with leaning to the left while engaging in fine motor activities, impacts on freedom of arm movements.

When sitting, Jai's trunk flexes forward, as a result of his low muscle tone, and due to the imbalance between his right and left sides, he consistently falls towards his left side. In an attempt to gain stability, Jai uses his existing compensatory movement patterns for keeping an upright position. Jai will also hold on to the sides of his chair or the table to maintain his sitting balance. As a result of these behaviours Jai is unable to use both hands freely, as one or both are needed to compensate for his trunk instability, and he is unable to move his arms in isolation from his trunk due to his shoulder fixation pattern. When provided with an appropriate-sized chair with lateral supports, Jai sits more symmetrically and is able to use both hands freely in activities (Figs 22.3 and 22.4).

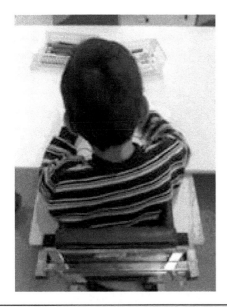

Fig. 22.3 More symmetrical trunk and head position, with both arms able to move freely when seated appropriately.

Where a child lacks postural stability in sitting, a seating system that provides support is required for times when the child wants to engage in handwriting activities. To this end, the seat should be appropriately sized to enable feet to be supported, with seat depth appropriate to leg length, and hips kept stable to enable the trunk to move over the pelvis as the child moves forward to the table and back into the chair. Lateral support may be provided by sides and arm rests, or contouring of the back rest/cushion (see Fig. 22.4). Children with more significant physical impairment may also require head support, and safety straps to assist them to maintain a safe, functional posture. The chair needs to be stable, not easily tipped, and the ease of accessing the chair and moving it in and out of the table needs to be considered.

The table needs to be appropriately sized for the chair and child, providing forearm support. An angled easel may assist the child to maintain an upright sitting posture and

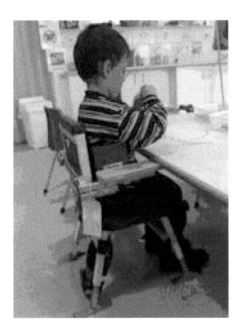

Fig. 22.4 Appropriate seating with lateral supports enables feet to be flat on the floor, hips and knees flexed, to create stability and optimize hand function.

provide a forward propping position. Therapeutic interventions to develop postural control and isolation of hand and arm movements can also be provided. However, it is important to remember that intervention for the development of handwriting or other refined hand activities cannot occur simultaneously with postural control interventions as one will be compromised at the expense of the other.

TOOL USE AND FINE MOTOR CONTROL

Handwriting requires unilateral hand function to grasp and manipulate the writing implement to form recognizable letters, as well as the bilateral hand function necessary for stabilization of the writing surface. Asymmetry and associated reactions can impair the ability of children with cerebral palsy to stabilize their work, turn pages, and use a ruler or other measurement or drawing tools.

Children with cerebral palsy may be impaired in their ability to grasp the writing implement, in their ability to isolate wrist and finger movements for manipulating and directing the tool with appropriate pressure, and in their development of necessary 'motor maps' for consistent letter formation. Limitations in motor control will result in reduced pencil control, which is evident in large or inconsistently sized and shaped letters, either too heavy or too light pencil pressure, or inconsistent line pressure. Significant motor impairments – such as those found in children at MACS levels III–IV (Eliasson et al 2006), who have difficulties manipulating objects – will be obvious, and adaptations to writing tools, external stabilization of work, and modified learning strategies will be required. The use of assistive technologies may also minimize the motor control required in writing.

Scenario 2: Tool use and fine motor control

Case 1: Jai

Jai's grasp of the pencil or crayon involves a whole hand action, although he can approximate a digital pencil grasp if reminded or if the tool is optimally positioned for grasp. His left arm moves into a flexion pattern with associated reactions, and reminders are needed to bring this hand down to stabilize himself and his activity. Stabilization of his paper is inconsistent, impacting on the quality of pencil control. Use of the pencil reflects stiff, stereotypical movement patterns that lack refinement or isolated finger or wrist control.

Assessment and monitoring of handwriting speed and legibility throughout the school years is important, particularly as students approach formal exams. At this stage, additional writing time for examinations may be needed, and use of portable note-takers or laptop computers, to enable optimal quality and quantity of written work.

A study on the development of a dynamic tripod grasp in children with hemiplegia found that children with right hemiplegia had a delayed and different developmental progression compared with those with left hemiplegia. Children with right hemiplegia moved from a whole-handed grasp of the writing tool to a two-finger pincer grip rather than using a tripod grasp (Molczanow 1974). Children with hemiplegia (right or left) have also been found to perform more slowly in handwriting tests, compared to normative samples, and their handwriting is less legible.

Even subtle impairments in fine motor control, such as those in children at MACS level I or II (Eliasson et al 2006), will impact on handwriting performance. Reduced dexterity and fine motor impairment will result in slower production, while difficulties with visual-motor control and kinaesthesia can impact on legibility (Harris and Livesey 1992). Children with hemiplegia frequently experience these subtle sensory-motor limitations on their 'non-affected' or dominant side. The potential impact on their handwriting and school performance as a result may not be fully appreciated.

A child with cerebral palsy may fatigue easily and this can have a detrimental influence on their handwriting when large quantities of work are required. It has been reported that children without disability demonstrate significant fatigue in the process of completing a ten-minute writing task (Parush et al 1998). Children with cerebral palsy are likely to experience motor fatigue in a much shorter time frame, although this has not been examined.

347

Case 2: Christian

Christian is a 16-year-old young man with left hemiplegia who attends a private secondary school where he is successfully pursuing an academic curriculum. His handwriting speed was found to be in the mildly impaired range when assessed using the Handwriting Speed Test (Wallen et al 1996). His writing comprised legible print script, formed with an appropriate pencil grasp. He had adequate isolated finger and hand movements for writing, but provided inconsistent paper stabilization of his work with his left hand. At this stage in his schooling, technology was advocated, and one-handed typing tuition recommended. Christian is able to write neatly, and complete assignments; however when lengthy assignments or essays are required he prefers to use a laptop to reduce the impact of fatigue by minimizing the motor requirements, particularly when reworking of early drafts is required. Christian is allowed additional time in exams to ensure that he is not penalized for the slowness of production. He continues to use a print script and has not developed a fluid, linked or cursive handwriting style.

As described, there are a number of limitations in body structure and function prevalent in children with cerebral palsy which can make handwriting a difficult task to master. In some situations, these limitations will be so significant that the production of manual handwriting will be impossible and alternative information and communication technologies (ICT) will be needed to compensate. ICT options include computers (laptops or desktops), portable note-takers (e.g. Alphasmart 2000, Dana, Neolite), and specialized software (e.g. for word prediction, or text reading). In many cases, however, ICT can and should be used to augment the manual skills of children with cerebral palsy, with the aim of enhancing the functionality of skills and ensuring success in communication attempts. Specialized assessment is recommended to ensure that ICT matches the child's abilities and needs, and is well supported, and that training needs for the individual's support workers are considered.

Principles of augmentation using ICT are evident in the case of Christian. In his case, a laptop is used to support the production of high quality written communication in specific instances where demands of time, quantity or repetition compromise his otherwise adequate manual handwriting skills.

VISION AND VISUAL-PERCEPTUAL SKILLS

Children with cerebral palsy are known to have associated visual deficits related to acuity, scanning, and visual field loss (e.g. hemianopia), as well as cortical visual impairments (Guzzetta et al 2001). Each of these can have an influence on handwriting performance and therefore needs to be identified and managed. Consistently missing information, or only completing work on one part of the page or board, may be signs of a visual field deficit, or ineffective scanning skills.

Scenario 4: Visual field deficit

Case 2: Christian
Christian has a left homonymous hemianopia which reduces his visual field awareness on this side. Functionally he has minimal impairment except for organization of his work on the page. This is particularly evident in maths where spatial alignment of work is needed for accuracy, and is also evident in his spacing of words along a line.

The child with cerebral palsy may need strategies to reinforce scanning across and down the page. These strategies may include working from a green edge to a red border, or the use of highlighters to focus attention on a particular area, or using a guide to isolate a small area of work to assist in locating and maintaining position on the page. Using paper with a grid (e.g. graph paper) can assist in spatial alignment of work. Additional time may also be required to enable the child with cerebral palsy to organize their eye movements to refine and guide their hand actions.

The presence of visual-perceptual difficulties is more prevalent in children with cerebral palsy than in their typically developing peers (Marozas and May 1985, Menken et al 1987, Reid and Drake 1990, Ito et al 1996, Stiers et al 2002, Burtner et al 2005). The combination of integrating visual information and developing the appropriate motor response to replicate a required form (often referred to as visual-motor integration) provides an additional challenge (Chu 1997, Stiers et al 2002). It is often at this complex level of visual-motor integration that children with cerebral palsy experience greatest difficulty.

Scenario 5: Perceptual-motor readiness

Case 1: Jai
Jai has visual impairments, and wears glasses to correct his problems with acuity. He inconsistently scans his environment, and needs cues to attend to visual forms. He recognizes and can name familiar shapes and forms. Jai tends to scribble in a circular and linear manner, and although he is able to copy lines and an immature circle, he is not yet forming recognizable, repeated shapes.

Jai's ability to recognize, match and name shapes accurately suggests that he has the necessary prerequisites for recognizing letters and words. However, his ability to direct his hands to form recognizable shapes is more challenging. This mismatch of abilities has the potential to frustrate his attempts to learn to write. The use of technology in the form of computers, specialized software and expanded keyboards enables Jai and other children with cerebral palsy to develop their early literacy skills, with minimal motor requirements. Specific interventions to develop handwriting, focusing on learning accurate letter formations, can then occur at a pace that does not compromise the development of literacy.

COGNITION, ATTENTION, AND ORGANIZATIONAL SKILLS

Handwriting is more than a motor task. It relies on a child's ability to focus and maintain his/her attention on the task, understand the cognitive elements of symbolic representation of sounds and words, sequence, generate ideas, translate ideas into text, and review performance. Memory skills are also needed to recall the accurate symbol to match sounds to form words.

Children who have hemiplegic cerebral palsy have been found to have limitations in their process skill ability (Van Zelst et al 2006) when undertaking activities of daily living. As the term 'process skill ability' refers to the ability to use knowledge, organize self and tools, and solve problems, it is likely that limitations in these abilities will also impact on the ability to perform handwriting tasks. While a detailed discussion of these issues is beyond the scope of this chapter, it is important to recognize the role that these skills play, and consider the impact they may have when assessing handwriting ability within the context of classroom demands and when developing interventions.

A cognitive process model described by Sturm and Koppenhaver (2000) was found to assist the development of written literacy in adolescents with developmental disabilities, and its principles could be applied to children and adolescents with cerebral palsy. Children's cognitive strengths can also be used to assist in their learning to write through the use of verbal and visual cueing to guide motor actions and spatial organization, memory mnemonics for letter formations, and checking strategies for self-correction of their work.

Handwriting has been found to correlate with other basic abilities in children in their first six years of schooling (Graham and Weintraub 1996). Children who are considered to be 'good' handwriters tend to perform well in other skills such as reading, spelling and mathematics. Handwriting speed has also been found to correlate with composing speed. Graham and Weintraub propose a number of reasons for this: children's need to focus on the mechanical aspects of writing may interfere with their ability to engage in higher order cognitive functions necessary for composition; overall speed of writing may be slower than speed of thinking, causing loss of consistency and sequencing of thoughts in the production of the text; children may experience difficulty shifting attention from the motor act of writing to the planning of thoughts and actions for the forthcoming text; and the motivation to write and develop skills may be diminished through a perceived lack of success. A child with cerebral palsy, therefore, who needs to expend more attention on execution of the motor aspects of handwriting than their typically developing peers, may experience difficulties in the related cognitive functions needed for generation of text. Alternatively, some children with cerebral palsy who appear to cope in a mainstream classroom alongside their typically developing peers may experience increased levels of fatigue due to additional cognitive load needed to perform motor tasks. It may then be necessary to reduce the motor requirements of handwriting in children with cerebral palsy to enable them to optimize their cognitive and attention abilities when the emphasis is on the production of composed text.

This becomes especially important for children with cerebral palsy who are neat, legible writers and high academic achievers.

Summary

A number of challenges are experienced by children with cerebral palsy which impact on their ability to develop neat, fluid and fast writing. This can impact on their ability to complete activities required for their participation at school, and social or legal written communications. Teachers play an important role in teaching children to write; however, if a child experiences difficulties in acquiring this skill, referral to an occupational therapist is warranted. Occupational therapists are able to analyse the requirements of the task, and the child's abilities, and develop appropriate intervention strategies. Information and communication technologies are opening up new alternative options for the production of written work; however, careful assessment is required to match the technology to the child, and their situation. Nevertheless, despite these options, handwriting remains an essential occupational task of school students.

REFERENCES

Amundson SJ (1995) *Evaluation Tool of Children's Handwriting: ETCH Examiner's Manual*. Homer AK: OT KIDS.

Benbow M (2006) Principles and practices of teaching handwriting. In: *Hand Function in the Child, 2nd edn.* Henderson A, Pehoski C, editors. St Louis: Mosby, pp 319–342.

Bonney MA (1992) Understanding and assessing handwriting difficulty; perspectives from the literature. *Aust Occup Ther J* 39: 7–15.

Bulwer-Lytton EGE (1839) *Richelieu* (act II, scene 2).

Burtner PA, Dukeminier A, Ben L, Qualls C, Scott K (2005) Visual perceptual skills and related school functions in children with hemiplegic cerebral palsy. *NZ J Occup Ther* 53: 24–29.

Case-Smith J (2002) Effectiveness of school-based occupational therapy intervention on handwriting. *Am J Occup Ther* 56: 17–25.

Cerebral Palsy Register (2005) Cerebral Palsy Register 2004. South Australian Clinical Genetics Service, Department of Genetic Medicine, Women's and Children's Hospital. Annual Report. Adelaide, Australia.

Chu S (1997) Occupational therapy for children with handwriting difficulties: a framework for evaluation and treatment. *Br J Occup Ther* 60: 514–520.

Cornhill H, Case-Smith J (1996) Factors that relate to good and poor handwriting. *Am J Occup Ther* 50: 732–739.

Dobbie L, Askov EN (1995) Progress of handwriting research in the 1980s and future prospects. *J Educ Res* 88: 339–351.

DuBois L, Klemm A, Murchland S, Ozols A (2004) Handwriting of children who have hemiplegia: a profile of abilities in children aged 8–13 years from parent and teacher survey. *Aust Occup Ther J* 51: 89–98.

Eliasson AC, Krumlinde Sundholm L, Rösblad B, Beckung E, Arner M, Öhrvall AM, Rosenbaum P (2006) The Manual Ability Classification System (MACS) for children with cerebral palsy: scale development and evidence of validity and reliability. *Dev Med Child Neurol* 48: 549–554.

Feder K, Majnemer A, Synnes A (2000) Handwriting: current trends in occupational therapy practice. *Can J Occup Ther* 67: 197–204.

Graham S, Weintraub N (1996) A review of handwriting research: progress and prospects from 1980 to 1994. *Educ Psychol Rev* 8: 7–87.

Guzzetta A, Fazzi B, Mercuri E, Bertuccelli B, Canapicchi R, van Hof-van Duin J, Cionni G (2001) Visual function in children with hemiplegia in the first years of life. *Dev Med Child Neurol* 43: 321–329.

Hammerschmidt SL, Sudsawad P (2004) Teachers' survey on problems with handwriting: referral, evaluation and outcomes. *Am J Occup Ther* 58: 185–192.

Harris SJ, Livesey DJ (1992) Improving handwriting through kinaesthetic sensitivity practice. *Aust Occup Ther J* 39: 23–27.

Ito J, Saijo H, Araki A, Tanaka H, Tasaki T, Cho K, Miyamoto A (1996) Assessment of visuoperceptual disturbance in children with spastic diplegia using measurements of the lateral ventricles on cerebral MRI. *Dev Med Child Neurol* 38: 496–502.

Johnson DJ, Carlisle JF (1996) A study of handwriting in written stories of normal and learning disabled children. *Reading Writing Interdisciplinary J* 8: 45–59.

Law M, Cooper B, Strong S, Stewart D, Rigby P, Letts L (1996) The person-environment-occupational model: a transactive approach to occupational therapy. *Can J Occup Ther* 63: 9–23.

Marozas DS, May DC (1985) Effects of figure-ground reversal on the visual-perceptual and visuo-motor performances of cerebral palsied and normal children. *Percept Mot Skills* 60: 591–598.

Menken C, Cermak SA, Fisher A (1987) Evaluating the visual-perceptual skills of children with cerebral palsy. *Am J Occup Ther* 41: 646–651.

Molczanow A (1974) The formation of manipulative activities on the example of writing in children with congenital right- and left-sided hemiplegia. *Neuropat Pol* 12: 181–185.

Murchland SR, Kernot J (2005) Unravelling handwriting: the handwriting abilities of children aged 8–13 years with hemiplegia. Project Report, Novita Children's Services, Adelaide, Australia.

Oliver CE (1990) A sensorimotor program for improving writing readiness skills in elementary-age children. *Am J Occup Ther* 44: 111–116.

Palisano R, Rosenbaum P, Walter S, Russell D, Wood E, Galuppi B (1997) Development and reliability of a system to classify gross motor function in children with cerebral palsy. *Dev Med Child Neurol* 39: 214–223.

Parush S, Pindak V, Hahn-Markowitz J, Mazor-Kersenty T (1998) Does fatigue influence children's handwriting performance? *Work* 11: 307–313.

Reid D, Drake S (1990) A comparative study of visual perceptual skills in normal children and children with diplegic cerebral palsy. *Can J Occup Ther* 57: 141–146.

Rigby P, Schwellnus H (1999) Occupational therapy decision making guidelines for problems in written productivity. *Phys Occup Ther Pediatr* 19: 5–27.

Schneck CM, Henderson A (1990) Descriptive analysis of the developmental progression of grip position for pencil and crayon control in nondysfunctional children. *Am J Occup Ther* 40: 893–900.

Schwellnus H, Lockhart J (2002) The development of the Tool for Optimizing Written Productivity (TOW-P). *Phys Occup Ther Pediatr* 22: 5–22.

Stiers P, Vanderkelen R, Vanneste G, Coene S, de Rammelaere M, Vandenbussche E (2002) Visual-perceptual impairment in a random sample of children with cerebral palsy. *Dev Med Child Neurol* 44: 370–382.

Sturm J, Koppenhaver DA (2000) Supporting writing development in adolescents with developmental disabilities. *Top Lang Disord* 20: 73–92.

Sudsawad P, Thrombly CA, Henderson A, Tickle-Dengen L (2002) Testing the effect of kinesthetic training on handwriting performance in first-grade students. *Am J Occup Ther* 56: 26–33.

Tomchek SD, Schneck CM (2006) Evaluation of handwriting. In: Henderson A, Pehoski C, editors. *Hand Function in the Child, 2nd edn.* St Louis: Mosby, pp 293–318.

Tseng MH, Cermak SA (1993) The influence of ergonomic factors and perceptual-motor abilities on handwriting. *Am J Occup Ther* 47: 919–925.

Van Zelst BR, Miller MD, Russo RN, Murchland SR, Crotty M (2006) Activities of daily living in children with hemiplegic cerebral palsy: a cross-sectional evaluation using the Assessment of Motor and Process Skills. *Dev Med Child Neurol* 48: 723–727.

Wallen M, Bonney M, Lennox L (1996) *The Handwriting Speed Test.* Adelaide: Helios Art and Book Co.

Weil M, Amundson SJC (1993) Biomechanical aspects of handwriting in the educational setting. *Phys Occup Ther Pediatr* 13: 57–66.

Weil MJ, Amundson SJC (1994) Relationship between visuomotor and handwriting skills of children in kindergarten. *Am J Occup Ther* 48: 982–988.

Ziviani J, Wallen M (2006) The development of graphomotor skills. In: Henderson A, Pehoski C, editors. *Hand Function in the Child, 2nd edn.* St Louis: Mosby, pp 217–236.

Handwriting intervention literature

AUTHORS	YEAR	TITLE	SOURCE	SUMMARY
Benbow M	2006	Principles and practices of teaching handwriting	In: A Henderson & C Pehoski (eds) *Hand Function and the Child: Foundations for Remediation.* 2nd edn. St Louis: Mosby, pp 255–281	A detailed description of a handwriting training programme covering motor and perceptual components of writing skill, handwriting training focusing on grip, and a kinaesthetic approach to teaching handwriting
Bonney M-A	1992	Understanding and assessing handwriting difficulty: perspectives from the literature	*Australian Occupational Therapy Journal* 39(3), 7–15	Literature review of papers concerned with handwriting performance, dysfunction, and assessment. Aims to provide a background to evaluate current occupational therapy assessment practice
Burton AW & Dacisak MJ	2000	Grip form and graphomotor control in pre-school children	*American Journal of Occupational Therapy* 54(1), 9–19	Pencil grip classification system. Effect of diameter on accuracy and pencil grip
Case-Smith J	2002	Effectiveness of school-based occupational therapy intervention on handwriting	*American Journal of Occupational Therapy* 56, 17–25	Intervention study which included teacher consultations and eclectic occupational therapy approaches individualized to each child's needs, found to improve student legibility of letters, but not speed (29 mainstream students aged 7–10 years with recognized handwriting difficulties but no underlying medical, visual or hearing disorder, compared to controls)
Chu S	1997	Occupational therapy for children with handwriting difficulties: a framework for evaluation and treatment	*British Journal of Occupational Therapy* 60(12), 514–520	Expert opinion describing a conceptual framework for evaluating and treating handwriting difficulties presented by children attending mainstream schools with specific developmental disorders
Cornhill H & Case-Smith J	1996	Factors that relate to good and poor handwriting	*American Journal of Occupational Therapy* 50(11), 732–739	In-hand manipulation skills found to have a significant association to handwriting ability

AUTHORS	YEAR	TITLE	SOURCE	SUMMARY
Dennis JL & Swinth Y	2001	Pencil grasp and children's handwriting legibility during different length writing tasks	*American Journal of Occupational Therapy* 55(2), 175–183	Endurance impacts on legibility. 46 children (typically developing, in 4th grade) wrote more legibly on the short task rather than the long task. Type of grip was not significant
Dobbie L & Askov EN	1995	Progress of handwriting research in the 1980s and future prospects	*Journal of Educational Research* 88(6), 339–351	Literature review of publications during 1980s to compare with earlier reviews of literature. Topics covered: nature of letter forms most efficiently and legibly produced; instructional methods most conducive to children's learning and perceptual-motor development and correlates of skill development in handwriting; effects of various body positions on writing performance; effects of speed and stress on the development of the handwriting product; effects of instructional sequences on the development of handwriting skill; nature of handwriting instruments and writing surfaces that facilitate learning to write; development of new handwriting scales and evaluative materials and means of helping teachers make better use of existing scales; use of mental models in forming letters during handwriting instruction; handwriting instruction for special-needs populations such as adult literacy and learning-disabled students, remedial education students, and those with neurological disorders
Feder K, Majnemer A & Synnes A	2000	Handwriting: current trends in occupational therapy practice	*Canadian Journal of Occupational Therapy* 67(3), 197–204	Survey of handwriting assessment and treatment approaches used by occupational therapists in Ontario, Canada. Eclectic treatment approach was favoured
Hammerschmidt SL & Sudsawad P	2004	Teachers' survey on problems with handwriting: referral, evaluation and outcomes	*American Journal of Occupational Therapy* 58, 185–192	Questionnaire survey of teachers of 1st–4th grade. 314 teachers responded, and indicated that legibility was the main criterion used to determine acceptability of students' handwriting
Harris SJ & Livesey DJ	1992	Improving handwriting through kinaesthetic sensitivity practice	*Australian Occupational Therapy Journal* 39(1), 23–27.	Intervention study comparing the effects of kinaesthetic acuity, kinaesthetic perception and memory programmes, and handwriting practice only upon the handwriting ability of children with poor handwriting in their early years of school. Results showed no apparent practice effect for handwriting practice alone for either group; strong practice effects for both methods of kinaesthetic programme for older children; and the perception and memory test also had a weaker effect for younger children

Oliver CE	1990	A sensorimotor program for improving writing readiness skills in elementary-age children	*American Journal of Occupational Therapy* 44(2), 111–116	Intervention study reporting results of a pilot with three groups of children with delayed writing readiness skills. Sensorimotor programme was supplemented by a daily programme in school administered by an adult. Group 1: n = 12 (9 boys), mean IQ = 94, mean age = 72 months Group 2: n = 6 (4 boys), mean IQ = 77 with significant difference between verbal > nonverbal skills, mean age = 67 months Group 3: n = 6 (2 boys), mean IQ = 65, mean age = 75 months Sensorimotor programme was most successful with children in special education classes (i.e. Groups 2 & 3), and within these combined groups boys made more progress than girls
Parush S, Pindak V, Hahn-Markowitz J & Mazor-Kersenty T	1998	Does fatigue influence children's handwriting performance?	*Work* 11, 307–313	Fatigue was found to impact on handwriting quality in 157 3rd-grade children over a ten-minute writing task
Rigby P & Schwellnus H	1999	Occupational therapy decision making guidelines for problems in written productivity	*Physical and Occupational Therapy in Paediatrics* 19(1), 5–27	Development of clinical decision making guidelines for occupational therapists working with school-aged children with cerebral palsy who have difficulty with handwriting performance. Discussion of how problems identified relate to interventions offered. Problems are grouped under areas of physical problems, cognitive problems and task performance problems. Interventions identified are classified in terms of aids and adaptations, instructional strategies, remedial strategies, and cognitive strategies
Schwellnus H & Lockhart J	2002	The development of the Tool for Optimizing Written Productivity (TOW-P)	*Physical and Occupational Therapy in Paediatrics* 22(2/3), 5–22	Description of the development of the TOW-P, pilot study and Canadian province-wide survey undertaken. Basis for developing consistent practice guidelines for occupational therapists working with school-aged children who experience handwriting difficulties
Sturm J & Koppenhaver DA	2000	Supporting writing development in adolescents with developmental disabilities	*Topics in Language Disorders* 20(2), 73–92	Descriptive paper illustrating the use of the cognitive process model to develop written literacy in adolescents with developmental disorders. Cognitive processes involved are planning (idea generation – involving goal-directed thinking, organization), translating (putting ideas into visual text, and maintaining continuity of ideas while creating new text), and reviewing (reviewing and evaluating what has been written). Intervention strategies, including use of maps and technology, are discussed

AUTHORS	YEAR	TITLE	SOURCE	SUMMARY
Sudsawad P, Thrombly CA, Henderson A & Tickle-Dengen L	2002	Testing the effect of kinesthetic training on handwriting performance in first-grade students	*American Journal of Occupational Therapy* 56(1), 26–33	Intervention study where 45 children were randomized into either a kinaesthetic training group, a handwriting practice group, or a no treatment group. At the end of the intervention period of six sessions within two weeks there were no significant differences between the groups, with all showing improvements in kinaesthesia, and handwriting legibility as judged by the teachers, but not on standardized measures of handwriting speed or legibility
Tseng MH & Cermak SA	1993	The influence of ergonomic factors and perceptual-motor abilities on handwriting	*American Journal of Occupational Therapy* 47(10), 919–925	Literature review of the research on the influence of pencil grip, pressure, and perceptual-motor factors on handwriting. Tactile-kinaesthetic, visual-motor, and motor planning appeared to have more influence on handwriting, while visual perception appeared to have little relationship
Weil M & Amundson SJC	1993	Biomechanical aspects of handwriting in the educational setting	*Physical and Occupational Therapy in Pediatrics* 13(2), 57–66	Annotated bibliography covering the aspects of pencil grasp, writing tools, writing paper
Ziviani J & Wallen M	2006	The development of graphomotor skills	In: A Henderson & C Pehoski (eds) *Hand Function and the Child: Foundations for Remediation.* 2nd edn. St Louis: Mosby, pp 184–193	General description of graphomotor competency, how it develops, with a focus on implement grasp and manipulation, nature, development and evaluation of drawing and writing

23
LEARNING TO PLAY: PROMOTING SKILLS AND QUALITY OF LIFE IN INDIVIDUALS WITH CEREBRAL PALSY

Erna Imperatore Blanche and Susan Hirsch Knox

Introduction

A query posted on the internet (www.cerebralpalsycentral.com) posed the following question:

> I have cerebral palsy and I am learning to play guitar. I am learning to strum while using one of the guitar picks that fits on your thumb. Here is my problem: I understand while strumming with your right hand you don't want to touch the guitar but to stop the slight trembling I have in my right hand I need to base a couple fingers on the guitar. Does anyone have any pointers to learn not to rest a couple fingers on the guitar? Does it really affect the sound of the music by resting a couple fingers on the guitar? Any special equipment I can try?
>
> Thanks,
>
> Kevin

From adjusting toys, to adapting bicycles, to running a baseball league, the main goal in occupational therapy intervention is to assist children with cerebral palsy (CP) to participate not only in productive activities but also in all the enjoyable experiences that life has to offer. The question of how to adjust the situation so that Kevin is able to play the guitar is an example of the complex nature of play in treatment, and raises the issue of being motivated to play as well as having the ability to engage in play.

The motivation to play is rooted in biology and is shaped by culture. The ability to choose activities that provide enjoyment and a sense of well-being is developed in play early in life and is well documented. Sutton-Smith (1997) describes play as having many rhetorics, including the ones he calls 'self' and 'progress'. Writers focusing on the rhetoric of self and the qualitative aspects of the experience of play describe it as being intrinsically motivated, enjoyable, absorbing, and often involving momentary suspension of reality, spontaneity, and an increased level of arousal (Huizinga 1950, Sutton-Smith and Kelly-Byrne 1982, Cohen 1987, Quarrick 1989, Csikszentmihalyi 1990). On the other hand, writers who focus on the productive aspects of play describe the benefits or outcomes of play as preparation for adult roles, learning, socialization, skill training, neurological and sensory development, and adaptation (Piaget 1952, Erikson 1963, Berlyne 1966, Vygotsky 1966, Bruner 1972, Groos 1976).

These two rhetorics or views of play – as a process that contributes to an outcome and as an experience that is an outcome in itself – are the two most easily included in the intervention process. In a study by Couch et al (1998) investigating how paediatric occupational therapists use play in intervention, 91 per cent of the therapists rated play as very important. For 95 per cent of the respondents, play was primarily used to elicit motor, sensory, or psychosocial outcomes; only 2 per cent used play as an outcome in itself. The therapists also primarily used adult-directed play as opposed to child-directed play.

This chapter is divided into two sections: the first section will focus on play in children with CP, and the second section will focus on the incorporation of play into the intervention process and the life of the child.

Play in children with CP

The impact of disability on participation in play and leisure has been extensively documented in the literature (Missiuna and Pollock 1991, Hestenes and Carroll 2000, Okimoto et al 2000). King et al (2004) identify 11 factors limiting children's participation in intrinsically motivated recreation and leisure activities that are not required for school. They organize these factors into a comprehensive model that includes environmental factors, family factors and child factors. The environmental factors include lack of support for the child and the family, physical barriers to access, and institutional barriers. Family factors include a family's recreational preferences, limited financial resources, and lack of time. Child factors include the child's developmental skills, their preferences, and their perception of self. These identified factors impact on the form, function and meaning of children's play.

FORM

The *form* of play is impacted by barriers in the child's abilities and motivations, their family's resources and preferences, and their access to varied materials and environments (Knox 2005). The literature focuses on these limitations as impacting play in terms of children's physical management of space and toys, as well as impacting the children's style of play in terms of decreased playfulness and social interactions (Finnie 1975, Mogford 1977).

Children with CP exhibit characteristics of play that impact the type of play they engage in and their level of playfulness (Okimoto et al 2000). For example, children with disabilities tend to spend more time in solitary play and onlooking behaviours (Hestenes and Carroll 2000), and are described as being less playful than their non-disabled peers (Okimoto et al 2000). These behaviours may relate to social limitations imposed by others rather than a child's personal characteristics. Children with CP often engage in adult- or peer-initiated play, and thus others shape and inadvertently limit their play experience. Studies focusing on social participation further illustrate this point as children who play with typically developing peers tend to show higher levels of interaction than those who play with peers with lower developmental play skills (Tanta et al 2005).

FUNCTION

The *function* of play relates to its purpose, such as contributing to development, learning or enculturation (Knox 2005). Because the form of play is often reduced, the function of play in children with CP may have limited value. The short-term benefits of play as part of the intervention process are widely understood. Play helps the child to stay motivated in the task at hand and helps the therapist to attain the treatment goals, often at the expense of the child's experience.

Less explored in the literature are the long-term benefits of play for overall sense of well-being. The literature supporting the long-term benefits of play in children with disabilities emphasizes its impact on the development of intrinsic motivation, self-competence, self-efficacy, and increased social acceptance (Miller and Reid 2003, Harris and Reid 2005). In addition, playfulness has been related to coping skills in non-disabled children (Saunders et al 1999).

MEANING

The *meaning* of play refers to the experience of play or state of mind (Knox 2005). The limitations in form and function may ultimately impact the meaning and the experience of play. The qualitative aspects of the experience of play include being intrinsically motivated, enjoying the process of the experience, being in control of the process of the activity, feeling free and flexible to start and stop the activity, experiencing the spontaneity of changing the process of the activity, and being physically or mentally active. Some play activities may also increase the person's level of arousal, include momentary suspension of reality, or include creativity. The experience of play in such situations contributes as much to its meaning as to its service as a context. Therefore if engagement in play is limited, the experiences derived from such an activity may also be reduced. For example, children with CP have limited access to the toys they can use. This will impact the type of play in which they engage and the type of social interaction they choose to have. These limitations may limit the meaning the child derives from play; however, if properly channelled, play as an intrinsic experience that is biologically based can re-surface.

Intrinsic motivation is an example of experience of play that provides meaning to the activity. Children with CP exhibit limitations in intrinsic motivation and inner drive (Mogford 1977). However, one can argue that these limitations in the experience of play may relate more to environmental factors, such as the toys that are presented to the child, than to the child's lack of interest. Most toys require precise fine motor skills which the child is not able to master, and hence such toys will result in decreased interest in participating. Recent research with virtual reality, in which the handling of the object is kept to a minimum, supports the argument that when the environment offers an opportunity for children with CP to engage in novel activities not requiring manual ability, they will exhibit the motivation to engage in the experience of play (Reid 2002, Harris and Reid 2005).

Evaluation of children's play

Evaluating a child's play skills is important for two reasons: first, play evaluations can be used to measure the developmental skills of the child and evaluate the progress that a child

TABLE 23.1
Play in children with cerebral palsy

	Form	Function	Meaning
Spastic quadriplegia	Manual abilities vary between MACS III and IV and very limited ability in level V Solitary play Limited exploration, physical play and object play Play preferences include computers, visual exploration, social interaction, and water play	Adaptive toys might bring the child from level IV to level III in certain activities of manual dexterity and increase interest in participation Preferred play can be used to facilitate development	Non-structured and sensory-rich activities can provide the experiential qualities of play. Other playful activities include computer games, virtual reality games, exposure to novelty, and increased sensory experiences such as water and nature walks
Diplegia	Manual abilities mainly MACS II and III Limited participation in physical activities that extend to the non-immediately available space Play preferences include sedentary activities, musical toys Sometimes avoidance of constructional toys	Play used to develop manual, cognitive and social abilities and to increase intrinsic motivation and sense of mastery	Play is a meaningful experience that reflects what the child enjoys and how it can be developed
Hemiplegia	Manual abilities mainly MACS I and II Reduced participation in group sports and bimanual play	Toys can be used to develop bimanual coordination and motor planning skills	Meaningful play activities may include exploration of space, social play
Athetosis	Depending on severity, manual abilities fluctuate between levels II and V Tends to watch rather than actively participate	Toys need to be adapted to facilitate interaction	Enjoys movement in space. Play can include vestibular stimulation in activities such as swinging, skiing, racing
Mild CP	Manual abilities MACS level I Play may be unstructured because of the child's difficulty in organizing actions in large spaces	Play can be used to increase function	Meaningful play experiences are similar to those of typically developing children. May want more intensive and less demanding activities

makes after the intervention; and second, understanding the child's play style will help the clinician to incorporate the experiences of that style into the intervention. The child's play can be evaluated in different ways including: observing the child in a environment that promotes choice, flexibility and spontaneity; interviewing the caretakers and/or the child to find out about the child's choices of activities; and using standardized tools. Evaluation of play also informs the therapist about the form, function, meaning and context of the

TABLE 23.2
Play assessments

Assessment	Purpose	Type	Age	Reliability and validity
Play History (Takata 1969, 1974)	Provides information on a child's daily activities; form and content of play; identifies age-appropriate play behaviour	Semi-structured interview and play observation	0–16 years	Behnke and Fetokovich (1984)
Knox Preschool Play Scale (Knox 1974, 1997, 2008)	Describes developmental skills as seen in play in four dimensions: space management, material management, pretence/symbolic, and participation	Play observation indoors and outdoors	0–6 years	Knox (1974) Bledsoe and Shepherd (1982) Harrison and Kielhofner (1986) Multiple studies summarized in Knox (2008)
Test of Playfulness (Bundy 1997, Skard and Bundy 2008)	Assesses the individual's degree of playfulness; four elements of playfulness: intrinsic motivation, internal control, ability to suspend reality, and framing	Observation of play; rating scale	18 months–adolescence	Multiple studies summarized in Bundy (1997) and Skard and Bundy (2008)
Pediatric Interest Profiles (Henry 2008)	Gathers information about play interests directly from the child or adolescent	Self-report questionnaire	3 forms Kid: 6–9 Pre-teen: 9–12 Adolescent: 12–21	Multiple studies summarized in Henry (2008)

individual child's play. Table 23.2 describes assessments developed by occupational therapists which are commonly used to assess play behaviour.

The following case illustrates the use of these assessments.

Brittany is a 4-year-old girl with left hemiplegia. She is ambulatory with an ankle-foot orthosis and she holds her left arm in a typical hemiplegic posture. She was evaluated on the Knox Preschool Play Scale (KPPS) and Play History (PH) with the following results.

Skills on the KPPS scatter widely due to the physical effects of her hemiplegia. In space management, her skills range from the 24- to 30-month level. She walks with the orthosis but does not run. She gets up and down from the floor and up and down stairs holding the railing but needing occasional assistance. She climbs over low objects with difficulty.

Her skills in material management are also affected, particularly in bilateral activities. They scatter from the 36- to 48-month level. She manipulates all objects easily with the right hand. With the left hemiplegic hand, she has a gross grasp with her forearm pronated and her wrist flexed. She uses the left hand occasionally to help support something. She catches a ball by trapping it against her body. She enjoys simple puzzles and construction and likes drawing. She is unable to cut without assistance but enjoys simple art projects with assistance.

Her skills on the pretence and participation dimensions are her highest, at the 48-month level. She has a vivid imagination and likes to play house, play 'therapist' and pretend to be one of the Disney 'princesses'. She is also beginning to dress-up. She plays cooperatively with her peers but likes to be in control of the situation. If the play becomes too complex or too physically demanding, she leaves and plays by herself. She enjoys stories, songs, and simple humour.

On the Play History, age-appropriate play was noted, with books, dolls, puzzles, drawing, and 'learning toys'. Her parents encouraged these types of play and assisted her when necessary. Types of play that were not evident or at lower levels were primarily in the gross motor area. She was also somewhat hypersensitive to toys of different textures. Her parents stated that they 'over-protected' her and were worried about her physical safety with gross motor play. In the garden at home they did not have swings or climbing toys and she did not do much outdoor play. Most of her gross motor activities consisted of home therapy programmes.

In her independent play, Brittany appeared quite playful; however, she appeared shy around unfamiliar peers and was slow to join activities. She was also reluctant to participate independently in gross motor activities in the clinic and would rely on the therapist or her parents to initiate activities and to assist her when she thought the activities would be difficult.

Through these assessments, the therapist was able to more easily identify and utilize Brittany's strengths in pretence and participation in order to motivate her to engage in the gross motor and bilateral activities that she needed. The therapist was also able to make suggestions to her parents to encourage more independent choices and participation in community activities.

Intervention in clinic/school settings

Play is a powerful and justifiable tool for treatment which can be used in occupational therapy in three ways: as a context for acquiring new skills; as a reward or motivation encouraging a child to interact with the tasks presented by a clinician; and as an experience that is valuable in itself and that may ultimately support a sense of well-being (Blanche 1997).

In this section, the intervention will be described as an implicit negotiation between the child and the therapist in which the child gets to enjoy play and the therapist meets their functional goals. Ultimately, including play will transform activities into enjoyable situations. In this way play will serve as a context for meeting functional goals, and participating in play will also be the ultimate goal.

Incorporating intrinsically motivated play requires identifying each person's motivations to engage in meaningful play. It also requires understanding how to incorporate the characteristics of play that make play a meaningful process oriented activity into the session and the life of the person. In other words, it requires looking beyond an activity that is labelled as play by its form and function, and instead exploring the meaning of play for each individual.

The six motivations to enter into intrinsically motivated enjoyable activities which are explored in this section are: restoring sense of well-being through quiet activities; exposing oneself to novelty; seeking short-term diversion through light-hearted spontaneous activities; increasing intensity of involvement in physically and/or mentally stimulating and demanding activities; enjoying the ability to master an activity; and creating novelty (Blanche 1999, 2002). This section will offer examples of how to incorporate the experience of play for the purpose of increasing manual abilities in children with CP. Experiences of play are described in relationship to intervention. The literature and examples of clinical practice will illustrate the concepts.

RESTORING SENSE OF WELL-BEING THROUGH QUIET ACTIVITIES
The motivation to enter into quiet activities that restore one's sense of well-being can be observed when a child has been challenged for a period of time. The following example illustrates this point.

Sarah, an occupational therapist, enjoyed treating Ben, an 8-year-old boy with limited manual abilities. He was cooperative, enjoyed the session and did not tire easily. On one occasion, Sarah in her enthusiasm inadvertently presented activities that challenged Ben's fine motor control beyond his skill level. Ben attempted the activity, failed, tried again, and with Sarah's help partially succeeded. At that point, to Sarah's frustration, Ben chose to play with bubbles, an activity that lent very little value to his goal of increasing hand manipulation skills.

This example illustrates that when children choose activities that appear to decrease their engagement, it can be an indication that the previous tasks presented to them were overly challenging and tiring. They may need that short period of time to restore themselves by performing a task that they like and which has no demands. In such situations, requiring the youngster to go back to the challenging tasks can diminish their sense of well-being and sense of accomplishment and diminish the long-term success of the intervention. In this situation Sarah recognized Ben's need to regain his sense of well-being and allowed the

363

simple activity to go on for a few minutes before asking him if he wanted to move on to the next activity.

EXPOSING ONESELF TO NOVELTY
Activities presented to children can be repetitious and monotonous. In the treatment session, therapists use the same toys to develop upper extremity mastery of specific movements. In daily life, the barriers to leisure and recreation that are present in the life of children with developmental disabilities (King et al 2004) may also result in monotonous daily activities.

Increasing novelty influences the level of arousal and attention and hence participation. Therefore, choosing toys for intervention should be based not only on meeting the therapist's goal of increasing manual abilities, but also on the child's interest in exploration. Studies exploring the use of virtual reality (Reid 2002, Miller and Reid 2003, Harris and Reid 2005) to increase self-efficacy and motivation support the importance of novelty in increasing participation and functional performance. Research using virtual reality games indicates that children with CP exhibit more behaviours indicative of volition when playing with virtual reality games, as measured using the Pediatric Volition Questionnaire (PVQ). The researchers provide three explanations for the higher score on the PVQ: the games offer more variation; the children cannot predict the virtual reality environment and therefore the games offer more challenge; and there is more competition (Harris and Reid 2005). These results are linked to non-controllable novelty in the activity. The richness that virtual reality can bring to intervention sessions is only starting to be explored. Further adaptation of this technology could result in games that increase fine motor dexterity, upper extremity mobility and coordination, motor planning, and visual perception, in a novel and exciting environment.

SEEKING SHORT-TERM DIVERSION THROUGH LIGHT-HEARTED SPONTANEOUS ACTIVITIES
Using play as a context or as a means towards an outcome can be maximized when therapists, instead of exclusively utilizing pre-planned challenging motor activities which a child with CP would seldom consider 'play', recognize the potential for play in spontaneous situations that occur during a clinic visit. Recognizing these situations as opportunities for free play that can still be used for the development of other outcomes of play – such as flexibility, intrinsic motivation and the ability to deal with unexpected events – will lead to more enjoyable and successful sessions (Blanche 1997, 2008).

INCREASING INTENSITY OF INVOLVEMENT IN PHYSICALLY AND/OR MENTALLY DEMANDING ACTIVITIES
The biological base of play is acknowledged in reference to individuals' tendency to seek intense, highly demanding and stimulating playful activities (Apter 1992, Zuckerman 1994). Examples of these activities include rock climbing, racing, parachuting, and boxing.

Individuals with disabilities have few opportunities to engage in these intensely stimulating and demanding activities but some of them may still have the desire. Increasing the amount of stimulation in a session can easily be accomplished by using a variety of intervention approaches, such as sensory integration, social interaction with peers, and virtual reality. Sensory integration offers tools to target these areas, especially in children who are under-responsive to input. These difficulties limit the functional abilities of the child as well as their level of arousal (Blanche et al 1995). The sensory input that children with CP best respond to may include large amounts of movement (Blanche and Nakasuji 2001). Once the child's level of arousal has been brought to an optimal level, challenging manual abilities is easier. The following example illustrates this point.

Don is a 4-year-old child with right hemiplegia functioning at MACS level II in terms of manual abilities. He exhibits difficulties in planning movement which affect both his gross motor and hand skills. Don is also hyporesponsive to stimulation and tends to take a long time to gear himself up to engaging in the therapeutic session. The therapist uses play to increase his level of arousal, and engages in a game of shark in which another child ('the shark') chases Don with a brush to 'bite' him. Don avoids the shark by climbing inside inner tubes placed on the floor. Both children take turns to play shark. When playing, Don uses adequate postural control and motor planning to climb over the inner tubes, uses the appropriate shoulder, elbow and forearm movements to brush his peer, and uses bilateral motor coordination to lift the inner tube over his head to prevent being caught.

The above example illustrates how increasing the intensity of the activity influences the child's arousal level and thus his engagement in activities that challenge motor control. When not playing, Don trips and falls often and has difficulty handling utensils. However, when playing 'shark', Don's motor abilities improve and with proper guidance his manual abilities improve.

Involving peers with higher level play skills also increases the level of involvement in children with delayed play skills. The results of a study conducted with children with delays in play development suggested that pairing these children with others with higher play skills increased initiation and response to initiation during play among children with delayed play skills (Tanta et al 2005).

ENJOYING THE ABILITY TO MASTER AN ACTIVITY
The experience of flow derived from the enjoyment of participating in a mastered activity has been extensively described by Csikszentmihalyi (1990). Children with CP seldom experience flow while participating in activities requiring motor involvement. In addition, because acquiring flow is not part of therapists' treatment goals, therapists often interrupt an activity to correct movements. Although correcting is necessary in intervention, over-doing it can be detrimental. A study by Germain and Dwyer (1988) supports this point. These authors studied the level of play in children with cerebral palsy under two conditions:

(1) handled, where the therapist facilitated postural responses while the child played; and (2) unhandled, where the children engaged in free play. They found that the children showed higher play skills in the unhandled condition. It was noted that when handled by a therapist, the children depended more on the therapist for direction and showed less self-initiated behaviour. The authors concluded that there is a delicate balance between giving the child enough support or assistance to facilitate play and giving too much. In situations where children are overcorrected they cannot experience the enjoyment derived from mastering a task.

Including unstructured toys that require little pre-established motor coordination but allow for free movement might be one way to involve the children in activities that target both the movement and the enjoyment of mastery. For example, shaving cream, finger paint, or bubbles can be utilized to start the session. These activities create the context for increasing manual abilities. For example, if playing with shaving cream is an activity the child wants, having the child supinate the hand so the shaving cream goes on the palm of the hand is one way of working on forearm supination. Or playing a game in which the rule is 'only the index can play now' in the shaving cream can help develop isolated finger movements and create flow in the activity.

CREATING NOVELTY

Creativity is another experience that therapists can include in the session and in the life of the child. Creativity can consist of telling stories, making up songs, or painting a picture. In the creative process, the child might be able to develop the motor skills required in the intervention. For example, in telling stories, the child could act the story with puppets and hence develop wrist and forearm movements. With painting a picture, the child can use crayons, finger paint, or adapted markers that create the need for the desired upper extremity movement and also increase the child's motivation.

Conclusion: valuing play in the life of the child

Developing playfulness in children contributes to their ability to incorporate meaningful activities into daily life. Morrison and Metzger (2001: 540) stated:

> The more playful child may generalize this flexible approach into environ-
> mental interaction beyond play and into other aspects of his or her life. For the
> child with a condition that impedes his or her ability to interact with the social
> or physical environment, a flexible (playful) approach may enable the child to
> succeed more frequently in these difficult situations.

The benefits of play in terms of contributing to quality of life and decreasing stress are widely recognized (Miller and Reid 2003, Harris and Reid 2005). Hence, play becomes important not only as a therapeutic tool but as an activity that can be fostered at home, at school, and in the community. However, because children with CP tend to spend large amounts of time in one-to-one situations with adults, one basic characteristic of play, intrinsic motivation, is reduced. At home they need adult intervention to engage in play. At school, they need others to initiate. Therefore, if we value play as part of life, it is important to create a context for play by attending to social and physical characteristics in the environment.

In terms of social characteristics, the adults interacting with the individual with CP need to value play as a meaningful experience that serves as context for the development of life skills as well as for self-fulfilment. The social interaction needs to be one in which there is opportunity for choice and self-initiation. Therapists need to know how to play and how to use playful strategies through speech, body language, and facial expressions (Bundy 1991, Parham 1992). Parents need to be able to access the community resources and take time to engage in play and leisure.

In creating a context for play it is also critical to consider the physical environment and the objects within it. There needs to be flexibility in the spaces, toys and equipment in order to foster play. Play spaces should offer a variety of experiences and allow for creativity, illusion, change, and chance. Children need to be able to control the space in terms of having objects, toys and people to move and change, and must also have freedom to move (Chandler 1997). When working with children with CP, the therapist may need to provide positioning equipment and adapt toys and play equipment in order for the child to access them optimally. Play can be enhanced through a variety of augmentative devices, ranging from very simple adaptations to complex electronic devices (Deitz and Swinth 1997). Parents can take advantage of community programmes that provide the experience of play and the opportunity for social interactions, including the use of adapted playgrounds, participation in special sports programmes and the use of toy libraries.

In summary, play offers the opportunity to develop new skills and to express the essence of who we are. Using its potential in intervention will allow the therapist and child to reach higher levels of manual dexterity and create a context for the child to explore who he/she truly is. The goal of intervention is to help people like Kevin to reach his goal of playing the guitar, and while playing the guitar he will also work on functional goals such as increasing motor abilities.

REFERENCES

Alessandrini N (1949) Play – a child's world. *Am J Occup Ther* 3: 9–12.
American Occupational Therapy Association (2000) Occupational Therapy Practice Framework: domain and process. *Am J Occup Ther* 56: 609–639.
Anderson J, Hinojosa J, Strauch C (1987) Integrating play in neurodevelopmental treatment. *Am J Occup Ther* 41: 421–426.
Apter M (1992) *The Dangerous Edge: The Psychology of Excitement.* New York: Free Press.
Ayres AJ (1972) *Sensory Integration and Learning Disorders.* Los Angeles: Western Psychological Services.
Ayres AJ (1979) *Sensory Integration and the Child.* Los Angeles: Western Psychological Services.
Bartlett DJ, Kneale Fanning JE (2003) Relationships of equipment use and play positions to motor development at eight months corrected age of infants born preterm. *Pediatr Phys Ther* 15: 8–15.
Behnke C, Fetokovich M (1984) Examining the reliability and validity of the play history. *Am J Occup Ther* 38: 94–100.
Bergen D (1988) *Play as a Medium for Learning and Development.* Portsmouth, NH: Heinemann.
Berlyne D (1966) Curiosity and exploration. *Science* 15: 25–32.
Blanche E (1997) Doing with, not doing to: play and the child with cerebral palsy. In: Parham D, Fazio L, editors. *Play in Occupational Therapy for Children.* St Louis, MO: Mosby, pp 202–218.

Blanche EI (1999) Why children like to play. In: Erhard R, editor. *Parent Articles about NDT*. San Antonio, TX: Therapy Skill Builders.

Blanche EI (2002) Play and process: adult play embedded in the daily routine. In: Roopnarine J, editor. *Conceptual, Social-cognitive, and Contextual Issues in the Field of Play*. Westport, CT: Ablex Publishing.

Blanche EI (2008) Doing with, not doing to: play and the child with cerebral palsy. In: Parham LD, Fazio L, editors. *Play in Occupational Therapy for Children, 2nd edn*. St Louis, MO: Mosby.

Blanche EI, Nakasuji B (2001) Sensory integration and the child with cerebral palsy. In: Smith-Roley S, Blanche EI, Schaaf RC, editors. *Understanding the Nature of Sensory Integration with Diverse Populations*. Tucson, AZ: Therapy Skill Builders.

Blanche EI, Botticelli TM, Hallway MK (1995) *Combining Neuro-developmental Treatment and Sensory Integration Principles – An Approach to Pediatric Therapy*. Tucson, AZ: Therapy Skill Builders.

Bledsoe N, Shepherd J (1982) A study of reliability and validity of a preschool play scale. *Am J Occup Ther* 36: 783–788.

Bruner J (1972) Nature and uses of immaturity. *Am Psychol* 27: 687–708.

Bundy A (1991) Play theory and sensory integration. In: Fisher AG, Murray EA, Bundy AC, editors. *Sensory Integration: Theory and Practice*. Philadelphia: F.A. Davis Co, pp 46–68.

Bundy A (1993) Assessment of play and leisure: delineation of the problem. *Am J Occup Ther* 47: 217–222.

Bundy A (1997) Play and playfulness: what to look for. In: Parham LD, Fazio L, editors. *Play in Occupational Therapy for Children*. St Louis, MO: Mosby, pp 52–66.

Caldwell B (1986) The significance of parent–child interaction in children's development. In: Gottfried AW, Brown CC, editors. *Play Interactions*. Lexington, MA: Lexington Books, pp 305–310.

Chandler B (1997) Where do you want to play? Play environments; an occupational therapy perspective. In: Chadler B, editor. *The Essence of Play*. Bethesda, MD: American Occupational Therapy Association, pp 159–174.

Clark F, Parham D, Carlson M, Frank G, Jackson J, Pierce D, Wolfe R, Zeke R (1991) Occupational science: academic innovation in the service of occupational therapy's future. *Am J Occup Ther* 4: 300–310.

Cohen D (1987) *The Development of Play*. London: Routledge.

Couch K, Dietz J, Kanny E (1998) The role of play in pediatric occupational therapy. *Am J Occup Ther* 2: 111–117.

Crowe T (1989) Pediatric assessments: a survey of their use by occupational therapists in northwestern school systems. *Occup Ther J Res* 9: 273–286.

Csikszentmihalyi M (1990) *Flow: The Psychology of Optimal Experience*. New York: Harper and Row.

Deitz J, Swinth Y (1997) Accessing play through assistive technology. In: Parham LD, Fazio L, editors. *Play in Occupational Therapy for Children*. St Louis, MO: Mosby, pp 219–232.

Eagle RS (1985) Deprivation of early sensorimotor experience and cognition in the severely involved cerebral-palsied child. *J Autism Dev Disord* 15: 269–283.

Erikson E (1963) *Childhood and Society*. New York: Norton.

Fabes RA, Martin CL, Hanish LD (2003) Young children's play qualities in same-, other-, and mixed-sex peer groups. *Child Dev* 74: 921–932.

Finnie N (1975) *Handling the Young Cerebral Palsied Child at Home, 2nd edn*. New York: E.P. Dutton & Co, Inc.

Germain A, Dwyer M (1988) Unpublished paper presented at the annual conference of the American Occupational Therapy Association, 17–20 April, Phoenix, AZ.

Graham MA, Bryant DM (1993) Developmentally appropriate environments for children with special needs. *Infants Young Child* 5: 31–42.

Groos K (1976) The play of animals: play and instinct, and the play of man: teasing and love play. In: Bruner J, Jolly A, Sylva K, editors. *Play: Its Role in Development and Evolution*. New York: Basic Books, pp 65–83.

Hanzlik JR (1989) The effect of intervention on the free-play experience for mothers and their infants with developmental delay and cerebral palsy. *Phys Occup Ther Pediatr* 9: 33–51.

Harkness L, Bundy A (2001) The test of playfulness and children with physical disabilities. *Occup Ther J Res* 21: 73–89.

Harris K, Reid D (2005) The influence of virtual reality play on children's motivation. *Can J Occup Ther* 72: 21–29.

Harrison H, Kielhofner G (1986) Examining reliability and validity of the preschool play scale with handicapped children. *Am J Occup Ther* 40: 167–173.

Henry A (2008) Assessment of play and leisure in children and adolescents. In: Parham LD, Fazio L, editors. *Play in Occupational Therapy for Children, 2nd edn*. St Louis, MO: Mosby.

Hestenes LL, Carroll DE (2000) The play interactions of young children with and without disabilities: individual and environmental influences. *Early Child Res Q* 15: 229–246.

Huizinga J (1950) *Homo Ludens*. Boston: Beacon Press.

King S, Teplicky R, King G, Rosenbaum P (2004) Family-centered service for children with cerebral palsy and their families: a review of the literature. *Semin Pediatr Neurol* 11: 78–86.

Knox S (1968) Observation and assessment of the everyday play behavior of the mentally retarded child. Unpublished master's thesis, University of Southern California, Los Angeles, California.

Knox S (1974) A play scale. In: Reilly M, editor. *Play as Exploratory Learning*. Beverly Hills: Sage Publications.

Knox S (1996) Play and playfulness in preschool children. In: Zemke R, Clark F, editors. *Occupational Science: The Evolving Discipline*. Philadelphia, PA: F.A. Davis, pp 81–88.

Knox S (1997) Development and current use of the Knox Preschool Play Scale. In: Parham LD, Fazio L, editors. *Play in Occupational Therapy for Children*. St Louis, MO: Mosby, pp 35–51.

Knox S (1999) Play and playfulness of preschool children. Unpublished doctoral dissertation. University of Southern California, Los Angeles, CA.

Knox S (2005) Play. In: Case-Smith J, editor. *Occupational Therapy for Children*. St Louis, MO: Mosby, pp 571–586.

Knox S (2008) Development and current use of the Knox Preschool Play Scale. In: Parham, LD, Fazio L, editors. *Play in Occupational Therapy for Children, 2nd edn*. St Louis, MO: Mosby.

Knox S, Mailloux Z (1997) Play as treatment and treatment through play. In: Chandler B, editor. *The Essence of Play*. Bethesda, MD: American Occupational Therapy Association.

Kogan KL, Tyler N, Turner P (1974) The process of interpersonal adaptation between mothers and their cerebral palsied children. *Dev Med Child Neurol* 16: 518–527.

Kuczynski M, Slonka K (1999) Influence of artificial saddle riding on postural stability in children with cerebral palsy. *Gait Posture* 10: 154–160.

Levitt S (1975) A study of the gross motor skills of cerebral palsied children in an adventure playground for handicapped children. *Child Care Health Dev* 1: 29–43.

Mactavish JB, Schleien SJ (2004) Re-injecting spontaneity and balance in family life: parents' perspectives on recreation in families that include children with developmental disability. *J Intellect Disabil Res* 48: 123–141.

Meyer A (1922) The philosophy of occupational therapy. *Arch Occup Ther* 1: 1–10.

Miller S, Reid D (2003) Doing play: competency, control, and expression. *Cyberpsychol Behav* 6: 623–632.

Missiuna C, Pollock N (1991) Play deprivation in children with physical disabilities: the role of the occupational therapist in preventing secondary disability. *Am J Occup Ther* 45: 882–887.

Mogford K (1977) The play of handicapped children. In: Tizard B, Harvey D, editors. *Biology of Play*. Philadelphia: J.B. Lippincott, pp 170–184.

Morrison C, Metzger P (2001) Play. In: Case-Smith J, Allen A, Pratt P, editors. *Occupational Therapy for Children, 4th edn*. St Louis, MO: Mosby, pp 528–544.

Okimoto A, Bundy A, Hanzlik J (2000) Playfulness in children with and without disability: measurement and intervention. *Amer J Occup Ther* 54: 734–782.

Parham D (1992) Strategies for maintaining a playful atmosphere during therapy. American Occupational Therapy Association, Sensory Integration Special Interest Section, *Newsletter* 15: 2–3.

Parham D, Fazio L, editors (1997) *Play in Occupational Therapy for Children*. St Louis, MO: Mosby.

Piaget J (1952) *Play, Dreams and Imitation in Childhood*. London: William Heinemann.

Pierce D (1991) Early object rule acquisition. *Am J Occup Ther* 45: 438–449.

Pierce D (1997) The power of object play. In: Parham LD, Fazio L, editors. *Play in Occupational Therapy for Children*. St Louis, MO: Mosby, pp 86–111.

Primeau L (1995) Orchestration of work and play within families. Unpublished dissertation, University of Southern California, Los Angeles, CA.

Primeau L, Clark F, Pierce D (1989) Occupational therapy alone has looked upon occupation: future applications of occupational science to pediatric occupational therapy. *Occup Ther Health Care* 6: 19–32.

Quarrick G (1989) *Our Sweetest Hours: Recreation and the Mental State of Absorption*. Jefferson, NC: McFarland and Co.

Rast M (1986) Play and therapy, play or therapy. In: *Play: A Skill for Life*. Rockville, MD: American Occupational Therapy Association.

Reid D (2002) Benefits of a virtual play rehabilitation environment for children with cerebral palsy on perceptions of self-efficacy: a pilot study. *Pediatr Rehabil* 5: 141–148.

Reid D (2004) The influence of virtual reality on playfulness in children with cerebral palsy: a pilot study. *Occup Ther Int* 11: 131–144.

Reilly M (1974) *Play as Exploratory Learning*. Beverly Hills, CA: Sage Publications.

Rubin K, Fein G, Vandenberg B (1983) Play. In: Mussin P, editor. *Handbook of Child Psychology, Vol IV*. New York: John Wiley and Sons, pp 694–774.

Saunders I, Sayer M, Goodale A (1999) The relationship between playfulness and coping in preschool children: a pilot study. *Am J Occup Ther* 53: 221–226.

Schaaf RC, Mulrooney LL (1989) Occupational therapy in early intervention: a family-centered approach. *Am J Occup Ther* 43: 745–753.

Sheridan MD (1975) The importance of spontaneous play in the fundamental learning of handicapped children. *Child Care Health Dev* 1: 3–17.

Skard G, Bundy A (2008) Play and playfulness: what to look for. In: Parham LD, Fazio L, editors. *Play in Occupational Therapy for Children, 2nd edn*. St Louis, MO: Mosby.

Sparling JW, Walker DF, Singdahlsen J (1984) Play techniques with neurologically impaired preschoolers. *Am J Occup Ther* 38: 603–611.

Sutton-Smith B (1997) *The Ambiguity of Play*. Cambridge, MA: Harvard University Press.

Sutton-Smith B, Kelly-Byrne D (1982) The phenomenon of bipolarity in play theories. In: Yawkey TD, Pellegrino AD, editors. *Child's Play: Developmental and Applied*. Hillsdale, NJ: Erlbaum

Takata N (1969) The play history. *Am J Occup Ther* 23: 314.

Takata N (1971) The play milieu – a preliminary appraisal. *Am J Occup Ther* 25: 281–284.

Takata N (1974) Play as a prescription. In: Reilly M, editor. *Play as Exploratory Learning*. Beverly Hills: Sage Publications, pp 209–246.

Tanta KJ, Deitz JC, White O, Billingsley F (2005) The effects of peer-play level on initiations and responses of preschool children with delayed play skills. *Am J Occup Ther* 59: 437–445.

Thomas AD, Rosenberg A (2003) Promoting community recreation and leisure. *Pediatr Phys Ther* 15: 232–246.

Vygotsky L (1966) Play and its role in the mental development of the child. *Soviet Psychology* 12: 62–76.

Weiss PL, Bialik P, Kizony R (2003) Virtual reality provides leisure time opportunities for young adults with physical and intellectual disabilities. *Cyberpsychol Behav* 6: 335–342.

White R (1959) Motivation reconsidered: the concept of competence. *Psychol Rev* 66: 297–333.

Zuckerman M (1994) *Behavioral Expressions and Biosocial Bases of Sensation Seeking*. Cambridge: Cambridge University Press.

24
ASSISTIVE TECHNOLOGY DEVICES IN COMPUTER ACTIVITIES

Helene Lidström and Maria Borgestig

Assistive technology devices – an opportunity for children with cerebral palsy

Computers are used by most people as multipurpose devices to support their efforts in education, at work and during leisure time. Information technology (IT) has especially had a great deal of influence on the lifestyle of today's children and youth, and its influence will probably increase in the future. Children with cerebral palsy (CP), just as typical children, need computer access in order to play games, send email, chat with their peers, and access information on the internet. However, a child with a disability may need adaptations in order to be able to use the computer for the same tasks as their peers.

Some children find it difficult to use a keyboard and a mouse, due to the fine motor skills required – typically individuals functioning at Manual Ability Classification System (MACS) levels III–V. Instead they may need to interface their computer with devices such as switches, a joystick, speech technology, or a head mouse (Lau and O'Leary 1993, Hawley 2002, Lancioni et al 2006). In addition, these children often need the computer to perform activities that are not ordinary computer-based activities, such as playing with toys, reading, calling a friend without handling a telephone, driving a power wheelchair, or controlling a CD-player. A computer can enable children with CP to participate in the same activities as their peers, but in a different and adapted way. Thus, information and communications technology (ICT) has the potential to be used by children with disabilities in ways that are meaningful and bring them satisfaction (Seymore 2005).

Children with CP have varying limitations in the form of physical, cognitive and visual impairments, which may reduce their performance in activities and their social participation. As functional limitations increase – Gross Motor Function Classification System (GMFCS) levels III, IV and V – so use and need of assistive technology devices (ATDs) also increase (Ostensjo et al 2005). Usually, children with severely impaired hand function become passive and unmotivated because of the lack of learning opportunities and/or possibilities to control their environment (Swinth 2001, Nilsson 2007). Therefore, ATDs are an important component of assessment and intervention when discussing how children with motor limitations can participate in play activities.

Identifying an object or an event of interest that motivates the child is a way of stimulating the child to be active and participate socially with others (Nilsson 2007). Even children classified as being at GMFCS and MACS levels IV–V can use a micro-switch to engage in many existing and developmentally challenging activities, such as playing with toys and

371

computer games and manipulating environment control systems (Lancioni et al 2001). Children as young as 9 months can use one switch for simple computer games (Glickman et al 1996).

It is not unusual for children with CP to have speech impairments in addition to motor limitations. For these children computer augmented communication devices provide the opportunity to express themselves (Salminen et al 2004b). For children with mild or severe motor limitations, but good cognitive ability, ATDs and computers offer enormous possibilities. Examples include independence in writing, listening to music, shopping, handling photos, and using an integrated control system to access their environment (e.g. TV control, door opener, electric wheelchair) (Ding et al 2003). By using a computer, children can experience feelings of equality (and sometimes advantage) as they are able to use technology in the same way as everyone else (Seymore 2005).

How to select the right device
It is well known that successful implementation of ATDs is not easy (Bain and Leger 1997, Coupley and Ziviani 2004). However, in support of ATD use, it is documented that students usually want to use more ICT in education than their current accessibility allows (Hemmingsson, Lidström and Nygård, accepted). Since the child's motivation for using ATDs is high, steps to increase their access should be emphasized. When planning ATD intervention a client-centred approach and a theoretical framework are important for success (Scherer 2000, Lenker and Paquet 2003). The Occupational Performance Process Model (CAOT 1997) is useful, with some modifications, for clarifying the steps of ATD prescription (see Fig. 24.1).

IDENTIFY ACTIVITY
The first step is to ask the child and family about the activities the child wants to do, or is required to do, throughout the day. It can be difficult to interview young children and children with communication disorders. In these cases, a parent, an assistant or a teacher may need to be the informant. However, having the child identify their own priorities is preferable. Talking Mats™ (Murphy and Cameron 2002) is an effective tool for interviewing children using pictures or symbols (CAOT 1997). It provides a structured framework for open questions and can be used across ages and abilities (see Fig. 24.2).

Open-ended questions – e.g. 'Have you thought about what you want to use the computer for?' 'What things have you seen other kids do on the computer that you would like to do?' 'What would be different if your child had an AT device?' – provide good information (Lidström and Zachrisson 2005). The Canadian Occupational Performance Measure (COPM) can also be used to identify issues that are important for the child; it can detect change in a child's self-perception of occupational performance over time (CAOT 1997).

SELECT THEORETICAL FRAMEWORK
Once an occupational performance issue is identified, rated and prioritized, the next step is to select a theoretical approach for intervention. When deciding on specific ATD

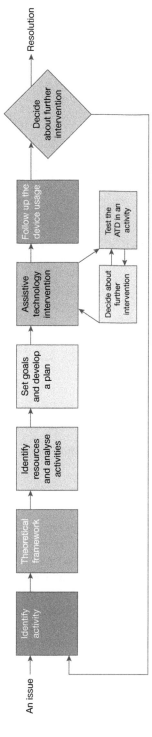

Fig. 24.1 The occupational therapy process and assistive technology devices (reproduced by permission of the Swedish Handicap Institute).

Source: Lidström and Zachrisson 2005.

373

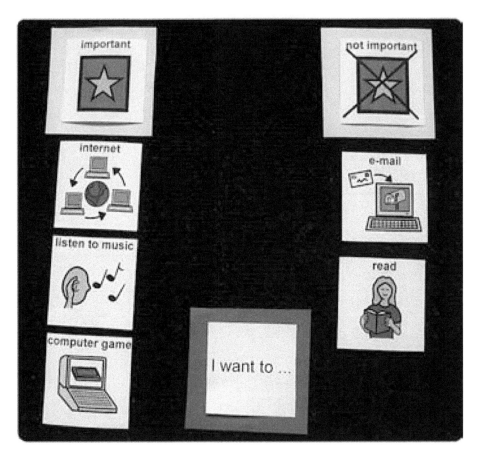

Fig. 24.2 Talking Mats, with symbols used to identify what activities the child wants to do with the computer.

Photo: Helene Lidström and Maria Borgestig.

interventions, biomechanical and learning theories are useful (McColl et al 1993). There are several models for AT prescriptions (Scherer and Craddock 2002, Lenker and Paquet 2003) but we have found the Bain Assistive Technology System (BATS) model especially useful (Bain and Leger 1997). This model emphasizes obtaining knowledge about: (1) the resources of the child; (2) the environments where the child will use the device and the support available for AT use in each environment; (3) the characteristics/limitations of a specific piece of AT; and (4) the chosen activity the assistive technology will support. By taking these factors into consideration, the therapist increases the possibility of finding a device that will match the child's needs in daily life.

IDENTIFY RESOURCES AND ANALYSE ACTIVITIES

After issues of computer use have been addressed, and resources and service in relation to ATDs have been identified, the therapist assesses the child's gross and fine motor functions to identify which body part is capable of producing the most accurate, reliable and controlled movements (Swinth 2001, Lidström and Zachrisson 2005). Since hand control is considered first, an important question to ask is: does the child have enough upper limb control to steer a joystick or a switch with their hand? Which hand and in which position? If it is not possible for the child to use an arm/hand/finger, perhaps the head or eyes can be used to control the device? Should the head movement be backwards or should the chin strike the switch? For some children, special movements in the wrist, elbow or foot can be used. Regardless of the body part used to steer, it is important for the child to have a stabilized secure sitting posture. The child's cognitive function and sight also need to be considered. Does the child understand the task and are they, for example, able to understand what they are seeing on the screen in order to select a new picture in a computer game?

For a better understanding of what demands the *activity* imposes on the child, the therapist needs to analyse the task by describing all of its steps. With increased severity of impairment, the computer can be adapted to do several steps in the chosen activity. For example, when pressing a single switch to write with a scanning system the computer compensates for the child's motor difficulties; however, the trade-off is that the activity will be more complicated, requiring more steps and more time. To simplify such an activity you can use the same device but choose an uncomplicated software programme, such as an easy game, which demands fewer presses on the switch and therefore requires less energy expenditure.

Factors in the social, cultural and physical environment, as well as circumstances in society, may influence the use of ATDs (Coupley and Ziviani 2004). Usage is most likely to increase when there are realistic expectations of what can be achieved and when there is social acceptance for using assistive technology among peers, family and teachers (Lidström and Zachrisson 2005).

A prerequisite is that the applied assistive technology together with the software gives the child a sense of control over the output from the computer. Some children are more comfortable with an uncomplicated device with less efficiency but more reliability. Often high technology devices have a higher risk of technical problems, which can have a negative effect on the child's experience.

SET GOALS AND DEVELOP A PLAN

It is important to specify and plan goals around different computer activities. For example, when selecting a device there is a great difference between playing computer games and writing a school essay. Thus, it is important that children, parents and/or professionals design clear goals together, on the basis of earlier prioritized computer activities. There are several assessments available that are useful in goal-setting, and in identifying steps to reach goals, such as the Goal Attainment Scale (GAS; Kiresuk et al 1994) and the COPM (Carswell et al 2004). According to the GAS one measurable goal would be: 'Philip sends an email message to his friends from his computer every day' (see Chapter 18 for more details of the GAS).

Once the goal is identified, a detailed plan needs to be outlined, and a timeline of steps for implementation of the ATD needs to be drawn up (Lidström and Zachrisson 2005). When an advanced technical device – for example, an eye gaze system – is chosen, the implementation phase could be long. A long-time perspective is also important for children with cognitive limitations (Nilsson 2007). When the aim is to teach the child with significant cognitive deficits to touch a micro-switch to activate a toy, it might take a long time for the child to understand that the toy is activated by his/her touch on the switch. In this case, it is advantageous to divide the long-term goal into short-term goals. Also, as children grow and gain higher levels of function, their interests often change. This is another reason to use goals achievable in a shorter time perspective (Swinth 2001).

Assistive Technology Intervention

Selecting the device
The prioritized activity affects the choice of device. There is a difference between having the child use arrow-keys for a high speed computer game, and accessing an entire keyboard for writing a school essay. In all cases, the exertion requirements of the child need to be considered when choosing an appropriate device. Measuring time requirements or counting the numbers of strikes to complete a task can, for example, be used to compare two devices (Lau and O'Leary 1993). This aspect is highly influenced by the child's voluntary and precise control of movement.

Often a child with significant functional limitations may use ATDs for more than one daily activity, such as driving a powered wheelchair as well as playing and doing schoolwork on the computer. A compromise might be needed between utilizing the same device for many different activities and using different types of ATDs for different activities during the day to avoid stress injuries.

The decision about ATDs is highly influenced by the child's cognitive capacity, but the decision about devices is mainly dependent on the child's ability to use their hands. MACS levels can be used to aid the choice of device. Children at most MACS levels will need some form of ATD, but to a different extent and with different types of adaptations. Typically, as the severity of the CP diagnosis increases, the need for ATDs also increases, due to poorer hand skills. However, since more complicated ATD use is related to both poor hand function and higher ATD demands on the child, in fact the determining factor is often the child's cognitive level.

Children classified as MACS level II are independent when handling objects in daily life, including computer activities. Yet, slowness and decreased function in one hand, as in the child with hemiplegic CP, may sometimes necessitate small adaptations (Steenbergen et al 1998). These could be changes in working strategy, or adaptations of a device and software. For a child with a hemiplegic arm/hand, the function 'stiff keys' can be useful when it is difficult to push two keys at the same time. More recent versions of many word-processing programs include these enlargement features as universal design. Often adaptations in the operating system and in the word processor are free of charge and relatively easy to make. For all younger children, a smaller keyboard without the numerical keypad may be preferable from an ergonomic perspective. It will make it easier for the child to reach both the keys and the mouse. For children who are partially sighted, enlarged menus and changing the background colour, typeface, and size of objects and icons on the screen may improve performance and should be considered for all children with vision impairments no matter what MACS level.

Children at MACS level III need adaptation and preparation in most activities requiring manual ability, so technical aids are important as well as ATDs. Keyboarding may be an alternative to handwriting for these children if speed and accuracy are a problem for them (Preminger et al 2004). In this case, an ordinary keyboard with reduced key repetition, an ordinary mouse with adjusted cursor speed, and the use of autotext (which expands short keywords into full phrases) might facilitate the speed and accuracy of written communication for the child. However, it is important to introduce ATDs at an early age since learning new activities takes a long time. ATDs are important for this group of children for play and leisure and will improve their ability to occupy themselves independently. Children at younger ages often start with one or two switches and progress to roller balls (see Fig. 24.3).

Children at MACS level IV need a lot of adaptations and personal support when handling objects in daily life. Thus ATDs are very important for almost all children in this group. Because they also have severe gross motor limitations, an ergonomically designed workplace is important. With plenty of training, the child's possibilities increase with age and they are able to use certain types of ATD more or less independently both for school work and leisure. Since these children have restrictions in controlling movements, it is difficult for them to use an ordinary keyboard and mouse. An enlarged keyboard with keys under the surface can be a good alternative (see Fig. 24.4).

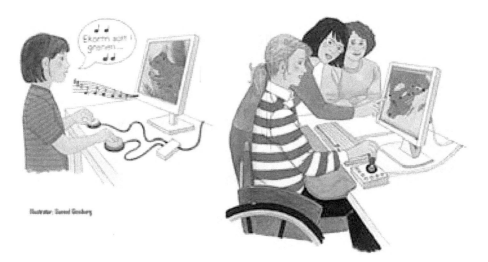

Fig. 24.3 A girl controlling the computer with two switches, and another girl with a joystick (reproduced by permission of the Swedish Handicap Institute).

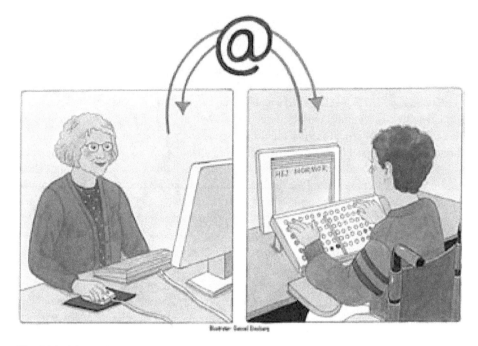

Fig. 24.4 A boy using his enlarged keyboard to send an email to his grandmother (reproduced by permission of the Swedish Handicap Institute).

To be able to make movements on screen children can use a special mouse to increase accuracy, like a joystick controlled by hand (see Fig. 24.5). For children who are not able to use a keyboard, an 'on-screen keyboard' can be used together with a joystick.

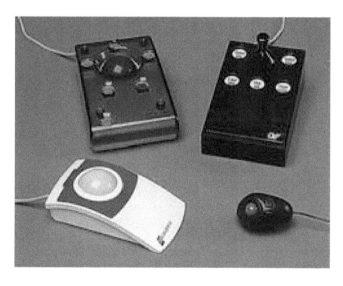

Fig. 24.5 Different types of mouse, roller balls and joysticks (reproduced by permission of the Swedish Handicap Institute).

Photo: Lars-Göran Jansson.

Further adaptations to the joystick may include an adapted grip and adjusted speed combined with a switch or autoclick function for mouse clicks, placed in a pretested position (see Fig. 24.6).

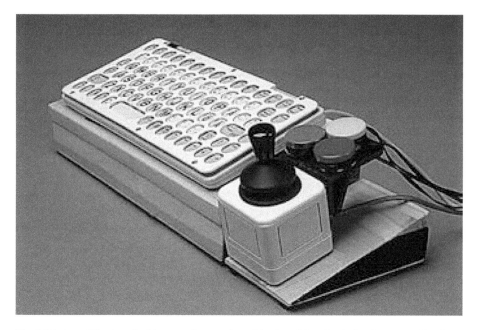

Fig. 24.6 A small keyboard with an overlay together with a joystick and switches for mouse click functions. This requires a limited working surface and the same height for the hands when working, alternating with keyboard and joystick (reproduced by permission of the Swedish Handicap Institute).

Photo: Lars-Göran Jansson.

If the child can use just one switch, they can write by using a scanning system and an 'on-screen keyboard'. Scanning is a method used by children who need beginning keyboard functions using switches for input (Simpson et al 2006). They can use one or two switches in row/column scanning in the panel on the screen, the 'on-screen keyboard'. Fig. 24.7 shows row/column scanning with a single switch.

Using word prediction is an excellent method of increasing the child's writing speed and efficiency, but it requires a higher level of cognitive function than other methods. When writing, a word prediction program will give the child word choices on screen to reduce the number of presses on the switch or the keyboard. Some children at this level may use devices other than switches. A joystick steered by the chin (see Fig. 24.8), a head mouse or an eye gaze system are all devices which can increase speed, accuracy and efficiency. When using a head mouse the child has a small reflector dot placed on their forehead. To move the mouse pointer on the screen the child moves their head. Eye gaze is a system with cameras, which can detect where the child looks on the screen. This means that the child can interact

A	B	C	D	E		A	B	C	D	E		A	B	C	D	E
F	G	H	I	J		F	G	H	I	J		F	G	H	I	J
K	L	M	N	O		K	L	M	N	O		K	L	M	N	O
P	Q	R	S	T		P	Q	R	S	T		P	Q	R	S	T
U	V	X	Y	Z		U	V	X	Y	Z		U	V	X	Y	Z

Fig. 24.7 In panel 1, the system starts row-scanning automatically and the first row is highlighted when the child presses the switch. In panel 2, the target row has been reached; pressing the switch will stop the row-scanning and select this row. In panel 3, the system scans through each column within the target row. The switch is pressed a third time to choose the target letter M.

Illustrator: Helene Lidström.

with programs by looking at objects on the screen without moving their head. Using head or eyes instead of hands will often decrease involuntary body movements for children with CP classified at MACS level IV. It will also be easier to focus on the screen when the child does not need to look down to press a switch by hand.

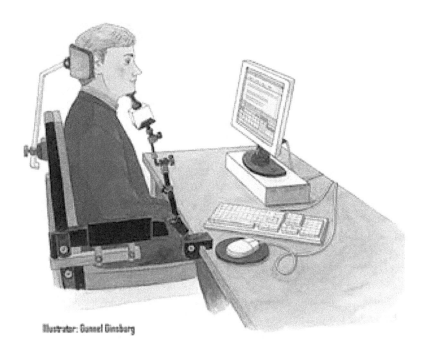

Illustrator: Gunnel Ginsburg

Fig. 24.8 A joystick is mounted on an adjustable arm to enable steering with the chin instead of the hand. The grip is adapted with a concave surface for the chin to lean on (reproduced by permission of the Swedish Handicap Institute).

380

Children classified at MACS level V may only be able to make a simple movement with the hand to push a switch to perform a computer activity (see Fig. 24.9). It is often easier for the child to press then lift the hand from the switch.

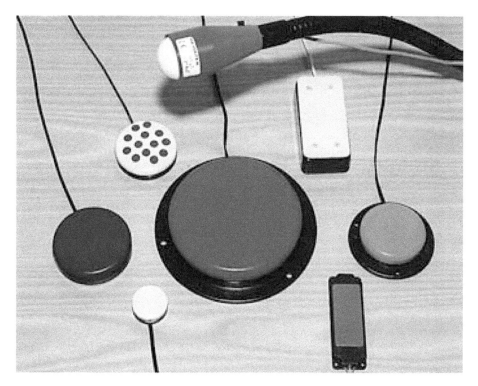

Fig. 24.9 Several types of switches (reproduced by permission of the Swedish Handicap Institute).
Photo: Sevim Yildiz.

The child's cognitive function and sight determine what it might be possible to achieve through ATDs. In special cases, when children with good cognitive function find it too difficult to push a switch by hand, another position for the switch has to be found – usually by the head (see Fig. 24.10).

Often the child can use one or two switches and 'on-screen keyboard'. There are also other interfaces available which activate the switch in other ways. With a sip and puff device the child can perform one or two actions just by using a mouthpiece for sipping or puffing. While the strength of this device is that it demands only a small sip or puff to activate, the weakness is that the child is unable to talk while operating the computer. Another activation option is to use an EMG device taped to the skin over a muscle group that the child can control voluntarily – the child can then activate the device by the muscle contraction. Other devices mentioned for use at MACS level IV may also be useful at this level, such as an eye gaze or scanning system, if the child's cognitive level is high enough.

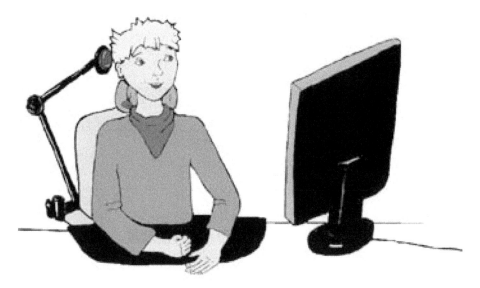

Fig. 24.10 A child pressing a switch by leaning the head to one side.

Illustrator: Hillevi Törmä.

Implementing the device

PRACTICE

Sometimes it is important to practise using the device in circumstances with fewer stimuli before using it in the natural environment, such as in the classroom. Starting with simple computer activities helps the child to concentrate on learning. At the same time the activities must be meaningful and motivate the child, particularly with younger children. Training should start with simple and enjoyable computer activities before introducing an activity such as scanning (Jones and Stewart 2004). For example, the task of learning how to scan can be divided into different steps to enable the process to be more easily understood by the child. Ultimately, the child needs to understand the whole scanning process, to follow the scanning selections and to activate a switch when the desired selection is highlighted.

Because many adaptations are often made to the workplace, to devices and to software programs, the child's need for assistance in the activity may require more individual time for training with the therapist/assistant before the ATD can be used in daily life.

Another way to grade an activity is to let the child do a part of the task – for example, an adult can move the mouse cursor and the child pushes a switch to make the mouse click. The adult then has the opportunity to give the child enough time to be able to perform the activity.

EDUCATION AND SUPPORT

Adaptations and software programs require education for the child's social network – e.g. assistants, teachers and parents – so that they can assist the child on a daily basis. For example, if the child is going to write with symbols, staff and family members in the environment need training in operating the on-screen communication keyboard, and information about how to get support when needed. When implementing a device in the child's environment a period of support must follow, especially when implementing computer-augmented communication. In this case, the use of a device by the child seems to be directly related to the amount of support provided (Salminen et al 2004a).

FOLLOW-UP

When the child has used ATDs in their daily life for some time there is a need for follow-up and re-evaluation. The timing of the follow-up depends upon how fast the child is expected to learn, and how complicated the ATD is. Often a longer period of time is required when AT is used as compensation for speech, language or cognitive problems (Scherer 2002). The follow-up should also include the child's level of satisfaction. The same assessments can be used for evaluation as for goal setting – i.e. 'Talking Mats'™ (see Fig. 24.2), COPM and GAS. In addition, the Quebec User Evaluation of Satisfaction with Assistive Technology (QUEST 2.0; Demers et al 2000, 2002) can be used; it is one of the few assessments to evaluate the user's satisfaction with the ATD provided.

The follow-up evaluation is crucial for deciding new directions for the child's computer skills. AT also gives an opportunity for increasing the child's development, which means that the re-evaluation process often identifies new needs and goals when earlier problems have been resolved. If the re-evaluation shows that the goal has not been reached or that the child's needs have changed, then you need, together with the family, to decide about further intervention. You may need to start the process over again from the beginning.

Conclusions

This chapter has demonstrated how assistive technology can provide children with CP with opportunities to actively participate in play and education in daily life. However, these opportunities are based on the premise that people in the child's environment have a working knowledge of computers and assistive technology, as well as knowing how different devices can fit the child's needs at different ages and different levels of function. As the amount of assistive technology increases, therapists need more knowledge about devices, equipment and software in order for them to be able to effectively and efficiently support children with CP, so that they have access to devices that can improve their quality of life.

REFERENCES

Bain BK, Leger D (1997) *Assistive Technology Interdisciplinary Approach*. New York: Churchill Livingstone.
CAOT (1997) *Enabling Occupation: An Occupational Therapy Perspective*. Toronto: Canadian Association of Occupational Therapists (CAOT) Publications.
Carswell A, McColl M, Baptiste S, Law M, Polatajko H, Pollock N (2004) The Canadian Occupational Performance Measure: a research and clinical literature review. *Can J Occup Ther* 71: 210–222.
Coupley J, Ziviani J (2004) Barriers to the use of assistive technology for children with multiple disabilities. *Occup Ther Int* 11: 229–243.
Demers L, Weiss-Lambrou R, Ska B (2000) Item analysis of the Quebec User Evaluation of Satisfaction with Assistive Technology (QUEST). *Assist Technol* 12: 96–105.

Demers L, Weiss-Lambrou R, Ska B (2002) The Quebec User Evaluation of Satisfaction with Assistive Technology (QUEST 2.0): an overview and recent progress. *Technol Disabil* 14: 101–105.

Ding D, Cooper R, Kaminski B, Kanaly J, Allegretti A, Chaves E, Hubbard S (2003) Integrated control and related technology of assistive devices. *Assist Technol* 15: 89–97.

Glickman L, Deitz J, Anson D, Stewart H (1996) The effect of switch control skills of infants and toddlers. *Am J Occup Ther* 50: 545–553.

Hawley M (2002) Speech recognition as an input to electronic assistive technology. *Br J Occup Ther* 65: 15–20.

Jones J, Stewart H (2004) A description of how three occupational therapists train children in using the scanning access technique. *Aust Occup Ther J* 51: 155–165.

Kiresuk T, Smith A, Cardillo J (1994) *Goal Attainment Scaling: Applications, Theory, and Measurement.* Hillsdale, NJ: Erlbaum Associates.

Lancioni GE, O'Reilly MF, Olivia D, Coppa M (2001) A micro-switch for vocalization responses to foster environment control in children with multiple disabilities. *J Intellect Disabil Res* 45: 271–275.

Lancioni GE, O'Reilly MF, Singh NN, Olivia D, Baccani L (2006) Micro-switch programs for students with multiple disabilities and minimal motor behavior: assessing response acquisition and choice. *Pediatr Rehabil* 9: 137–143.

Lau C, O'Leary S (1993) Comparison of computer interface devices for persons with severe physical disabilities. *Am J Occup Ther* 47: 1022–1030.

Lenker JA, Paquet VL (2003) A review of conceptual models for assistive technology outcomes research and practice. *Assist Technol* 15: 1–15.

Lidström H, Zachrisson G (2005) *Aktiv med dator – möjligheter för personer med rörelsehinder* [To be active through the computer – opportunities for people with disabilities]. Klippan: Ljungbergs Tryckeri.

McColl MA, Law M, Steward D (1993) *Theoretical Basis of Occupational Therapy: An Annotated Bibliography of Applied Theory in the Professional Literature.* Thorofare, NJ: Slack Inc.

Murphy J, Cameron L (2002) Let your mats do the talking. Speech and language therapy in practice. The AAC Research Group at the University of Stirling. http://www.talkingmats.com/research-publications.htm

Nilsson L (2007) Driving to learn. Dissertation, Department of Health Sciences Division of Occupational Therapy and Gerontology, Lund University.

Ostensjo S, Brogren Carlberg E, Vøllestad N (2005) The use and impact of assistive devices and other environmental modifications on everyday activities and care in young children with cerebral palsy. *Disabil Rehabil* 27: 849–861.

Preminger F, Weiss P, Weintraub N (2004) Predicting occupational performance: handwriting versus keyboarding. *Am J Occup Ther* 58: 193–201.

Salminen A-L, Petrie H, Ryan S (2004a) Impact of computer augmented communication on the daily lives of speech-impaired children. Part I: Daily communication and activities. *Technol Disabil* 16: 157–167.

Salminen A, Ryan S, Petrie H (2004b) Impact of computer augmented communication on the daily lives of speech-impaired children. Part II: Services to support computer augmented communication. *Technol Disabil* 16: 169–177.

Scherer M (2000) *Living in the State of Stuck. How Assistive Technology Impacts the Lives of People with Disabilities.* Cambridge, MA: Brookline Books.

Scherer M (2002) *Assistive Technology: Matching Device and Consumer for Successful Rehabilitation.* Washington, DC: American Psychological Association.

Scherer M, Craddock G (2002) Matching Person & Technology (MPT) assessment process. *Technol Disabil* 14: 125–131.

Seymore W (2005) ICT and disability: exploring the human dimensions of technological engagement. *Technol Disabil* 17: 195–204.

Simpson H, Koester H, LoPresti E (2006) Evaluation of an adaptive row/column scanning system. *Technol Disabil* 18: 127–138.

Steenbergen B, Veringa A, de Haan A, Hulstijn W (1998) Manual dexterity and keyboard use in spastic hemiparesis: a comparison between the impaired hand and the good hand on a number of performance measures. *Clin Rehabil* 12: 64–72.

Swinth Y (2001) Assistive technology: computers and augmentative communication. In: Case-Smith C, editor. *Occupational Therapy for Children.* St Louis, MO: Mosby.

25
PARTICIPATION – THE ULTIMATE CHALLENGE

Jenny Ziviani and Margaret Wallen

Children with cerebral palsy face enduring health-related issues that can impact on their engagement in everyday activities and restrict their participation in a range of life situations (Lepage et al 1998). Performance of activities and the ability to participate in home, school and leisure pursuits are influenced by a child's capabilities and are mediated by personal and environmental factors (Majnemer and Mazer 2004, Morris et al 2005). In the International Classification of Functioning, Disability and Health (ICF), the World Health Organization (2001) has stressed the importance of participation as a health outcome. For children in particular, participation facilitates the development and refinement of skills, promotes physical and psychological health, supports engagement in collaborative activities with others, and enhances meaning in life (King et al 2003). Although there is a growing body of literature about participation for children and youth, there is little information about the experience of participation in the context of developmental difficulties, such as those experienced by children with cerebral palsy.

The objectives of this chapter are to:

1   Present a framework for understanding the individual and environmental factors impacting children's participation.
2   Describe the participation of children with cerebral palsy.
3   Review how participation can be evaluated.
4   Explore the factors which impact on the ability of children with cerebral palsy to participate in family, school and community arenas.

Participation

The literal definition of participation is 'taking part' in something (*Macquarie Dictionary* 2002). Conceptually, however, participation is both a process and an outcome. As a process, participation is the act of engaging in everyday activities within physical, socio-cultural, economic and institutional environments. Implicit in this concept is the assumption that participation has temporal and spatial qualities, as well as personally ascribed meaning. A thorough understanding of the meaning of participation requires therapists to consider dimensions of participation such as 'with whom' and 'where' activities take place as well as children's activity enjoyment and preferences (Law 2002).

The concept of participation as the ultimate health outcome for people with disabilities has been advanced by the World Health Organization (2001) in their International Classification of Functioning, Disability and Health (ICF). The introduction of the ICF heightened our appreciation of the dynamic and interdependent nature of disability (Majnemer and Mazer 2004). Participation is defined in the ICF as involvement within a life situation (WHO 2001). Participation in day-to-day activities is an important aspect of children's health, well-being and development. Being a performer rather than an onlooker contributes to children's physical and psychosocial development (Law et al 2004). Yet for children with disability it is their performance which can be a limiting factor. In this context children's upper limb function is one element of a complex interplay of factors which enables the performance of everyday activities necessary for successful participation.

Fig. 25.1 depicts participation as the outcome of a child, environment and occupation interaction. The arrows from participation back to the child and environment represent the self-perpetuating and growth potential of successful participation. Participation is also conceived as a continuum whereby a child might move from being an onlooker to being fully

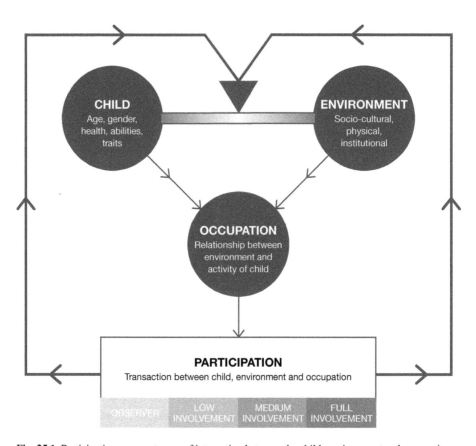

Fig. 25.1 Participation as an outcome of interaction between the child, environment and occupation.

involved, depending on enabling factors. Specifically, there are key environmental features (cultural, physical, institutional, social) and child attributes (age, gender, health, traits) which influence the way children will participate in specific occupations in family, school and community contexts. As a result of participation children can benefit with respect to physical, social and emotional health, skill development, academic/vocational outcomes, and general life satisfaction. Children may also be more motivated to continue to seek participation as they achieve benefits in these areas.

Participation and children with cerebral palsy

Understanding how children with cerebral palsy participate in family and community life, and the factors that influence this participation, will assist us to develop interventions, services and policies to optimize this important health outcome (Law et al 2004). Little is currently known about the extent and quality of participation, the meaning attributed to it by children with cerebral palsy and their families/caregivers, or overall satisfaction with the levels of participation attained. Much more is known about the factors that influence participation and how the participation of children with cerebral palsy compares with that of children without disabilities.

The literature base in cerebral palsy is growing. Majnemer and Mazer (2004) examined the cerebral palsy research published in 1992 compared with 2002. Reports of research increased from 26 to 77 articles, with a proportionally greater increase for intervention research – from 28 per cent to 53 per cent. Only two of the 77 studies published in 2002, however, measured participation as an outcome, so our knowledge is drawn from studies of participation in children with physical disabilities generally. Many of these studies contain large proportions of children with cerebral palsy in their study populations (e.g. 41 per cent (Hemmingson and Borell 2002); 51 per cent (Brown and Gordon 1987, Law et al 2004)). As there appears to be no difference in participation between the children with cerebral palsy and the other diagnostic groups in these studies (Law et al 2004), we can cautiously extrapolate the information gleaned about participation to children with cerebral palsy.

It is reasonable to conclude that children with cerebral palsy have participation limitation. As long ago as 1987 Brown and Gordon compared the activity patterns of 6- to 19-year-old children with (N = 239) and without (N = 519) disabilities. Fifty-one per cent of the sample had cerebral palsy. Compared with their non-disabled peers, children with disability had less variety in daily life and lived life at a slower tempo. They spent more time in quiet recreation and dependent activity, and less time in social engagements and energy-using activities.

More recent studies of children with cerebral palsy echoed these results. A Swedish birth-cohort study examined the participation of 233 5- to 8-year-old children with cerebral palsy (Beckung and Hagberg 2002). They found that 46 per cent of the cohort had moderate, severe or complete participation restriction in mobility, 66 per cent in education, and 39 per cent in social relations. Similarly a Norwegian study (Ostensjo et al 2003) of 95 children with cerebral palsy aged 2 to 7 years reported that most children had scores greater than two standard deviations below the norm-referenced mean in the mobility, self-care and social function domains of the Pediatric Evaluation of Disability Inventory (PEDI). While the

PEDI is primarily a measure of activity, these findings do have implications for participation in a range of social domains.

Law and colleagues' comprehensive study of 427 Canadian children with physical disabilities aged 6 to 12 years has added substantially to our knowledge of participation (2004, 2006). The Children's Assessment of Participation and Enjoyment (CAPE; King et al 2004) was used to measure participation in activities outside school-mandated activities. Law and colleagues (2005, 2006) found participation rates for children with disabilities in formal or organized activities (e.g. music lessons, sport) to be lower and less intense than participation in informal activities, and also substantially lower when compared with a comparison group of children without disabilities.

Further, Law and colleagues (2005, 2006) reported that typically developing children participated in leisure activities more frequently than children with disabilities and were involved in significantly more informal activities (e.g. reading or doing puzzles). Despite this, they described participation of children with physical disabilities in informal activities as extensive (Law et al 2006), which is in contrast to the common belief that children with disability have notably restricted participation. Maher and colleagues (2007) posit that this participation in informal activities might relate more to sedentary pursuits. Law and colleagues (2005, 2006) concluded that their results might be due to the comprehensive ability of the CAPE to draw out participation in this population as compared with previous instruments. Alternatively their findings might also represent the adoption of more inclusive services and facilities in Canada in recent years.

Schenker and colleagues (2005) used the School Function Assessment (Coster et al 1998) to explore school participation and found that children with cerebral palsy had significantly lower levels of participation than did a concurrent cohort of students without disability. The playground during recess was the environment in which children with cerebral palsy achieved the lowest participation score. This has implications for restrictions to these children's opportunities for social engagement. The ability to move around independently, to communicate effectively and to use hands in a skilled manner all influence successful participation in the school context.

This snapshot of research provides us with evidence that participation of children with cerebral palsy can be restricted across school and out-of-school settings. More information is required about additional aspects of participation; for instance, what is the meaning of participation for these children and how satisfied are they with the type and extent of their participation?

What are the factors that influence the participation of children with cerebral palsy?

A number of factors (intrinsic and extrinsic to the child) are known to be powerful mediators of ability and participation. Gross motor function, for instance, an intrinsic factor, has a strong relationship to participation (Beckung and Hagberg 2002, Ostensjo et al 2003). Arm and hand function, however, and their association with participation have received very little attention in the cerebral palsy literature (Ostensjo et al 2003). Although we assume that upper limb function is essential for the successful completion of many tasks, we do not have a good understanding of its association with participation. The Swedish study (Beckung and Hagberg 2002) mentioned earlier is the only study to directly examine the relationship between upper limb ability and participation. Using a classification system of bimanual motor function developed for this study, upper limb function, along with IQ and gross motor function (measured using the Gross Motor Function Classification System, GMFCS), was found to be one of the most important predictors of the degree of participation restriction. Of the neuro-impairments measured, these researchers also found that severe or complete restriction of participation was generally associated with: IQ less than 50, epilepsy, visual impairment, and infantile hydrocephalus. The classification tool used in this study for measuring upper limb ability was developed based on similar principles to the GMFCS and for similar research and clinical purposes, and was the precursor to a promising new tool, the Manual Abilities Classification System (MACS; Eliasson et al 2006).

Schenker and colleagues (2005) demonstrated that, for children with disabilities, being able to complete physical functional activities was a stronger predictor of participation at school (measured using the School Function Assessment (SFA)), than cognitive/behavioural functional ability. Law and colleagues (2005) also identified that the strongest predictor of participation in informal activities was increased physical functional ability. There is convincing evidence, therefore, that motor abilities and completion of physical functional activities have an impact on the important outcome of participation. Schenker's regression model (Schenker et al 2005) to examine the factors predicting participation at school contained a reasonable amount of unexplained variance (18–31 per cent) – an important reminder that other factors are also involved in explaining participation. Law and colleagues (2004), for instance, identified children's activity preferences as being the strongest predictor of participation in formal activity (Law et al 2004, 2005). An important intrinsic factor associated with decreased participation was the child's age; in particular, children over 12 years participated less than younger children (Law et al 2005). A number of extrinsic factors were also associated with participation – family participation in recreational, social and cultural activities, family income and cohesiveness, educational background, and accessibility of the physical environment were all positive influences.

A powerful example of the contribution which can be made by cerebral palsy registers is a study by Hammal and colleagues (2004). They examined participation in a cohort of children identified through a cerebral palsy register in the north of England. Factors associated with reduced participation were: severity of intellectual impairment, the presence of epilepsy, walking and communication difficulties, visual impairment, and feeding difficulties. The influence of poor nutritional status, which can coexist with feeding difficulties, has been clearly associated with decreased participation (Samson-Fang et al 2002). As might be expected, children with hemiplegic cerebral palsy generally had the highest levels of participation amongst the cohort but, according to the regression modelling completed by these researchers, upper limb function did not influence participation (Hammal et al 2004). An interesting finding of this study was that year of birth was associated with educational exclusion. This finding was thought to be related to educational policy implementation which promoted educational inclusion, and, if this is right, it demonstrates the impact of socio-political change on participation of children with cerebral palsy.

A fascinating finding was that the substantially reduced participation experienced by children living in the most deprived area compared with children in the most affluent area was similar to the reduction in participation experienced by children with severe intellectual impairment. Thus, socioeconomic background can influence participation through its relationship with access to services, quality of health care, and parent education, as well as financial resources. These are all factors for which equity needs to be achieved for the well-being of all children with disability.

As well as identifying factors that are associated with participation, some researchers have specifically identified barriers to participation as perceived by people with disabilities and their caregivers. Mihaylov and colleagues' (2004) literature review revealed that there was very little research which sought the perceptions of children with cerebral palsy or of their families. Participants in the few existing studies identified a wide range of physical and non-physical environmental factors as influencing participation. Some factors were obvious, such as access to services and the physical environments of the home, community and school. Others, however, including financial issues (assets and benefits), the natural environment (e.g. noise, temperature), friendships, social inclusion/exclusion and the attitudes of others, also influenced participation.

Hemmingson and Borell's study (2002) is an important example of research which sought students' perceptions of the barriers to their participation at school. The School Setting Interview was completed with 10- to 19-year-old students with physical disability (41 per cent had cerebral palsy). Twenty-six of the 34 interviewees (76 per cent) experienced unmet needs in relation to environmental access in their school lives. Of all the potential barriers, including access around the school, furniture and assistive devices, the largest category of unmet needs pertained to occupational form – a social dimension of the environment. Occupational form is defined as 'rule bound sequences of action or a way of doing something that is generated and stored in society' (Hemmingson and Borell 2002: 58). That is, occupational form relates to how activities are organized and carried out. Examples identified by the students included: failure to adapt tasks for students with disabilities, insufficient time to complete tasks, and the need to move between different classrooms. This finding provides an important insight into the diversity of factors impacting on school participation and the need to consider issues beyond the obvious ones of attitude and architectural barriers.

It is interesting to note that the factors associated with participation represent the entire scope of the ICF model. The severity of a health condition, the presence and degree of impairment of body functions and structures, and the degree of activity limitation, as well as a vast array of social and physical environmental factors and personal factors, all influence participation. This makes the pursuit of the ultimate outcome of participation a substantial challenge. We need to know more about children's coping style, motivation and aspirations, about family functioning and cohesiveness, about health and community service influences, and about attitudes affecting the individual and policy development – amongst a myriad of other factors (Law et al 2004) – in order to allow us to intervene to enhance the participation of children with cerebral palsy.

The measurement of participation

Objective measures which quantify participation, changes in participation and satisfaction with participation are necessary, regardless of the strategies that stakeholders adopt to enhance participation. Objective measurement facilitates appropriate service planning and resource allocation, and, importantly, can motivate children and families in the pursuit of enhanced quality of life through participation (Majnemer and Mazer 2004). Tools to assist young people and families to identify barriers and facilitators to participation will also be invaluable in the quest for promoting self-advocacy for participation.

The increasing focus of rehabilitation research is to operationalize outcomes not only at the level of activity but also at a participation level. It is sobering to discover how few measures exist to determine participation in home, school and community for children with disabilities in general and cerebral palsy specifically (Sakzewski et al 2007). This is in sharp contrast to the number of excellent measures, such as the Pediatric Evaluation of Disability Inventory (PEDI; Haley et al 1992), which target activity.

Participation is related to the roles of children so most assessments of participation focus on specific environments such as school, home or leisure environments. One assessment, however, which takes a global approach to examining participation is the Assessment of Life Habits (LIFE-H; Fougeyrollas et al 1998, 2004). The LIFE-H was developed to gather information pertaining to the life habits of young people (aged 5 to 13 years). The developers defined life habits as regular activities (personal care, mobility, housing, nutrition, fitness, and communication) and social roles (recreation, community, education, responsibility, family relations, and interpersonal relations) that allow young people to achieve their potential in society. In a review of instruments that use child or family self-assessment of activity and participation for children with cerebral palsy, the LIFE-H was considered to have the most comprehensive coverage of content of the ICF domains (Morris et al 2005).

LIFE-H adopts a questionnaire format in which the level of accomplishment is recorded for a number of life habits (e.g. preparing a snack, participating in social activities with parents) along with the level of assistance required for these habits to occur. Respondents (who can be child, parent or other) are also asked to indicate the degree of satisfaction they have with this level of engagement. Most of the research to date on the LIFE-H has been undertaken by the test developers. Validity is supported by review of content by experts in the field as well as concurrent validation with measures such as PEDI and WeeFIM. The assessment has high internal consistency (ranging between 0.90 and 0.97), and adequate to excellent intra-rater (ICC 0.82–0.96), inter-rater (ICC 0.62–0.91), and test-retest (ICC 0.67–0.73) reliabilities (Fougeyrollas et al 1998, 2004). As such this measure has the potential to support both clinical practice and research.

Three assessments of participation in daily life roles in specific environments will now be briefly summarized: the School Function Assessment (SFA); the Children Helping Out: Responsibilities, Expectations and Supports (CHORES; Dunn 2004); and the Children's Assessment of Participation and Enjoyment (CAPE). These have been selected because they target children's participation in key life areas (school, home and recreation).

The SFA (Coster et al 1998) looks at both participation and activity performance at school. It consists of three sections: participation, task supports, and activity performance.

The participation section measures the child's level of participation in six school settings: general or social education classroom; playground; transportation to and from school; bathroom; transitions to and from class; and mealtimes. The task support section measures assistance given and adaptations made which contribute to the child's school-related functions. These functions include physical tasks and cognitive/behavioural tasks. Finally, the performance section measures performance in more detail in school-related functional tasks such as using school material, following school rules and communicating needs. This assessment has been widely used for children with a range of disabilities, not specifically cerebral palsy. The assessment follows an interview format and children's performance is rated according to specified criteria.

Numerous studies have examined the content and construct validity of the SFA. Internal consistency has been reported as excellent (0.92–0.98), inter-rater reliability as adequate (ICC 0.68–0.73), and test-retest reliability as excellent (ICC 0.82–0.98) (Davis et al 2003). It can take up to two hours to complete the SFA in its entirety, which may limit its usefulness in some settings; however, it can be broken down into components. The SFA has had almost ten years of published use in a wide range of settings (clinical and research), making it one of the more robust measures of school function currently available.

Assessment of participation at home is not well established. One measure which endeavours to undertake this task is the Children Helping Out: Responsibilities, Expectations and Supports (CHORES; Dunn 2004). Separate performance and assistance scores enable examination of changes in children's responsibilities for household tasks as they mature, and the work of families to promote participation. The CHORES is a 33-item parent-report survey with 12 items forming a Self-Care subscale and 21 items forming a Family Care subscale. Two types of responses are elicited for each item: a dichotomous yes/no response for performance of each household task, and a seven-point Likert scale for level of assistance (ranging from 7 = own initiative to 1 = not expected to do task). The CHORES was standardized using a sample of 32 parents of children with and without disabilities who were aged 6 to 11 years. This measure focuses more on activity than participation, however, and further test development and evaluation of the psychometric properties of the CHORES are needed if it is to become a useful measure in practice.

The Children's Assessment of Participation and Enjoyment (CAPE) and Preferences for Activities in Children (PAC) (King et al 2004) have been developed for use with children and youth (with and without disabilities). The CAPE and PAC address participation in recreational, active physical, social, skill-based and self-improvement/educational activities, outside school time. The CAPE was specifically designed to be a measure of participation and as such does not seek information on the human or environmental supports required to facilitate participation. The measure examines formal and informal activities and is completed by the child/youth, with assistance if needed. The range of activities in which the child participates and the frequency of participation are recorded, thereby providing a measure of both activity diversity and intensity. Further, the child is asked with whom they typically do each activity, where this occurs and how much they enjoy it. As a result the CAPE provides three outcome measures: overall participation, domain scores reflecting participation in formal and informal activities, and scores reflecting participation in five types

392

of activities (recreational, active physical, social, skill-based and self-improvement/educational).

Validation of the CAPE is based on expert review, literature and factor analytic studies. Internal consistency is reported to be 0.42 in the formal domain and 0.76 in the informal domain. Test-retest reliability is generally adequate (ICC 0.64–0.86 for overall participation; 0.67–0.77 for diversity; 0.72–0.81 for intensity). While relatively new, the CAPE promises to be an extremely useful measure which targets participation and can be used with children with cerebral palsy.

The PAC is an important adjunct to the CAPE as it identifies children's preferences for different activities. As such it provides the clinician with information about which activities are motivating for children in the attainment of participatory goals.

The assessment of participation is obviously an area that requires ongoing attention if we are to measure status, set goals and monitor outcomes relating to participation. The establishment of participation as an important health outcome means that its adequate measurement cannot be overlooked.

What can be done to influence participation and ensure children with cerebral palsy and their families are satisfied with their degree of participation?

This book concerns itself with the management of upper limb function in children with cerebral palsy, a long-standing treatment priority for therapists (Eliasson 2005). Upper limb function is an integral and important part of physical function, and physical function is strongly associated with participation. Beckung and Hagberg (2002) demonstrated that manual abilities are a strong predictor of participation. We assume that improving upper limb function will facilitate the engagement of children in a range of occupationally relevant roles such as those of school child, family member, sibling, friend, and player. We do not yet have the evidence to show that improving upper limb function is sufficient to increase the level of participation in everyday activities for children with cerebral palsy (Morris et al 2006). Individual attributes such as motivation, and the interplay with social and physical environmental factors, also need to be considered when attending to participation (Hammal et al 2004, Mihaylov et al 2004).

Our knowledge of factors influencing participation, viewed within the ICF (WHO 2001), allows us to plan strategies to enhance participation which incorporate the individual, the activity and the environment. The focus of rehabilitation is shifting away from a child-focused impairment-oriented practice to one which promotes participation and the elements that will achieve this; an approach which demands we view children with cerebral palsy within their familial and community contexts (Palisano et al 2004). At the level of the individual with cerebral palsy, the concept of participation blends neatly with other current practice philosophies (Palisano et al 2004). A top-down, occupational performance focus guides us to identify children's preferences and then to target the barriers to achieving these. This can involve: enhancing the skills necessary for participation, employment of adaptive techniques, task modification, and exploitation of the rapidly developing array of assistive technology. A family-focused orientation facilitates our consideration of the child within their family, including family resources, coping, motivation and preferences (Eriksson

2005). Armed with our knowledge of the 'bigger picture' issues impacting on participation it is incumbent upon policy makers and service providers to meet international expectations regarding the ultimate outcome of health-care provision as guided by the ICF (WHO 2001).

REFERENCES

Beckung E, Hagberg G (2002) Neuroimpairments, activity limitations, and participation restrictions in children with cerebral palsy. *Dev Med Child Neurol* 44: 309–316.

Brown M, Gordon WA (1987) Impact of impairment on activity patterns of children. *Arch Phys Med Rehabil* 68: 828–832.

Coster W, Deeney TA, Haltiwanger JT, Haley SM (1998) *School Function Assessment.* San Antonio, TX: Therapy Skill Builders.

Davis PL, Soon PL, Young M, Clausen-Yamaki A (2003) Validity and reliability of the School Function Assessment in elementary school students with disabilities. *Phys Occup Ther Pediatr* 24: 23–43.

Dunn L (2004) Validation of the CHORES: a measure of school-aged children's participation in household tasks. *Scand J Occup Ther* 11: 179–190.

Eliasson AC (2005) Improving the use of hands in daily activities: aspects of the treatment of children with cerebral palsy. *Phys Occup Ther Pediatr* 25: 37–60.

Eliasson AC, Krumlinde Sundholm L, Rösblad B, Beckung E, Arner M, Öhrvall AM, Rosenbaum P (2006) The Manual Ability Classification System (MACS) for children with cerebral palsy: scale development and evidence of validity and reliability. *Dev Med Child Neurol* 48: 549–554.

Eriksson L (2005) The relationship between school environment and participation for students with disabilities. *Pediatr Rehabil* 8: 130–139.

Fougeyrollas P, Noreau L, Bergeron H, Cloutier R, Dion SA, St-Michel G (1998) Social consequences of long term impairments and disabilities: conceptual approach and assessment of handicap. *Int J Rehabil Res* 21: 127–141.

Fougeyrollas P, Noreau L, Lepage C (2004) *Assessment of Life Habits.* Quebec: INDCP.

Haley SM, Coster WJ, Ludlow LH, Haltiwanger JT, Andrellos PJ (1992) *Pediatric Evaluation of Disability Inventory (PEDI).* Boston, MA: New England Medical Center Hospitals.

Hammal D, Jarvis SN, Colver AF (2004) Participation of children with cerebral palsy is influenced by where they live. *Dev Med Child Neurol* 46: 292–298.

Hemmingson H, Borell L (2002) Environmental barriers in mainstream schools. *Child Care Health Dev* 28: 57–63.

King G, Law M, King S, Rosenbaum P, Kertoy MK, Young NL (2003) A conceptual model of the factors affecting the recreation and leisure participation of children with disabilities. *Phys Occup Ther Pediatr* 23: 63–90.

King G, Law M, King S, Hurley P, Hanna S, Kertoy M, Rosenbaum P, Young N (2004) *Children's Assessment of Participation and Enjoyment (CAPE) and Preferences for Activities of Children (PAC).* San Antonio, TX: Harcourt Assessment, Inc.

Law M (2002) Participation in the occupations of everyday life. *Am J Occup Ther* 56: 640–649.

Law M, Finkelman S, Hurley P, Rosenbaum P, King S, King G, Hanna S (2004) Participation of children with physical disabilities: relationships with diagnosis, physical function, and demographic variables. *Scand J Occup Ther* 11: 156–162.

Law M, King G, Rosenbaum P, Kertoy M, King S, Young N, Hanna S, Hurley P (2005) Final report to families and community partners on the Participate study findings. Hamilton, Ontario: CanChild Centre for Childhood Disability Research.

Law M, King G, King S, Kertoy M, Hurley P, Rosenbaum P, Young N, Hanna S (2006) Patterns of participation in recreational and leisure activities among children with complex physical disabilities. *Dev Med Child Neurol* 48: 337–342.

Lepage C, Noreau L, Bernard P, Fougeyrollas P (1998) Profile of handicap situations in children with cerebral palsy. *Scand J Occup Ther* 30: 263–272.

Maher CA, Williams MT, Olds T, Lane A (2007). Physical and sedentary activity in adolescents with cerebral palsy. *Dev Med Child Neurol* 49: 450–457.

Majnemer A, Mazer B (2004) New directions in the outcome evaluation of children with cerebral palsy. *Semin Pediatr Neurol* 11: 11–17.

Mihaylov SI, Jarvis SN, Colver AF, Beresford B (2004) Identification and description of environmental factors that influence participation of children with cerebral palsy. *Dev Med Child Neurol* 46: 299–304.

Morris C, Kurinczuk JJ, Fitzpatrick R (2005) Child or family assessed measures of activity performance and participation for children with cerebral palsy: a structured review. *Child Care Health Dev* 31: 397–407.

Morris C, Kurinczuk JJ, Fitzpatrick R. Rosenbaum P (2006) Do the abilities of children with cerebral palsy explain their activities and participation? *Dev Med Child Neurol* 48: 954–961.

Ostensjo S, Carlberg EB, Vollestad NK (2003) Everyday functioning in young children with cerebral palsy: functional skills, caregiver assistance, and modifications of the environment. *Dev Med Child Neurol* 45: 603–612.

Palisano RJ, Snider LM, Orlin MN (2004) Recent advances in physical and occupational therapy for children with cerebral palsy. *Semin Pediatr Neurol* 11: 66–77.

Sakzewski L, Boyd R, Ziviani J (2007) A systematic review of the clinimetric properties of participation measures for 5–13 year old children with cerebral palsy. *Dev Med Child Neurol* 49: 232–240.

Samson-Fang L, Fung E, Stallings VA, Conaway M, Worley G, Rosenbaum P, Calvert R, O'Donnell M, Henderson RC, Chumlea WC, Liptak GS, Stevenson RD (2002) Relationship of nutritional status to health and societal participation in children with cerebral palsy. *J Pediatr* 141: 637–643.

Schenker R, Coster W, Parush S (2005) Participation and activity performance of students with cerebral palsy within the school environment. *Disabil Rehabil* 27: 539–552.

WHO (2001) *International Classification of Functioning, Disability and Health.* Geneva: World Health Organization.

26
THE EVIDENCE-BASE FOR UPPER EXTREMITY INTERVENTION FOR CHILDREN WITH CEREBRAL PALSY

Christine Imms

The intention of this chapter is to promote evidence-based practice in the management of the upper extremity. A summary of the best available evidence for the treatment of the upper extremity in children with cerebral palsy is presented to guide clinical practice and provide directions for future research.

Evidence-based practice is the integration of the best available research evidence with clinical expertise, the client's preferences and values, and clinical circumstances (Sackett et al 2000, Law 2002). The skilled evidence-based practitioner considers research evidence in context. He/she is able to evaluate the quality of research reported in the literature (thus discarding poor quality research) and is also able to interpret the value of research findings to individuals or specific circumstances – making reasoned, evidence-based adjustments of the results for their likely effect within a given circumstance. This includes determining how or whether the evidence can be applied to an individual. Evidence-based practice is a six-step process that can be used to ensure that clinical practice is relevant and appropriate.

The six steps of evidence-based practice

1 Reflect on your practice and ask clinical questions
Readers of this book are likely to be asking a variety of questions related to upper extremity intervention. What upper extremity intervention should be offered – botulinum toxin A injections or surgery? When should constraint-induced movement therapy be used versus an alternative? Which children benefit from surgery? Does cognitive orientation to daily occupational performance work? How should the outcomes of intervention be measured? What do children want? What do children and families experience as helpful? We all have clinical questions. How, or whether, we answer them is important.

2 Structure a searchable clinical question and search for evidence
Structuring your question to identify the population, intervention and outcomes of interest will ensure that you know what you are really asking and facilitate searching for the answer efficiently. Using structured search strategies (Richardson et al 1995) within multiple electronic databases – for example, Medline, CINAHL, AMED, the Cochrane Library – will increase the likelihood that relevant research is located (Lovarini et al 2006).

3 Appraise the evidence

There is considerable emphasis in medical literature on only using high level evidence. Levels of evidence such as those proposed by Sackett et al (1996) focus on systematic reviews and randomized controlled trials (RCT) as Level I and II evidence (that is, high level) to determine whether interventions are effective. The commonly used hierarchies for classifying intervention studies typically rate single subject design research, in which there can be a considerable amount of control, as Level IV, along with case studies and single group designs. The American Academy of Cerebral Palsy and Developmental Medicine (AACPDM), in contrast, have included randomized single subject designs as Level I evidence (Butler et al 2003). For research involving children who have cerebral palsy this is important, as the vast differences in children's presentation and responses to intervention pose considerable difficulty in conducting large randomized controlled trials (RCT) with homogeneous groups. Well conducted single subject design research can provide good evidence for treatment protocols.

As well as hierarchies for intervention research there are other levels of evidence for diagnostic, prognostic or cost-effectiveness research which identify the appropriate designs for research pertaining to those issues (Phillips et al 2001): an RCT would certainly be inappropriate. In addition, there are many clinical and research questions that should not be investigated using quantitative methods at all, but rather require a qualitative approach. Qualitative research has no hierarchy. Regardless of type or level, it is important that a particular research design is not automatically equated with good quality.

The quality of the research dictates whether a systematic review, randomized controlled trial or single subject design study provides useful evidence related to intervention effectiveness. Research appraisal is based on knowledge of sound methodologies for the type of research question being addressed, as well as being able to read, understand and interpret the results. There are a number of appraisal forms and guidelines available to assist in appraising the validity of research (for example, Law et al 1998a,1998b, Jackson 2004).

When good quality research evidence is located, the results must be interpreted. Readers (clinicians) need to consider both statistical significance and clinical importance, perhaps determining the clinical importance of the results for themselves when the researcher does not discuss it (for practical support in learning these skills, see Herbert et al 2005). Researchers, on the other hand, must commit to good quality research and, once conducted, translate their findings from statistical or analytical jargon to practice-based utility, assisting the user of the evidence to make the connections between the findings and what might happen in practice as a result. This requires reporting of both point estimates of effect (mean or median differences) and confidence intervals (or other estimate of variation) which allow the reader to understand the precision of the estimate. It also requires discussion of what score change represents a clinically meaningful change on each of the important outcome measures within the study.

The aim of randomization or matching within intervention trials is to have groups that are unbiased and comparable on the important dependent and demographic variables prior to intervention, so that any difference between groups at the end of the trial can be reasonably ascribed to the intervention (Herbert et al 2005). But randomization may not result in comparability, especially in small trials, which are common in research involving children with cerebral palsy. There may be important differences between groups at baseline that are not found to be statistically significant, perhaps because the trial is small. The reader must judge whether any difference between groups on baseline scores, especially the primary outcome, is clinically important. If it is, then only looking at differences between the groups at endpoints is not always appropriate; the reader may need to make a judgement about the difference in the change scores between groups. Having said this, however, it may be that groups that are clinically different at baseline might actually represent groups of individuals who would respond differently to the intervention under investigation – they may be more severe, or less severe, older or younger, and therefore the groups may not be truly comparable anyway.

4 Integrate useful evidence from different sources and apply findings to practice
It is the clinician's role to determine when good quality research evidence is applicable to individual clients. This requires integration of clinical experience along with careful evaluation of the client's clinical state, consideration of his/her personal circumstances, and discussion of the evidence with families and clients (Sackett et al 2000). In this way the best form of intervention can be determined. Providing the best intervention for an individual may involve a change, or even cessation, of practice, or require clinician education and training, gathering of resources, or referral of individuals to services where resources are available.

5 Evaluate the effect of any change of practice
Determining whether individual clients have benefited from an intervention is an ongoing requirement which can only be met if we measure, at baseline and follow-up, the impairment, activity or participation elements expected to change as a result of the intervention. Routine reliable measurement of outcomes within clinical practice provides the basis for the final critical stage of evidence-based practice.

6 Report on the effect of a change of practice
This stage leads to the production of evidence: researching clinical practice and contributing to the knowledge base. This stage also ensures that evidence-based practice becomes the self-directed learning spiral it is intended to be (Hammel et al 2002). As suggested by the scholarship of practice model (Hammel et al 2002; see Fig. 26.1), this learning spiral provides the potential effect of aligning research and practice much more closely.

Evidence for treatment effect in upper extremity interventions for children with cerebral palsy
Management of the upper extremity does not happen in isolation from the child, the family or the service setting. In addition, other goals and requirements, such as those related to the lower limbs or communication needs, must be considered. Children with cerebral palsy have complex and multiple needs, so decisions about which intervention to use, and when, must be made as efficiently as possible.

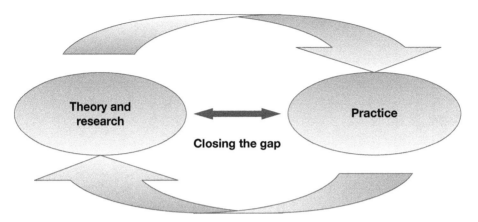

Fig. 26.1 Scholarship of practice model.

Source: Adapted with permission from Hammel J, Finlayson M, Kielhofner G, Helfrich C, Peterson E (2001) Educating scholars of practice: an approach to preparing tomorrow's researchers. *Occupational Therapy in Health Care* 15: 157–176.

The following review of the evidence supporting upper extremity interventions is based on literature located through comprehensive searches of the Medline, CINAHL, AMED, Cochrane Library, OTseeker and PEDro databases in March/April 2006 (updated in May 2007). The search strategies included varying index and key-word terms for cerebral palsy, the upper extremity and child or adolescent. Only English language articles published after 1990 were retrieved. Levels of evidence were classified according to the evidence review guidelines of the American Academy for Cerebral Palsy and Developmental Medicine (Butler et al 2005). Butler et al's levels of evidence classify systematic reviews of RCTs and large RCTs as Level I, smaller RCTs and systematic reviews of cohort studies as Level II, cohort studies with concurrent control groups as Level III, and case series or cohort studies without control groups as Level IV. In this review, papers reporting expert opinion or those that were non-systematic literature reviews were excluded (Level V). Reviews were deemed systematic and were included if an explicit research question was identified, a clear and comprehensive search was conducted, with clear inclusion/exclusion criteria for included studies provided, and the quality of each included trial was evaluated. Level IV studies were considered where there was limited higher level evidence.

The search located two systematic reviews that investigated multiple types of interventions for children with cerebral palsy, nine systematic reviews of specific interventions and 17 controlled trials of interventions to promote upper extremity outcomes. All systematic reviews and controlled trials were appraised for the strength of their internal validity, using tools with established validity and reliability: the PEDro scale for controlled trials (Maher et al 2003) and the Overview Quality Assessment Questionnaire for systematic reviews (Oxman and Guyatt 1991, Hoving et al 2001). The studies have been grouped according to their primary purpose and are summarized in Table 26.1.

TABLE 26.1
Quality of evidence and activity level outcomes for upper extremity interventions: Level I, II and III studies only

Intervention	Level of evidence	First author & year	N	Quality rating	Outcome	Effect size
BoNT-A	I	Reeuwijk 2006	$N_s = 12$	17/18	Studies are 3 RCTs and 9 uncontrolled trials. Insufficient evidence – see Level II studies below for evidence published since review	–
	I	Wasiak 2004	$N_s = 2$	16/18	Insufficient evidence – see Level II studies below for evidence published since review	–
	II	Corry 1997	$N_t = 7$, $N_c = 7$	9/10	Treatment conditions: BoNT-A vs control. Statistically significant reduction in muscle stiffness (resonant frequency) at 2 & 12 weeks in group receiving BoNT-A in comparison to placebo	±
BoNT-A + therapy	II	Russo 2007	$N_t = 21$, $N_c = 22$	8/10	Treatment conditions: BoNT-A+ OT vs OT alone. Both groups improved but no significant difference between groups on AMPS at 3 or 6 months. GAS scores were significantly greater for group 1 at 3 months only. No significant change in PEDI – self care	0–6 months[†] AMPS motor = –0.08 AMPS process = 0.28 GAS = 0.23 PEDI-SC = 0.04
	II	Wallen 2007	$N_{t1} = 20$ $N_{t2} = 20$ $N_{t3} = 17$ $N_{t4} = 15$	7/10	Treatment conditions: T_1 = BoNT-A+ OT; T_2 =BoNT-A; T_3 = OT; T_4 = Control. No significant difference between any group on Melbourne, QUEST, PEDI at 3 or 6 months. Significant difference between Group 1 & 4 only on COPM performance & satisfaction at 3 & 6 months and GAS at 3 months. Data presented for Groups 1 & 3 for comparison with other studies	0–6 months[†] COPM perf = 0.36 COPM sat = 0.12 GAS = 0.02 QUEST (n = 7, & 6) = –0.15 Melbourne (n = 10 & 10) = 0.40
	II	Lowe 2006	$N_t = 21$, $N_c = 21$	8/10	Treatment conditions: BoNT-A + OT vs OT alone. All children improved significantly. BoNT-A + OT improved faster & gained more than OT alone group. BoNT-A + OT group significantly improved in QUEST at 1 & 3 months but not 6 months. Average treatment effects across all time points were significant for QUEST, GAS (family & therapist), COPM, and PEDI functional skills	0–6 months[§] QUEST = 7.7 GAS (family) = 7.5 GAS (therapist) = 14.0 COPM perf = 0.8 COPM sat = 0.8 PEDI function = 1.9
	II	Speth 2005	$N_t = 10$, $N_c = 10$	7/10	Treatment conditions: BoNT-A + OT/PT vs OT/PT alone. Significantly reduced wrist tone at 2 weeks & 9 months in BoNT-A + OT/PT group compared with OT/PT alone. No significant differences on Melbourne or PEDI	±

	Level	Study	N	Score	Findings	±
	II	Greaves 2004	$N_t = 10$ $N_c = 10$	8/10	Treatment conditions: BoNT-A + OT vs OT alone. No significant difference between groups on COPM, GAS, Peabody or QUEST at 16 weeks. All children improved significantly at 6 & 16 weeks on COPM, GAS, Peabody & QUEST. Clinically important improvement on COPM in BoNT-A + OT group	0–12 weeks[†] Melbourne = 1.06 GAS (therapist) = –0.22 COPM perf = 0.28 COPM sat = 0.09
	II	Boyd 2004	$N_t = 15$ $N_c = 15$	9/10	Treatment conditions: BoNT-A + OT vs OT alone. Significantly greater improvement on Melbourne in BoNT-A + OT group compared with OT alone. No difference between groups on COPM or GAS. Significant changes in BoNT-A + OT group 0 to 12 weeks on PEDI, COPM & GAS. Clinically important change in COPM in both groups	
	II	Fehlings 2000	$N_t = 14$ $N_c = 15$	6/10	Treatment conditions: BoNT-A + OT vs OT alone. Significant improvement in QUEST (primarily weight bearing domain) in BoNT-A + OT group compared to OT alone	0–1 month[†] QUEST = 0.99
Casting/ splinting	I	Autti-Ramo 2006	$N_s = 5$	N/A	Systematic review of systematic reviews. $N_s = 2$ UE reviews (Boyd 2001 & Teplicky 2002 presented below)	–
	I	Teplicky 2002	$N_s = 21$	6/18	$N_s = 6$ UE studies: 2 were RCTs. Evidence for casting to increase range and reduce tone. Limited evidence related to improved hand function	–
	II	^Law 1991	$N_{t1} = 19$ $N_{t2} = 17$ $N_{t3} = 18$ $N_{t4} = 18$	6/10	Treatment conditions: T_1 = intense NDT + casting; T_2 = regular NDT + casting; T_3 = intense NDT; T_4 = regular NDT. No significant difference between groups at 6 or 9 months on Peabody; significant difference on QUEST at 6 months between those wearing casts and those not	0–6 months^ (cast vs no cast) Peabody = 0.17 QUEST = 0.53
CIMT	I	Hoare 2007	$N_s = 3$	16/18	Weak positive evidence; see included studies below	–
	II	Charles 2006	$N_t = 11$ $N_c = 11$	6/10	Treatment conditions: CIMT vs control. No significant difference between groups at any time point on Jebsen or Bruininks, but significant interaction effects at 3 weeks: CIMT group changed more (CIMT group had poorer scores at baseline and better scores at 3 weeks)	0–3 weeks[§] Jebsen = 0.32 Bruininks = 0.40
	II	DeLuca 2002; 2006; Taub 2004	$N_t = 9$ $N_c = 9$	5/10	Treatment conditions: CIMT vs control. No significant difference between CIMT & traditional therapy groups on QUEST dissociated movement subscale at 3 weeks. Other outcomes lacked established validity & reliability	0–3 weeks[†] QUEST = 0.91
	II	Willis 2002	$N_t = 12$ $N_c = 13$	3/10	Treatment conditions: forced use vs control. Study included some children with cerebral palsy. Non-valid administration of Peabody administered without supporting rationale or evidence	–

TABLE 26.1 (continued)

Quality of evidence and activity level outcomes for upper extremity interventions: Level I, II and III studies only

Intervention	Level of evidence	First author & year	N	Quality rating	Outcome	Effect size
	III	Eliasson 2005	$N_t = 21$ $N_c = 20$	5/10	Treatment conditions: modified CIMT vs traditional therapy. No significant difference between groups. Within group differences favour CIMT group on AHA	0–2; 0–6 months§ AHA (0–2 m) = 1.16 AHA (0–6 m) = 0.72
Conductive education	I	Darrah 2004	$N_s = 15$	14/18	10 studies examined fine motor, or functional outcomes related to UE abilities. Of 185 outcomes, 21 were statistically significant, 10 were in favour of CE (rather than control); 4 of these were UE outcomes	—
	III	Stiller 2003	$N_{t1} = 7$ $N_{t2} = 8$ $N_{t3} = 4$	4/10	Treatment conditions: T_1 = CE; T_2 = intense therapy; T_3 = special education; no significant difference between groups; all groups improved on some outcomes; CE better on hand use and eye–hand, intense therapy group better on manual dexterity of the Peabody	0–5 weeks Peabody† Grasping = 0.55 Hand use = –0.85 Eye–hand = –0.35 Manual dex = 0.92
Functional therapy	II	Ketelaar 2001	$N_t = 28$ $N_c = 27$	5/10	Treatment conditions: functional therapy vs physical therapy based on neuro-physiological principles. Partially randomized trial. Not specifically a UE intervention. Significant improvement on self-care skills and caregiver assistance in the functional therapy group	0–18 months§ Self-care domains PEDI function = 0.34 PEDI caregiver = 0.9
Multiple/ combined	I	Boyd 2001	$N_s = 5$	16/18	Reviewed UE interventions: 3 RCTs (Law 1991, 1997, Fehlings 2000) analysed for treatment effect on QUEST with negligible effect sizes in Law studies (1991, 1997) & moderate–large effects for Fehlings	—
	I	Steultjens 2004	$N_s = 17$	17/18	Reviewed OT interventions to improve daily activities. 7 RCTs, 1 controlled trial, 9 others. Largest effect for sensorimotor intervention to improve sensory perception (Bumin 2001). Concluded insufficient evidence	—
	II	^Law 1991	$N_{t1} = 19$ $N_{t2} = 17$ $N_{t3} = 18$ $N_{t4} = 18$	6/10	Treatment conditions: T_1 = intense NDT + casting; T_2 = regular NDT + casting; T_3 = intense NDT; T_4 = regular NDT. No significant difference between groups at 6 or 9 months on Peabody or QUEST	0–6 months^ Int. NDT + cast vs rest Peabody = 0.25 QUEST = 0.18

		N	Quality rating		Effect sizes
II	Law 1997	$N_t = 25$ $N_c = 25$	6/10	Treatment conditions: NDT + casting vs regular OT. Crossover trial. Power adequate. No significant difference between groups on Peabody, QUEST, COPM. Statistically & clinically significant differences in both groups over time. Those wearing casts > 19.5 hrs/wk improved more	0–4 months[†] Peabody = −0.03 QUEST = −0.15 COPM perf = 0.71 COPM sat = 0.73
NDT					
I	Brown 2001	$N_s = 17$	14/18	Of 4 studies explicitly measuring UE outcomes, none reported statistically significant beneficial effect of NDT	—
I	Butler 2001	$N_s = 21$	17/18	Of 5 studies explicitly measuring UE outcomes 4 report no significant benefit from NDT; 1 Level IV study found improved UE movement time	—
II	^Law 1991	$N_{t1} = 19$ $N_{t2} = 17$ $N_{t3} = 18$ $N_{t4} = 18$	6/10	Treatment conditions: T_1 = intense NDT + casting; T_2 = regular NDT + casting; T_3 = intense NDT; T_4 = regular NDT. No significant differences between groups at 6 or 9 months on Peabody or QUEST	0–6 months^ Intense vs regular NDT Peabody = 0.1 QUEST = 0.13
NMES					
II	Ozer 2006	$N_{t1} = 8$ $N_{t2} = 8$ $N_{t3} = 8$	6/10	Treatment conditions: T_1 = NMES; T_2 = bracing; T_3 = NMES + bracing. Group 3 had statistically significant improvements on Melbourne and grip strength that were not sustained beyond 1 month post-treatment	≈
Surgery					
II	Smeulders 2006	$N_s = 9$	16/18	Systematic review of surgery for thumb in palm deformity: no RCT or clinical trials located; 9 prospective Level IV trials evaluated, all deemed poor quality	—

Notes:

1 *Quality ratings*: rating of systematic reviews using Overview Quality Assessment Questionnaire (Oxman and Guyatt 1991, Hoving et al 2001): rating of randomized trials using PEDro rating scale (not partitioned).

2 *Abbreviations*: N/A = not applicable; N_s = number of studies; N_t = number in treatment group; N_c = number in control group; RCT = randomized controlled trial; UE = upper extremity; vs = versus; OT = occupational therapy; BoNT-A = botulinum toxin A; CIMT = constraint-induced movement therapy; modified constraint-induced movement therapy or forced use therapy studies; NDT = neurodevelopmental therapy; CE = conductive education; NMES = neuromuscular electrical stimulation; AMPS = Assessment of Motor and Process Skills; Peabody = Peabody Developmental Fine Motor Scale; AHA = Assisting Hand Assessment; QUEST = Quality of Upper Extremity Skills Test; GAS = Goal Attainment Scale; COPM = Canadian Occupational Performance Measure; PEDI = Pediatric Evaluation of Disability Inventory; Melbourne = Melbourne Assessment of Unilateral Upper Limb Function; Jebsen = Jebsen Test of Hand Function; Bruininks = Bruininks Oseretsky Test of Motor Proficiency.

3 *Effect sizes*: ± medians reported therefore effect size not calculated; [†] standardized mean difference calculated using change scores in RevMan 1.0.3 using published and unpublished data; [§] published data; ≈ data not reported clearly – unable to determine effect; ^ Law et al 1991 study findings are presented in 3 sections – casting, combined and NDT with reviewer-calculated between-group effect size (Thalheimer and Cook 2002) calculated using data available.

SYSTEMATIC REVIEWS OF MULTIPLE INTERVENTIONS

In 2001 Boyd et al published a systematic review of research investigating the management of upper extremity dysfunction in children with cerebral palsy. Up to that time there were few randomized trials to review and the strongest evidence (largest treatment effect) was found for occupational therapy plus botulinum toxin A (BoNT-A) (Fehlings et al 2000) and for casting plus neurodevelopmental therapy (Law et al 1991). Both of these trials will be discussed below. In 2004, Steultjens et al published a systematic review of the efficacy of occupational therapy interventions to promote performance of daily activities by children with cerebral palsy. The review included studies of orthoses, advice regarding assistive devices, parental counselling, training of sensory-motor functions and/or skills and comprehensive therapy. Some included studies were common to both the Boyd et al and Steultjens et al systematic reviews. Steultjens et al found only one study comparing different upper extremity orthotics to be of sufficiently high quality (Exner and Bonder 1983) and thus the review found inconclusive evidence for a positive effect of occupational therapy.

EVIDENCE FOR EFFECT OF BOTULINUM TOXIN A INJECTIONS

Since the publication of two systematic reviews (Wasiak et al 2004, Reeuwijk et al 2006) which both found insufficient evidence related to the effectiveness of BoNT-A injections in the upper limb, the results of five more randomized trials have become available (Boyd 2004, Greaves 2004, Lowe et al 2006, Russo et al 2007, Wallen et al 2007). Each of these trials examined the effect of occupational therapy plus BoNT-A in comparison to occupational therapy alone, and Wallen et al also included groups receiving BoNT-A alone and a true control group. The strength of these RCTs is in the overall quality of the designs, each of which demonstrated good to high internal validity (see Table 26.1). Limitations remain in terms of small study sizes and heterogeneous groups, although Lowe et al, Russo et al and Wallen et al each demonstrated adequate power.

While each randomized trial has demonstrated the positive effect of BoNT-A on reducing muscle tone or muscle stiffness (body function outcomes; WHO 2001), there are equivocal results related to improved outcomes at the activity level. The three trials that reported adequate power each demonstrated increased goal achievement in their BoNT-A plus occupational therapy groups compared with occupational therapy alone (Lowe et al 2006, Russo et al 2007) or a control group (Wallen et al 2007). Quality of movement also improved more in the BoNT-A plus occupational therapy group in Lowe et al's study but not in Wallen et al, and likewise with self-care. In each of these three studies as well as in Greaves (2004) and Boyd (2004), the groups receiving BoNT-A plus occupational therapy and the groups receiving occupational therapy alone made significant gains after treatment in their primary activity level outcomes (see Table 26.1). In contrast, Speth et al (2005) in a smaller trial did not find statistically or clinically important differences between the group receiving BoNT-A in addition to physical and occupational therapy and the group receiving physical and occupational therapy alone, in either quality of movement or self-care function.

Importantly, five of these six new trials demonstrated significant positive gains from occupational therapy alone, with one trial showing definitive additional benefits from BoNT-A (Lowe et al 2006) and two showing additional benefits of BoNT-A in the short term

(Russo et al 2007, Wallen et al 2007). The key elements that were described in the trials that provided well-defined, structured post-injection therapy included individual goal setting, task training (related to goals set) and specific interventions related to components of upper limb function such as strength training, application of orthotics to provide prolonged stretch, or coordination training (Boyd 2004, Greaves 2004, Lowe et al 2006). The trials demonstrating significant changes in activity measures, within groups, provide evidence of the importance of the process of goal setting within therapy and of providing general activity or motor training as well as specific task practice in achieving outcomes of relevance and importance to children, families and therapists.

EVIDENCE FOR EFFECT OF CASTING OR ORTHOSES

There is limited high level evidence for the effectiveness of casting or orthotic application to the upper extremity. The two reviews located (Teplicky et al 2002, Autti-Ramo et al 2006) primarily included Level IV studies and only two RCTs (Law et al 1991, 1997). The RCTs (Law et al 1991, 1997) combined casting with differing intensities of neurodevelopmental therapy (NDT) and compared the combined intervention with differing intensities of NDT alone (Law et al 1991) or with a regular occupational therapy programme alone (Law et al 1997). The 1991 study found differences between groups in favour of intense NDT plus casting. There was also a significant difference immediately after treatment between those who wore casts and those who did not, regardless of NDT intensity. No statistically significant or clinically important differences between intense NDT plus casting and regular occupational therapy were detected in the 1997 study. Important statistical and clinical differences were found for both groups over time as measured by the Quality of Upper Extremity Skills Test (QUEST), the Peabody Developmental Motor Scales – Fine Motor Scale (Peabody FM) and the Canadian Occupational Performance Measure (COPM). These results again support the effectiveness of therapy focusing on functional goals for children with cerebral palsy. Casting appeared to confer an advantage to children in both the studies.

Upper extremity lycra garments are also available for children with cerebral palsy. To date only single subject design (Corn et al 2003) or small case series studies (Nicholson et al 2001, Knox 2003) have been undertaken. These methods are useful for testing or describing new intervention methods but they do not provide generalizable evidence of effectiveness. In addition, Knox reported a 50 per cent dropout rate due to difficulties associated with wearing the garments, and both Corn et al and Nicholson et al reported reduced independence in some children while wearing the garments.

EVIDENCE FOR EFFECT OF CONSTRAINT-INDUCED MOVEMENT THERAPY

Constraint-induced movement therapy (CIMT), as described in Chapter 20, is characterized by two components: constraint of the unimpaired arm/hand; and intensive therapy for the impaired arm. Fourteen different studies of CIMT were identified. A systematic review of the effect of CIMT for children with cerebral palsy (Hoare et al 2007) found only three clinical trials (Level II and III) and 11 single group, before and after trials or case reports (Level IV). Of these, the ability to evaluate the quality of one Level II clinical trial (DeLuca

2002, Taub et al 2004, DeLuca et al 2006) was affected by the inconsistent reporting between the doctoral thesis (DeLuca 2002) and the published paper (Taub et al 2004). This trial also included a number of outcome measures without established validity and reliability. The Level III report, a non-randomized trial (Eliasson et al 2005) of modified CIMT, demonstrated a small positive increase in rate of improvement in the group wearing a constraint in comparison to the control group on the Assisting Hand Assessment (Krumlinde-Sundholm and Eliasson 2003). The other Level II study (Sung et al 2005) examined a forced-use protocol but had a number of methodological weaknesses and ambiguous reporting which limited interpretation of any findings. All of the Level IV studies suggested that there were positive outcomes for children as measured by at least one of a variety of impairment or activity level outcomes. The Level IV studies, however, are limited by their lack of control and the selection of the outcome measures, many of which lacked evidence of validity or reliability. These are significant issues and their impact on the estimate of the treatment effect should not be underestimated. Since the publication of this systematic review, Charles et al (2006) have reported that while there was no significant difference between their CIMT and control groups, children within the CIMT group improved more on fine motor outcomes. In conclusion, there is weak evidence for the positive effect of CIMT from the studies available so far.

Notably, the research into the effect of CIMT or modifications of CIMT is characterized by huge variation in the application of the intervention. Across the 14 studies of CIMT five different types of constraint and five different therapy regimes were identified. As well as variations in the two key elements of CIMT (constraint and therapy) there is also significant variation in the frequency of constraint wearing, intensity of training and the environmental context in which therapy is provided. Based on the existing evidence, it is currently very difficult for the clinician to understand whether CIMT is an intervention worth pursuing and, if so, how it should be applied. While it might be tempting to suggest that almost any combination of variables results in a positive effect, this has not been demonstrated. Nor has there been a careful evaluation of, or examination of, potentially harmful effects, including those related to restraining the unimpaired arm of a young child during critical periods of development. There are, however, at least five clinical trials underway that will provide more evidence to guide future practice (see Table 26.2). We may also then be able to determine which children will benefit from this new intervention and at what stages of their development.

EVIDENCE FOR THE EFFECT OF STRENGTH TRAINING
Despite growing interest in investigating the effect of strength training in the lower extremities (Dodd et al 2002) there is little evidence that upper extremity strength training is being examined. One means which is theoretically proposed to increase strength, and as a result improve functional performance, is neuromuscular electrical stimulation (NMES) of muscles (Kerr et al 2004). Kerr et al's (2004) systematic review of electrical stimulation in cerebral palsy found insufficient evidence to support the proposal that stimulation increases strength in either the lower or upper limb. Only two of the studies included in Kerr et al's review related to upper extremity interventions, and strength was not measured in

either study. There were, however encouraging improvements in hand function following upper extremity NMES. Ozer et al (2006) have since published their three-group RCT which found that combining NMES (to the wrist and finger extensors) with dynamic bracing resulted in a short-term gain in strength and quality of movement that was greater than in the groups that received only NMES or only the brace.

EVIDENCE FOR THE EFFECT OF SURGERY

In 2006 a systematic review of the effectiveness of surgery to correct thumb-in-palm deformity in children and adults with cerebral palsy was published (Smeulders et al 2006). All of the nine trials included in this systematic review were Level IV studies and therefore lacked control or comparative groups. The authors found that all nine studies were open to significant risk of bias, with no blinding of assessors, inadequate inclusion of outcomes with demonstrated reliability and validity and inadequate control of co-interventions. Bearing in mind that the study designs may lead to an overestimate of the effectiveness of surgery, the results suggested positive outcomes, with improved appearance and gains in functional grasps demonstrated in many studies (Smeulders et al 2006).

Investigations of other upper limb surgical techniques for children with cerebral palsy were characterized by the same issue of low level study design. The studies reported tendon transfers (Eliasson et al 1998, El-Said 2001, Schwartz 2005) or re-routing (Bunata 2006), wrist arthrodesis (Rayan and Young 1999, Hargreaves et al 2000) or a range of surgical procedures (Dahlin et al 1998, Nylander et al 1999). The strongest of these studies were those that used prospective case series designs with explicit standardized, objective measurement of outcomes both before and after surgery (for example, Eliasson et al 1998, Bunata 2006, Kreulen et al 2006).

The upper limb surgical studies, like many interventions for children with cerebral palsy, appear to be limited by the need to provide individualized surgical procedures, making the development of tight research protocols and random allocation to treatment group problematic. There does appear, however, to be some potential for standardized surgical procedures, or groups of procedures, in some instances (Bunata 2006, Kreulen et al 2006, Smeulders et al 2006). There is also the possibility that children act as their own controls through the use of an extended baseline period. This would, however, only offer short-term comparisons, and the success or otherwise of surgery requires long-term follow-up. Likewise, contractures, deformities and loss of function require time to declare themselves. Allowing a comparison or control group to wait for either outcome is ethically dubious; but so is failing to demonstrate convincingly that an intervention as invasive as surgery is clinically worthwhile.

EVIDENCE FOR THE EFFECT OF TASK PRACTICE AND FOCUSING ON GOAL ACHIEVEMENT

Two recent theoretical papers have highlighted the importance of practice for improvement of task performance and hand use (Valvano 2004, Eliasson 2005). The increased use of the Goal Attainment Scale (GAS; Kiresuk et al 1994) as an outcome measure and intervention protocols aimed at achieving specific activity-based goals suggests that both researchers and clinicians are rapidly integrating the theory into practice. In the past, research specifically examining the effect of task practice on upper extremity function has been limited to a few single subject Level IV studies. Each of these studies contributes some knowledge to the theory, and the studies suggest that quality of upper extremity movement or control is improved when practice is task- or object-based, rather than exercise-based (van der Weel et al 1991, Beauregard et al 1998, Volman et al 2002). Functional therapy has also been described and examined in single subject (Lammi and Law 2003) and single group studies (Ekström et al 2005) and a randomized trial (Ketelaar et al 2001). Among key components of the functional therapy described by each of these authors is the setting of task-based goals and a focus on practice of the task in natural settings. Each of these studies demonstrated improved performance on the Pediatric Evaluation of Disability Inventory (PEDI) self-care domains, which include many tasks requiring the use of the upper extremity. In addition to these studies of varying functional therapies, there is evidence from the studies investigating the effect of BoNT-A injections and occupational therapy that intervention protocols that included goal-focused task practice were effective (Boyd 2004, Greaves 2004, Lowe et al 2006, Wallen et al 2007).

Along with traditional methods of providing task practice, studies are emerging which investigate whether the intense practice embedded within virtual reality technology can improve upper extremity skills. Reid's (2002a, 2002b) pilot work, although very preliminary and limited by the outcomes selected to measure change, provides impetus for continued consideration of a technology that has been rapidly absorbed into the lives of Western children.

EFFECT OF INTERVENTIONS NOT SPECIFIC TO THE UPPER EXTREMITY
Good quality systematic reviews have been conducted on both neurodevelopmental therapy (Brown and Burns 2001, Butler and Darrah 2001) and conductive education (Darrah et al 2004). Each review found inconclusive results, with many of the included studies being under-powered or poorly conducted. In addition, where significant differences were found between groups, half tended to favour the intervention of interest and half favoured the various control groups. Outcomes related to upper extremity skills did not significantly support either neurodevelopmental therapy or conductive education.

Since publication of the systematic review of conductive education, Stiller et al (2003) have compared conductive education with intensive therapy or special education services to improve gross and fine motor skills. This was a very small trial, with group sizes of seven, eight and four respectively, and no statistically significant differences were found. Improvements in the Gross Motor Function Measure, the PEDI and the Peabody-FM were spread across the groups. For example, the intensive therapy group improved more on the Manual Dexterity scale of the Peabody and the conductive education group improved more on Hand Use and Eye–Hand Coordination (see Table 26.1).

A search conducted within the clinical trials registers (www.clinicaltrials.gov) identified two randomized trials which are underway in Canada which propose to examine interventions that, while not specific to the upper extremity, are relevant to upper extremity functions and outcomes. One trial, led by D. Cameron at the University of Toronto, will examine the effect of cognitive orientation to occupational performance (CO-OP) in comparison to a contemporary treatment approach on whether children gain and maintain the skills they set as goals (see Chapter 17 for a description of CO-OP). The second trial, led by M. Law at McMaster University, will compare interventions targeted at the child (child-focused), with those targeted at adapting or changing the task or environment (context-focused), and examine their effect across each level of the ICF (WHO 2001).

INTERVENTIONS EMERGING WITHIN THE RESEARCH LITERATURE
Much of the current research literature has focused on investigating the effect of interventions for children with hemiplegia as a distinct group. CIMT and its variants as well as BoNT-A are good examples of interventions either designed for (CIMT), or predominantly investigated in (BoNT-A), children with hemiplegia. The application of CIMT particularly has given rise to discussions regarding the relative effectiveness of unimanual and bimanual training, especially as smooth and effective performance of many tasks requires the hands to work together. Arising from their investigations of CIMT, Charles and Gordon have proposed a new intervention, called hand-arm bimanual intensive training (HABIT), which utilizes the element of massed practice provided within CIMT but which focuses on bimanual coordination (Charles and Gordon 2006). This intervention is currently under investigation (Gordon et al 2007) (see Table 26.2). Sheppard et al (2007) have also recently reported on a bilateral training method for children with hemiplegia. They investigated bilateral isokinematic training which utilizes the principle of entrainment, such that during training both hands/arms are performing the same action at the same time within rhythmical and repetitive tasks. This investigation of bilateral isokinematic training in children was developed following positive findings in adults after stroke. Sheppard et al's investigation was preliminary, utilizing a single subject design which demonstrated some positive gains in frequency of use of the impaired arm as measured using study-specific outcomes.

OUTCOMES USED IN UPPER EXTREMITY RESEARCH
One of the important limitations of all the research conducted in the area of intervention efficacy for children with cerebral palsy is the availability of valid, reliable measures. Researchers to date have often had to rely on measures that inadequately capture the phenomena of interest or which were not developed for children with neurological impairments. In these circumstances researchers may resort to developing study-specific measures. Some research groups follow established procedures for test development, such as classical test theory or item response theory, resulting in increased confidence in the data generated from the measures. This represents a significant time and resource commitment. There remain a number of measures that were developed for specific research projects that have not had their psychometric properties examined. Unfortunately this limits their ongoing utility and the confidence with which we interpret study outcomes.

Across the studies identified in this review the focus of outcome measurement has been at impairment and activity levels. This review has found no good evidence that upper extremity intervention improves participation, as no study has measured it well. Achievement of goals may indicate increased participation; however, this is dependent on the goals set, and most examples provided in the literature appear to represent activity goals. In the past five to ten years there has been an increase in the choice of outcome measures for both clinicians and researchers, and there are now measures that capture impairment, activity and participation outcomes that would be relevant following many upper extremity interventions (see Chapter 12).

Assessments and outcome measures must be both valid (actually measuring what they are designed to measure) and reliable – that is, stable when no change has occurred, or when different raters score the same performance. Regardless of an outcome's established reliability, the actual reliability of scores achieved by children on a specific assessment depends on the rater reliability of the individual administering the test. Both clinicians and researchers can establish their own reliability by ensuring that they undertake appropriate training in test administration and then determining their ability to score consistently when no change has occurred in a child's performance.

Future directions

Clinical Practice

For children with hemiplegia, there is a growing body of good evidence that BoNT-A combined with therapy, and to a lesser extent (modified) CIMT, is effective in improving upper extremity movement quality and use of the hands. Fig. 26.2 provides a visual comparison of treatment effect from six studies which measured quality of upper extremity movement using the QUEST and provided parametric data. This figure must be interpreted cautiously as the interventions differ and so do the times at which outcomes were measured. That BoNT-A plus occupational therapy is effective for young children with hemiplegia and moderate spasticity appears clear, and it may be time for evidence-based clinical practice guidelines to be developed by the key researchers in this field. Alternative indications for the use of BoNT-A with other children – for example, for cosmetic improvement, or for gains in ease-of-care – have not yet been addressed thoroughly by research.

Although many studies demonstrated some positive effects, small study samples, varying severity and wide age ranges all influence our ability to select particular interventions for individual children. The youngest child included in a BoNT-A or CIMT study was aged 7 months; however, children were more typically older than 2 years. Few studies have really addressed appropriate upper extremity interventions for infants.

One of the clearest messages from the recent literature has been a more holistic focus of intervention. That is, intervention and outcome measurement now more frequently consider the person–environment–occupation dynamic rather than only attempting to remove the positive symptoms of cerebral palsy, for example hypertonicity. Researchers are planning therapy using knowledge of motor skills acquisition and refinement. There is important evidence that intervention based on these principles is effective. This was seen in the gains in goal achievement made in functional therapy (Ketelaar et al 2001) and by many children in control groups within the BoNT-A studies (Boyd 2004, Greaves 2004, Lowe et al 2006, Wallen et al 2007), and in Law et al's (1997) study comparing casting plus neurodevelopmental therapy with traditional occupational therapy. The findings suggest

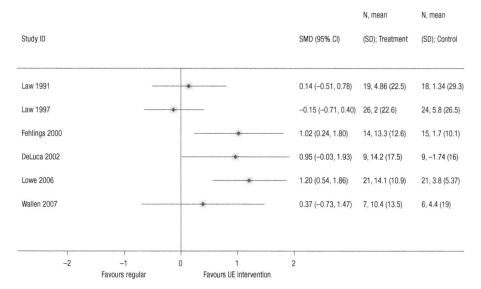

Study ID	SMD (95% CI)	N, mean (SD); Treatment	N, mean (SD); Control
Law 1991	0.14 (−0.51, 0.78)	19, 4.86 (22.5)	18, 1.34 (29.3)
Law 1997	−0.15 (−0.71, 0.40)	26, 2 (22.6)	24, 5.8 (26.5)
Fehlings 2000	1.02 (0.24, 1.80)	14, 13.3 (12.6)	15, 1.7 (10.1)
DeLuca 2002	0.95 (−0.03, 1.93)	9, 14.2 (17.5)	9, −1.74 (16)
Lowe 2006	1.20 (0.54, 1.86)	21, 14.1 (10.9)	21, 3.8 (5.37)
Wallen 2007	0.37 (−0.73, 1.47)	7, 10.4 (13.5)	6, 4.4 (19)

Fig. 26.2 Mean change in quality of movement scores following upper extremity intervention versus regular therapy. All outcomes are QUEST and calculations are change scores from baseline to time specified below.

SMD = standardized mean difference calculated in Stata Statistical Software 9 (2005) using published and unpublished data. UE = upper extremity; SD = standard deviation; N = sample size; Intervention = upper extremity intervention as specified below; Control = regular therapy.

Law 1991	Law et al 1991: intense neurodevelopmental therapy + cast *versus* regular neurodevelopmental therapy at 6 months
Law 1997	Law et al 1997: intense neurodevelopmental therapy + cast *versus* regular occupational therapy at 4 months
Fehlings 2000	Fehlings et al 2000: botulinum toxin A + occupational therapy *versus* regular occupational therapy at 1 month
DeLuca 2002	DeLuca 2002: constraint induced movement therapy *versus* regular therapy at 3 weeks
Lowe 2006	Lowe et al 2006: botulinum toxin A + occupational therapy *versus* occupational therapy alone at 3 months
Wallen 2007	Wallen et al 2007: botulinum toxin A + occupational therapy *versus* occupational therapy alone at 3 months

that short bursts of goal-focused intervention may be very effective and clinically applicable across a range of services.

SUMMARY OF RESEARCH GAPS AND FUTURE DIRECTIONS

Research into upper extremity interventions for children with cerebral palsy is growing rapidly, and Table 26.2 describes some of the exciting forthcoming research. The following points are offered for consideration for further investigation.

1   *There is a need for empirical support for the assumption that intervention focused at impairment and activity levels actually changes the participation of children with cerebral palsy.* This is especially important for those children at Levels I, II and perhaps

III of the Manual Ability Classification System (MACS; see Introduction) as intervention is often focused on reduction of impairment at these levels. Conversely, children at Levels IV and V may benefit from targeted impairment-focused interventions, such as surgery or BoNT-A, for pain management, improved appearance or ease-of-care, as well as some functional gains. Improved activity and participation, however, are more likely to be gained through careful attention to environmental and occupation-based factors. Further research to support therapeutic endeavours in each of these areas is also necessary.

2 *Long-term efficacy of short-term, intensive bursts of therapy to promote acquisition of specific skills*. The promising research in both BoNT-A and CIMT, and the emergent ideas within cognitive orientation to occupational performance and other task-oriented approaches, all point to the effectiveness of bursts of therapy focused on specific skill acquisition or goal achievement. The long-term efficacy of short bursts of therapy both for goal achievement and health maintenance (such as managing contractures or maintaining general health and fitness), as well as for ongoing life quality and satisfaction, needs to be evaluated.

3 *Further research of specific interventions*. Each of the chapters describing intervention approaches within this book will have referred to research that is required – for example, investigation of how outcomes vary according to intensity of CIMT, or after repeated BoNT-A injections. One glaring gap in upper extremity intervention research is that of strength training, an area showing significant promise in the lower extremity. However, upper extremity function is more complex than lower extremity function and similar outcomes should not be assumed.

4 *The missing age groups*. Very little research has been undertaken on upper extremity intervention for infants with cerebral palsy. Clearly they are a complex group, with issues related to timing of diagnosis and the need for families to manage the early months. However, our understandings of neuronal development within the critical first two years of life mean that we must study this group. Likewise, adolescents and adults have been neglected, although recent research is beginning to examine issues specific to those groups (for example, Skold et al 2004).

5 *Outcome measurement*. Development of outcome measures that truly capture phenomena of interest is required. But perhaps the most urgent requirement at present is to identify, or develop, valid, reliable measures that are also responsive to change.

Summary

The driving forces for evidence-based practice were managing information overload and a rapidly changing knowledge base (Sackett et al 2000, Law 2002). In addition, the shift in community expectations from practitioner-as-expert to client-centred practice promotes family and child involvement in decisions and an expectation that health-care decisions will be made with explicit knowledge; that is, evidence. Current health practices require us to be able to engage clients in informed decision making. This includes being able to translate research findings and evidence for individual families – interpreting the likely effect of disease, intervention, or prevention for the individual. There is skill in this process. Families

TABLE 26.2
Ongoing clinical trials of upper extremity intervention for children with cerebral palsy

Intervention	First author	Aim	Outcome focus	Identified
Acupuncture	Duncan	2 group RCT: acupuncture + conventional therapy vs conventional therapy for 12–72 mth-olds		USCTR
Bimanual training	Gordon	2 group randomized crossover trial for 4–16 y/o		USCTR
BoNT-A	Gill	2 group RCT: BoNT-A vs Baclofen for UE spasticity for > 18 y/o		USCTR
	Novak	3 group RCT: BoNT-A + intense therapy, BoNT-A + regular therapy, BoNT-A + home programme	A, P	ACTR
	Olesch	2 group RCT: BoNT-A + OT vs OT only: repeat injection trial for 18 mth–5 y/o	BF, A, P	PC
	Thorley	2 group RCT: BoNT-A to thumb + orthoses & home programme; placebo + casting & home programme	BF, A	ACTR
CIMT	Boyd	2 group RCT of CIMT vs bimanual training for 5–15 y/o	BF, A, P	ACTR
	Taub	2 group RCT of CIMT vs conventional motor training for 2–6 y/o		USCTR
	Wallen	2 group RCT of modified CIMT vs standard occupational therapy for 18 mth–8 y/o	BF, A, P	PC
Combined	Eliasson	2 group RCT: BoNT-A+ CIMT vs BoNT-A + OT for 5–15 y/o		PC
	Hoare	2 group RCT: BoNT-A+ CIMT vs BoNT-A + OT for 18 mth–6 y/o	A, P	ACTR
EMG	Sanger	Single group observational study	BF	USCTR
Strength training	Lamvik	RCT: groups not specified		USCTR
Surgery	James	3 group RCT: UE standard tendon surgery vs BoNT-A vs regular therapy for 5–15 y/o		USCTR
Virtual reality	Reid	2 group RCT: virtual reality vs standard OT &/or PT for 8–10 y/o	BF, A	PC
Task practice	Vu	2 group randomized crossover trial: LE strength training followed by UE dexterity vs UE dexterity followed by LE strength training for 6–14 y/o	A, P	ACTR

Notes:

1 *Identification of trials*: ACTR = Australian Clinical Trial Register [http://www.actr.org.au/]; International Standard Randomised Controlled Trial Number Register [http://www.controlled-trials.com/isrctn/search.asp]; USCTR = US clinical trials register [http://www.clinicaltrials.gov/]; PC = personal communication.

2 *Abbreviations*: BF = ICF body function domain; A = ICF activity domain; P = ICF participation domain; vs = versus; y/o = year-olds; mth = month; LE = lower extremity; UE = upper extremity; RCT = randomized controlled trial; OT = occupational therapy; PT = physiotherapy; BoNT-A = botulinum toxin A; CIMT = constraint-induced movement therapy or modified constraint-induced movement therapy.

do come asking for specific interventions such as BoNT-A, CIMT or surgery. Empowering families to access and understand the evidence, mesh this with clinical experience and make truly informed decisions is an integral part of the evidence-based practitioner's role.

Client-centred practice also requires us to involve families and children in setting our research agendas in order to ensure we are researching issues that are of critical importance to them. Using consumers as research partners is not yet prevalent in paediatric research. The Working Together for Change project (Ostroff et al 2006) from the CanChild Centre for Disability Research is however exploring paediatric models of partnership in research and should be able to inform us in the future.

Hand use is extremely complex, being influenced by many factors both within the child and in the environment (see Eliasson 2005, fig. 1). At present our focus on conducting systematic research to understand both whether and why an intervention is effective is limited by traditional designs and data analysis procedures. Development or use of complex statistical models may assist. So, too, may an acceptance of more varied research methods that can inform practice. As an example, qualitative enquiry can expose the reasoning and experiences of therapists, families and children who participate in interventions. Granlund and Björk-Åkesson (2005) describe a continuum of research methods spanning 'pure analytical designs' which study one phenomenon at a time to 'pure integrative systemic designs'. Integrative designs examine complex phenomena taking into account multiple factors with the aim of understanding patterns and interrelationships between factors within groups of children. Research paradigms that explicate the complexities of the upper extremity and hand use of children with cerebral palsy are now required.

REFERENCES

Autti-Ramo I, Suoranta J, Anttila H, Malmivaara A, Makela M (2006) Effectiveness of upper and lower limb casting and orthoses in children with cerebral palsy. *Am J Phys Med Rehabil* 85: 89–103.

Beauregard R, Thomas JJ, Nelson DL (1998) Quality of reach during a game and during a rote movement in children with cerebral palsy. *Phys Occup Ther Pediatr* 18: 67–84.

Boyd RN (2004) The central and peripheral effects of botulinum toxin-A in children with cerebral palsy. PhD dissertation, La Trobe University, Melbourne.

Boyd RN, Morris ME, Graham HK (2001) Management of upper limb dysfunction in children with cerebral palsy: a systematic review. *Eur J Neurol* 8: 150–166.

Brown T, Burns S (2001) The efficacy of neurodevelopmental treatment in paediatrics: a systematic review. *Br J Occup Ther* 64: 235–244.

Bunata RE (2006) Pronator teres rerouting in children with cerebral palsy. *J Hand Surg* 31.

Butler C, Darrah J (2001) Effects of neurodevelopmental treatment (NDT) for cerebral palsy: an AACPDM evidence report. *Dev Med Child Neurol* 43: 778–790.

Butler C, Chambers H, Goldstein M, Adams R, Darrah J, Leach J (2003) Evaluating research in developmental disabilities: a conceptual framework for reviewing treatment outcomes. http: www.aacpdm.org/home.html (accessed 7 March 2005).

Butler C, Chambers H, Goldstein M, Harris S, Leach J, Campbell S, Adams R, Darrah J, Msall ME, Edgar T, McDonnell M, Samson-Fang L, Abel M (2005) Evaluating research in developmental disabilities: a conceptual framework for reviewing treatment outcomes. http://www.aacpdm.org/index?service=page/treatmentOutcomesReport (accessed May 2005).

Charles J, Gordon AM (2006) Development of hand-arm bimanual intensive training (HABIT) for improving bimanual coordination in children with hemiplegic cerebral palsy. *Dev Med Child Neurol* 48: 931–936.

Charles J, Wolf SL, Schneider JA, Gordon AM (2006) Efficacy of a child-friendly form of constraint-induced movement therapy in hemiplegic cerebral palsy: a randomized control trial. *Dev Med Child Neurol* 48: 635–642.

Corn K, Imms C, Timewell G, Carter C, Collins L, Dubbeld S, Schubiger S, Froude E (2003) Impact of second skin lycra splinting on the quality of upper limb movement in children *Br J Occup Ther* 66: 464–472.

Corry IS, Cosgrove AP, Walsh EG, McClean D, Graham HK (1997) Botulinum toxin A in the hemiplegic upper limb: a double-blind trial. *Dev Med Child Neurol* 39: 185–193.

Dahlin LB, Komoto-Tufvesson Y, Salgeback S (1998) Surgery of the spastic hand in cerebral palsy. Improvement in stereognosis and hand function after surgery. *J Hand Surg [Br]* 23: 334–339.

Darrah J, Watkins B, Chen L, Bonin C (2004) Conductive education intervention for children with cerebral palsy: an AACPDM evidence report. *Dev Med Child Neurol* 46: 187–203.

DeLuca SC (2002) Intensive movement therapy with casting for children with hemiparetic cerebral palsy: a randomized controlled crossover trial. PhD dissertation, University of Alabama at Birmingham, Birmingham, AL.

DeLuca SC, Echols K, Law CR, Ramey SL (2006) Intensive pediatric constraint-induced therapy for children with cerebral palsy: randomized, controlled, crossover trial. *J Child Neurol* 21: 931–938.

Dodd KJ, Taylor NF, Damiano DL (2002) A systematic review of the effectiveness of strength-training programs for people with cerebral palsy *Arch Phys Med Rehabil* 83: 1157–1164.

Ekström L, Johansson E, Granat T, Carlberg EB (2005) Functional therapy for children with cerebral palsy: an ecological approach. *Dev Med Child Neurol* 47: 613–619.

Eliasson AC (2005) Improving the use of hands in daily activities: aspects of treatment of children with cerebral palsy. *Phys Occup Ther Pediatr* 25: 37–60.

Eliasson AC, Ekholm C, Carlstedt T (1998) Hand function in children with cerebral palsy after upper-limb tendon transfer and muscle release. *Dev Med Child Neurol* 40: 612–621.

Eliasson AC, Krumlinde-Sundholm L, Shaw K, Wang C (2005) Effects of constraint induced movement therapy in young children with hemiplegic cerebral palsy: an adapted model. *Dev Med Child Neurol* 47: 266–275.

El-Said NS (2001) Selective release of the flexor origin with transfer of flexor carpi ulnaris in cerebral palsy. *J Bone Joint Surg* 83: 259–262.

Exner CE, Bonder BR (1983) Comparative effects of three hand splints on bilateral hand use, grasp and arm-hand posture in hemiplegic children: a pilot study. *Occup Ther J Res* 3: 75–92.

Fehlings D, Rang M, Glazier J, Steele C (2000) An evaluation of botulinum-A toxin injections to improve upper extremity function in children with hemiplegic cerebral palsy. *J Pediatr* 137: 331–337.

Gordon AM, Schneider JA, Chinnan A, Charles JR (2007) Efficacy of a hand-arm bimanual intensive therapy (HABIT) in children with hemiplegic cerebral palsy: a randomized controlled trial. *Dev Med Child Neurol* 49: 830–838.

Granlund M, Björk-Åkesson E (2005) Participation and general competence: do type and degree of disability really matter? In: Traustadottir R, Gustavsson A, Tøsselbro J, Sandvin JT, editors. *Change, Resistance and Reflection: Current Nordic Disability Research.* Lund, Sweden: Studentlitteratur.

Greaves SM (2004) The effect of botulinum toxin A injections on occupational therapy outcomes for children with spastic hemiplegia. PhD dissertation, La Trobe University, Bundoora.

Hammel J, Finlayson M, Kielhofner G, Helfrich C, Peterson E (2002) Educating scholars of practice: an approach to preparing tomorrow's researchers. *Occup Ther Health Care* 15: 157–176.

Hargreaves DG, Warwick DJ, Tonkin MA (2000) Changes in hand function following wrist arthrodesis in cerebal palsy. *J Hand Surg [Br]* 25: 193–194.

Herbert RD, Jamtvedt G, Mead J, Hagen KB (2005) *Practical Evidence-based Physiotherapy.* Edinburgh: Elsevier.

Hoare BJ, Wasiak J, Imms C, Carey L (2007) Constraint induced movement therapy in the treatment of the upper limb in children with cerebral palsy. *Cochrane Database Syst Rev* 2: CD004149.

Hoving JL, Gross AR, Gasner D, Kay T, Kennedy C, Hondras MA, Haines T, Bouter LM (2001) A critical appraisal of review articles on the effectiveness of conservative treatment for neck pain. *Spine* 26: 196–205.

Jackson R (2004) Gate checklist for intervention studies. http://www.health.auckland.ac.nz/population-health/epidemiology-biostats/epiq/ (accessed April 2005).

Kerr C, McDowell B, McDonough S (2004) Electrical stimulation in cerebral palsy: a review of effects on strength and motor function. *Dev Med Child Neurol* 46: 205–213.

Ketelaar M, Vermeer A, 't Hart H, van Petegem-van Beek E, Helders PJM (2001) Effects of a functional therapy program on motor abilities of children with cerebral palsy. *Phys Ther* 81: 1534–1545.

Kiresuk TJ, Smith A, Cardillo JE (1994) *Goal Attainment Scaling: Applications, Theory and Measurement.* Hillsdale, NJ: Erlbaum Associates.

415

Knox V (2003) The use of lycra garments in children with cerebral palsy: a report of a descriptive clinical trial. *Br J Occup Ther* 66: 71–77.

Kreulen M, Smeulders MJC, Veeger HEJ, Hage JJ (2006) Movement patterns of the upper extremity and trunk before and after corrective surgery of impaired forearm rotation in patients with cerebral palsy. *Dev Med Child Neurol* 48: 436–441.

Krumlinde-Sundholm L, Eliasson A (2003) Development of the Assisting Hand Assessment: a Rasch-built measure intended for children with unilateral upper limb impairments *Scand J Occup Ther* 10: 16–26.

Lammi BM, Law M (2003) The effects of Family-Centred Functional Therapy on the occupational performance of children with cerebral palsy. *Can J Occup Ther* 70: 285–297.

Law M (2002) *Evidence-based Rehabilitation*. Thorofare, NJ: Slack Incorporated.

Law M, Cadman D, Rosenbaum P, Walter S, Russell D, DeMatteo C (1991) Neurodevelopmental therapy and upper-extremity inhibitive casting for children with cerebral palsy. *Dev Med Child Neurol* 33: 379–387.

Law M, Russell D, Pollock N, Rosenbaum P, Walter S, King G (1997) A comparison of intensive neuro-developmental therapy plus casting and a regular occupational therapy program for children with cerebral palsy. *Dev Med Child Neurol* 39: 664–670.

Law M, Stewart D, Letts L, Polluck N, Bosch J, Westmorland M (1998a) Guidelines for critical review form – qualitative studies. http://www-fhs.mcmaster.ca/rehab/ebp/

Law M, Stewart D, Letts L, Polluck N, Bosch J, Westmorland M (1998b) Guidelines for critical review form – quantitative studies. http://www-fhs.mcmaster.ca/rehab/ebp/

Lovarini M, Wallen M, Imms C (2006) Searching for evidence in pediatric occupational therapy using free versus subscription databases: a comparison of outcomes. *Phys Occup Ther Pediatr* 26: 19–38.

Lowe K, Novak I, Cusick A (2006) Low-dose/high concentration localised botulinum toxin A improves upper limb movement and function in children with hemiplegic cerebral palsy. *Dev Med Child Neurol* 48: 170–175.

Maher CG, Sherrington C, Herbert RD, Moseley AM, Elkins M (2003) Reliability of the PEDro scale for rating quality of randomised controlled trials. *Phys Ther* 83: 713–721.

Nicholson JH, Morton RE, Attfield S, Rennie D (2001) Assessment of upper limb function and movement in children with cerebral palsy wearing lycra garments. *Dev Med Child Neurol* 43: 384–391.

Nylander G, Carlstrom C, Adolfsson L (1999) 4.5 year follow-up after surgical correction of upper extremity deformities in spastic cerebral palsy. *J Hand Surg [Br]* 24: 719–723.

Ostroff B, Law M, Pantich M, Gaffney JB, Barbadoro S (2006) Working together for change. http://www.communityfaculty.ca/ (accessed 18 May 2006).

Oxman AD, Guyatt G (1991) Validation of an index of the quality of review articles. *J Clin Epidemiol* 44: 1271–1278.

Ozer K, Chesher SP, Scheker LR (2006) Neuromuscular electrical stimulation and dynamic bracing for the management of upper-extremity spasticity in children with cerebral palsy. *Dev Med Child Neurol* 48: 559–563.

Phillips B, Ball C, Sackett DL, Badenoch D, Straus S, Haynes B, Dawes M (2001) Oxford Centre for Evidence-based Medicine levels of evidence. http://www.cebm.net/downloads/Oxford_CEBM_Levels_5.rtf (accessed March 2006).

Rayan GM, Young BT (1999) Arthrodesis of the spastic wrist. *J Hand Surg* 24: 944–952.

Reeuwijk A, van Schie PEM, Becher JG, Kwakkel G (2006) Effects of botulinum toxin type A on upper limb function in children with cerebral palsy: a systematic review. *Clin Rehabil* 20: 375–387.

Reid DT (2002a) Benefits of a virtual play rehabilitation environment for children with cerebral palsy on perceptions of self-efficacy: a pilot study *Pediatr Rehabil* 5: 141–148.

Reid DT (2002b) The use of virtual reality to improve upper-extremity efficiency skills in children with cerebral palsy: a pilot study. *Technol Disabil* 14: 53–61.

Richardson W, Scott MD, Wilson MC, Nishikawa J, Hayward R (1995) The well-built clinical question: a key to evidence-based decisions. *ACP J Club* 123: A12–A13.

Russo RN, Crotty M, Miller MD, Murchland S, Flett P, Haan E (2007) Upper limb botulinum toxin A injection and occupational therapy in children with hemiplegic cerebral palsy identified form a population register: a single-blind randomized controlled trial. *Pediatr* 119: e1149–e1158.

Sackett DL, Rosenberg WMC, Gray JAM, Haynes RB, Richardson WS (1996) Evidence-based medicine: what it is and what it isn't. *BMJ* 312: 71–72.

Sackett DL, Strauss SE, Richardson WS, Rosenberg W, Haynes RB (2000) *Evidence-based Medicine: How to Practice and Teach EBM*. Edinburgh: Churchill Livingstone.

416

Schwartz DA (2005) Strategies for facilitation of tendon transfers for enhanced wrist extension in cerebral palsy: a case report. *Br J Hand Ther* 10: 10–16.

Sheppard L, Mudie H, Froude E (2007) An investigation of bilateral isokinematic training and neurodevelopmental therapy in improving use of the affected hand in children with hemiplegia. *Phys Occup Ther Pediatr* 27: 5–25.

Skold A, Josephsson S, Eliasson AC (2004) Performing bimanual activities: the experiences of young persons with hemiplegic cerebral palsy. *Am J Occup Ther* 58: 416–425.

Smeulders M, Coester A, Kreulen M (2006) Surgical treatment for the thumb-in-palm deformity in patients with cerebral palsy. *Cochrane Database System Rev* 19: CD004093.

Speth LAWM, Leffers P, Janssen-Potten YJM, Vles JSH (2005) Botulinum toxin A and upper limb functional skills in hemiparetic cerebral palsy: a randomized trial in children receiving intensive therapy. *Dev Med Child Neurol* 46: 468–473.

Steultjens EMJ, Dekker J, Bouter LM, van de Nes JCM, Lambregts BLM, van den Ende CHM (2004) Occupational therapy for children with cerebral palsy: a systematic review. *Clin Rehabil* 18: 1–14.

Stiller C, Marcoux BC, Olson RE (2003) The effect of conductive education, intensive therapy, and special education services on motor skills in children with cerebral palsy. *Phys Occ Ther Pediatr* 23: 31–50.

Sung IY, Ryu JS, Pyun SB, Yoo SD, Song WH, Park MJ (2005) Efficacy of forced use therapy in hemiplegic cerebral palsy. *Arch Phys Med Rehabil* 86: 2195–2198.

Taub E, Landesman Ramey S, DeLuca SC, Echols K (2004) Efficacy of constraint-induced movement therapy for children with cerebral palsy with asymmetric motor impairment. *Pediatr* 113: 305–312.

Teplicky R, Law M, Russell D (2002) The effectiveness of casts, orthoses and splints for children with neurological disorders. *Infants Young Child* 15: 42–50.

Thalheimer W, Cook S (2002) How to calculate effect sizes from published research articles: a simplified methodology. In: Somerville, MA. Work-Learning Research, Inc. http://work-learning.com/effect_sizes.htm (accessed March 2005).

Valvano J (2004) Activity-focused motor interventions for children with neurological conditions. *Phys Occ Ther Pediatr* 24: 79–107.

van der Weel FR, van der Meer AL, Lee DN (1991) Effect of task on movement control in cerebral palsy: implications for assessment and therapy. *Dev Med Child Neurol* 33: 419–426.

Volman MJM, Wihnroks A, Vermeer A (2002) Effect of task context on reaching performance in children with spastic hemiparesis. *Clin Rehabil* 16: 684–692.

Wallen M, O'Flaherty SJ, Waugh MA (2007) Functional outcomes of intramuscular Botulinum Toxin type A and occupational therapy in the upper limbs of children with cerebral palsy: a randomised controlled trial. *Arch Phys Med Rehabil* 88: 1–10.

Wasiak J, Hoare BJ, Wallen M (2004) Botulinum toxin A as an adjunct to treatment in the management of the upper limb in children with spastic cerebral palsy. *Cochrane Database Syst Rev* 3.

WHO (2001) *International Classification of Functioning, Disability and Health.* Short version. Geneva: World Health Organization.

Willis JK, Morello A, Davie A, Rice JC, Bennett JT (2002) Forced use treatment of childhood hemiparesis. *Pediatr* 110: 94–96.

417

APPENDIX

Assessments used to measure hand function, activities and participation of children with cerebral palsy

Heidi Sanders

Assessment of Life Habits for Children (LIFE-H 1.0)
Authors: L. Noreau, P. Fougeyrollas and C. Lepage
Purpose: Descriptive
Age range: 5–13 years with disabilities
Psychometrics:

- *Standardization:* Content validity study included children with myelomeningocele. Samples for further studies included children with cerebral palsy
- *Validity:* Content and criterion studies reported
- *Reliability:* Internal: moderate to high; test-retest: moderate; intra-rater: moderate to high; inter-rater: moderate to high

Ordering information:
 INDCP
525 boul Wilfred-Hamel Est, A-08
Quebec, QC, Canada, GIM 2S8
418-529-9141X6202

Assisting Hand Assessment (AHA)
Authors: L. Krumlinde-Sundholm, M. Holmefur and A.-C. Eliasson
Purpose: Descriptive and evaluative; criterion-referenced test
Age range: 18 months to 12 years with hemiplegic cerebral palsy or brachial plexus palsy
Psychometrics:

- *Standardization:* Developed with Rasch measurement with children 18 months to 12 years of age. Children with hemiplegic cerebral palsy included in samples
- *Validity:* Construct validity studies reported
- *Reliability:* Intra-rater: high, SEM: 1.2; inter-rater: high, SEM: 1.5; internal consistency: high

Ordering information:
Handfast AB
Fogdevreten 2b
Se 171 77 Stockholm, Sweden
www.ahanetwork.se

Bruininks-Oseretsky Test of Motor Proficiency, Second Edition (BOT2)

Authors: R.H. Bruininks and B.D. Bruininks
Purpose: Descriptive and evaluative; norm-referenced test
Age range: 4–21 years
Psychometrics:

- *Standardization:* Normative sample of 1520 children, 4–21 years of age, in 230 sites located in 38 states, with representation by gender, race/ethnicity, socioeconomic status, geographic region, and children with disabilities based upon US Census
- *Validity:* Construct, discriminative and criterion validity studies reported; specific validation for children with cerebral palsy not reported
- *Reliability:* Test-retest: moderate to high; inter-rater: high

Ordering information:
American Guidance Service
4201 Woodland Road
Circle Pines, MN 55014-1796
1-800-328-256

Canadian Occupational Performance Measure (COPM)

Authors: M. Law, S. Baptiste, A. Carswell, M.A. McColl, H. Polatajko and N. Pollock
Purpose: Descriptive and evaluative; individually determined
Age range: All developmental levels, through family or caregiver response when needed
Psychometrics:

- *Standardization:* Validity and reliability study samples from 300 clients and 219 occupational therapists throughout Canada. Standardized procedures, not norm-referenced
- *Validity:* Content, criterion and construct validity studies reported
- *Reliability:* Test-retest: moderate to high; internal consistency: low to moderate

Ordering information:
The Canadian Association of Occupational Therapists
CTTC Building, Suite 2300
1125 Colonel By Drive
Ottawa, Ontario K1S 5R1
613-523-2268

Child Occupational Self Assessment, Version 2.0 (COSA)
Authors: J. Keller, A. Kafkes, S. Basu, J. Federico and G. Kielhofner
Purpose: Descriptive
Age range: 8–17 years
Psychometrics:

- *Standardization:* Developed using Rasch measurement. Samples included children with neurological, developmental and mental health diagnoses. Children with cerebral palsy were included
- *Validity:* Construct validity studies reported
- *Reliability:* Internal consistency: high to moderate

Ordering information:
The Model of Human Occupation Clearinghouse
Department of Occupational Therapy
AHS (MC 811)
University of Illinois at Chicago
1919 W. Taylor Street
Chicago, Illinois 60612

Children Helping Out: Responsibilities, Expectations and Supports (CHORES)
Author: L. Dunn
Purpose: Descriptive
Age range: 6–11 years
Psychometrics:

- *Standardization:* Standardized using a sample of 32 parents of children with and without disabilities who were aged 6 to 11 years, from Maine and Massachusetts, United States. Diagnoses included cerebral palsy
- *Validity:* Content and construct validity studies reported
- *Reliability:* Test-retest: high

Ordering information:
Copies can be obtained through the author:
Louise Dunn
louise.dunn@hsc.utah.edu
1-801-585-9356

Children's Assessment of Participation and Enjoyment (CAPE)
Authors: G. King, M. Law, S. King, P. Hurley, P. Rosenbaum, S. Hanna, M. Kertoy and
 N. Young
Purpose: Descriptive
Age range: 6–21 years
Psychometrics:

- *Standardization:* Longitudinal research study of 427 children, 6–15 years of age, with physical disabilities, from the province of Ontario, Canada, with representation by gender, socioeconomic status and ethnicity of parent. Diagnoses included cerebral palsy
- *Validity:* Content and construct validity studies reported
- *Reliability:* Internal consistency: low to moderate; test-retest: low to moderate; inter-rater: low to high

Ordering information:
Harcourt Assessment, Inc.
19500 Bulverde Road
San Antonio, TX 78259
1-800-211-8378

Evaluation Tool of Children's Handwriting (ETCH)
Author: S.J. Amundson
Purpose: Descriptive and evaluative; criterion-referenced test
Age range: 6–12 years
Psychometrics:

- *Standardization:* Preliminary normative sample of first graders
- *Validity:* Discriminative and construct validity studies reported
- *Reliability:* Inter-rater reliability: low to high; test-retest: high

Ordering information:
O.T. KIDS
PO Box 1118
Homer, Alaska 99603
(907) 235-0688

Functional Independence Measure for Children (WeeFIM) II
Authors: M.E. Msall, M. McCabe, S. Braun, B.T. Rogers, N.R. Lyons and L.C. Duffy
Purpose: Descriptive and evaluative; norm-referenced test
Age range: 6 months to 7 years (children with no disabilities); 6 months to 12 years (children
 with disabilities)
Psychometrics:

- *Standardization*: Normative sample of over 500 children without disabilities and 705 children with disabilities with representation by gender, ethnicity/race, socioeconomic status, and disabilities including cerebral palsy
- *Validity*: Content and concurrent validity studies reported; responsiveness reported in children with cerebral palsy following early intervention or selective dorsal rhizotomy
- *Reliability*: Test-retest: high; inter-rater: moderate to high

Ordering information:
Uniform Data System for Medical Rehabilitation
270 Northpointe Parkway
Ste 300
Amherst, New York 14228
(716) 817-7800 (ext. 23)

Jebsen-Taylor Test of Hand Function
Authors: R.H. Jebsen, N. Taylor, R.B. Treischmann, M.J. Trotter and L.A. Howard
Purpose: Evaluative; norm-referenced test
Age range: 6–90 years
Psychometrics:

- *Standardization:* Normative sample of approximately 330 children, aged 6–19 years with no identified disability, in the Pacific Northwest region of the US; 20 children with stable hand disabilities, including cerebral palsy and rheumatoid arthritis, were evaluated to determine test-retest reliability
- *Validity:* Content, criterion and construct validity studies reported for adults; no report of validity studies for children with or without disabilities
- *Reliability:* Test-retest in sample of children with stable hand disabilities: high

Ordering information:
Sammons Preston
P.O. Box 5071
Bolingbrook, IL 60440-5071
1-800-323-5547

Knox Preschool Play Scale
Authors: S.A. Knox, N. Bledsoe and J. Shepard
Purpose: Descriptive and evaluative
Age range: Birth to 6 years
Psychometrics:

- *Standardization:* No normative data collected. Pilot tested with children with cognitive delay and correlated with children's developmental ages
- *Validity:* Concurrent and discriminative validity studies reported
- *Reliability:* Test-retest: high; inter-rater: high

Ordering information:
Cannot order. Information available in:
Parham, LD and Fazio, LS (1997) *Play in Occupational Therapy for Children*. St Louis, MO: Mosby

Melbourne Assessment of Unilateral Upper Limb Function

Authors: M. Randall, L. Johnson and D. Reddihough
Purpose: Descriptive and evaluative; criterion-referenced test
Age range: 5–15 years with neurological impairment
Psychometrics:

- *Standardization*: Sample of 11 children with cerebral palsy, 11 children with traumatic brain injury, in Melbourne
- *Validity*: Content, criterion and construct validity studies reported
- *Reliability*: Internal consistency: moderate to high; test-retest: high; inter-rater: high; intra-rater: high

Ordering information:
Occupational Therapy Department
Royal Children's Hospital, Melbourne
Flemington Road, Parkville 3052
Victoria, Australia
(03) 9345 540

Pediatric Evaluation of Disability Inventory (PEDI)

Authors: S.M. Haley, W.J. Coster, L.H. Ludlow, J.T. Haltiwanger and P.J. Andrellos
Purpose: Descriptive and evaluative; norm-referenced test
Age range: 6 months to 7.5 years
Psychometrics:

- *Standardization:* Normative sample of 412 children from the Northeast US, with representation by ethnicity
- *Validity:* Content, construct, concurrent and discriminative validity studies reported; clinical validation studies included children with cerebral palsy, developmental delay, traumatic brain injury, and children admitted to a paediatric trauma centre
- *Reliability:* Inter-rater: moderate to high with SEM of 0.54–1.75 for the normative sample and 1.55–5.20 for clinical samples

Ordering information:
Boston University
Health & Disability Research Institute
635 Commonwealth Avenue
Boston, MA 02215-1605
(617) 353-3277

Pediatric Volitional Questionnaire

Authors: S. Basu, A. Kafkes, R. Geist and G. Kielhofner
Purpose: Descriptive and evaluative
Age range: 2–7 years
Psychometrics:

- *Standardization:* Developed using Rasch measurement. Sample did include children with cerebral palsy
- *Validity:* Construct and criterion validity studies reported
- *Reliability:* No studies reported

Ordering information:
The Model of Human Occupation Clearinghouse
Department of Occupational Therapy
AHS (MC 811)
University of Illinois at Chicago
1919 W. Taylor Street
Chicago, Illinois 60612

Quality of Upper Extremities Skills Test (QUEST)

Authors: C. DeMatteo, M. Law, D. Russell, N. Pollock, P. Rosenbaum and S. Walter
Purpose: Descriptive and evaluative; criterion-referenced test
Age range: 18 months to 8 years
Psychometrics:

- *Standardization:* Normative sample of 71 children, aged 18 months to 8 years, in Ontario, Canada, diagnosed with spastic cerebral palsy and with spasticity present in the wrist and hand during movement
- *Validity:* Construct, criterion and responsiveness validity studies reported
- *Reliability:* Test-retest: moderate to high; inter-rater: moderate to high

Ordering information:
CanChild Centre for Childhood Disability Research
Institute for Applied Health Sciences
McMaster University
1400 Main Street West, Room 408
Hamilton, Ontario
Canada L8S 1C7
1-905-525-9140 (ext. 27850)

School Assessment of Motor Processing Skills (AMPS)
Authors: A.G. Fisher and K. Bryze
Purpose: Descriptive and evaluative; criterion-referenced
Age range: 3–12 years
Psychometrics:

- *Standardization:* Reliability and validity samples included children with developmental disabilities, as well as a cross-cultural study of children residing in the US and in Brazil
- *Validity:* Construct, criterion and person response validity studies reported
- *Reliability:* Inter-rater: moderate to high

Ordering information:
info@AMPSIntl.com

School Function Assessment (SFA)
Authors: W. Coster, T. Deeney, J. Haltwanger and S. Haley
Purpose: Evaluative
Age range: Kindergarten to sixth grade
Psychometrics:

- *Standardization*: Normative sample of 363 students with disabilities and 315 regular education students from the US and Puerto Rico, with representation by gender, ethnicity/race, socioeconomic status, disabling conditions and urban/suburban/rural areas
- *Validity*: Content and construct validity studies reported
- *Reliability*: Internal consistency: high; test-retest: moderate to high; inter-rater: moderate

Ordering information:
Harcourt Assessment
19500 Bulverde Rd
San Antonio, TX 78259
1-800-211-8378

Short Child's Occupational Profile
Authors: P. Bowyer, M. Ross, O. Schwartz, G. Kielhofner and J. Kramer
Purpose: Descriptive and evaluative
Age range: 2–21 years with a range of disabilities
Psychometrics:

- *Standardization:* Currently being validated using Rasch analysis. The sample includes children of varying ages and diagnoses, including cerebral palsy
- *Validity:* Construct validity study reported; study of psychometric properties in process
- *Reliability:* Study of psychometric properties in process

Ordering information:
(not yet available for purchase)
The Model of Human Occupation Clearinghouse
Department of Occupational Therapy
AHS (MC 811)
University of Illinois at Chicago
1919 W. Taylor Street
Chicago, Illinois 60612

Test of Playfulness (TOPS)
Authors: A.C. Bundy, P. Metzger and B. McNicholas
Purpose: Descriptive and evaluative
Age range: 2–10 years
Psychometrics:

- *Standardization:* Initial validity and reliability study sample of 68 typically developing children and 9 children with developmental delays (ambulatory and verbal), Caucasian and from middle socioeconomic status in the Eastern US and Canada
- *Validity:* Concurrent and construct validity studies reported
- *Reliability:* Inter-rater: high

Ordering information:
Cannot order. Information available in:
Parham, LD and Fazio, LS (1997) *Play in Occupational Therapy for Children.* St Louis, MO: Mosby

Tool for Optimizing Written Production (TOW-P)
Authors: P. Rigby and H. Schwellnus
Purpose: Descriptive
Age range: School-aged children
Psychometrics:

- *Standardization:* Study samples included 300 children from Canada with written productivity concerns. Samples included children with physical, learning and developmental disabilities. Children with cerebral palsy were included
- *Validity:* No studies reported
- *Reliability:* No studies reported

INDEX

Note: page numbers in *italics* refer to figures and tables. 'CP' refers to cerebral palsy.

ABILHAND-Kids 190, 192
acetylcholine 213, *214*
acromioclavicular joint 82
actin 104
action perception theory 3
activity
    preferences 389
    simplification 290
activity-based practice 314–15
adductor pollicis brevis, release 207, *208,* 209
amputees, cortical maps 15–16
anaesthesia/analgesia, botulinum toxin A
        administration 219
ankle joint, fixed contracture 103
anterior intraparietal cortex (AIP) 35–6, 128
anticipatory control 147
arm
    abductor muscles *88*
    movement patterns in reaching/grasping
        112–13, *115*
        cerebral palsy 113–14, *116*
    movements for handwriting 344
    muscles 92–4
Assessment of Life Habits (LIFE-H) 391, 418
assessments of hand function 176–95, 418–26
    biomechanical prerequisites of functioning
        193
    classifications 178
    expectations 191
    functional activity performance 191–2
    object manipulation skilfulness 192–3
    organizing frameworks 187–8, *189,* 190–1
    outcomes *186*
    perceptions 191
    psychometric properties 182–5
    reliability 182–3
    scores 181
        use 179–80
    tests 177–82

criterion-referenced 179, 181–2
discriminative/descriptive 179, 180–1
evaluative measures 179
instrument evaluating framework *186*
norm-referenced 178, 180–1
predictive measures 179
purpose 179, *186*
reliability 182–3
reliability coefficient 184
responsiveness to change 183
scores 179–80, 181
screening 179
standard errors of measurement 183–5
types 178–9
use 180–2
validity 182, 183
use 190
validity 182, 183
Assisting Hand Assessment 190, 193, 418
assistive technology devices 371–83
    activity analysis 375
    activity identification 372, *374*
    adaptations 376–81
    control over output 375
    follow-up 383
    goal setting 375–6
    implementing 382–3
    interventions 376–83
    joystick 378–9
    keyboards 376–7, *378, 379*
        on-screen 379, *380,* 381, *382*
    mouse 378
    occupational therapy 372, *373*
    plan development 376
    resource identification 375
    selection of device 372, *373,* 374–81
    switches 381, *382*
    theoretical framework selection 372, 374
athetosis, play *360*
attention, handwriting 350–1
augmented feedback 252–3, *254*
axillary nerve 95–6

axiohumeral muscles 90
axioscapular muscles 82, *83–5,* 85–6

Bain Assistive Technology System (BATS) model
    374
basal ganglia 27–8
    congenital lesions 27–8
    implicit learning measures 47
    ordinal sequence learning 54
    temporal sequence learning 51, 52
bathing *333*
biceps brachii 86, *87*
    botulinum toxin injection 223, *224*
bimanual coordination 160–72
    assessment instruments 194
    Assisting Hand Assessment 193
    asymmetric control 166, *167*
    constraint-induced therapy 169–72
    decoupling of movement of extremities 164
    development 160–1
    HABIT rehabilitation 169–72
    hemiplegic cerebral palsy 161–6, *167, 168*
    homologous task performance 164–6
    ICF classification 232
    joint angle displacement of elbow/shoulder 163
    neural control 160–1
    non-homologous task performance 164–6
    rehabilitation 169–72
    spatial interference 161
    task difficulty 166, *168*
    temporal interference 161
    temporal synchronization 162–3
    training 409
    trunk anticipatory control 161
    unimanual movement comparison 164
bimanual fine motor function system (BFMF) 66
biofeedback 252–3, *254*
    motor learning 268–9
    muscle control 233
biomechanical anchoring 111–12
biomechanical prerequisites of hand functioning
    193
blindness, cerebral palsy 124
body function interventions 235–6
body structure interventions 235–6
BOTOX 215–16
    reconstitution 217
botulinum toxin 9, 213–27
    diagnostic muscle blockade 199
    serotypes 213
botulinum toxin A
    anaesthesia/analgesia 219
    antibody formation risk 222
    complications 226
    evidence from systematic reviews *400–1, 404–5,*
        409
    goal setting 219–20

goal-focused task practice intervention 408
hand therapy combined use 227
indications 226–7
injection 217–19
    frequency 222
    localization 218
    repeated 222
    specific muscles 222–4, *225–6*
    speed 218–19
mechanism of action 213, *214,* 216
needle/syringe size 218–19
with occupational therapy 244, *247–8,* 249,
    400–1, 404–5, 410
pharmacology/pharmacokinetics 213, *214,*
    215–16
precautions 222
pre-operative 234
reconstitution 217
results 226–7
selection of children 221–2
self-care impact of treatment 335
structure 215
systematic reviews *400–1,* 404–5, 409
target muscle selection 220, *221*
bow tying 330
Box and Block test 192
brachial plexus 95, 97
brachialis muscle 92
brachioradialis muscle
    botulinum toxin injection 223
    rerouting 204
brain
    activity modulation during precision grip
        33–4
    auditory area 15
    developing 14–15
        neural system competition 19
    malformations 67, *68*
    muscle relationship *102*
    pathologies in cerebral palsy 67–9
    repetitive finger movements 28, *29*
    topography 68–9
    visual area 14, 15
brain lesions
    corticospinal organization 72–3
    defective 68–9
    dorsal stream-related dysfunction 129–30
    early and organization of hand function 70
brain plasticity 13–22
    immature brain 126
    neuroimaging 13–14
    young damaged brain 19–20
Bruininks–Oseretsky Test of Motor Proficiency
    316, 419
buckles *331*
bupivacaine, diagnostic muscle blockade 199
buttons 330, *331,* 332

428

Canadian Occupational Performance Measure
     (COPM) 10, 191–2, 281, 419
   assistive technology devices 375, 383
   casting with neurodevelopmental therapy 405
   goal-setting 288
capacity
   decreased 301
   sense of 299
carers, assistive technology education 382–3
carpi radialis, flexor 92
   botulinum toxin injection 224, 225
   Z-lengthening 206
carpi ulnaris
   extensor transfer 206
   flexor 92–3
     adhesions 103
     botulinum toxin injection 224, 225
     sarcomeres 104
     transfer 205, 206
carpometacarpal joint (CMC) 91
casts/casting
   change schedules 239
   with neurodevelopmental therapy 236, 237–8,
     401, 403, 405
   post-botulinum toxin A treatment 249
   restraint 312–13
   serial 236, 237–8, 239
     pre-operative 234
   systematic reviews 401, 405
central group of muscles 95
central nervous system (CNS) plasticity, CIMT 309,
     311
central sulcus, epsilon and omega signs 69, 70
cerebellum, temporal sequence learning 52–3
cerebral palsy
   ataxic 62, 65, 126
     lesions 69
   choreoathetotic 64, 65
   definition 61, 162
   diagnostic guidelines 69
   dyskinetic 62, 64–5
     lesions 68–9
   dystonic 64–5
   functional severity 65–6
   growth curves 66, 67
   neurological classification 61, 62, 63–6, 67
   neuroradiology 67–73, 74, 75
   registers 389
   spastic 62, 63
     bilateral 63, 66, 68
     functional severity 65–6
     unilateral 63–4, 66, 68
   subtypes 62
   upper extremity involvement 66, 68
     neuroradiological correlates 69–70
chemodenervation, upper extremity 213
chewing, problems 325

Child Occupational Self Assessment (COSA) 420
child-centred goals, goal-oriented training 287
childhood 299–300
   interests 300–1
   values 300
Children Helping Out: Responsibilities,
     Expectations and Supports (CHORES)
     391, 392, 420
Children's Assessment of Participation and
     Enjoyment (CAPE) 388, 391, 392–3, 421
Child's Occupational Self-Assessment 302, 305
choice reaction time 44
cingulate motor area (CMA) 25, 26
   precision grip 32–3
   self-initiated movements 38
clavicle 82
client-centred practice 414
clothing, adaptive 332, 335
cognition, handwriting 350–1
cognitive effort, motor learning 264
cognitive function, handwriting 340
cognitive orientation to daily occupational
     performance (CO-OP) 276–83
   case study 280–3
   child-chosen goals 278
   cognitive strategies 277, 279
   domain-specific strategies 279, 280
   dynamic performance analysis 278
   enabling principles 279
   evidence for 409
   generalization and transfer of strategies 277–8
   global strategy 279
   guided discovery 279
   intervention session format 280
   key features 278–80
   objectives 277
   parental involvement 280
   significant other involvement 280
   transfer of learning 278
cognitive process model 350
cognitive processes, task-related 261
cognitive processing, handwriting 341–2
cognitive strategies
   CO-OP 277, 279
   domain-specific 279
   global 279
cognitive–perceptual deficit 260
collagen, muscle content 105
communication
   computer-augmented devices 372, 383
   computers 348
   EMG device 381
   ICT 348
   participation impact 389
   written 339–51, 353–6
computers
   assistive technology devices 371–83

communication function 348
control over output 375
training 382
conductive education *402,* 408–9
confidence, functional limitations 301
constraint-induced movement therapy (CIMT) 19,
       308–17
   activity-based practice 314–15
   in adults 308–9
   age appropriateness 311–12
   assessments 316
   core concept 316–17
   day-camp programmes 315
   duration 315
   environment 315
   evidence for *401,* 405–6, 409, 410
   forced use 309, *310–11, 311–13*
   frustration for children 313
   goals 316
   HABIT 169–72
   inclusion criteria 309, 311
   intensity 313
   motor learning 315
   outcome 316
   practice 313–15
   principles 308
   programme intensity 312–13
   repetitive task practice 314
   restraint
       duration 312–13
       types 309, 312
       without therapy 309
   shaping 313–14
   structured practice 313–14
   systematic reviews *401,* 405–6, 409
contextual interference (CI) effect 266
continuous guidance 268
contractures
   ankle 103
   dynamic 231–2
   fixed 103, 231–2
   wrist and finger *101*
corobrachialis muscle *87,* 89
corpus callosum, spatial interference 161
cortex
   activity
       precision grip 33–4
       static hold 32, *33*
   lateral premotor *25, 26,* 51
   lesions 68
   parietal 128
   posterior frontal 51, 52
   prefrontal in explicit ordinal sequence learning
       48–9
   prehension control 35–8
   primary somatosensory 69, *70*
   Rolandic 71, 73, *75*

synaptic plasticity 15–16
   see also frontal cortex; motor cortex; primary
       motor cortex (M1); primary sensorimotor
       cortex (M1S1)
cortical circuits
   development in hemiplegia 19
   reorganization with constraint-induced
       movement therapy 309
cortical control of hand function 25–40
cortical maps 15–16
   sensory experiences 140
corticomotoneuronal connections 32
corticomotoneuronal fibres 27
corticomotoneuronal projections, finger movements
       31–2
corticospinal neurons, excitability in precision grip
       34
corticospinal pathways 19
corticospinal projections *26,* 27
   bilateral 72
   contralateral 75
   ipsilateral 75
       from contra-lesional hemisphere 72, 73, *74,*
       75
   organization 72–3
   TMS assessment 71
corticospinal tract *26,* 27
   axons 27, 38
   fibres 38
   lesions 38–9
   precision grip 32
cutaneous afferent nerves
   manipulation 134–5
   sensory feedback 136
cutting food 326

daily activities
   goal-oriented training 286–96
   independence 3–4
   self-care 320–36
   see also dressing; eating
declarative memory systems, medial temporal lobe
       49
deformity patterns 220, *221,* 231–2
   classification 232
   dynamic 231
   growth differences 232
   static 231
deltoid muscle *88, 89,* 90
developmental disuse 160
diffusion tensor imaging (DTI) 13, *14*
   motor cortex plasticity 17
digitorum profundus, flexor 93
   botulinum toxin injection 224, *225*
digitorum superficialis, flexor, botulinum toxin
       injection 224, *225*
digits *see* finger(s)

diparesis 66
diplegia 66
  handwriting 341
  play *360*
  visual disorders 124
disability, classification systems 4, *5,* 6–7
distal interphalangeal joints (DIP) 92
dorsal premotor cortex 128
dorsal stream 128–9
  disorders in children 129–31
dressing 326–32
  case study 330, 332
  fasteners 330–2
  gross motor function 329
  undressing 327, 329–32
dynamic performance analysis (DPA) 278
dynamic systems theory 2–3, 109
dynamic tripod grasp 347
dyskinetic cerebral palsy 28
dyslexia, handwriting 342
Dysport 215
dystonia 101

eating
  advanced skills 324–5
  basic skills 323–4
  case study 326
  children with CP 325–6
  cutting food 326
  finger feeding 325
  impact of difficulties on participation 389
  self-feeding behaviour 114
  skill acquisition 323–6
education
  assistive technology for child's social network 382–3
  see also school
efficacy, sense of 299
  decreased 301
elbow joint 91
  angle displacement in bimanual coordination 163
  botulinum toxin A injection 223, *224*
  casts 236
  deformities 200, 203
  flexion deformity 200, 223
  fusion 203
  hyperpronation 200, 203
  operative procedures 200, *201,* 203
electrical stimulation
  functional 233, 249
  muscle 233
  post-operative 234
  threshold 249
  see also neuromuscular electrical stimulation (NMES)
electromyographic biofeedback 252–3, *254*

electromyography (EMG) 14
  botulinum toxin A injection localization 218
  diagnostic evaluation 199
electromyography (EMG) device for communication 381
environment
  adaptation 9–10
  constraint-induced movement therapy 315
  handwriting 342
  interrelationship 299
epilepsy, participation impact 389
equipment, adaptive
  assistive technology devices 371, 376–81
  computer interface 371
  handwriting 348
  joystick 378–9
  mouse 378
  play 367
  seating for postural control 111–12, 345, *346*
  self-care 335
  switches 381, *382*
  see also keyboards
error detection capacity 268
Evaluation Tool of Children's Handwriting (ETCH) 344, 421
evidence-based practice 396–414
  appraisal of evidence 397–8
  change of practice evaluation/reporting 398
  integration of evidence 398
  outcomes in research 409–10, 412
  reflection 396
  research quality 397
  six steps 396–8
  structuring question/search strategy 396
  treatment effects of interventions 398–9, *400–3,* 404–10
  validity of studies 399, 410
evidence-based studies, reliability 410
extensor digiti minimi muscle 93
extensor digitorum muscle 93
extensor indicis muscle 93
eye gaze 379–80
eye movements, abnormal 126
eye–hand coordination, visual function 127

facilitation task, ordinal sequence learning 46
family
  involvement in research 414
  participation enhancement 393
family-centred services 10–11
  goal-oriented training 286–7
fasteners 330–2
fatigue, handwriting 347, 348, 350–1
feedback
  augmented 267
  bandwidth 268
  computer-assisted 268

431

concurrent 268
continuous 268
fine motor skill acquisition 270
motor learning 263–4, 267–9
   organizing *271, 272*
feed-forward control 147
feeding *see* eating
fine motor control, handwriting 346–8
fine motor skills
   computer use 371
   learning 270
finger(s)
   closing in grasping 134
   contraction *101*
   dynamic flexion 206
   flexor muscles 92–3
   pre-shaping activity 152
   surgery *201,* 206–7, 210
   see also thumb; thumb deformities
finger deformities 206–7, *208,* 209–10
   botulinum toxin injection 224, *225*
   fixed contractures 207
   swan neck 210
finger feeding 325
finger grip, adult 324–5
finger movements
   control 154
   control development 154
   repetitive simple/complex 28, *29,* 30
finger pads, cutaneous receptors 135
fingertip forces 30, *31*
fist 148
fixed extensor muscle strategy 110
force
   control 152, *154*
   scaling 154
   see also grip force
force generation
   children with cerebral palsy 156–7
   grasping 152, 154
   hemiparesis 137
forced-use therapy 117, 309, *310–11,* 311–13
forearm
   botulinum toxin injection 224, *225*
   extensor muscles 93–4
   flexor muscles 92–3
   muscles 92–4
   operative procedures *201,* 203–4
   pronation deformities 203–4, 224, *225*
fork use 325, 326
frontal cortex
   posterior and temporal sequence learning 51, 52
   precision grip 34
fronto-parietal area, precision grip 32, 34
functional activity performance 191–2
functional electrical stimulation 249
   muscle control 233

Functional Independence Measure for Children
   421–2
functional limitations 301
functional movements, cognitive processes
   292
Functional Repertoire of the Hand Model
   (FRH model) 190, 290
functional therapy *402,* 408, 410
function-oriented intervention 230

gastrocnemius muscle, spastic 103
general anaesthesia, muscle relaxation 103
glenohumeral joint 79, *81*
   adductor muscles *88*
   biceps role 86
   extensor muscles *87*
   flexor muscles *87*
   rotator muscles *89*
gloves, restraint 312
goal(s)
   achievement 407–8
   child-centred 287
   child-chosen for CO-OP 278
   constraint-induced movement therapy 316
   evaluation 294–5
   selection 286–9
   treatment in MACS 7
   WHO global goals for botulinum toxin injection
      220
Goal Attainment Scale (GAS) 191, 288–9,
   292
   assistive technology devices 375, 383
   goal evaluation 294–5
   task performance 407–8
goal-oriented training 286–96
   activity simplification 290
   assessment for goal setting 288–9
   capacity of person 290
   case studies 288, 291, 293–4, 294–5
   child-centred goals 287
   environment assessment 290, 291
   evidence 407–8
   family-centred service 286–7
   goals
      evaluation 294–5
      selection 286–9
   intervention 292–4
   personal perspective 291
   process *289*
   self-care 335, 336
   task performance analysis 289–92, 291
   transfer of learning 295
GOAL–PLAN–DO–CHECK strategy 279, 280,
   281
goal-setting
   assistive technology devices 375–6
   botulinum toxin A 219–20

Canadian Occupational Performance Measure 288
grasping
  development 149, *150*, 151–2, *153*, 154
    children with cerebral palsy 155–7
  dorsal stream role 128–9
  dynamic tripod 347
  dynamics 147–8
  eating skills acquisition 323–5
  force generation 152, 154
  functional 149, *151*
  handwriting implement 346
  hemiplegia 155
  interventions to improve 114–15, 117–18
  patterns 148
  postural control 112–15, *116*, 117–19
  reaching out 35–8
  segregation from reaching 128
  self-directed 148
  trunk movement patterns 112–13
    cerebral palsy 113–14
  trunk restraint in training 117, *118*
  vision role 134
grey matter
  lesions 68
  motor skill learning 18–19
grip
  afferent fibre recording 135
  eating skills 324–5
  formation *36*
  patterns 8
  pre-precision 148
  see also precision grip
grip force 135
  regulation impairment 136
  sensation in anticipatory control 136
  sensory feedback for recalibration 136
  sensory input 142
grip–lift force synergy *156*
  training effect in cerebral palsy 155, *156*
grip–lift phase, corticospinal neuron excitability 34
grip–lift synergy 31
grip–lift task 30–1
grooming 333–4
gross motor function
  dressing 329
  participation predictor 389
  self-care deficit 320
Gross Motor Function Classification System (GMFCS) 4, *6*, 7, 66, 178
  postural deficit classification 110, 343
growth deformities 232
guidance techniques
  fine motor skill acquisition 270
  motor learning 269
guided discovery 279

hair care *333*, 334
hand
  botulinum toxin injection 224, *225, 226*
  deformities 224, *225, 226*
  dominance 28, *29*
  intrinsic muscles 94
  motor control 103
  object-related actions 290
  roles in Functional Repertoire of the Hand Model 290
  spatial relationship 135
  surgery 9
  transport 36–7
  see also bimanual coordination
hand function
  ability 3–4
  development 7–8
  organization after early brain lesions 70
  refined 134–8
  see also assessments of hand function
hand therapy, botulinum toxin A injection combined use 227
hand to mouth movements 324
  training 325
Hand–Arm Bimanual Intensive Training (HABIT) 169–72, 409
handwriting 339–51, *353–6*
  arm movements 344
  attention 350–1
  case studies 344–5, *346*, 347, 348, 349
  cognition 350–1
  cognitive processing 341–2
  CP impact 341–2
  environment 342
  fatigue 347, 348, 350–1
  fine motor control 346–8
  hemiplegia 341, 347
  interventions *353–6*
  legibility 347
  letter formation 346
  motor control 346–8
  muscle tone 342–3
  occupational therapy 340, 342
  organizational skills 350–1
  participation support 342–51
  performance components 340–2
  postural control 342–6
  skill correlation with other basic skills 350
  speed 347, 348
  success 340
  tool use 346–8
  visual field abnormalities 349
  visual/visual-perceptual skills 348–50
  visuo-motor transformation deficits 349
head
  control in eating 324, 325

reach trajectory 114, *116*
  yaw angle *115*
hemiparesis 65
  congenital
    hand movements 73, *74, 75*
    transcranial magnetic stimulation 72–3
  force-matching 137
hemiplegia 65
  bimanual coordination 160–72, 161–6, *167,*
    168
  causes 161–2
  congenital 38
    motion coherence thresholds *131*
  constraint-induced movement therapy 308–17
  cortical circuit development 19
  corticospinal pathways development 19
  fingertip force synergy difficulties 38
  grasping 155
  handwriting 341, 347
  ipsilateral motor cortex pathways 15
  mirror movement 19
  motor function with intense training 19
  paretic arm size 103
  participation in daily activities 6
  play *360*
  postural control 155
  reaching 155
  sitting deviant posture 155
  visual disorders 124, 125–6
hemispheric dissociation 75
holistic approach 410
House Scale, Modified 232
House Thumb position classification 193, 199
humerus 79
  casts 236
hygiene 333–4
hypertonia 101
hypertonicity, evaluation of effects 221, *222*
hypothenar group of muscles 94

immediate serial recall (ISR) 44–5
  metrical patterns of movement sequence 50
  ordinal/temporal sequence learning 51
immobilization, post-operative 234
independence in daily life 3–4
index finger movement
  grasp development 149
  imitation by neonates 148–9
infants, research needs 412
inferior parietal cortex, sequence representation 48
information and communication technologies (ICT)
  348, 371
information processing, motor learning 262–3
infraspinatus muscle 89–90
in-hand manipulation, skill development 149, 151
instructions, motor learning 269
intellectual impairment, participation impact 389, 390

interests, childhood 300–1
International Classification of Functioning,
  Disability and Health (ICF: WHO) 1–2,
  187–8, *189,* 190
  activity performance 188, *189*
  bimanual ability 232
  Body Structure and Function 232
  capacity 187–8, *189*
  framework for health and disability 277
  handwriting 339
  intervention levels 9
  participation 386
  performance 187–8, *189*
intraparietal areas, precision grip 34
intraventricular haemorrhage 68
  visual disorders 124–5
intrinsic motivation, play 359, 363–6
IQ
  ordinal sequence learning correlation 54–5
  participation predictor 389
Item Response Theory 179

Jebsen and Taylor Test of Hand Function 8, 190,
  192, 199, 422
  constraint-induced movement therapy 316
Joe Cool™ splints *242,* 243
joystick 378–9
  steered by the chin 379, *380*

keyboards 376–7, *378, 379*
  on-screen 379, *380,* 381, *382*
kinaesthesia 347
kinesion-taping 243
knife use 325, *326*
knowledge of performance (KP) 267
knowledge of results (KR) 267
Knox Preschool Play Scale (KPPS) 361, 422–3

language disorder, handwriting 342
laptops, communication function 348
lateral premotor cortex (PM) 25, *26*
  temporal sequence learning 51
latissimus dorsi muscle *83,* 90
  botulinum toxin A injection 222–3
  transfer 200, *202*
learned helplessness 301, 311
learning disability, self-care deficit 320
letter formation 346
levator scapulae *84,* 86
limb neglect 141–2
long-term depression (LTD) 13
long-term potentiation (LTP) 13
Lycra garments 239, 405

magnetic resonance imaging (MRI) 13, *14*
magnetic resonance imaging, functional (fMRI) 13,
  14

congenital hemiparesis 73, *74, 75*
   motor skill learning 18
   precision grip 34
   upper extremity functions 71
manipulation
   cutaneous afferent nerves 134–5
   vision in development 127
Manual Ability Classification System (MACS) 4, *5,*
      6–7, 66, 178
   assessment use 194
   CO-OP 280
   daily activities 320–1
   levels 6–7, 321
   treatment goals 7
M-band *104, 105*
medial temporal lobe, declarative memory systems
      49
median nerve 96, *98*
Melbourne Assessment of Unilateral Upper Limb
      Function 190, 193, 199, 423
memory
   declarative systems 49
   short-term capacity 55
mesial premotor region 48
metacarpophalangeal joints 91
   casts 236
   fusion 207
micro-switches 371–2
mirror movements, ipsilateral corticospinal
      pathways in hemiplegia 19
mitts, restraint 312
Model of Human Occupation (MOHO) 10, 302, *303*
Modified House Scale 232
motion analysis, diagnostic evaluation 199
motion coherence thresholds 129, *130, 131*
motoneurons, hand muscle 27
motor behaviour, resilience 261
motor control
   development 147
   handwriting 346–8
   selective 231
motor cortex
   areas *25, 26*
   motor skill learning 18
   ordinal sequence learning 47–8
   plasticity 17
   see also primary motor cortex (M1); primary
      sensorimotor cortex (M1S1)
motor deficit, spastic cerebral palsy 63–4
motor development theories 2–4, *5,* 6–7
motor evoked potentials (MEPs) 71
   congenital hemiparesis 72–3
motor function *see* gross motor function
motor learning 115, 117, 260–73
   associative phase 263
   autonomous phase 263, 293
   blocked practice 266–7

cognitive effort 264
cognitive phase 263
conceptual algorithm 271–3
constant practice 265
constraint-induced movement therapy 315
definition 261
enhancement 264
error detection capacity 268
feedback 263–4, 267–9
   organizing *271,* 272
feedback-related variables 267–9
guidance techniques 269
information processing 262–3
instructions 269
learning–performance distinction 261
motor stage 293
movement analysis *271,* 272
outcome measure *271,* 273
physical assistance 269
practice 263–4
   organizing *271,* 272
   part-task 265
   random 266–7
   schedules 266–7
   structure 264–7
   variable 265
   whole-task 265
process 260, 261–3
response programming 262, 263
response selection 262, 263
skill assessment *271,* 273
stages 263
stimulus identification 262
task selection *271,* 272
three-stage model 292–3
verbal-cognitive stage 292
see also cognitive orientation to daily
      occupational performance (CO-OP)
motor maps, letter formation 346
motor performance
   motor learning 261
   sensory deficit effects 142
motor skills
   acquisition 277, 292–3
      therapy planning 410
   early learning phase 18
   fine 8
   intense training 19
   learning new 17–19
   self-care 335
   task-oriented approach 109–10
motor system
   impairments 260–1
   see also gross motor function
mouse 378
movement
   cognitive processes 292

elastic forces 148
functional 292
learned strategies 8
passive forces 148
quality 8
object handling 192–3
selectivity reduction 260
movement analysis, motor learning *271, 272*
Movement Assessment Battery for Children 190
movement patterns
grasping 112–13
cerebral palsy 113–14
predetermined 109–10
reaching 112–13
cerebral palsy 113–14
spasticity 231
stereotyped 341
movement sequence
metrical patterns 49–50
ordinal structure 43, 45
dissociation of implicit/explicit 45–7
learning 45–9
procedural learning 43
temporal sequence type 49–50
temporal structure 49–52
movement sequence learning 43–56
2 × N task 45, 48, 49
developmental aspects 53–4
explicit 43–4, 45, 55
ordinal neural correlates 48–9
implicit 43–4
IQ correlation 55
ordinal 47–8
temporal 50
individual differences 54–5
neuropsychology 43–56
ordinal
dissociation from temporal 50–1
implicit 47–8
IQ correlation 54–5
STRR studies 53–4
paradigms 44–5
temporal
dissociation from ordinal 50–1
neural correlates 51–3
working memory 55
movement therapy *see* constraint-induced
movement therapy (CIMT)
multi-electrode electroencephalography (MEG) 14
muscle
activity selective control 233
adhesions with muscle fibres 103
agonist/antagonist coactivation 233
agonist/antagonist imbalance 233
antagonist 233
architecture 102–3
brain relationship *102*

central group 95
electrical stimulation 233
fixed extensor strategy 110
intracellular alterations 105
sarcomere reduction 104
spasticity 101–7
strengthening programmes 234, 243–4,
245–6
post-botulinum toxin A treatment 249
upper extremity
distal 92–4
proximal 82, *83–5,* 85–6, *87–9,* 89–90
weakness 233
see also named muscles
muscle blockade, diagnostic 199
muscle fibres
adhesions 103
types 1 and 2 106
muscle re-education training 233
muscle tone
disordered 341
handwriting 342–3
musculocutaneous nerve 95, 97
musculoskeletal surgery *see* surgery
musicians, age at training commencement 17
myosin 104, 105, 106
myosin heavy chain (MyHC) 106

necktie 330–1
neglect 142
neonates, index finger movement imitation
148–9
neoprene orthoses 239, *242,* 243
neural circuits, development 19
neural control of hand movements 28, *29,* 30–9
neural plasticity, use-dependent 15, 19–20
neurodevelopmental training (NDT) 9, 234, 235
assumptions 235
with casting 236, *237–8, 401, 403,* 405
evidence for *401, 403,* 404, 405, 408, 410
systematic review 404, 408, 410
upper limb reaching 115
neuromuscular blockade, upper extremity 213
neuromuscular electrical stimulation (NMES) 233,
249, *250–1,* 252
electrode placement 252, *253*
evidence for *403,* 406–7
post-operative 234
neuronal group selection theory 3
neuropsychology of movement sequence learning
43–56
Nine-Hole Peg test 192
nose care *333*
novelty, play 364
nutritional status, participation impact 389
nystagmus 126
see also optokinetic nystagmus

object location, prehension 36–7
object manipulation
  development 149, *150,* 151–2, *153,* 154
  skilfulness 192–3
object properties, prehension 35–6
object release development 149
Occupational Performance Process Model 372, *373*
occupational therapy
  assistive technology devices 372, *373*
  with botulinum toxin A 244, *247–8,* 249, *400–1,*
    404–5, 410
  evidence for *400–1,* 404–5, 410, *411*
  goal-focused task practice intervention 408
  handwriting 340, 342
  post-operative hand therapy 211
  self-care impact 335
  systematic reviews *400–1,* 404–5, 410, *411*
Occupational Therapy Intervention Model (OTIPM)
  10
occupations
  participation level 299
  volition 298, 301
ocular dominance columns 14
operation span task, working memory 55
opportunities, lacking for children with disability
  300–1
optokinetic nystagmus 126
  hemiplegia 125
organizational skills, handwriting 350–1
orthopaedic intervention
  musculoskeletal surgery 198–211
  see also botulinum toxin
orthoses 239, *240–2,* 243
  dynamic 239
  interventions 243
  systematic reviews *401,* 404, 405
outcome measures 412
  assessments of hand function *186*
  constraint-induced movement therapy 316
  motor learning *271,* 273
  research 409–10, 412

palmaris longus muscle 92
  botulinum toxin injection 224
parents
  assistive technology education 382–3
  CO-OP strategies 279–80
  goal-oriented training 286–7
parietal cortex, prehension under visual guidance
  128
parietal lobules 128
participation 385–94
  activity preferences 389
  assessment 391–3
  barriers 390
  children with CP 387–90
  concept 386–7

definition 385
  enhancement strategies 393–4
  factors influencing 388–90, 393
  limitations 387–8
  measurement 391–3
  predictors 389
  research needs 411–12
  school 388, 390
passive motion range in general anaesthesia 103
Peabody Development Test 8
  casting with neurodevelopmental therapy 405
pectoralis major muscle *83,* 90
  botulinum toxin A injection 222–3
  Z-lengthening 200, *202*
pectoralis minor muscle *83,* 85
Pediatric Activity Card Sort (PACS) 281
Pediatric Evaluation of Disability Inventory (PEDI)
  288, 322, 423
  participation 387–8
Pediatric Volitional Questionnaire (PVQ) 302, *304,*
  364, 424
Pedi-Comfy splints *242,* 243
Perceived Efficacy and Goal Setting (PEGS) 288
perceptual-motor readiness 349
Performance Quality Rating Scale (PQRS) 281, 283
periventricular leukomalacia 68
  visual disorders 124–5
periventricular white matter lesions 68, 75
personal causation
  childhood 299–300
  low sense of 301
personal constraints, Functional Repertoire of the
  Hand Model 290
Person–Environment–Occupation (PEO) model
  289, 291
phantom hand 16
physical assistance, motor learning 269
physical therapy, post-operative hand therapy 211
physiological cross-sectional area (PCSA) 102–3
pinch strength 142
play 357–67
  assessments *361*
  Assisting Hand Assessment 193
  benefits 366–7
  case study 361–2, 363, 365
  children with CP 358–9, *360*
  enjoying ability to master activity 365–6
  equipment 367
  evaluation 359–62
  experience 359
  exposing self to novelty 364
  form 358
  function 359
  intensity of involvement in demanding activities
    364–5
  intervention in clinic/school settings 362–6
  meaning 359

motivation 357–8
   intrinsic 359, 363–6
   novelty creation 366
   peers with higher level skills 365
   restoring sense of well-being 363
   short-term diversion 364
   social interaction 359, 367
   unstructured toys 366
   value 366–7
   volition 364
Play History (PH) 361
pollicis brevis
   adductor, botulinum toxin injection 224, *226*
   extensor 93–4
      plication 209
pollicis longus
   abductor 94
      plication 209
   extensor 93
      plication 209, *210*
   flexor 93
      botulinum toxin injection 224, *225*
      fixed contractures 207, *209*
positioning devices 111–12
positron emission tomography (PET) 14
posterior frontal cortex (PFC), temporal sequence
     learning 51, 52
postural control 109–19
   anticipatory adjustments 110
   extrinsic support 112
   Goal Attainment Scale 292
   grasping 112–15, *116,* 117–19
   handwriting 342–6
   hemiplegia 155
   improvement during movement 111
   positioning devices 111–12
   prehension 148
   reaching 112–15, *116,* 117–19, 148
   seating 111–12, 345, *346*
   sitting 110
   therapeutic interventions 346
postural deficit 111
   classification 110
postural support, orthotic interventions 239,
     243
precentral gyrus, motor hand area *29,* 30
precision grip 30–4
   brain activity modulation 33–4
   cortical control 32–4
   development 31–2, 148, 149, 152, 154
     children with cerebral palsy 155–6
   sensation impact 142–3
precision grip–lift task 30–1
Preferences for Activities in Children (PAC) 392,
     393
prefrontal cortex, explicit ordinal sequence learning
     48–9

prehension 35–8
   cortical control 35–8
   development 35
   motor control development 147
   postural control 148
   visual guidance 128
   visuo-motor transformation 35–8
premotor region, mesial 48
pressure sensitivity 139
presupplementary motor area (preSMA), temporal
     sequence learning 51, 52
primary motor cortex (M1) *25,* 26
   cortico-spinal projections 69–70
   ipsilateral in precision grip 34
   ordinal sequence learning 47
   repetitive finger movements 30
   temporal sequence learning 52
   transcranial magnetic stimulation 70–1
   upper extremity involvement in CP 69
primary sensorimotor cortex (M1S1), upper
     extremity functions 71
procedural learning, ordinal sequence learning 55
process skill ability 350
pronator quadratus 93
pronator teres muscle 92
   botulinum toxin injection 224, *225*
   operative procedures 203–4
proprioceptive afferent nerves 135–6
proximal interphalangeal joints (PIP) 92
psychometric measures 182–5

quadriplegia 66
   play *360*
   reaching 155
Quality of Upper Extremity Skills Test (QUEST)
     190, 193, 424
   casting with neurodevelopmental therapy 405
   constraint-induced movement therapy 316

radial nerve 95, *96,* 97
radiology, diagnostic evaluation 199
radioulnar joint 91
randomization 397–8
randomized controlled trials (RCT) 397
   validity 399
range of motion (ROM)
   casting effects 236, *237–8,* 239
   growth differences 232
   measurement 221–2
   passive in general anaesthesia 103
   splinting 239
Rasch analysis 179, 195
rater reliability 184
reaching
   development 151–2, *153*
     children with cerebral palsy 154–5
   dorsal stream role 128–9

dynamics 147–8
hemiplegia 155
interventions to improve 114–15, 117–18
motor control development 147
postural control 112–15, *116,* 117–19, 148
quadriplegia 155
segregation from grasping 128
trunk movement patterns 112–13, *115*
cerebral palsy 113–14, *116*
trunk restraint in training 117, *118*
vision in development 127, 134
reach-to-grasp movements *36*
reaction time 44
reflex–hierarchical theory 235
rehabilitation
sensory ability 142
upper extremity pre-/post-operative 233–4
reliability
coefficient 184
evidence-based studies 410
of tests 182–3
repetitive multi-sensory training programme 143
repetitive task practice 314
research quality 397
restraint
duration 312–13
physical, gentle intermittent 312
trunk in reaching/grasping training 117, *118*
types 309, 312
without therapy 309
reticulospinal pathway 28
rhomboid major muscle *85,* 86
rigidity 101
Rolandic cortex 71
activating 73, *75*
rotation 151
rubrospinal tract 28

sarcomeres, spastic muscles 104
sashes, tying *331*
scapula
depressor muscles *83*
elevator muscles *82*
protractor muscles *84*
retractor muscles *85*
rotator muscles *83–4*
scapulohumeral muscles 86, *87–9,* 89–90
school
assessment measures 388, 389, 390, 391–2, 425
participation 388, 390
School Assessment of Motor Processing Skills
(AMPS) 425
School Function Assessment 388, 389, 391–2, 425
School Setting Interview 390
seating, adapted for postural control 111–12, 345,
346
segment alignment 111–12

selective posterior rhizotomy, self-care impact of
treatment 335
self-care 320–36
acquisition 322–34
age variability in children 320
assessment 321–2
deficits 320
dressing 326–32
eating skills 114, 323–6
goal-oriented training 335, 336
grooming 333–4
guidelines for treatment 336
hygiene 333–4
management 321–2
motor skills 335
toileting 334
training 335, 336
self-directed grasp 148
self-feeding behaviour 114
Semmes–Weinstein monofilaments 139
sensation 134–44
anticipatory control of grip force 136
hand function in children with cerebral palsy
138–40, *141,* 142–4
precision grip 142–3
refined hand function 134–8
standardized measures 138
upper limb functional outcome 233
sensibility testing 199
sensorimotor development 148–9
sensorimotor organization 70–1
limitations 347
sensory assessment, children with cerebral palsy
138
sensory deficit 260
adaptive strategies 142
cerebral palsy type 140
limb neglect 141–2
motor performance effects 142
sensory function, children with cerebral palsy
138–40, *141*
sensory inputs
feedback for force modification 143
interventions 233
movement initiation 142–3
sensory interventions 233
Sensory Profile 139
sensory–motor integration, refined hand function
136–8
sensory–perceptual–motor training 143
sequence *see* movement sequence
serial reaction time task (SRTT) 44, 45
ordinal sequence learning 46, 47–8, 51, 53–4
procedural learning 55
temporal sequence learning 50, 51
serratus anterior muscle *84,* 85
shaping 313–14

439

shoe laces *331*
Short Child Occupational Profile (SCOPE) 302, *306*, 425–6
short-term memory capacity, ordinal sequence learning 55
shoulder joint
    angle displacement in bimanual coordination 163
    botulinum toxin A injection 222–3
    movement 81
    operative procedures 200, *201–2*
    osteotomy 200
    rotation deformities 200, *201*
Shriners Hospital Upper Extremity Evaluation (SHUEE) 193
sip and puff device 381
sitting
    deviant posture in hemiplegia 155
    independent 110
    postural control 110
    see also seating, adapted
skill acquisition 412
skill assessment, motor learning *271*, 273
slings, restraint 312
Smallest Detectable Difference (SDD) 184–5
snaps 330, *331*
SNARE proteins *214*, 216
social interaction, play 359, 367
socioeconomic status, participation impact 390
soleus muscle, spastic 103
somatosensory cortex, primary 69, *70*
somatosensory system plasticity 15–16
spasticity 101–7, 260
    handwriting 341
    movement patterns 231
speech impairment, computer-augmented communication devices 372
splinting 239, *240–2*, 243
    dynamic *242*
    protective post-operative 234
    serial pre-operative 234
    static *242*
spoon use 324
standard errors of measurement (SEM) 183–5
standing balance, static 143
static hold, cortical activity 32, *33*
sternoclavicular joint 79, 81
    movement 82
    muscles 82, *83–5*, 85–6
strengthening/strength training 234, 243–4, *245–6*
    evidence *401*, 406–7
    post-botulinum toxin A treatment 249
stretch reflex 101, *102*
stretching 236, *237–8*
stroke
    hand coordination *37*
    neural reorganization 19
subclavius muscle *83*, 85

subscapularis muscle 89
    Z-lengthening 200, *202*
supplementary motor area (SMA) *25, 26*
    precision grip 32–3
    self-initiated movements 38
    temporal sequence learning 51, 52
supraspinatus muscle *88*, 89
surgery
    candidate selection 200
    elbow joint 200, *201*, 203
    evidence for *403*, 407
    fingers *201*, 206–7, 210
    forearm *201*, 203–4
    hand 9
    hand therapy 211
    indications 200
    musculoskeletal 198–211
    operative procedures 200, *201–2*, 203–7, *208*, 209–10
    post-operative care 210–11
    selective posterior rhizotomy 335
    shoulder joint 200, *201–2*
    standardized procedures 407
    thumb *201*, 207, *208*, 209, *210*
    thumb-in-palm deformity 207, *208*, 209, *210*, *403*, 407
    wrist joint *201*, 204–6
    Z-plasty for thumb deformities 207, *208*, 209
Surveillance of CP in Europe (SCPE) 61, 66
swallowing problems 325
swan neck deformities 210
switches 381, *382*
synaptic activity, motor skill learning 18
synaptic connectivity 13
    strengthening 19
systematic reviews 397
    botulinum toxin A *400–1*, 404–5
    casting *401*, 405
    multiple interventions 404
    occupational therapy *400–1*, 404–5
    orthoses *401*, 404, 405
    validity 399

tactile sensibility 143
Talking Mats™ 372, *374*, 383
Tardieu assessment of range of motion 221–2
task parameters 290, 291
task performance
    discrepancy 4
    practice 407–8
task-oriented approach 109–10
teachers, assistive technology education 382–3
teeth brushing *333*, 334
temporal lobe, medial 49
teres major muscle *88*, 90
    transfer 200, *202*
Test of Playfulness (TOPS) 426

Test of Sensory Functions in Infants 139
tetraplegia 66
thenar group of muscles 94
therapy, intensive bursts 412
thumb, cutaneous receptors 135
thumb deformities 206–7, *208, 209–10*
  flexion 207, 224, *225*
  Z-plasty 207, *208,* 209
thumb-in-palm deformity
  botulinum toxin injection 224, *226*
  orthoses 243
  surgery 207, *208,* 209, *210, 403,* 407
titin 105
toileting 334
Tool for Optimizing Written Production (TOW-P)
  342, *343,* 426
tool use, handwriting 346–8
transcranial magnetic stimulation (TMS)
  congenital hemiparesis 72–3
  precision grip 32
  sensorimotor organization assessment 70–1
translation 151
trapezius muscle *83,* 86
treatment models 10
tri modal spectroscopic (TMS) imaging 14
triceps muscle 92
  long head *88,* 90
trunk
  compensatory role in reaching 117
  displacement 114, *116*
  excessive movement restriction 117–18
  movement patterns in reaching/grasping 112–13,
    115
    cerebral palsy 113–14, *116*
  reach trajectory 114, *116*
  restraint in reaching/grasping training 117, *118*
  yaw angle *115*
two-point discrimination 139

ulnar nerve 95, *99*
ultrasonography, botulinum toxin A injection
    localization 218
undressing 327, 329–32
unimanual movement 164
  constraint-induced therapy 169
  homologous task performance 164–6
  non-homologous task performance 164–6
  training 169
upper extremity
  chemodenervation 213
  conservative treatments 234–54
  deformities 231–2
    classification 232
  development 147–57
  diagnostic evaluation 199
  distal joints 91–2
  distal muscles 92–4

evidence for treatment effect in CP 398–9,
    400–3, 404
evidence-base for interventions 396–414
function 3–4
  classification 232
  impairment relationship 230–3
  participation predictor 389
  rate-limiting factors 232–3
history taking 198–9
impairments and function relationship 230–3
innervation 95–9, *96*
interventions
  evidence base 396–414
  holistic focus 410
  ongoing trials *413*
  research gaps 411–12
  volition development support 302, *303*
involvement in CP 66
normal anatomy 79–99
outcomes in research 409–10, 412
physical examination 198–9
proximal joints 79, 81–2
proximal muscles 82, *83–5,* 85–6, *87–9,* 89–90
rehabilitation 233–4
restraint without training 309
sensation 233
volition impact on intervention 301
  see also arm; elbow joint; finger(s); forearm;
    hand; shoulder joint; thumb; wrist joint
upper extremity rating scale (UERS) 199
use-dependent plasticity 15, 19–20

validity 182–3
  evidence-based studies 399, 410
values, childhood 300
ventral intraparietal region 37
vestibulospinal pathway 28
virtual reality games 364
vision
  hand action/manipulation 127
  hand function 134
visual attention in hemiplegia 125
visual cortex
  critical periods 19
  ocular dominance columns 14
  visual information transformation 128
visual development 127
visual disorders with brain lesions/CP 124–6
visual dominance 127
visual field abnormalities
  handwriting 349
  hemiplegia 125, 126
visual function, eye–hand coordination 127
visual guidance 127
visual impairment 124–31
  participation impact 389
visual pathway, classical/occipito-parietal 128

visual skills, handwriting 348–50
visual ventral/dorsal stream 128–9
  disorders in children 129–31
visuo-motor control 347
visuo-motor transformation deficits 129
  handwriting 349
volition 298–306
  assessment tools 302
  case study 302, *304–6,* 306
  development support 302, *303*
  functional limitations 301
  nature of 298–9
  occupations 298, 301
  origins 298
  play 364
  upper extremity intervention 301
volume-based morphometry 13, *14*

walking difficulties, participation impact 389
washing hands/face 333–4
weakness, children with cerebral palsy 156–7, 260
Wee Functional Independence Measure (WeeFim)
  199, 321–2
well-being, play 363

white matter, periventricular lesions 68
Williams syndrome 129
word prediction 379
working memory, movement sequence learning
  55
World Health Organization (WHO)
  global goals for botulinum toxin injection 220
  see also International Classification of
      Functioning, Disability and Health
      (ICF: WHO)
wrist joint 91
  botulinum toxin injection 224, *225*
  contraction *101*
  fixed contractures 204
  fusion 205
  motor control 103
  muscle 93
  operative procedures *201,* 204–6
  palmar flexion 204–5
  tendon transfer 204, 205–6

Zancolli scale 193, 232
Z-band *104,* 105
zippers 330, *331,* 332

442

Milton Keynes UK
Ingram Content Group UK Ltd.
UKHW020345310724
446199UK00002B/48

9 781898 683537